Stedman's
OPHTHALMOLOGY
WORDS

FOURTH EDITION

Stedman's

OPHTHALMOLOGY
WORDS

FOURTH EDITION

Wolters Kluwer | Lippincott Williams & Wilkins
Health

Philadelphia • Baltimore • New York • London
Buenos Aires • Hong Kong • Sydney • Tokyo

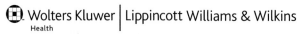

Wolters Kluwer | Lippincott Williams & Wilkins
Health

Philadelphia · Baltimore · New York · London
Buenos Aires · Hong Kong · Sydney · Tokyo

Publisher: Julie K. Stegman
Senior Product Manager: Eric Branger
Associate Managing Editor: Cecilia González
Typesetter: Brighid Willson
Printer & Binder: Malloy Litho, Inc.

Printed in the United States of America

Fourth Edition, 2007

Library of Congress Cataloging-in-Publication Data

Stedman, Thomas Lathrop, 1853–1938.
    Stedman's ophthalmology words. — 4th ed.
        p.   ; cm.
    Includes bibliographical references.
    ISBN-13: 978-0-7817-8175-6 (pbk.)
    ISBN-10: 0-7817-8175-2 (pbk.)
    1. Ophthalmology—Terminology.   I. Title. II. Title: Ophthalmology words.
    [DNLM: 1. Ophthalmology—Terminology—English.   WV 15 S812s
2007]
RE20.S7 2007
617.7001'4—dc22

                                                    2006032242

01
1 2 3 4 5 6 7 8 9 10

Contents

Acknowledgments

An important part of our editorial process is the involvement of medical transcriptionists—as advisors, reviewers, and/or editors.

We extend special thanks to Jeanne Bock, CSR, MT, and to Patty White for editing the manuscript and for helping resolve many difficult questions. We are grateful to our Editorial Advisory Board members, including Robin Koza; Nicole Peck, CMT; Shemah Fletcher; Wendy Ryan; Janet West; and Kathy Rockel, who were instrumental in the development of this reference. They recommended sources and shared their valuable judgment, insight, and perspective.

Our appreciation goes to Pat Forbis and Robin Koza, who enhanced the A–Z content for this edition. We also extend thanks to Darcy Johnson for working on the appendices. Additional thanks to Helen Littrell for performing the final prepublication review. Other important contributors to this edition include Jo-Ann Clarke, who gathered the sample reports.

And, as always, Barb Ferretti played an integral role in the process by reviewing the content files for format, updating the content, and providing a final quality check.

As with all our *Stedman's* word references, this resource incorporates the suggestions and expertise of our many contacts in the medical transcriptionist community. Thanks to all of our advisory board participants, reviewers, and editors; AAMT meeting attendees; and others who have written us with requests and comments—keep talking, and we'll keep listening.

Editor's Preface

Approximately 12 years ago I had the opportunity to work in the ophthalmology clinic of a large teaching hospital in the Midwest. When I began that job, I thought I had a fair knowledge base in ophthalmology, but I soon learned otherwise. I spent the first six months in that MT position delving into ophthalmology references and picking the brains of the residents. During my 18-month stint at that job, I gained a real appreciation for the complexities of the human eye and for the specialists who dedicate themselves to helping those with ophthalmologic diseases and abnormalities. Because of that background, I knew there is a need for accurate references in this unique medical specialty and, therefore, I was very excited to have an opportunity to work on *Stedman's Ophthalmology Words*.

You will find that *Stedman's Ophthalmology Words, Fourth Edition*, contains a vast number of new terms, including the names of pieces of equipment and procedures to correct eye conditions. There are also an increased number of terms related to the subspecialties of pediatric ophthalmology, neuroophthalmology, and endocrinology-related eye disorders.

The appendix section of this book is a unique and informative resource in its own right. We have included a substantial collection of anatomical illustrations and cross-section of sample reports. Also contained in the appendix are common terms heard in ophthalmologic procedures, a listing of drugs used in the specialty of ophthalmology, and a table of cranial nerves.

This preface would not be complete without thanking everyone involved in the process of bringing this word book together. I extend my thanks to the reviewers who culled journals, texts, and the Internet to find the terms included in this book; to the transcriptionists who requested this book and sent in their own lists of terms; and to the entire Stedman's team for listening to transcriptionists everywhere and making this word book possible. I also extend special thanks to Patty White, Cecilia González, and Barb Ferretti for their valuable assistance.

Jeanne Bock, CSR, MT

Publisher's Preface

Stedman's Ophthalmology Words, Fourth Edition, offers an authoritative assurance of quality and exactness to the wordsmiths of the healthcare professions—medical transcriptionists, medical editors and copyeditors, health information management personnel, court reporters, and the many other users and producers of medical documentation.

In *Stedman's Ophthalmology Words, Fourth Edition*, users will find protocols, diagnoses, and therapeutic procedures, new techniques, lab tests, clinical research terms, as well as abbreviations with their expansions pertinent to ophthalmology. The appendix sections, substantially enhanced over the previous edition, provide anatomical illustrations with useful captions and labels; a table of cranial nerves; sample reports; common terms by procedure; and drugs by indication.

This new edition contains more than 4,000 new terms. The extensive A–Z list was developed from manufactures' literature, scientific reports, books, journals, CDs, and Web sites (please see list of References on page xvii).

We at Lippincott Williams & Wilkins strive to provide you with the most up-to-date and accurate word references available. Your use of this Word Book will prompt new editions, which we will publish as often as updates and revisions justify. We welcome your suggestions for improvements, changes, corrections, and additions—whatever will make this Stedman's product more useful to you. Please complete the postage-paid card in this book for future suggestions and recommendations, or visit us online at www.stedmans.com.

Explanatory Notes

Medical transcription is an art as well as a science. Both approaches are needed to correctly interpret the dictation of a physician, whose language is a product of education, training, and experience. This variety in medical language means that there are several acceptable ways to express certain terms, including jargon. *Stedman's Ophthalmology Words, Fourth Edition*, provides variant spellings and phrasings for many terms. These elements, in addition to complete cross-indexing, make *Stedman's Ophthalmology Words, Fourth Edition*, a valuable resource for determining the validity of terms as they are encountered.

Alphabetical Organization

Alphabetization of main entries is letter by letter as spelled, ignoring punctuation, spaces, prefixed numbers, or other characters. For example:

emergent ray of light
Emerson 1-piece segment bifocal
EMI

Terms beginning or ending with Greek letters show the Greek letters spelled out and listed alphabetically. For example:

alpha, α
   a. agonist
   a. angle

In subentry alphabetization, the abbreviated singular form or the spelled-out plural form of the noun main entry word is ignored.

Format and Style

All main entries are in boldface to expedite locating a sought-after term, to enhance distinction between main entries and subentries, and to relieve the textual density of the pages.

Irregular plurals and variant spellings are shown on the same line as the singular or preferred form of the word. For example:

papilla, pl. **papillae**
anular, annular

Hyphenation

As a rule of style, multiple eponyms (e.g., Elschnig-O'Brien forceps) are hyphenated. Also, hyphens have been added between a manufacturer and one or more eponyms (e.g., Storz-Walker retinal detachment unit). Please note that in many cases, hyphenation is a question of style, not of accuracy, and thus is a matter of choice.

Possessives

Possessive forms have been dropped in this reference for the sake of consistency and conformance with the guidelines of the American Association for Medical Transcription (AAMT) and other groups. Please note, however, that in many cases, retaining the possessive, like hyphenating, is a question of style, not of accuracy, and thus is a matter of choice. To form the possessive of a word, simply add the apostrophe or apostrophe "s" to the end of the word.

Cross-indexing

The word list is in an index-like main entry–subentry format that contains two combined alphabetical listings:

(1) A *noun* main entry–subentry organization, which is typical of the A–Z section of medical dictionaries like *Stedman's*:

Clayman
  C. guide
  C. intraocular lens
  C. lens-holding forceps

malformation
  Arnold-Chiari m.
  arteriovenous m.
  iris m.

(2) An *adjective* main entry–subentry organization, which lists words and phrases as you hear them. The main entries are the adjectives or modifiers in a multiword term. The subentries are the nouns around which the terms are constructed and to which the adjectives or modifiers pertain:

central
  c. abrasion
  c. amaurosis
  c. anisocoria

intraretinal
  i. bleeding
  i. hemorrhage
  i. space

This format provides the user with more than one way to locate and identify a multiword term. For example:

involutional
  i. blepharoptosis

blepharoptosis
  involutional b.

recurrent
  r. opacification

opacification
  recurrent o.

It also allows the user to see together all terms that contain a particular descriptor, as well as all types, kinds, or variations of a noun entity. For example:

rectus
  r. muscle of eyeball
  r. muscle pulley
  superior r.

seborrheic
  s. blepharitis
  s. debris
  s. keratosis

Wherever possible, abbreviations are separately defined and cross-referenced. For example:

SEBR
  spontaneous eye blink rate

spontaneous
  s. eye blink rate (SEBR)

rate
  spontaneous eye blink r. (SEBR)

References

In addition to the lists of our MT Editorial Advisory Board members (from their daily transcription work), we used the following sources for new terms in *Stedman's Ophthalmology Words, Fourth Edition.*

Books

The AAMT Book of Style, 2nd Edition. Modesto, CA: AAMT, 2002.

Bartlett, Jimmy D. *Ophthalmic Drug Facts 2006.* Baltimore: Lippincott Williams & Wilkins, 2006.

Garg, Ashok, Suresh K. Pandey, David F. Chang, Pandelis A. Papadopoulos, and Anthony J. Maloof. *Advances in Ophthalmology.* Tunbridge Wells, Kent, UK: Anshan Ltd, 2005.

Holz, Frank G., and Richard F. Spaide. *Medical Retina (Essentials in Ophthalmology).* The Netherlands: Springer-Verlag, 2005.

Lance, L. L. *Quick Look Drug Book (2006).* Baltimore: Lippincott Williams & Wilkins, 2006.

Nelson, Leonard B., and Scott E. Olitsky. *Harley's Pediatric Ophthalmology, 5th Edition.* Baltimore: Lippincott Williams & Wilkins, 2005.

Rapuano, Christopher J. *Year Book of Ophthalmology.* Philadelphia: Elsevier/Mosby, 2005.

Stedman's Medical Dictionary, 28th Edition. Baltimore: Lippincott Williams & Wilkins, 2006.

Wills Eye Hospital, Derek Y. Kunimoto, Kunal D. Kanitkar, Mary Makar, and Mark A. Friedberg. *The Wills Eye Manual: Office and Emergency Room Diagnosis and Treatment of Eye Disease, 4th Edition.* Baltimore: Lippincott Williams & Wilkins, 2004.

Wilson, M. Edward, Suresh K. Pandey, and Rupal H. Trivedi. *Pediatric Cataract Surgery.* Baltimore: Lippincott Williams & Wilkins, 2005.

Journals

American Journal of Ophthalmalogy. Philadelphia: Elsevier/Mosby, 2005–2006.

Evidence-Based Ophthalmology. Baltimore: Lippincott Williams & Wilkins, 2005.

Ophthalmology. San Francisco: American Academy of Ophthalmology, 2006.

Ophthalmology Times. Cleveland: Advanstar Communications, 2005–2006.

Optometry and Vision Science. Baltimore: Lippincott Williams & Wilkins, 2005–2006.

Retina. Baltimore: Lippincott Williams & Wilkins, 2005

Newsletters

The Latest Word

Let's Talk Terms

Web Sites

www.djo.harvard.edu

www.eyecancer.com/

www.nei.nih.gov

www.revophth.com/

www.wilmer.jhu.edu/

www.glaucomatoday.com/pages/0101/07.html

www.stronghealth.com/services/strongvision/technology/Zyoptix.cfm

www.miscpaper.com/ophthalmictests.htm

www.centerwatch.com/patient/drugs/area13.html

www.drugs.com/recent-additions.html

www.accessdata.fda.gov

www.hpisum.com

www.mtdesk.com/lstTrAcry.shtml

Images

Agur, A. M. R., and M. J. Lee. *Grant's Atlas of Anatomy, 10th Edition*. Baltimore: Lippincott Williams & Wilkins, 1999.

Battista, K. From C. *Oatis Kinesiology: The Mechanics and Pathomechanics of Human Movement*. Baltimore: Lippincott Williams & Wilkins, 2003.

Caldwell, S. From *Stedman's Medical Dictionary, 27th Edition*. Baltimore: Lippincott Williams & Wilkins, 2000.

Hadry. N. O. From *Stedman's Medical Dictionary, 27th Edition*. Baltimore: Lippincott Williams & Wilkins, 2000.

LifeART Nursing Collection 3, CD-ROM. Baltimore: Lippincott Williams & Wilkins.

LifeART Pediatrics Collection 1, CD-ROM. Baltimore: Lippincott Williams & Wilkins.

LifeART Super Anatomy Collection 2, CD-ROM. Baltimore: Lippincott Williams & Wilkins.

LifeART Super Anatomy Collection 4, CD-ROM. Baltimore: Lippincott Williams & Wilkins.

LifeART Super Anatomy Collection 7, CD-ROM. Baltimore: Lippincott Williams & Wilkins.

LifeART Super Anatomy Collection 9, CD-ROM. Baltimore: Lippincott Williams & Wilkins.

Ward, L. From J. Fuller and J. Schaller-Ayers. *A Nursing Approach, 2nd Edition*. Philadelphia: J. B. Lippincott Company, 1994.

A

accommodation
A band
crofilcon A
cyclofilcon A
cyclosporin A
dimefilcon A
droxifilcon A
A esotropia
A exotropia
focofilcon A
hefilcon A
Intron A
A measurement
Muro Opcon A
A pattern
pentafilcon A
perfilcon A
phemfilcon A
silafocon A
A syndrome
tetrafilcon A
ultraviolet A (UVA)
A wave

AA

accommodative amplitude
amplitude of accommodation

AACE

acute acquired comitant esotropia

AACG

acute angle-closure glaucoma

AAO

American Academy of Ophthalmology
American Academy of Optometry

AAOE

American Academy of Ophthalmic
Executives

AAP

achromatic automated perimetry

AAPOS

American Association for Pediatric
Ophthalmology and Strabismus

Aarskog syndrome
Aase syndrome
A+ Autoscan portable A-scan
ab

ab externo
ab externo filtering operation
ab externo trabeculectomy
ab interno approach

Abbe

A. refractometer
A. value

abdominal migraine

abducens

a. internuclear neuron
a. nerve fascicle
a. nerve palsy
a. nerve paralysis
a. nucleus
a. oculi
a. paresis

abduct
abduction

absence of a.
congenital absence of a.
a. deficit

abductor muscle
aberrant

a. degeneration
a. regeneration
a. regeneration of nerve
a. reinnervation of oculomotor
nerve

aberrated

a. acuity chart
a. eye

aberration

angle of a.
anterior surface a.
chromatic a.
chromatic lens a.
color a.
coma a.
corneal lens a.
coupling of a.
crystalline lens a.
curvature a.
dioptric a.
distantial a.
distortion a.
higher order wavefront a.
lateral a.
lens a.
longitudinal a.
low total spherical a.
meridional a.
monochromatic a.
newtonian a.
oblique a.
ocular total higher order a.
(OTHA)
optic a.
optical a.
positive spherical a.
pseudophakic spherical a.
reduction of a.
refractive a.
regeneration a.

aberration *(continued)*
spatially resolved wavefront a.
spheric a.
spherical lens a.
visual a.
aberrometer
Hartmann-Shack wavefront a.
state-of-the-art a.
Tracey a.
Wasca a.
wavefront a.
Z-View a.
Zywave II a.
aberrometry
clinical applications of a.
postoperative a.
preoperative a.
Shack-Hartmann a.
ABES
American Board of Eye Surgeons
abetalipoproteinemia
hereditary a.
ability
Neale analysis of reading a.
reading a.
Abiotrophia defectiva
abiotrophy
retinal a.
ABK
aphakic bullous keratopathy
ablation
aspheric custom a.
broad-beam a.
cross-cylinder a.
customized hyperopic a.
decentered a.
eccentric a.
excimer laser subepithelial a.
hyperopic a.
laser a.
off-center a.
panretinal a.
peripheral retinal a.
pituitary a.
a. planner topography
topography-guided a.
toric a.
treatment zone laser a.
wavefront-guided a.
a. zone
ablepharia
ablepsia, ablepsy
ABMD
anterior basement membrane dystrophy
abnormal
a. harmonious retinal
correspondence
a. head posture

a. nearwork-induced transient
myopia
a. ocular condition
a. staining pattern
a. unharmonious retinal
correspondence
a. vasculature
abnormality
angle of a.
color vision a.
congenital a.
cornea a.
cranial nerve a.
cytogenetic a.
developmental anterior segment a.
eyelash a.
eyelid a.
facial movement a.
intraretinal microvascular a. (IRMA)
macular a.
microvascular a.
neuroophthalmologic a.
ocular surface a.
optic nerve congenital a.
punctal a.
retinal thickness a.
saccadic a.
skeletal a.
structural a.
vascular a.
vertebrobasilar vascular a.
vitreoretinal interface a.
ABO
American Board of Ophthalmology
abrade
abrader
cornea a.
Abraham
A. iridectomy laser lens
A. iridotomy
A. peripheral button iridotomy lens
A. YAG laser lens
abrasion
central a.
conjunctival a.
a. of cornea
corneal a. (CA)
traumatic corneal a.
abrin
abscess, pl. **abscesses**
cerebral a.
choroidal a.
corneal a.
fulminant a.
lacrimal a.
orbital subperiosteal a.
psoriatic corneal a.
retrobulbar a.
a. ring

A

ring a.
scleral tunnel a.
stitch a.
subperiosteal a.
suture a.
vitreous a.
abscission
corneal a.
absence of abduction
absent
a. lens
a. retina
a. vitreous
Absidia corymbifera
absinthe
absolute
a. accommodation
a. glaucoma
a. hemianopia
a. hemianopsia
a. hyperopia
a. intensity threshold acuity
near point a.
a. risk reduction
a. scotoma
a. strabismus
a. threshold
absorbable
a. gelatin film
a. implant
a. suture
absorbance
absorbency
absorptance
radiant a.
absorption
fluorescent treponemal antibody a.
a. line
abtorsion
AC
accommodative convergence
anterior chamber
Eye Drops AC
AC eye drops
AC tube inserter ·
Visine AC
a.c.
before meals
AC/A
accommodative convergence-
accommodation
acanthamebiasis

Acanthamoeba
A. *castellanii*
A. cyst
A. endophthalmitis
A. keratitis
A. keratitis pseudodendrites
A. *polyphaga*
acanthocytosis
acantholysis
acanthoma fissuratum
acanthosis nigricans
acarica
blepharitis a.
ACC
anterior central curve
acc
accommodation
accelerometer
access
braille a.
large print a.
accessoriae
glandulae lacrimales a.
accessory
a. fiber
a. lacrimal gland
a. lacrimal gland of Wolfring
lens a.
a. nucleus
a. nucleus of optic tract
optical a.
a. organ of eye
a. visual apparatus
a. visual structure
accidental
a. image
a. mydriasis
accommodating IOL
accommodation (A, acc)
absolute a.
a. accuracy
amplitude of a. (AA)
binocular a.
breadth of a.
bright-field a.
convergence a.
a. of crystalline lens
dark-field a.
defective a.
a. disorder
esodeviation a.
esotropia a.
excessive a.

NOTES

accommodation *(continued)*
a. of eye
far point of a. (FPA, p.r.)
fusion with a.
Helmholtz theory of a.
a. insufficiency
iridoplegia a.
light and a. (L&A)
near-point a.
near point of a. (NPA, p.p.)
negative a.
open-loop a.
paralysis of a.
a. paresis
pinhole a.
position a.
positive a.
punctum proximum of a.
pupils equal, reactive to light and a. (PERLA)
pupils equal, round, reactive to light and a. (PERRLA)
range of a.
reflex a.
a. reflex
relative a.
residual a.
a. response
reticule a.
a. rule
spasm of a.
a. spasm
steady-state a.
subnormal a.
tonic a.
accommodation-convergence ratio
accommodative
a. adaptation
a. amplitude (AA)
a. arching theory
a. asthenopia
a. convergence (AC)
a. convergence-accommodation (AC/A)
a. convergence-accommodation ratio
a. cyclophoria
a. effort syndrome
a. esodeviation
a. esophoria
a. esotropia
a. implant
a. insufficiency (AI)
a. IOL
a. palsy
a. pupillary reflex
a. response
a. spasm
a. squint
a. stimulus

a. strabismus
a. target
accommodometer
Accugel lens
Accu-Line surgical marking pen
AccuMap multifocal objective perimeter
accumulated lead exposure
accumulation
age-related lipid a.
lipid a.
accuracy
accommodation a.
Accurate Surgical and Scientific Instruments (ASSI)
Accurus
A. 2500 probe
A. vitreoretinal surgical system
Accutane
Accutome
A. black diamond blade
A. black diamond clear cornea keratome
A. LRI diamond knife
A. side-port diamond knife
Accuvac smoke evacuation attachment
aceclidine
acellular
a. dermal allograft
a. dermis
a. diurnal allograft
a. matrix
acephalgic migraine
acephalic migraine
ACES
American College of Eye Surgeons
acetaldehyde
acetaminophen
a. with codeine
a. with hydrocodone
acetate
anecortave a.
aqueous uranyl a.
cellulose a.
cortisone a.
Cortone A.
dexamethasone a.
fluorometholone a.
glatiramer a.
hydrocortisone a.
medroxyprogesterone a.
paramethasone a.
phenylmercuric a.
potassium a.
prednisolone a.
sodium a.
zinc a.
acetazolamide
acetic acid
acetohexamide

acetonide
    fluocinolone a.
    intravitreal triamcinolone a.
    triamcinolone a.
acetoxycycloheximide (AXM)
acetoxyphenylmercury
aceturate
    diminazene a.
acetylcholine
    a. chloride
    a. intraocular
    a. receptor deficiency
acetylcholinesterase deficiency
acetylcysteine
N-**acetyl-beta-D-glucosaminidase**
ACG
    angle-closure glaucoma
ACHIEVE
    Adolescent and Child Health Initiative to
    Encourage Vision Empowerment
      ACHIEVE study
achloropsia
achromat
achromatic
    a. automated perimetry (AAP)
    a. axis
    a. doublet
    a. objective
    a. spectacle lens
    a. threshold
    a. vision
achromatism
achromatopsia, achromatopsy
    atypical a.
    central a.
    cerebral a.
    complete a.
    cone a.
    incomplete a.
    rod a.
    typical a.
    X-linked a.
achromatopsia
achromatopsic
achromia
achromocytosis
acid
    acetic a.
    aminocaproic a.
    boric a.
    a. burn
    ethylene diamine tetraacetic a.
      (EDTA)

    folinic a.
    hyaluronic a.
    hydrobromic a. (HBr)
    hydrochloric a.
    a. maltase deficiency
    meibum oleic a.
    phosphonoformic a.
    phosphoric a.
    polyunsaturated fatty a. (PUFA)
    ribonucleic a. (RNA)
    sorbic a.
    tranexamic a.
acid-fast
    a.-f. bacillus (AFB)
    a.-f. stain
acidophilic adenoma
acid-resistant penicillin
acid-Schiff
    periodic a.-S. (PAS)
acinar
    a. dropout
    a. lacrimal gland
Acinetobacter calcoaceticus
acinus, pl. **acini**
    lacrimal gland a.
ACIOL
    anterior chamber intraocular lens
      ACIOL implant
aCL
    anticardiolipin
ACM
    anterior chamber maintainer
acne
    a. ciliaris
    a. rosacea
    a. rosacea blepharoconjunctivitis
    a. rosacea conjunctivitis
    a. rosacea corneal ulcer
    a. rosacea keratitis
    a. rosacea meibomianitis
acnes
    Propionibacterium a.
acorea
acorn-shaped eye implant
acoustic
    a. nerve
    a. neuroma
    a. spot
acoustical
    a. shadowing
    a. sonolucent
acquired
    a. abducens nerve lesion

NOTES

acquired *(continued)*
    a. alexia
    a. astigmatism
    a. cataract
    a. color defect
    a. cranial nerve lesion
    a. distichiasis
    a. dyschromatopsia
    a. entropion
    a. esotropia
    a. fixation nystagmus
    a. gustolacrimal reflex
    a. Horner syndrome
    a. hyperopia
    a. immune response
    a. immunodeficiency syndrome
    (AIDS)
    a. jerk nystagmus
    a. melanosis
    a. myopathic ptosis
    a. nevus
    a. ocular motor apraxia
    a. pendular nystagmus
    a. prepapillary venous loop
    a. retinoschisis
    a. superior oblique palsy
    a. syphilis
    a. toxoplasmosis retinitis
acquisita
    epidermolysis bullosa a.
ACR
    Clear Eyes ACR
acritochromacy
acrocephalosyndactyly of Apert
acrodermatitis enteropathica
acrylate
    silicone a.
acrylic
    a. foldable intraocular lens
    a. hydroxyapatite implant
    a. lens implant
    a. separator
AcrySof
    A. foldable intraocular lens
    A. haptic lens
    A. IQ IOL
    A. MA60 lens
    A. Natural intraocular lens
    A. Natural IOL
    A. ReSTOR apodized diffractive
    optic posterior chamber intraocular
    lens
    A. single-piece IOL
ACS
    Alcon closure system
    automated corneal shaper
    ACS needle
ACT
    alternate cover test

actinic
    a. conjunctivitis
    a. hyperplasia
    a. keratitis
    a. keratosis
    a. prurigo
    a. retinitis
Actinobacillus actinomycetemcomitans
Actinomadura madurae
Actinomyces israelii
Actinomycetales
actinomycetemcomitans
    Actinobacillus a.
actinomycin D
action
    evasive a.
    mechanism of a.
    mode of a.
    primary a.
    secondary a.
activation
    endothelial cell a.
    T-cell a.
activator
    plasminogen a.
    recombinant tissue plasminogen a.
    tissue plasminogen a. (TPA, tPA)
    urokinase-type plasminogen a.
    (UPA)
active
    a. emmetropization
    a. force generation test
    a. pterygium
activity, pl. **activities**
    activities of daily vision scale
    (ADVS)
    intrinsic sympathomimetic a.
    laser a.
    mitochondrial enzyme a.
    near-vision a.
    ristocetin cofactor a.
actomyosin ATPase
actual degree of independence
acuity
    absolute intensity threshold a.
    Bailey-Lovie distance visual a.
    best corrected visual a.
    best spectacle-corrected visual a.
    (BSCVA)
    best uncorrected visual a.
    binocular visual a.
    a. card procedure
    central visual a.
    a. of color vision (VC)
    contrast a.
    corrected visual a. (Va_{cc})
    detection a.
    distance visual a. (DVA)
    dynamic visual a.

functional visual a.
grating a.
high-contrast distance visual a.
(HCDVA)
identification a.
Jaeger a.
line of visual a.
low-contrast distance visual a.
(LCDVA)
luminance a.
mean a.
minimum perceptible a.
minimum separable a.
monocular visual a.
near visual a. (NVA)
numerical visual a.
perceptible a.
postoperative visual a.
potential visual a.
preoperative visual a.
resolution a.
separable a.
Snellen visual a.
spatial a.
spectacle-corrected visual a.
stereoscopic a.
Teller visual a.
true visual a. (TVA)
uncorrected visual a. (UCVA)
Vernier visual a.
visibility a.
visual a.
visual discriminatory a. (VDA)
a. visual projector

Acular
A. drops
A. LS ophthalmic solution
A. Ophthalmic
A. P.F.

aculeiform cataract
Acuson
A. 128 apparatus
A. ultrasound

acute
a. acquired comitant esotropia
(AACE)
a. angle-closure glaucoma (AACG)
a. anular outer retinopathy
a. atopic conjunctivitis
a. catarrhal conjunctivitis
a. catarrhal rhinitis
a. chalazion
a. chronic glaucoma

a. congestive conjunctivitis
a. congestive glaucoma
a. contagious conjunctivitis
a. dacryocystitis
a. diffuse serous choroiditis
a. disc edema
a. epidemic conjunctivitis
a. febrile neutrophilic dermatosis
a. follicular conjunctivitis
a. hemorrhagic conjunctivitis
a. hydrops
a. idiopathic blind spot enlargement
syndrome (AIBSES)
a. idiopathic demyelinating optic
neuritis
a. lymphoblastic leukemia
a. macular neuroretinopathy (AMN)
a. multifocal placoid pigment
epitheliopathy
a. multifocal posterior placoid
pigment epitheliopathy (AMPPPE)
a. orbitopathy
a. papilledema
a. pharyngoconjunctival fever
a. primary angle-closure glaucoma
(APACG)
a. red eye (ARE)
a. retinal necrosis (ARN)
a. retinal necrosis syndrome
a. spastic entropion
a. sterile inflammation
a. viral conjunctivitis
a. zonal occult outer retinopathy
(AZOOR)

acute-onset endophthalmitis
Acuvue
A. Advance contact lens
A. bifocal contact lens
A. brand toric contact lens
A. 1-day disposable lens
A. disposable contact lens
A. Etafilcon A lens
A. toric contact lens
A. 2-week UV-blocking disposable
lens

acyclic nucleoside analog
acyclovir
adacrya
Adams
A. desaturated D15 test
A. operation
A. operation for ectropion

NOTES

adaptation
    accommodative a.
    color a.
    dark a.
    light a.
    photopic a.
    prism a.
    retinal a.
    saccadic a.
    scotopic a.
    sensorial a.

adapter
    Ceralink slit lamp laser a.
    large spot slit lamp a.
    Sheehy-Urban sliding lens a.
    Volk Minus noncontact a.
    Volk retinal scale a.
    Volk ultra field aspherical lens a.
    Volk yellow filter a.
    Zeiss cine a.

adaptive immunity

adaptometer
    color a.
    Feldman a.
    Goldmann-Weekers dark a.

adaptometry
    dark a.

AdatoSil silicone oil

ADCC
    autosomal dominant congenital cataract

add
    near a.
    a. power

adduct

adduction
    a. impairment
    a. lag

adductor muscle

adenine arabinoside

adenocarcinoma
    necrotic a.

adenoid cystic carcinoma

adenologaditis

adenoma
    acidophilic a.
    basophilic a.
    chromophobe a.
    endocrine-inactive a.
    Fuchs a.
    invasive a.
    parathyroid a.
    pituitary a.
    pleomorphic a.
    prolactin-secreting a.
    sebaceous a.
    a. sebaceum

adenomectomy
    medical a.

adenophthalmia

adenosine monophosphate (AMP)

adenoviral
    a. conjunctivitis
    a. keratoconjunctivitis

adenovirus (ADV)
    a. 3, 7, 8, 19
    a. conjunctivitis
    a. monoclonal antibody
    a. type 34

adequacy
    blink a.

adherence syndrome

adherens
    leukoma a.
    macula a.
    zonula a.

adherent
    a. cataract
    a. lens
    a. leukoma
    a. plaque

adhesion
    cell a.
    chorioretinal a.
    cicatricial a.
    leukocyte a.
    thermal a.
    vitreoretinal a.

adhesive
    biodendrimer a.
    Brown sterile a.
    cyanoacrylate tissue a.
    Nexacryl tissue a.
    a. syndrome
    tissue a.

Adie
    A. syndrome
    A. tonic pupil

adiposa
    blepharoptosis a.
    cataracta a.
    ptosis a.

adipose
    a. body
    a. tissue

adiposus
    arcus a.

aditus orbitae

adjunct
    a. anesthetic agent
    nonsurgical a.
    surgical a.

adjunctive
    a. mitomycin C
    a. MMC

adjustable suture

adjuster
>Seibel paracentesis valve a.
>Serdarevic suture a.

adjustment
>early postoperative suture a. (EPSA)
>intraoperative suture a. (ISA)
>late postoperative suture a. (LPSA)
>postoperative a.
>suture a.

adjuvant
>a. microwave thermotherapy
>a. therapy

Adler operation

administration
>intracameral a.
>intraocular a.
>intravitreal a.
>oral a.
>parenteral a.
>peribulbar a.
>periocular a.
>retrobulbar a.
>route of a.
>subconjunctival a.
>sub-Tenon a.
>systemic a.

adnata
>alopecia a.

adnatum
>ankyloblepharon filiforme a.

adnexal

adnexum, pl. **adnexa**
>adnexa oculi

adolescent
>a. cataract
>A. and Child Health Initiative to Encourage Vision Empowerment (ACHIEVE)

adrenal
>a. disorder
>a. hypertension

adrenaline

adrenalone

adrenergic
>a. agonist
>a. drug

adrenochrome deposit

adrenoleukodystrophy

adrenomedullin

Adson forceps

adsorbate

adtorsion

adult
>a. foveomacular retinal dystrophy
>a. inclusion conjunctivitis
>a. medulloepithelioma
>a. nucleus
>a. vitelliform macular dystrophy

adult-onset
>a.-o. cataract
>a.-o. diabetes mellitus (AODM)
>a.-o. foveomacular dystrophy (AOFMD)
>a.-o. vitelliform macular dystrophy

adumbration

ADV
>adenovirus

advanced
>A. Glaucoma Intervention Study (AGIS)
>A. Medical Optics (AMO)
>a. pellucid marginal degeneration
>A. Relief Visine
>A. Shape Technology Refractive Algorithm (ASTRA)
>a. visual instrument system

advancement
>capsular a.
>conjunctival a.
>a. flap
>levator a.
>a. procedure
>tendon a.

advancing
>a. age
>a. wave-like epitheliopathy (AWE)

AdvanTec Legacy

Advent pachymeter

adverse event

ADVS
>activities of daily vision scale
>ADVS score

Aebli corneal section scissors

aegyptius
>*Haemophilus a.*

AEO
>apraxia of eyelid opening

aerial
>a. haze
>a. image

aerogenes
>*Enterobacter a.*

Aeromonas hydrophila

aerosol keratitis

Aerosporin

NOTES

aeruginosa
    Pseudomonas a.
AES
    antielevation syndrome
Aesculap
    A. argon ophthalmic laser
    A. excimer laser
Aesculap-Meditec
    A.-M. excimer laser
    A.-M. MEL60 system
aesthesiometer (*var. of* esthesiometer)
AFB
    acid-fast bacillus
afferent
    a. nerve
    a. pupillary defect (APD)
    a. visual pathway
    a. visual symptom
afferentiation
AFI
    amaurotic familial idiocy
afocal
    a. optical system
    a. telescope
africanum
    Mycobacterium a.
aftercataract bur
aftereffect
afterimage
    complementary a.
    negative a.
    positive a.
    a. test
afterimagery
afternystagmus, after-nystagmus
afterperception
aftervision
AG
    Amsler grid
against-the-rule (ATR)
    a.-t.-r. astigmatism
agar
    chocolate a.
    nonnutrient a.
    Sabouraud dextrose a.
Agarwal irrigating phaco chopper
age
    advancing a.
    gestational a.
    postconceptual a.
agenesis
    colossal a.
    congenital punctal a.
agent
    adjunct anesthetic a.
    alpha-2-adrenergic agonist a.
    alternate coupling a.
    antiallergy a.
    antibacterial a.
    antifibrinolytic a.
    antifibrotic a.
    antifungal a.
    antiinfective a.
    antiinflammatory a.
    antimicrobial a.
    antiviral a.
    bacterial a.
    corticosteroid-sparing a.
    coupling a.
    cytoskeletal a.
    fungal a.
    glaucoma a.
    hemostatic a.
    high viscosity a.
    hyperosmotic a.
    hypotensive a.
    intraocular anesthetic a.
    ocular hypotensive a.
    osmotic a.
    parasitic a.
    pharmaceutical a.
    reversal a.
    systemic hyperosmolar a.
    tonicity a.
    topical hyperosmolar a.
    topical ocular antihypertensive a.
    viscoadaptive a.
    viscoelastic a.
    viscosity-increasing a.
    VisionBlue ophthalmic a.
    wetting a.
ageotropic nystagmus
age-related
    a.-r. cataract
    a.-r. decrement
    a.-r. degenerative retinoschisis
    a.-r. disciform macular degeneration
    a.-r. eye disease
    A.-r. Eye Disease Study (AREDS)
    a.-r. lipid accumulation
    a.-r. macular degeneration (AMD, ARMD)
    a.-r. maculopathy (ARM)
    a.-r. ptosis
agglutination
    lid a.
    plasmoid a.
agglutinin
    Ricinus communis a.
    Ulex europaeus a. 1 (UEA-1)
aggravating condition
aggregate
    cellular a.
aggregation
    lymphocytic a.
aggressive histologic subtype
aging
    Canadian Study of Health and A.

AGIS
Advanced Glaucoma Intervention Study
AGL-400
Mira AGL-400
aglaucopsia
Agnew
A. canaliculus knife
A. canthoplasty
A. keratome
A. operation
A. tattooing needle
Agnew-Verhoeff incision
agnosia
apperceptive a.
color a.
optic a.
topographic a.
visual a.
visual-spatial a.
agonist
adrenergic a.
alpha a.
alpha-adrenergic a.
a. muscle
P2Y2 a.
topical androgen a.
agonist-antagonist relationship
Agricola lacrimal sac retractor
AGV
Ahmed glaucoma valve
AGV pars plana clip
Ahlström syndrome
AHM
anterior hyaloid membrane
Ahmed
A. device
A. drainage seton
A. glaucoma biplate valve
A. glaucoma drainage tube
A. glaucoma valve (AGV)
A. glaucoma valve implantation
A. glaucoma valve tube
A. shunt tube
A. tube extender
A. valve implant
AI
accommodative insufficiency
AIBSES
acute idiopathic blind spot enlargement
syndrome
AICA
anterior inferior cerebellar artery
AICA syndrome

Aicardi syndrome
aid
canalicular visualization a.
low-vision a.
magnification a.
optical low vision a.
AIDS
acquired immunodeficiency syndrome
Longitudinal Study of Ocular
Complications of AIDS (LSOCA)
Studies of the Ocular
Complications in AIDS (SOCA)
AIDS-related
AIDS-r. complex (ARC)
AIDS-r. cytomegalovirus
AIDS-r. eye disease
AIDS-r. keratitis
AIDS-r. retinitis
Aimark perimetry
aiming beam
AION
anterior ischemic optic neuropathy
air
a. bag-associated trauma
a. bubble
a. bubbling
a. cell
a. chamber
a. cystotome
A. Force test grid target
a. injection cannula
intraocular a.
intraorbital a.
a. pump
a. rifle
air-block glaucoma
air-bubble dissection technique
air-fluid exchange
AIRLens contact lens
air-puff
a.-p. contact tonometer
a.-p. noncontact tonometer
Airy
A. cylindric lens
A. disc
AK
astigmatic keratotomy
Akahoshi
A. acrylic intraocular lens forceps
A. acrylic IOL loading forceps
A. hybrid combo prechopper
A. hydrodissection cannula
A. implantation forceps

NOTES

A

Akahoshi *(continued)*
 A. nucleus completer
 A. nucleus manipulator
 A. nucleus ring sustainer
 A. nucleus separator
 A. nucleus splitter
 A. phaco prechopper
 A. prechopper forceps
 A. Universal prechopper
Akarpine Ophthalmic
AK-Beta
AK-Chlor Ophthalmic
AK-Cide
 AK-C. Ophthalmic
 AK-C. Suspension
AK-Con-A
AK-Con ophthalmic
AK-Dex Ophthalmic
AK-Dilate ophthalmic solution
Aker lens pusher
AK-Fluor
AK-Homatropine Ophthalmic
akinesia
 Nadbath a.
 O'Brien a.
 orbital a.
 retrobulbar a.
 Scheie a.
 supraorbital a.
 Van Lint a.
akinesis
 pupillary sphincter a.
akinetic
akinetopsia
 cerebral a.
AK-Lor
AK-Mycin
AK-NaCl
AK-Nefrin ophthalmic solution
AK-Neo-Cort
AK-Neo-Dex Ophthalmic
aknephascopia
Akorn OcuCaps
AK-Pentolate
AK-Poly-Bac
 A.-P.-B. Ointment
 A.-P.-B. Ophthalmic
AK-Pred Ophthalmic
AKPro Ophthalmic
AK-Rinse
AK-Spore
 AK-S. H.C. Ophthalmic Ointment
 AK-S. H.C. Ophthalmic Suspension
 AK-S. Solution
AK-Sulf
 AK-S. Forte
 AK-S. Ophthalmic
AK-Taine
AK-Tate

AK-T-Caine
AK-Tetra
AKTob Ophthalmic
AK-Tracin Ophthalmic
AK-Trol Suspension
Akura partial depth astigmatic keratotomy marker
Akwa
 A. Tears
 A. Tears lubricant eye drops
 A. Tears lubricant ophthalmic ointment
 A. Tears solution
AK-Zol
AL
 axial length
Alabama
 A. tying forceps
 A. University utility forceps
alacrima
Alamar blue redox reaction
Alamast
ala minor ossis sphenoidalis
Åland
 Å. Island albinism
 Å. Island eye disease
Alan-Thorpe lens
Albalon
 A. Liquifilm
 A. Liquifilm Ophthalmic
Albalon-A Ophthalmic
Albamycin
albedo retinae
albendazole
Albenza
Albers-Schönberg disease
albescens
 retinitis punctata a.
 retinopathy punctata a.
albicans
 Candida a.
albinism
 Åland Island a.
 autosomal dominant oculocutaneous a.
 autosomal recessive ocular a. (AROA)
 localized a.
 minimal pigment oculocutaneous a.
 Nettleship-Falls X-linked ocular a.
 ocular a.
 oculocutaneous a.
 partial a.
 punctate oculocutaneous a.
 tyrosinase-negative type oculocutaneous a.
 tyrosinase-positive type oculocutaneous a.
 yellow-mutant oculocutaneous a.

albino
albinoidism
    oculocutaneous a.
    punctate oculocutaneous a.
albinotic fundus
albipunctate fundus
Albright disease
albuminuric
    a. amaurosis
    a. retinitis
Alcaligenes xylosoxidans
alcohol
    benzyl a.
    fluorometholone a.
    lanolin a.
    phenethyl a.
    polyvinyl a. (PVA)
    a. well
alcoholic amblyopia
Alcon
    A. Accurus vitrectomy cutter
    A. AcrySof SA30AL single-piece
    lens
    A. A-OK crescent knife
    A. A-OK ShortCut knife
    A. A-OK slit knife
    A. applanation pneumatonograph
    A. aspiration
    A. aspirator
    A. closure system (ACS)
    A. cryoextractor
    A. cryophake
    A. cryosurgical unit
    A. CU-15 4-mil needle
    A. Digital B 2000 ultrasound
    A. disposable drape
    A. EyeMap EH-290 corneal
    topography system
    A. hand cautery
    A. ICaps
    A. I knife
    A. indirect ophthalmoscope
    A. Infiniti system
    A. irrigating/aspirating unit
    A. irrigating needle
    A. 20,000 Legacy unit
    A. MA30BA optic AcrySof lens
    A. 10,000 Master unit
    A. microsponge
    A. phacoemulsification unit
    A. portable autokeratometer
    A. reverse cutting needle

    A. Saline Especially for Sensitive
    Eyes Solution
    A. spatula needle
    A. Surgical instrument
    A. suture
    A. taper cut needle
    A. taper point needle
    A. tonometer
    A. ultrasound pachometer
    A. vitrectomy probe
    A. vitrector
AL/CR
    axial length-corneal radius
    AL/CR ratio
ALD
    average lens density
Alder anomaly
Alder-Reilly phenomenon
aldose reductase
Alexander-Ballen retractor
Alexander law
alexia
    acquired a.
    literal a.
    optical a.
    pure a.
    subcortical a.
alexic
Alezzandrini syndrome
alfa-2a
    interferon a.-2a
alfa-2b
    interferon a.-2b
Alfonso
    A. cutting platform
    A. diamond corneal transplant
    blade
    A. nucleus forceps
    A. nucleus ophthalmic trisector
    A. pediatric eyelid speculum
Alfonso-McIntyre nucleus spoon
Alger
    A. brush
    A. brush rust ring remover
Alges bifocal contact lens
algorithm
    Advanced Shape Technology
    Refractive A. (ASTRA)
    Canny edge a.
    commercial segmentation a.
    dry eye a.
    fast optic disc a.
    FastPac a.

NOTES

algorithm *(continued)*
    Fourier a.
    6-step a.
    Swedish interactive thresholding a.
    (SITA)
    Zernike a.
algorithmic formulation
Alhazen theory
alignment
    entry-site a. (ESA)
    ocular a.
    primary gaze a.
Alio
    A. capsulorrhexis forceps
    A. enclavation forceps
    A. iridectomy forceps
    A. MICS capsulorrhexis forceps
Alio-Prats irrigating stinger
aliquot
alizarin
    a. red S dye
    a. red stain
ALK
    automated laser keratomileusis
alkali
    a. burn
    a. burn of cornea
    a. burn to eye
alkaline burn
alkaloid
    belladonna a.
    dissociated a.
    ergot a.
    miotic a.
    undissociated a.
alkaptonuria
Alkeran
alkylating agent therapy
alkyl ether sulfate
all
    A. Clear AR
    A. Pupil II indirect ophthalmoscope
allachesthesia
    optical a.
Allegra
Allegretto
    A. Wave excimer laser
    A. Wave excimer laser system
    A. Wave Topolyzer
allele
Allen
    A. cyclodialysis
    A. figure
    A. figure acuity testing
    A. operation
    A. orbital implant
    A. preschool card
    A. stereo separator
Allen-Schiötz tonometer

Allen-Thorpe
    A.-T. goniolens
    A.-T. gonioscopic prism
    A.-T. lens
Aller-Chlor
Allerest eye drops
Allergan
    A. AMO Array S155 lens
    A. Enzymatic Cleaner
    A. Humphrey laser
    A. Humphrey lensometer
    A. Humphrey perimeter
    A. Humphrey photokeratoscope
    A. Humphrey refractor
    A. Medical Optics photokeratoscope
allergen
    conjunctival a.
allergic
    a. blepharitis
    a. blepharoconjunctivitis
    a. condition
    a. conjunctivitis
    a. conjunctivitis quality of life
    questionnaire
    a. eye disease
    a. keratoconjunctivitis
    a. ocular disease
    a. pannus
    a. phlyctenulosis
    a. response
    a. rhinitis
allergica
allergy
    ocular a.
AllerMax Oral
Allescheria boydii
allesthesia
    visual a.
alligator scissors
Allis forceps
AlloDerm
allogeneic retinal epithelial cell
allograft
    acellular dermal a.
    acellular diurnal a.
    application of acellular diurnal a.
    a. corneal rejection
    epithelium-deprived orthotopic
      corneal a.
    keratolimbal a. (KLA)
    limbal a.
    living-related conjunctival limbal a.
    (lr-CLAL)
allografting
    limbal cell a.
allokeratoplasty
allopathic keratoplasty
allophthalmia
alloplastic donor material

allopurinol
alloxan diabetes
all-PMMA intraocular lens
Allport
    A. cutting bur
    A. operation
all-*trans*-retinal
Alocril ophthalmic solution
Alomide
    A. drops
    A. ophthalmic solution
alone
    lens a.
alopecia
    a. adnata
    a. leprotica
    a. orbicularis
Alpern cortex aspirator/hydrodissector
alpha
    a. agonist
    a. angle
    a. antagonist
    A. Chymar
    a. crystallin
    a. herpes virus
alpha-2a
alpha-2-adrenergic
    a.-2-a. agonist agent
    a.-2-a. agonist agent, ophthalmic
alpha-adrenergic agonist
alpha$_1$-antitrypsin
alphabet keratitis
alpha-chymotrypsin cannula
alpha-chymotrypsin-induced glaucoma
AlphaCor
    A. artificial cornea
    A. hydrogel synthetic cornea
Alphadrol
Alphagan P
alpha-methyldopa
alpha-methyl-*p*-tyrosine
ALPI
    argon laser peripheral iridoplasty
Alport syndrome
Alrex ophthalmic suspension
Alström
    A. disease
    A. syndrome
Alström-Hallgren syndrome
Alström-Olsen syndrome
ALT
    argon laser trabeculopexy
alteplase

alteration
    retinal pigmentation a.
altered
    a. tear composition
    a. tear distribution
Alternaria alternata
alternata
    Alternaria a.
alternate
    a. coupling agent
    a. cover test (ACT)
    a. cover-uncover test
    a. day esotropia
    a. day strabismus
    a. fixation
    a. hyperdeviation
alternating
    a. amblyopia
    a. esotropia
    a. exophoria
    a. exotropia
    a. Horner syndrome
    a. hypertropia
    a. hypotropia
    a. light test
    a. mydriasis
    a. oculomotor hemiplegia
    a. strabismus
    a. sursumduction
    a. tropia
alternation
alternative
    bladeless a.
    photoreceptor transplantation
      ineffective a.
    Soft Mate Enzyme A.
alternocular
altitudinal
    a. field
    a. hemianopia
    a. hemianopsia
    a. scotoma
    a. visual field defect
    a. visual field loss
ALTK
    automated lamellar therapeutic
    keratoplasty
    ALTK system microkeratome
ALTP
    argon laser trabeculoplasty
Alumina implant
aluminum
    a. chloride

NOTES

aluminum *(continued)*
    a. eye shield
    a. oxide implant
Alvis
    A. curette
    A. fixation forceps
    A. foreign body spud
    A. operation
Alvis-Lancaster sclerotome
AM
    myopic astigmatism
AMA
    American Medical Association
amacrine
    a. cell
    a. cell somata
Amadeus
    A. epikeratome
    A. microkeratome
amaurosis
    albuminuric a.
    Burns a.
    cat's-eye a.
    central a.
    a. centralis
    cerebral a.
    congenital a.
    a. congenita of Leber
    diabetic a.
    a. fugax
    gaze-evoked a.
    gutta a.
    intoxication a.
    Leber congenital a.
    a. nystagmus
    a. partialis fugax
    pressure a.
    reflex a.
    saburral a.
    sympathetic a.
    toxic a.
    uremic a.
amaurotic
    a. cat's eye
    a. familial idiocy (AFI)
    a. mydriasis
    a. nystagmus
    a. pupil
    a. pupillary paralysis
ambient light exposure
amblyogenic period
amblyopia
    alcoholic a.
    alternating a.
    ametropic a.
    anisometric a.
    anisometropic a.
    arsenic a.
    astigmatic a.

    axial a.
    color a.
    crossed a.
    deprivation a.
    eclipse a.
    esotropic a.
    ethyl alcohol a.
    a. ex anopsia
    exertional a.
    functional a.
    hysterical a.
    idiopathic a.
    index a.
    irreversible a.
    macular suppression a.
    meridional a.
    microstrabismic a.
    moderate a.
    nocturnal a.
    nutritional a.
    occlusion a.
    organic a.
    pattern distortion a.
    postmarital a.
    postoperative a.
    quinine a.
    receptor a.
    reflex a.
    refractive a.
    relative a.
    reverse a.
    sensory a.
    strabismic a.
    superimposed a.
    suppression a.
    tobacco a.
    tobacco-alcohol a.
    toxic a.
    traumatic a.
    A. Treatment Study (ATS)
    uremic a.
    visual-deprivation a.
    West Indian a.
amblyopic eye
amblyoscope
    major a.
    Worth a.
ambulatory vision
AMD
    age-related macular degeneration
    exudative AMD
AMDF
    American Macula Degeneration
    Foundation
amebiasis
amebic keratitis
ameboid
    a. keratitis
    a. ulcer

amelanotic
   a. choroidal melanoma
   a. lesion
   a. melanoma
ameliorate
ameloblastic neurilemoma
America
   Eye Bank Association of A.
   (EBAA)
   Laser Institute of A. (LIA)
   Prevent Blindness A. (PBA)
   Vision Council of A. (VCA)
American
   A. Academy of Ophthalmic
   Executives (AAOE)
   A. Academy of Ophthalmology
   (AAO)
   A. Academy of Ophthalmology's
   Preferred Practice Pattern
   guidelines
   A. Academy of Optometry (AAO)
   A. Academy of Pediatric
   Ophthalmology and Strabismus
   A. Association for Pediatric
   Ophthalmology and Strabismus
   (AAPOS)
   A. Board of Eye Surgeons
   (ABES)
   A. Board of Ophthalmology (ABO)
   A. College of Eye Surgeons
   (ACES)
   A. Hydron
   A. Hydron instrument
   A. leishmaniasis
   A. Macula Degeneration Foundation
   (AMDF)
   A. Medical Association (AMA)
   A. Medical Optics (AMO)
   A. Medical Optics Baron lens
   A. National Standards Institute
   (ANSI)
   A. National Standards Institute
   standard
   A. Optical (AO)
   A. Optical Hardy-Rand-Rittler color
   plate
   A. Optometric Association (AOA)
   A. Society of Cataract and
   Refractive Surgery (ASCRS)
   A. Society of Contemporary
   Ophthalmology (ASCO)
   A. Society of Ocularists

   A. Society of Ophthalmic Plastic
   and Reconstruction Surgery
   A. Society of Retina Specialists
   (ASRS)
   A. Surgical Instrument Company
   (ASICO)
Ames test
ametrometer
ametropia
   axial a.
   curvature a.
   defocus-induced a.
   index a.
   position a.
   refractive a.
   transient a.
ametropic amblyopia
Amicar
Amies
   A. transport medium with charcoal
   A. transport medium without
   charcoal
amifloxacin
amikacin
Amikin
amine
   vasoactive a.
amino acid metabolism
aminoaciduria cataract
aminocaproic acid
aminoglutethimide
aminoglycoside with cefazolin
aminophylline
aminopyridine
4-aminoquinoline
aminosteroid
amiodarone-related vision loss
amiodarone toxicity
amitriptyline
Ammon
   A. blepharoplasty
   A. canthoplasty
   A. dacryocystotomy
   A. filament
   A. fissure
   A. operation
   A. scleral prominence
ammonia alkali burn
ammonium
   a. hydroxide alkali burn
   a. lactate
AMN
   acute macular neuroretinopathy

NOTES

amnesic color blindness
amniocentesis
AmnioGraft wound dressing
amniotic
    a. band syndrome
    a. cell
    a. fluid
    a. membrane
    a. membrane transplantation
AMO
    Advanced Medical Optics
    American Medical Optics
        AMO Array foldable intraocular lens
        AMO Array multifocal ultraviolet-absorbing silicone posterior chamber intraocular lens
        AMO Array SA40N multifocal IOL
        AMO Clariflex IOL
        AMO Endosol Extra
        AMO HPF 500 pump
        AMO Ioptex Model ACR 360 foldable acrylic lens
        AMO PhacoFlex II foldable intraocular lens
        AMO PhacoFlex lens and inserter
        AMO Prestige advanced cataract extraction system
        AMO Prestige Phaco System
        AMO Sensar intraocular lens
        AMO Series 4 phaco handpiece
        AMO Set-Up
        AMO Sovereign compact WhiteStar system
        AMO Vitrax viscoelastic solution
        AMO YAG 100 laser
amobarbital
amodiaquine
Amoils epithelial scrubber
amorphic lens
amorphous
    a. corneal deposit
    a. corneal dystrophy
amoxicillin
amoxicillin/clavulanate
AMP
    adenosine monophosphate
Amphadase
amphetamine
amphiphilic drug
amphodiplopia
amphotericin B
amphoterodiplopia
amplification
amplitude
    a. of accommodation (AA)
    accommodative a. (AA)
    a. analysis

    artificial eye a.
    binocular a.
    b-wave a.
    cone b-wave a.
    cone and rod a.
    convergence a.
    a. of convergence
    a. deficit
    divergence a.
    flicker a.
    a. of fusion
    fusional convergence a.
    fusional divergence a.
    fusion with a.
    increased vertical fusional a.
    peak-to-peak a.
    rod b-wave a.
    rod-cone a.
    vertical fusional vergence a.
AMPPPE
    acute multifocal posterior placoid pigment epitheliopathy
ampulla, pl. **ampullae**
    a. canaliculi lacrimalis
    a. ductus lacrimalis
    a. of lacrimal canal
    a. of lacrimal canaliculus
    a. of lacrimal duct
amputation of scleral flap
amputator
    Smith intraocular capsular a.
Amsler
    A. aqueous transplant needle
    A. chart
    A. corneal graft
    A. grid (AG)
    A. operation
    A. scleral marker
    A. test
Amsoft lens
Amvisc
    A. Plus
    A. Plus solution
amyloid
    a. body
    a. cellulitis
    a. corneal degeneration
    a. deposit
    a. P component
    serum a. A
    subcutaneous a.
amyloidosis
    conjunctival a.
    corneal a.
    localized a.
    orbital a.
    primary familial a.
    secondary a.
    systemic a.

Amytal
ANA
    antinuclear antibody
Anacel
anaclasis
anaerobic
    a. medium
    a. ocular infection
anaglyph test
Anagnostakis operation
analgesia
    surface a.
analog, analogue
    acyclic nucleoside a.
    prostaglandin a.
    thymidine a.
analphalipoproteinemia
analysis, pl. **analyses**
    amplitude a.
    astigmatic vector a.
    bivariate a.
    Cochran-Mantel-Haenszel a.
    corneal topographic a.
    cost-effective a.
    digital image a.
    endothelial cell a.
    Fourier harmonic a.
    gelatino-lattice corneal dystrophy a.
    image a.
    immunochromatography a.
    infrared image a.
    latency a.
    linkage a.
    logistic discriminant a.
    morphometric a.
    multivariate logistic regression a.
    Neale reading a.
    pedigree a.
    photograph reading a.
    Rasch a.
    retinal thickness a. (RTA)
    risk factor a.
    sensitivity a.
    test-retest a.
    Topcon noncontact morphometric a.
    total eye a.
    univariant a.
    a. of variance (ANOVA)
    vector a.
    wavefront a.
    Western immunoblotting a.
analyzer
    automatic a.

Dicon ocular blood flow a.
Eye Scan corneal a.
Friedmann visual field a.
GDx nerve fiber a.
Humphrey field a. (HFA)
Humphrey field a. II
Humphrey Instruments vision a.
Humphrey lens a.
Humphrey visual field a.
nerve fiber layer a.
Ocular blood flow a.
ocular response a.
Paradigm ocular blood flow a.
P55 Pachymetric A.
profile a.
retinal thickness a. (RTA)
scanning retinal thickness a.
Tomey retinal function a.
vision a.
anamorphosis
anaphoria
anaphylactic
    a. conjunctivitis
    a. reaction
    a. shock
anaphylaxis
anastigmatic lens
anastomosis, pl. **anastomoses**
    chorioretinal venous a.
    occult chorioretinal a.
    retinal-choroidal a.
anatomic
    a. equator
    a. strabismus
    a. success
anatomical anomaly
anatomy
    facial a.
    intracanalicular a.
    intracranial a.
    intraocular a.
    intraorbital a.
    macular a.
    topographic a.
anatropia
anatropic
anaxon
ANCA
    antineutrophil cytoplasmic antibody
Ancef
anchor
    a. hook
    a. suture

NOTES

anchorage
 plug a.
anchor/fixation
 Searcy a./f.
anchoring suture
Ancobon
Andersen syndrome
Anderson-Kestenbaum procedure
Androgen Tear
anecortave acetate
Anectine
Anel
 A. operation
 A. probe
 A. syringe
anemia
 aplastic a.
 macrocytic a.
 Mediterranean a.
 normocytic hypochromic a.
 pernicious a.
 sickle cell a.
anemone cell tumor
anencephaly
Anergan
anergy
anesthesia
 cornea a.
 endotracheal a.
 exam under a. (EUA)
 general a.
 hypotensive a.
 infraorbital a.
 intracameral a.
 intraorbital a.
 modified Van Lint a.
 a. needle
 needleless regional a.
 O'Brien a.
 orbital a.
 peribulbar a.
 retrobulbar a.
 sub-Tenon parabulbar a.
 topical a.
 Van Lint a.
anesthetic
 general a.
 inhalation a.
 local a.
 a. ointment
 postoperative topical a.
 topical a.
anetoderma
 Jadassohn-type a.
aneuploidy
aneurysm
 arteriovenous a.
 basilar artery a.
 berry a.

carotid a.
cavernous sinus a.
cerebral artery a.
cirsoid a.
communicating artery a.
fusiform a.
giant a.
IC-PC artery a.
internal carotid-posterior
 communicating artery a.
intracavernous a.
intracranial a.
Leber miliary a.
miliary a.
ophthalmic artery a.
a. of orbit
orbital a.
racemose a.
a. of retinal arteriole
retinal artery a.
saccular a.
suprasellar a.
aneurysmal bone cyst
Angelman syndrome
Angelucci
 A. operation
 A. syndrome
angiitis
 frosted branch a.
angio-Behçet disease
angioblastic meningioma
angiodiathermy
angioedema
angioendotheliomatosis
 neoplastic a.
Angiofluor Lite
angiogenesis
 cascade-induced a.
angiogenic
 a. cascade
 a. sprout
angiogram
 fluorescein a.
angiograph
 Heidelberg retina a.
angiographer
 fluorescein a.
angiography
 anterior segment fluorescein a.
 (ASFA)
 carotid a.
 cerebral radionuclide a.
 computed tomographic a.
 digital subtraction indocyanine
 green a. (DS-ICGA)
 fluorescein a. (FA)
 fluorescein angiography/indocyanine
 green a. (FA/ICGA)
 ICG a.

indocyanine green a. (ICGA)
intravenous fluorescein a. (IVFA)
IV retinal fluorescein a.
magnetic resonance a. (MRA)
orbital a.
quantitative fluorescein a.
retinal a.
vertebral a.

angioid
a. disc
a. retinal streak

angiokeratoma
a. corporis diffusum
a. corporis diffusum universale
diffuse a.

angioma
cavernous a.
conjunctival a.
episcleral a.
nerve head a.
orbital a.
racemose a.
retinal a.
spider a.
von Hippel a.

angiomatosis
cerebroretinal a.
encephalofacial a.
encephalotrigeminal a.
meningocutaneous a.
a. of retina
a. retinae
retinal a.
retinocerebellar a.
Sturge-Weber encephalotrigeminal a.

angiopathia retinae juvenilis
angiopathic retinopathy
angiopathy
cerebral amyloid a.

angiophakomatosis
angiosarcoma
orbital a.

angioscopy
fluorescein fundus a.

angioscotoma
angioscotomata
angioscotometry
angiosis streak
angiospasm
angiospastic retinopathy
angiotensin
angle
a. of aberration

a. of abnormality
alpha a.
a. of anomaly
anomaly a.
anterior chamber a.
a. of anterior chamber
a. of aperture
apical a.
ASSI Phaco Chopper 90-degree a.
biorbital a.
cerebellopontine a. (CPA)
chamber a.
contact a.
convergence a.
a. of convergence
critical a.
deformity a.
a. of deviation
a. of direction
disparity a.
divergent cut a.
drainage a.
a. of eccentricity
elevation a.
a. of emergence
filtration a.
a. of Fuchs
gamma a.
a. of incidence
incident a.
iridial a.
iridocorneal a.
a. of iris
Jacquart a.
kappa a.
lambda a.
large kappa a.
lateral a.
limiting a.
medial a.
meter a.
minimum separable a.
minimum visible a.
minimum visual a.
a. narrowing
ocular a.
optic a.
pantoscopic a.
a. of polarization
posterior a.
prism a.
a. recession
a. of reflection

NOTES

angle *(continued)*
    a. of refraction
    refraction a.
    a. in Rieger anomaly
    space of iridocorneal a.
    squint a.
    a. of squint
    a. structure
    a. surgery
    tarsal a.
    temporal catchment a.
    visual a.
    water-contact a.
    wetting a.
    a. width
    zipped a.
angle-closure glaucoma (ACG)
angled
    a. capsule forceps
    a. Connor wand
    a. discission hook
    a. iris hook and IOL dialer
    a. iris retractor
    a. iris spatula
    a. left/right cannula
    a. lens loupe
    a. manipulator
    a. nucleus removal loupe
    a. probe
    a. sapphire knife
    a. suction tube
2-angled polypropylene loop
angle-fixated lens
angle-recession glaucoma
angle-supported lens
angling
    pantoscopic a.
Angosky syndrome
Ångstrom
    Å. law
    Å. unit
angular
    a. aqueous sinus plexus
    a. blepharitis
    a. blepharoconjunctivitis
    a. conjunctivitis
    a. distance
    a. gyrus
    a. junction of eyelid
    a. line
    a. vein
angularis
    blepharitis a.
    vena a.
angulated iris spatula
angulation
    haptic a.
angulus
    a. iridis

    a. iridocornealis
    a. oculi lateralis
    a. oculi medialis
anhydrase
    carbonic a. (CA)
    a. glycerol
anicteric
aniridia
    autosomal recessive a.
    congenital sporadic a.
    a. in newborn
    a. ring
    sporadic a.
    traumatic a.
Anis
    A. irrigating vectis
    A. lens-holding forceps
    A. microforceps model 2-848
    A. radial marker
    A. staple lens
    A. suture placement marker
aniseikonia
    field-dependent a.
    spectacle-induced a.
    a. symptom
aniseikonic lens
anisoaccommodation
anisochromatic
anisochromia
anisocoria
    benign a.
    central a.
    a. contraction
    essential a.
    physiologic a.
    seesaw a.
    simple a.
    simple-central a.
anisometric amblyopia
anisometrope
    hypermetropic a.
anisometropia
    axial a.
    myopic a.
    refractive a.
anisometropic amblyopia
anisophoria
    induced a.
anisotropal
anisotropy map
ankyloblepharon
    external a.
    a. filiforme adnatum
anlage
    lacrimal duct a.
Ann
    A. Arbor Hodgkin disease staging classification
    A. Arbor stage

annular (*var. of* anular)
annulus (*var. of* anulus)
anomaloscope
 Kamppeter a.
 Nagel a.
 Pickford-Nicholson a.
 a. plate test (APT)
 Spectrum color vision meter
  712 a.
anomalous
 a. disc
 a. fixation
 a. retinal correspondence (ARC)
 a. trichromatism
 a. trichromatopsia
 a. vessel
anomaly
 Alder a.
 anatomical a.
 angle of a.
 a. angle
 angle in Rieger a.
 anterior chamber cleavage a.
 Axenfeld a.
 Axenfeld-Rieger a. (ARA)
 Chédiak-Higashi a.
 Chédiak-Steinbrinck-Higashi a.
 coloboma a.
 coloboma, heart defects, atresia
  choanae, retarded growth, genital
  hypoplasia, and ear a.'s
  (CHARGE)
 congenital a.
 craniofacial a.
 developmental a.
 excavated optic disc a.
 facial a.
 Klippel-Feil a.
 lacrimal angle duct a.
 location a.
 microscopic a.
 morning glory optic disc a.
 ocular a.
 oculocephalic vascular a.
 optic disc a.
 orbital venous a.
 osseous a.
 Peters a.
 Rieger a.
 Steinbrinck a.
anomia
 color a.
anophoria

anophthalmanopia
anophthalmia
 consecutive a.
 primary a.
 secondary a.
anophthalmic
 a. implant
 a. socket
anophthalmos
 congenital a.
anopsia
 amblyopia ex a.
anotropia
ANOVA
 analysis of variance
anoxia
ANSI
 American National Standards Institute
 ANSI standard
antagonist
 alpha a.
 beta-adrenergic a.
 contralateral a.
 folic acid a.
 inhibitional palsy of contralateral a.
 ipsilateral a.
 thromboxane receptor a.
$_H$**1-antagonist**
antazoline
 naphazoline and a.
 a. phosphate and naphazoline HCl
Antazoline-V Ophthalmic
antecedent trauma
antenatal testing
anterior
 a. axial developmental cataract
 a. axial embryonal cataract
 a. axonal embryonal cataract
 a. basal membrane
 a. basement membrane dystrophy
  (ABMD)
 camera oculi a.
 a. capsular opacification
 a. capsulectomy
 a. capsule hydrodissector
 a. capsule management
 a. capsule shagreen
 a. capsule staining
 a. capsulorrhexis
 a. capsulotomy
 a. central curve (ACC)
 a. cerebral artery
 a. chamber (AC)

NOTES

anterior *(continued)*
a. chamber angle
a. chamber angle width
a. chamber cleavage anomaly
a. chamber cleavage syndrome
a. chamber depth
a. chamber of eyeball
a. chamber hemorrhage
a. chamber inflammation
a. chamber intraocular lens (ACIOL)
a. chamber intraocular lens implant
a. chamber IOL
a. chamber irrigating vectis
a. chamber irrigator
a. chamber lymphoma
a. chamber maintainer (ACM)
a. chamber paracentesis
a. chamber phacoemulsification
a. chamber reaction
a. chamber refractive surgery
a. chamber shallowing
a. chamber sinus
a. chamber stability
a. chamber synechia scissors
a. chamber tap
a. chamber trabecula
a. chamber tube
a. chamber washout
a. chamber washout cannula
a. choroiditis
a. ciliary artery
a. ciliary vein
a. compressive optic neuropathy
a. conjunctival artery
a. conjunctival vein
a. corneal curvature
a. corneal dystrophy
a. corneal epithelium of cornea
a. corneal staphyloma
a. corneal surface
a. cylinder
a. embryotoxon
a. epithelium corneae
a. ethmoidal artery
a. eye segment analysis system
a. focal point
a. hyaloidal fibrovascular proliferation
a. hyaloid membrane (AHM)
a. hydrophthalmia
a. inferior cerebellar artery (AICA)
a. ischemic optic neuritis
a. ischemic optic neuropathy (AION)
a. keratoconus
lamina elastica a.
a. lens capsule
a. lenticonus

limiting lamina a.
a. limiting lamina
a. limiting lamina of cornea
a. limiting layer of cornea
a. limiting ring
a. lip
a. loop traction
a. megalophthalmos
a. mosaic crocodile shagreen
a. ocular segment
a. optic chiasmal syndrome
a. optic zone
a. optic zone diameter
a. peripheral curve
a. polar cataract
a. pole
a. pole of eye
a. pole of eyeball
a. pole of lens
a. proliferative vitreoretinopathy (APVR)
a. puncture
a. pyramidal cataract
a. scleritis
sclerochoroiditis a.
a. sclerochoroiditis
a. sclerotomy
a. segment dysgenesis
a. segment examination
a. segment of eye
a. segment of eyeball
a. segment fluorescein angiography (ASFA)
a. segment inflammation
a. segment ischemia
a. segment necrosis
a. segment sleeve
a. stromal micropuncture
a. stromal puncture
a. subcapsular cataract (ASC)
a. surface aberration
a. surface of cornea
a. surface of iris
a. symblepharon
a. synechia
a. uveitis
a. vented gas forced fusion system
a. visual pathway
a. visual pathway dysfunction
a. visual pathway glioma
a. vitrectomy
a. vitrectorhexis
a. vitreous
a. vitreous face
anterograde degeneration
anteroposterior
a. axis
a. axis of Fick
Anthony orbital compressor

anthracis
>   *Bacillus a.*

antiacetylcholine
>   a. receptor antibody
>   a. receptor antibody assay

anti-ACh receptor antibody
antiadrenergic drug
antiallergy
>   a. agent
>   a. therapy

antiangiogenesis injection
antibacterial agent
antibiotic
>   bacteriocidal a.
>   bacteriostatic a.
>   broad-spectrum a.
>   a. eye drops
>   fluoroquinolone a.
>   fortified a.
>   intravitreal a.
>   postoperative a.
>   prophylactic a.
>   a. prophylaxis
>   subconjunctival a.

antibody, pl. **antibodies**
>   adenovirus monoclonal a.
>   antiacetylcholine receptor a.
>   anti-ACh receptor a.
>   anticardiolipin a.
>   anti-CD 154 monoclonal a.
>   antilens protein a.
>   antilipoarabinomannan-B a.
>   antineutrophil cytoplasmic a.
>   (ANCA)
>   antinuclear a. (ANA)
>   antiphospholipid a.
>   antirecoverin a.
>   antiretina a.
>   apolipoprotein E a.
>   chromogranin a.
>   complement-fixing a.
>   cytokeratin 7, 20 a.
>   cytotoxic a.
>   diolipin a.
>   ELISA a.
>   glial fibrillary acidic protein a.
>   HIV-specific a.
>   homotropic a.
>   humanized anti-Tac monoclonal a.
>   immunodominant a.
>   indirect fluorescent a.
>   monoclonal a.
>   neurofilament triplets a.

>   neuron-specific enolase a.
>   pancytokeratin a.
>   perinuclear antineutrophil
>   cytoplasmic a. (pANCA)
>   S-100 protein a.
>   stimulatory a.
>   synaptophysin a.
>   treponemal a.

anticardiolipin (aCL)
>   a. antibody

anticataract drug
anti-CD 154 monoclonal antibody
anticholinergic drug
anticomplement immunofluorescence
antielevation syndrome (AES)
antifibrinolytic agent
antifibrotic agent
antifungal
>   a. agent
>   a. therapy

antigen
>   Australia a.
>   early a.
>   EBV-associated a.
>   EBV nuclear a.
>   epithelial membrane a. (EMA)
>   extractable nuclear a.
>   fluorescent-antibody-to-membrane a.
>   (FAMA)
>   HLA-A29 a.
>   HLA-B5 a.
>   HLA-B7 a.
>   HLA-B15 a.
>   HLA-B27 a.
>   HLA-DR4 a.
>   human leukocyte a. (HLA)
>   ICAM-1 a.
>   Kveim a.
>   major histocompatibility a.
>   nuclear a.
>   rheumatoid-associated nuclear a.
>   transplantation a.
>   viral capsid a.

antigen-1
>   leukocyte function associated a.-1
>   (LFA-1)

antigen-presenting cell
antiglaucoma
>   a. surgery
>   a. therapy

antiglial fibrillary acidic protein
Antihist-1
antihistamine

NOTES

anti-Hu syndrome
antiinfective agent
antiinflammatory agent
antilens protein antibody
antilipoarabinomannan-B antibody
Antilirium
antimalarial drug
antimetabolite
antimetropia
antimicrobial
    a. agent
    a. drug
    a. treatment
antimonate
    meglumine a.
antimongoloid slant
antineutrophil cytoplasmic antibody
  (ANCA)
antinuclear antibody (ANA)
antiophthalmic
antioxidant
    a. enzyme
    a. supplement
antipericyte autoantibody
antiphospholipid (aPL)
    a. antibody
    a. syndrome
antirecoverin antibody
antireflection coating
antirejection drug
antiretina antibody
antiretroviral therapy
antistaphylococcal penicillin
antisuppression exercise
antitonic
antitorque suture
anti-VEGF
    a.-VEGF antibody fragment
    a.-VEGF injection
antiviral
    a. agent
    a. therapy
antixerophthalmic
antixerotic
Antley-Bixler syndrome
Anton
    A. symptom
    A. syndrome
Anton-Babinski syndrome
antonina
    facies a.
Antoni pattern
antrophose
anular, annular
    a. bifocal contact lens
    a. cataract
    a. corneal graft
    a. corneal graft operation
    a. infiltrate

    a. keratitis
    a. macular dystrophy
    a. plexus
    a. ring
    a. scleritis
    a. scotoma
    a. staphyloma
    a. synechia
    a. ulcer
anulus, annulus
    a. ciliaris
    a. of conjunctiva
    a. iridis
    a. iridis major
    a. iridis minor
    a. tendineus communis
    a. of Zinn
Anxanil
anxiety
    surgery-related a.
AO
    American Optical
    AO lens
    AO Reichert Instruments
      applanation tonometer
    AO Reichert Instruments binocular
      indirect ophthalmoscope
    AO Reichert Instruments Ful-Vue
      diagnostic unit
    AO Reichert Instruments lensometer
    AO Reichert Instruments Project-O-
      Chart
    AO rotary prism
    AO Vectographic Project-O-Chart
      slide
AOA
    American Optometric Association
AoDisc Neutralizer
AODM
    adult-onset diabetes mellitus
AOFMD
    adult-onset foveomacular dystrophy
AoSept
    A. Clear Care
    A. Disinfectant
    A. Lens Holder and Cup
APACG
    acute primary angle-closure glaucoma
A-pattern
    A-p. esotropia
    A-p. exotropia
    A-p. strabismus
APD
    afferent pupillary defect
Apert
    acrocephalosyndactyly of A.
    A. syndrome
aperture
    angle of a.

A

a. disc
numeric a.
numerical a. (NA)
orbital a.
palpebral a.
pupillary a.
a. ratio
apex, pl. **apices**
corneal a.
a. fracture
orbital a.
petrous a.
A. Plus excimer laser
a. of prism
prism a.
tumor a.
aphakia
binocular a.
extracapsular a.
monocular a.
pediatric a.
aphakic
a. bullous keratopathy (ABK)
a. contact lens
a. correction
a. cystoid macular edema
a. detachment
a. eye
a. glasses
a. glaucoma
a. pupillary block
a. refraction
a. spectacles
aphasia
Broca a.
optic a.
visual a.
aphose
aphotesthesia
aphotic
apical
a. angle
a. clearance
a. cone
a. orbital inflammation
a. radius
a. tumor
a. zone
a. zone of cornea
apices (*pl. of* apex)
apiospermum
Scedosporium a.

aPL
antiphospholipid
aplanatic
a. focus
a. lens
aplanatism
aplasia
chiasmal a.
lacrimal nucleus a.
macular a.
a. of optic nerve
optic nerve a.
punctum a.
retinal a.
aplastic anemia
apochromatic
a. lens
a. objective
apocrine
a. gland
a. hidrocystoma
apodized
a. diffractive IOL
a. diffractive lens
apolipoprotein
a. E
a. E antibody
a. E gene polymorphism
a. E genotyping
Apollo
A. conjunctivitis
A. disease
aponeurogenic ptosis
aponeurosis
aponeurotic ptosis
apoplectic
a. glaucoma
a. retinitis
apoplexy
occipital a.
pituitary a.
a. of pituitary
retinal a.
apoptosis
apostilb
apotripsis
apparatus
accessory visual a.
Acuson 128 a.
ciliary a.
dioptric a.
experimental a.

NOTES

apparatus *(continued)*
    Frigitronics nitrous oxide
      cryosurgery a.
    Golgi a.
    Howard-Dolman a.
    lacrimal a.
    a. lacrimalis
    a. suspensorius lentis
appearance
    beaten bronze a.
    beaten copper a.
    beaten metal a.
    bleb a.
    cobblestone a.
    cushingoid a.
    dendritiform a.
    dropped-socket a.
    feathery a.
    fluffy a.
    granular a.
    leonine a.
    mottled a.
    optic nerve head a.
    salt-and-pepper a.
    silent cornea a.
    snake-like a.
    spongy a.
    squashed-tomato a.
    sunset-glow a.
appendage of eye
apperceptive
    a. agnosia
    a. prosopagnosia
applanation
    a. pressure
    tension by a. (TAP)
    a. tension (AT)
    a. tonometer
    a. tonometry (AT)
applanator
    Johnston LASIK flap a.
applanometer
applanometry
application
    a. of acellular diurnal allograft
    autologous serum a.
    diathermy a.
    pilot a.
    topical a.
applicator
    beta therapy eye a.
    cotton-tipped a.
    Gass dye a.
apposition
    central choroidal a. (CCA)
    wound a.
approach
    ab interno a.
    Berke a.

    bleb grading a.
    Caldwell-Luc a.
    convex iris a.
    fornix a.
    limbal a.
    Lynch a.
    multimodal a.
    nasal a.
    pars plana a.
    shotgun a.
    superior a.
    transcaruncular-transconjunctival a.
    transpunctal endocanalicular a.
apraclonidine
    a. HCl
    a. hydrochloride
    a. ophthalmic solution
apraxia
    acquired ocular motor a.
    Cogan congenital oculomotor a.
    congenital ocular motor a.
      (COMA)
    constructional a.
    eyelid a.
    a. of eyelid opening (AEO)
    a. of gaze
    a. of lid opening
    ocular motor a.
    oculomotor a.
Apresoline
A-Probe
    Soft-Touch A-P.
APT
    anomaloscope plate test
APT-5 Color Vision Tester
APVR
    anterior proliferative vitreoretinopathy
Aquaflex contact lens
AquaFlow collagen glaucoma drainage device
AquaLase
    A. cataract removal system
    A. liquefaction device
    A. solution
AquaSense IOL
Aquasight lens
AquaSite
    A. ophthalmic solution
    A. PF
Aquasonic 100 gel
Aqua-Tears
aqueductal stenosis
aqueous
    a. chamber
    a. communication
    a. concentration level
    a. crystalline penicillin G
    a. double-tubed valve shunt
    fibrinous a.

a. flare
a. fluid
a. humor
a. humor drainage
a. humor eye
a. humor flow
a. humor production
a. inflow
a. influx phenomenon
a. layer of tear film
a. misdirected glaucoma
a. misdirection
a. misdirection syndrome
a. outflow
a. paracentesis
plasmoid a.
a. protein concentration
a. suppressant
a. tap
a. tear deficiency (ATD)
a. tear layer
a. transplant needle
a. tube shunt
a. uranyl acetate
a. vein

Aquify
A. long-lasting comfort drops
A. MPS

aquocapsulitis

aquosus
humor a.

AR
autorefraction
All Clear AR
AR 1000 refractor

ARA
Axenfeld-Rieger anomaly

Arabic eye test

arabinoside
adenine a.

arachnoid
a. hemorrhage
a. sheath

arachnoidal cyst

arachnoiditis
chiasmal a.
opticochiasmatic a.
optochiasmatic a.

Aralen Phosphate

arborescent
a. cataract
a. keratitis

arborization
pattern a.
a. pattern

ARC
AIDS-related complex
anomalous retinal correspondence
unharmonious ARC

arc
a. and bowl perimeter
a. of contact
nuclear a.
a. perimetry
a. scotoma
a. staining
xenon a.

arcade
inferior retinal a.
inferior temporal a.
inferotemporal a.
limbal a.
major vascular a.
superior vascular a.
temporal vascular a.
vascular a.

arc-flash conjunctivitis

arch
orbital a.
Salus a.
superciliary a.
supraorbital a.

Archer lesion

architecture
eyelid a.
iris a.
nasal a.

arciform density

arcitome
Hanna a.

arcuate
a. Bjerrum scotoma
a. commissure
a. course
a. field defect
a. incision
a. nerve fiber bundle
a. retinal fold
a. staining
a. transverse keratotomy

arcus, pl. arcus
a. adiposus
a. cornealis
a. juvenilis
a. lipoides

NOTES

arcus *(continued)*
    a. palpebralis inferior
    a. palpebralis superior
    a. senilis
    a. superciliaris
    unilateral a.
Arden grating
ARE
    acute red eye
area, pl. **areae, areas**
    aspheric lenticular a.
    Bjerrum a.
    Brodmann a.
    a. centralis
    a. of conscious regard
    cortical oculomotor a.
    corticooculocephalogyric a.
    a. of critical definition
    fusion a.
    macular a.
    medial superior temporal visual a.
    middle temporal visual a.
    mirror a.
    MST visual a.
    MT visual a.
    Panum fusion a.
    papillary a.
    parastriate a.
    pretectal a.
    spindle-shaped a.
    visual association a.
AREDS
    Age-Related Eye Disease Study
areflexia
    pupillary a.
areflexical mydriasis
areolar
    a. central choroiditis
    a. choroidopathy
ArF
    argon fluoride
    ArF excimer laser
    ArF excimer laser system
argamblyopia
argema
argon
    a. blue laser
    a. fluoride (ArF)
    a. fluoride excimer laser
    a. green laser
    a. laser coagulator
    a. laser endophotocoagulation
    a. laser iridectomy
    a. laser peripheral iridoplasty
      (ALPI)
    a. laser photocoagulation
    a. laser retinal treatment
    a. laser therapy

    a. laser trabeculopexy (ALT)
    a. laser trabeculoplasty (ALTP)
argon-pumped tunable dye laser
Argyll
    A. Robertson instrument
    A. Robertson operation
    A. Robertson pupil (ARP)
    A. Robertson pupil sign
argyria
argyrism
argyrosis
    ocular a.
arida
    conjunctivitis a.
Arion sling
Aristocort
Aristospan
Arlt
    A. disease
    A. epicanthus repair
    A. eyelid repair
    A. lens
    A. lens loupe
    A. line
    A. operation
    A. pterygium
    A. recess
    A. scoop
    A. sinus
    A. trachoma
    A. triangle
ARM
    age-related maculopathy
arm
    q a.
    Wiltmoser optical a.
Armaly cup/disc ratio
Armaly-Drance technique
ARMD
    age-related macular degeneration
    dry ARMD
    risk factors in ARMD
    wet ARMD
ARN
    acute retinal necrosis
    ARN syndrome
Arnold
    zygomatic foramen of A.
Arnold-Chiari malformation
AROA
    autosomal recessive ocular albinism
ARP
    Argyll Robertson pupil
array
    color filter a. (CFA)
    A. multifocal intraocular lens
    ordered a.
    radial vessel a.

A

ARRON
autoimmune-related retinopathy and optic neuropathy
ARRON syndrome
arrow-shaft silicone punctal plug
Arrowsmith corneal marker
Arroyo
A. dacryostomy
A. encircling suture
A. forceps
A. implant
A. keratoplasty
A. operation
A. protector
A. sign
A. tenotomy
A. trephine
Arruga
A. capsule forceps
A. cataract extraction
A. dacryostomy
A. elevator retractor
A. encircling suture
A. expressor
A. implant
A. keratoplasty
A. lacrimal trephine
A. lens
A. needle holder
A. operation
A. orbital retractor
A. protector
A. tenotomy
Arruga-Nicetic ophthalmology forceps
arsenic amblyopia
arterial
a. circle
a. circle of greater iris
a. circle of lesser iris
a. dissection
a. hypertension
a. macroaneurysm
a. occlusive change
a. occlusive disease
arteriogram
carotid a.
arteriography
cerebral a.
arteriolar
a. attenuation
a. narrowing
a. nicking

a. sclerosis
a. sheathing
arteriole, arteriola
aneurysm of retinal a.
attenuated retinal a.
a. communication
copper-wire a.
inferior macular a.
macular a.
narrowed a.
narrowing of retinal a.
perifoveal a.
precapillary a.
retinal a.
silver-wire a.
superior macular a.
arteriosclerosis (AS)
cerebral a.
a. of retina
arteriosclerotic
a. ischemic optic neuropathy
a. retinopathy
arteriosus
arteriovenous (AV)
a. adventitial sheathotomy
a. aneurysm
a. communication
a. crossing defect
a. malformation
a. nicking
a. pattern
a. ratio
a. strabismus syndrome
arteritic anterior ischemic optic neuropathy
arteritis
cranial a.
giant cell a. (GCA)
occlusive retinal a.
occult temporal a.
pseudotemporal a.
temporal a. (TA)
artery
anterior cerebral a.
anterior ciliary a.
anterior conjunctival a.
anterior ethmoidal a.
anterior inferior cerebellar a. (AICA)
basilar a.
branch retinal a. (BRA)
calcarine a.
carotid a.

NOTES

31

artery *(continued)*
    central retinal a. (CRA)
    cerebellar a.
    cerebral a.
    ciliary a.
    cilioretinal a.
    conjunctival a.
    copper-wire a.
    corkscrew a.
    dolichoectatic anterior cerebral a.
    episcleral a.
    ethmoidal a.
    hyaline a.
    hyaloid a.
    hypophysial a.
    inferior nasal a.
    inferior temporal a.
    inferonasal a.
    inferotemporal a.
    infraorbital a.
    internal carotid a.
    intracavernous carotid a.
    lacrimal a.
    long posterior ciliary a.
    middle cerebral a.
    ophthalmic a.
    optic a.
    parietooccipital a.
    persistent hyaloid a.
    posterior cerebral a.
    posterior ciliary a.
    posterior conjunctival a.
    posterior ethmoidal a. (PEA)
    retinal a.
    retrobulbar a.
    short posterior ciliary a.
    superior nasal a.
    superior temporal a.
    supraorbital a.
    tarsal a.
    temporal a.
    temporooccipital a.
    thrombosed a.
    vertebrobasilar a.
    zygomaticoorbital a.
artery-to-vein ratio (A/V)
arthrokinetic nystagmus
arthroophthalmopathy
    hereditary progressive a.
Arthus reaction
artifact
    degraded image a.
    high-gain a.
    image a.
artifact-free
    a.-f. recording
    a.-f. scan
artifactiously
artifactual

artificial
    a. anterior chamber
    a. cornea
    a. diabetes
    a. divergence procedure
    a. divergency surgery
    a. eye
    a. eye amplitude
    a. eye motility
    a. intelligence
    a. iris diaphragm implant
    a. lens
    a. pupil
    a. silicone retina
    a. silicone retina microchip
    a. silk keratitis
    a. tears (AT)
    a. tear supplementation
    a. UV radiation
    a. vision
Artisan
    A. iris-fixated phakic IOL
    A. lens implantation
    A. lens implantation for myopia
    A. myopia lens
ARVO
    Association for Research in Vision and Ophthalmology
Arxxant
AS
    arteriosclerosis
As
    astigmatism
ASC
    anterior subcapsular cataract
A-scan
    A+ Autoscan portable A-s.
    contact A-s.
    DGH 5000 A-s.
    Jedmed A-s.
    Jedmed/DGH A-s.
    Ultra-Image A-s.
    Ultrascan Digital 2000 contact ultrasound A-s.
    A-s. ultrasonogram
    A-s. ultrasonography
Ascaris lumbricoides
ascent phase
Ascher
    A. aqueous influx phenomenon
    A. glass-rod phenomenon
    A. syndrome
    A. vein
Aschner
    A. phenomenon
    A. reflex
Aschner-Dagnini reflex
Asch septal forceps

ASCO
American Society of Contemporary
Ophthalmology
ASCR
autologous stem cell rescue
ASCRS
American Society of Cataract and
Refractive Surgery
aseptic
a. endophthalmitis
a. injection technique
Aseptron II
ASFA
anterior segment fluorescein angiography
AsH
hyperopic astigmatism
ash-leaf
a.-l. sign
a.-l. spot
ASICO
American Surgical Instrument Company
ASICO capsulorrhexis forceps
ASICO multiangled diamond knife
AsM
myopic astigmatism
aspartoacylase
aspartylglycosaminuria
aspergillosis uveitis
Aspergillus
A. *flavus*
A. *fumigatus*
A. *niger*
A. *terreus*
aspheric
a. cataract lens
a. contact lens
a. cornea
a. custom ablation
a. implant
a. lenticular area
a. optic design
a. spectacle lens
aspherical ophthalmoscopic lens
aspheric-viewing lens
aspirate
vitreoretinal a.
aspirating/irrigating vectis
aspirating lid speculum
aspiration
Alcon a.
cataract a.
a. of cortex
fine-needle a.

a. flow rate
irrigation and a. (I&A)
a. of lens
a. technique
trabecular a.
vitreous a.
aspirator
Alcon a.
Castroviejo orbital a.
Cavitron a.
Cooper a.
Kelman a.
Legacy Series 2000
Cavitron/Kelman
phacoemulsifier a.
Nugent soft cataract a.
Stat a.
aspirator/hydrodissector
Alpern cortex a./h.
ASRS
American Society of Retina Specialists
assay
antiacetylcholine receptor
antibody a.
chemiluminescence a.
enzyme-linked immunosorbent a.
(ELISA)
immunofluorescent a.
Leber hereditary optic atrophy
reverse dot-blot a.
Lowry a.
mucous a.
Raji cell a.
Southern blot hybridization a.
TUNEL a.
urinary GAG a.
urinary glycosaminoglycan
measurement a.
in vitro toxicology a.
assessment
driving a.
fixation a.
fluorescein tear clearance a.
Hirschberg reflex a.
intraoperative frozen section a.
Jacko Low Vision Interaction A.
(JLVIA)
ocular hemodynamic a.
preoperative risk a.
quantitative haze a.
ASSI
Accurate Surgical and Scientific
Instruments

NOTES

ASSI *(continued)*
    ASSI Accu-line surgical marking pen
    ASSI air injection cannula
    ASSI capsulorrhexis forceps
    ASSI fixation hook
    ASSI IOL inserter forceps
    ASSI Phaco Chopper 90-degree angle
    ASSI Polar-Mate coagulator
    ASSI serrefine
    ASSI triple marker
    ASSI tubing introducer forceps
    ASSI universal lens folding forceps

assignment
    lens a.

assistant
    certified paraoptometric a. (CPOA)

association
    American Medical A. (AMA)
    American Optometric A. (AOA)
    CHARGE a.
    A. for Research in Vision and Ophthalmology (ARVO)
    A. of Technical Personnel in Ophthalmology (ATPO)
    teratogenic a.

associative prosopagnosia

Ast
    astigmatism

astemizole

asteroid
    a. body
    a. hyalitis
    hyaloid a.
    a. hyalosis

asteroides
    Nocardia a.

asthenocoria

asthenometer

asthenopia
    accommodative a.
    muscular a.
    nervous a.
    neurasthenic a.
    retinal a.
    tarsal a.

asthenopic

astigmagraph

astigmatic
    a. amblyopia
    a. axis
    a. clock
    a. control
    a. dial
    a. dial chart
    a. image
    a. image blur
    a. keratotomy (AK)

    a. keratotomy enhancement
    a. lens
    a. marker
    a. refractive error
    a. vector analysis

astigmatism (As, Ast)
    acquired a.
    a. against the rule
    against-the-rule a.
    asymmetric a.
    ATR a.
    central a.
    complex a.
    compound hyperopic a.
    compound myopic a.
    congenital a.
    corneal a.
    a. correction
    direct a.
    hypermetropic a.
    hyperopic a. (AsH)
    induced a.
    inverse a.
    irregular a.
    keratometric a.
    lenticular a.
    mixed a.
    myopic a. (AM, AsM)
    oblique a.
    a. of oblique pencils
    pathological a.
    penetrating keratoplasty a.
    physiologic a.
    postoperative irregular a.
    pterygium-induced a.
    radial a.
    refractive a.
    regular a.
    residual a.
    reversed a.
    secondary a.
    simple hyperopic a.
    simple myopic a.
    surgically induced a.
    suture-out a.
    symmetrical a.
    topographic a.
    total a.
    a. with the rule
    with-the-rule a.
    WTR a.

astigmatome
    Terry a.
    Terry-Schanzlin a.

astigmatometer, astigmometer
astigmatometry, astigmometry
astigmatoscope, astigmoscope
astigmatoscopy, astigmoscopy
astigmia

astigmic
astigmometer (*var.* *of* astigmatometer)
astigmometry (*var.* *of* astigmatometry)
astigmoscope (*var.* *of* astigmatoscope)
astigmoscopy (*var.* *of* astigmatoscopy)
ASTRA
    Advanced Shape Technology Refractive
    Algorithm
A-strabismus
AstraMax stereo topographer
astringent ophthalmic solution
astrocytic
    a. glioma
    a. hamartoma
astrocytoma
    juvenile pilocytic a.
    pilocytic a.
    retinal a.
asymmetric
    a. astigmatism
    a. fold
    a. folds of eyes
    a. papilledema
    a. refractive error
    a. surgery
asymmetry
    chromatic a.
    facial a.
asymptomatic optic neuritis
AT
    applanation tension
    applanation tonometry
    artificial tears
Atabrine
Atarax
ataxia
    cerebellar a.
    cone dystrophy-cerebellar a.
    familial episodic a.
    familial paroxysmal a.
    Friedreich a.
    hereditary cerebellar a.
    Marie a.
    ocular a.
    optic a.
    Pierre-Marie a.
    spinocerebellar a.
    vestibulocerebellar a.
ataxia-telangiectasia syndrome
ataxic nystagmus
ATD
    aqueous tear deficiency
at distance and at near (D/N)

atenolol
Athens suture spreader
atheroembolism
atheroma
atherosclerosis
    diffuse a.
    ischemic a.
atherosclerotic ischemic neuritis
athetosis
    pupillary a.
Atkin lid block
Atkinson
    A. block
    A. corneal scissors
    A. 25-G short curved cystotome
    A. peribulbar needle
    A. retrobulbar needle
    A. sclerotome
    A. single-bevel blunt-tip needle
    A. technique
    A. tip peribulbar needle
Atlas
    A. corneal topographer
    Humphrey A. 991
    A. ophthalmic laser
    A. 995 topographer
Atlas-Elite laser
atonic
    a. ectropion
    a. entropion
    a. epiphora
atopic
    a. cataract
    a. conjunctivitis
    a. eczema keratoconjunctivitis
    a. line
atopy
atovaquone
ATPase
    actomyosin ATPase
ATPO
    Association of Technical Personnel in
    Ophthalmology
ATR
    against-the-rule
    ATR astigmatism
Atraloc suture
atresia
    a. iridis
    retinal a.
    tilting lens a.
atretoblepharia
atretopsia

NOTES

Atropair
atrophia
  a. bulbi
  a. bulborum hereditaria
  a. choroideae et retinae
  a. dolorosa
  a. gyrata
  a. striata et maculosa
atrophic
  a. age-related macular degeneration
  a. degenerative maculopathy
  a. excavation
  a. heterochromia
  a. hole
  a. polychondritis
  a. rhinitis
  a. scar formation
atrophy
  autosomal dominant optic a.
  autosomal recessive optic a.
  band optic a.
  Behr optic a.
  bow-tie optic a.
  bulbous a.
  cavernous optic a.
  central areolar choroidal a.
  central gyrate a.
  cerebral a.
  choriocapillaris a.
  chorioretinal a.
  choroidal epithelial a.
  choroidal gyrate a.
  choroidal myopic a.
  choroidal secondary a.
  choroidal vascular a.
  congenital optic a.
  consecutive optic a.
  diabetic optic a.
  diffuse inflammatory eyelid a.
  dominant optic a.
  essential iris a.
  essential progressive atrophy of a.
  flat chorioretinal a.
  Fuchs a.
  geographic retinal a.
  glaucomatous a.
  gray a.
  growth retardation, alopecia,
    pseudoanodontia, and optic a.
    (GAPO)
  gyrate a.
  helicoid peripapillary a.
  hemifacial a.
  hereditary optic a.
  heredodegenerative a.
  heredofamilial optic a.
  infantile optic a.
  iris a.
  ischemic choroidal a.

ischemic optic a.
juvenile optic a.
Kjer dominant optic a.
Leber hereditary optic a.
linear subcutaneous a.
morning glory optic a.
myopic choroidal a.
neuritic a.
neurogenic iris a.
nummular a.
olivopontocerebellar a. (OPCA)
optical a.
optic disc a.
a. of optic nerve
optic nerve a.
opticoacoustic nerve a.
patchy a.
periorbital fat a.
peripapillary choroidal a.
peripheral chorioretinal a.
peripheral retinal a.
pigment a.
pigmented paravenous
  chorioretinal a.
pigmented paravenous
  retinochoroidal a.
postinflammatory a.
postpapilledema a.
primary optic a.
progressive bifocal chorioretinal a.
progressive choroidal a.
progressive encephalopathy with
  edema, hypsarrhythmia and
  optic a. (PEHO)
progressive hemifacial a.
progressive optic a.
retinal pigment epithelial a.
retinochoroidal a.
Schnabel optic a.
Schweninger-Buzzi macular a.
secondary inverse optic a.
segmental iris a.
senile a.
sex-linked recessive optic a.
simple optic a.
subcutaneous fat a.
tabetic optic a.
traumatic a.
uveal a.
atropine
  a. conjunctivitis
  Isopto A.
  a. penalization
  prednisolone and a.
  a. sulfate
atropinism
atropinization
Atropisol

ATS
Amblyopia Treatment Study
attachment
Accuvac smoke evacuation a.
desmosomal cellular a.
pathometer a.
specular a.
vitreoretinal a.
zonular a.
attack
transient ischemic a. (TIA)
attention
a. reflex
a. reflex of pupil
attentional dyslexia
attentiveness
visual a.
attenuated retinal arteriole
attenuation
arteriolar a.
focal a.
Atwood loupe
atypia
cellular a.
atypical
a. achromatopsia
a. coloboma
a. facial pain
a. microbacteria
a. monochromat
a. mycobacteria
Aubert phenomenon
audiovisual
auditory
a. oculogyric reflex
a. perceptual disability
a. stimulus
augmentation
periorbital volume a.
Augmentin
aura
migraine with a.
migraine without a.
A. Nd:YAG photodisruptor
aural
a. nystagmus
a. scotoma
Aureomycin
aureus
methicillin-resistant
Staphylococcus a. (MRSA)
Staphylococcus a.
auriasis

auricular glaucoma
aurochromoderma
Aurolate
Aurora luminous acuity chart
Australia
A. antigen
Fellow of the Royal College of
Surgeons of A. (FRCSA)
Glaucoma Foundation of A.
Australian Corneal Graft Registry
autism
visual a.
auto
A. Ref-keratometer ARK-900
autorefractor and retinoscopy
A. Ref-keratometer instrument
autoantibody
antipericyte a.
circulating antipericyte a.
autoenucleation
autofluorescence
fundus a.
autofunduscope
autofunduscopy
autogenous
a. dermis fat graft
a. donor material
a. hard palate eyelid spacer
a. keratoplasty
autograft
conjunctival a.
conjunctival-limbal a.
free conjunctival a.
free skin a.
full-thickness a.
limbal-conjunctival a.
rotating corneal a.
skin a.
split-thickness a.
autografting
conjunctival rotation a.
limbal a.
autoimmune
a. corneal endotheliopathy
a. demyelination
autoimmune-related retinopathy and optic neuropathy (ARRON)
autokeratometer
Alcon portable a.
autokeratometry
autokeratoplasty
auto-kerato-refractometer
Topcon KR-7500 a.-k.-r.

NOTES

37

autokinesis visible light
autokinetic
- a. effect
- a. nystagmus
- a. visible light phenomenon

autologous
- a. blood injection
- a. chondrocyte transplantation
- a. ipsilateral rotating penetrating keratoplasty
- a. oral mucosal epithelium sheet
- a. plasmin enzyme
- a. serum application
- a. serum eye drops
- a. stem cell rescue (ASCR)

autolysis
automated
- a. capsulotomy
- a. corneal shaper (ACS)
- a. corneal shaper microkeratome
- a. hemisphere perimeter
- a. lamellar keratectomy
- a. lamellar therapeutic keratoplasty (ALTK)
- a. laser keratomileusis (ALK)
- A. Quantification of After-Cataract automated analysis system
- a. refraction
- a. refractor
- a. static threshold perimetry
- a. threshold microperimetry
- a. tissue delamination technique
- a. trephine
- a. visual field
- a. vitrectomy
- a. vitrector

automatic
- a. analyzer
- a. infrared optometer
- a. refractor
- a. tonometry
- a. trephine
- a. twin syringe injector

autonomic
- a. nervous system
- a. nervous system disorder

Autonomous Technologies laser
autopatch
- intralamellar a.

autoperimetry
- short wavelength a.

autophagic vacuole
autophthalmoscope
autophthalmoscopy
Auto-Plot
autopsy eye database
autorefraction (AR)
autorefractometer refraction

autorefractor
- 6600 a.
- Burton BAR-7 a.
- Canon R-50+ a.
- handheld a.
- Hoya AR-570 a.
- Nikon Retinomax K-Plus a.
- Retinomax 2 a.
- Retinomax cordless hand-held a.
- Subjective A.
- SureSight a.
- table-mounted a.
- Tomey a.
- Topcon RM8000B table-mounted a.
- Welch Allyn SureSight a.

autorefractor/keratometer
- Retinomax K-Plus a./k.

autoregulation
autoshaped lamellar keratomileusis
autosomal
- a. dominant congenital cataract (ADCC)
- a. dominant cystoid macular edema
- a. dominant drusen
- a. dominant hereditary optic neuropathy
- a. dominant oculocutaneous albinism
- a. dominant ophthalmoplegia
- a. dominant optic atrophy
- a. dominant retinitis pigmentosa
- a. dominant vitellus rupture
- a. recessive aniridia
- a. recessive hereditary optic neuropathy
- a. recessive ocular albinism (AROA)
- a. recessive ophthalmoplegia
- a. recessive optic atrophy

autotopographer
- Tomey a.

auxiliary
- a. fiber
- a. lens

auxometer
AV
- arteriovenous
  - AV crossing
  - AV crossing defect
  - AV nicking
  - AV pattern
  - AV strabismus syndrome

A/V
- artery-to-vein ratio

avascular
- a. corneal stroma
- a. keratitis
- a. peripheral retina
- a. plaque

avascularity
Avastin
Avellino dystrophy
average
    a. lens density (ALD)
    a. retinal image quality
Avit handpiece
avium
    Mycobacterium a.
avoidance
    hazard a.
Avonex
avulsion
    a. of caruncula lacrimalis
    corneal a.
    a. of eyelid
    facial nerve a.
    optic nerve head a.
    scleral a.
a-wave test
AWE
    advancing wave-like epitheliopathy
awl
    lacrimal a.
    Mustarde a.
axanthopsia
axe
    19-gauge irrigating a.
Axenfeld
    A. anomaly
    A. follicular conjunctivitis
    A. nerve loop
    A. suture
    A. syndrome
Axenfeld-Krukenberg spindle
Axenfeld-Rieger
    A.-R. anomaly (ARA)
    A.-R. syndrome
axes (*pl. of* axis)
axial
    a. amblyopia
    a. ametropia
    a. anisometropia
    a. chamber
    a. cornea
    a. CT scan
    a. curvature map
    a. curvature mapping
    a. embryonal cataract
    a. fusiform developmental cataract
    a. growth
    a. hyperopia
    a. illumination

    a. length (AL)
    a. length-corneal radius (AL/CR)
    a. length-corneal radius ratio
    a. length of eye
    a. myopia
    a. partial childhood cataract
    a. point
    a. proptosis
    a. ray of light
    a. rigidity
    a. tomography
    a. view
axicon
    inverse a.
    quartic a.
axis, pl. **axes**
    achromatic a.
    anteroposterior a.
    astigmatic a.
    axis external a.
    a. bulbi externus
    a. bulbi internus
    corneal polarization a. (CPA)
    cylinder a.
    a. of cylindric lens (x)
    Fick a.
    a. of Fick
    a. fixation
    flat a.
    frontal a.
    geometric a.
    hypothalamic-pituitary-thyroid a.
    lens a.
    a. lentis
    longitudinal a.
    ocular a.
    a. oculi externa
    a. oculi interna
    optic a.
    optical a.
    a. opticus
    orbital a.
    principal optic a.
    pupillary a.
    red-green a.
    sagittal a.
    secondary a.
    steep a.
    tritan a.
    vertical a.
    visual a.
    x a.
    y a.

A

NOTES

Axisonic II ultrasound
AXM
    acetoxycycloheximide
axometer
axon
    fiber layer of a.
    nerve fiber a.
    preganglionic parasympathetic a.
    retinal ganglion cell a.
axonal loss
axonometer
axoplasm
axoplasmic
    a. flow
    a. stasis
Azar
    A. curved cystotome
    A. lens

    A. lens-holding forceps
    A. lens-manipulating hook
    A. lid speculum
azatadine
azathioprine
azelastine
    a. HCl
    a. hydrochloride ophthalmic solution
azidamfenicol
azidothymidine (AZT)
azithromycin
azlocillin
AZOOR
    acute zonal occult outer retinopathy
Azopt
azotemic retinitis
AZT
    azidothymidine

B

amphotericin B
bacitracin, neomycin, and
  polymyxin B
B cell
Fumidil B
B measurement
B scan
ultraviolet B (UVB)
B wave

BAB

blood-aqueous barrier

baby Barraquer needle holder
Baciguent
bacillary layer
bacillus, pl. **bacilli**

acid-fast b. (AFB)
B. anthracis
B. cereus
gonococcal b.
Koch-Weeks b.
pneumococcal b.
B. pyocyaneus
streptococcal b.
B. subtilis
tubercle b.
Weeks b.

bacitracin

b., neomycin, and polymyxin B
b., neomycin, polymyxin B, and
  hydrocortisone
zinc b.
b. zinc

back

b. optic zone radius (BOZR)
b. surface debris (BSD)
b. surface toric
b. surface toric contact lens
b. vertex power (BVP)

backcrack
backcracking
background

b. diabetic retinopathy (BDR)
b. illumination
b. luminance
tigroid b.

Backhaus

B. clamp
B. towel clip

back-scattered light
backscattering
bacteria

Gram-negative b.
Gram-positive b.
saprophytic b.

bacterial

b. agent
b. blepharitis
b. blepharoconjunctivitis
b. collagenase
b. conjunctivitis
b. contamination
b. corneal binding
b. culture
b. dacryoadenitis
b. endophthalmitis
b. infection
b. infectious corneal infiltrate
b. infectious corneal ulcer
b. keratitis
b. pathogen
b. superinfection
b. uveitis

**bactericidal permeability-increasing
  protein (BPI)**
bacteriocidal antibiotic
bacteriostatic antibiotic
Bacteroides

B. fragilis
B. melaninogenicus

Bacticort
Bactrim
Badal stimulus system
Baer nystagmus
Baerveldt

B. filtering procedure
B. glaucoma implant
B. glaucoma implant tube
B. seton implant
B. shunt
B. shunt tube

bag

capsular b.
mercury b.
palpebral adipose b.
small capsular b.

bagginess of eye
baggy eyelid
Bagolini

B. lens
B. striated glasses test

Baikoff lens
Bailey

B. chalazion forceps
B. foreign body remover
B. lacrimal cannula

Bailey-Lovie

B.-L. distance visual acuity
B.-L. logMar chart
B.-L. near test

B

Bailey-Lovie *(continued)*
    B.-L. test chart
    B.-L. visual acuity chart
Bailliart
    B. goniometer
    B. ophthalmodynamometer
Baird chalazion forceps
BAK
    benzalkonium chloride
Baker equation
balafilcon A contact lens
balance
    Humphriss binocular b.
    meridional b.
    muscular b.
balanced
    b. saline solution
    b. salt solution (BSS)
    b. translocation
Baldex
Balint syndrome
ball
    ice b.
    pinky b.
    retinal ice b.
    super pinky b.
8-ball
    8-b. hemorrhage
    8-b. hyphema
ballast
    prism b.
Baller-Gerold syndrome
Ballet
    B. disease
    B. sign
ballistic protective lens
balloon
    b. buckle
    b. catheter dilatation
    b. catheter dilation
    b. dacryoplasty
    b. degeneration
    endocapsular b.
    Honan b.
    Lincoff b.
ballottement
    ocular b.
Balo
    concentric sclerosis of B.
balsam
    Canada b.
Baltimore
    B. Eye Survey
    B. Pediatric Eye Disease Study
Bamatter syndrome
Banaji
    B. irrigation cannula
    B. LASIK irrigating cannula

band
    #40 b.
    A b.
    cellophane-like b.
    ciliary body b.
    circling b.
    encircling b.
    fascia b.
    H b.
    keratitis b.
    b. keratitis
    b. keratopathy
    M b.
    Mach b.
    b. optic atrophy
    retinal demarcation b.
    scleral expansion b.
    silicone circling b.
    Storz b.
    traction b.
    Watzke b.
    Z b.
    zonular b.
bandage
    binocular b.
    Borsch b.
    Elastoplast b.
    monocular b.
    pressure b.
    b. scissors
    b. soft contact lens
bandelette
    keratitis b.
bandpass function
band-shaped
    b.-s. keratitis
    b.-s. keratopathy
Bangerter
    B. iris spatula
    B. method of pleoptics
    B. muscle forceps
    B. pterygium operation
bank
    eye b.
    Lions Doheny Eye and Tissue
      Transplant B.
    national stem cell b.
    New England Eye B.
    stem cell b.
banking
    venule b.
Bannayan syndrome
Banophen Oral
Bansal
    B. LASIK cannula
    B. LASIK forceps
Baquacil
bar
    Berens prism b.

horizontal prism b.
prism b.
b. prism
b. reader
vertical prism b.
Bárány
    B. caloric test
    B. sign
Barbie retractor
barbital
Bardet-Biedl syndrome
Bard-Parker
    B.-P. blade
    B.-P. forceps
    B.-P. keratome
    B.-P. knife
    B.-P. razor
    B.-P. trephine
Bard sign
bare
    b. lymphocyte syndrome
    b. sclera excision
    b. scleral technique
bared sclera
bare-needle phacoemulsification
baring
    b. of blind spot
    b. of sclera
Barkan
    B. double cyclodialysis operation
    B. goniolens
    B. gonioscopic lens
    B. goniotomy knife
    B. goniotomy lens
    B. goniotomy operation
    B. infant implant
    B. light
    B. membrane
Barlow syndrome
Barnes
    B. Hind ComfortCare soaking and wetting solution
    B. Hind contact lens cleaning and soaking solution
    B. Hind Gas Permeable Daily Cleaner
Baron lens
barrage
    double-row diathermy b.
Barraquer
    B. applanation tonometer
    B. cannula
    B. cilia forceps

B. conjunctival forceps
B. corneal dissector
B. corneal utility forceps
B. corneoscleral scissors
B. curved holder
B. enzymatic zonulolysis operation
B. eye shield
B. eye speculum
B. hemostatic mosquito forceps
B. implant
B. irrigator spatula
B. keratomileusis
B. keratomileusis operation
B. keratoplasty knife
B. lens
B. method
B. microkeratome
B. needle
B. needle carrier
B. needle holder
B. needle holder clamp
B. operating room tonometer
B. sable brush
B. sweep
B. trephine
B. vitreous strand scissors
B. wire speculum
B. zonulolysis
Barraquer-Colibri
    B.-C. forceps
    B.-C. speculum
Barraquer-von Mandach capsule forceps
Barr body
barrel
    b. card convergence
    b. distortion
Barré sign
Barrett hydrodelineation cannula
Barrier
    B. drape
    B. sheet
barrier
    blood b.
    blood-aqueous b. (BAB)
    blood-eye b.
    blood-ocular b.
    blood-optic nerve b.
    blood-retinal b. (BRB)
    blood-vitreous b.
    epithelial b.
    ocular b.
    posterior capsular zonular b.

NOTES

Barron
    B. disposable artificial anterior
      chamber
    B. donor corneal punch
    B. epikeratophakia trephine
    B. marking corneal punch
    B. radial vacuum trephine
Barron-Hessburg corneal trephine
Bartel spectacles
Bartonella henselae
bartonellosis
    ocular b.
Bartter syndrome
basal
    b. cell
    b. cell carcinoma (BCC)
    b. cell carcinoma of eyelid
    b. cell carcinoma of medial
      canthus
    b. cell nevus
    b. cell nevus syndrome
    b. coil
    b. encephalocele
    b. epithelial nerve
    b. ganglia disease
    b. ganglia lesion
    b. ganglion
    b. iridectomy
    b. junction
    b. lamina
    b. lamina of choroid
    b. lamina of ciliary body
    b. laminar deposit (BLD)
    b. laminar drusen
    b. layer
    b. linear drusen
    b. ophthalmoplegia
    b. phoria
    b. tear secretion
basalis
    b. choroideae lamina
    b. corporis ciliaris lamina
basaloid cell
base
    cilia b.
    b. curve (BC)
    b. down
    b. in (BI)
    b. out (BO)
    prism b.
    sloughing b.
    b. up (BU)
    vitreous b.
baseball lens
Basedow disease
base-down (BD)
    b.-d. prism

base-in
    b.-i. prism
    b.-i. reserve
baseline
    b. IOP
    b. thickness measurement
    b. vision
basement
    b. membrane (BM)
    b. membrane of choroid
    b. membrane of corneal epithelium
    b. membrane disorder
    b. membrane dystrophy
base-out
    b.-o. prism
    b.-o. reserve
basic
    b. esotropia
    b. exotropia
    b. secretion test
basilar
    b. artery
    b. artery aneurysm
    b. impression
    b. migraine
basin of inferior orbital fissure
basket
    Schultz fiber b.
basket-style scleral supporter speculum
basophilic
    b. adenoma
    b. intranuclear inclusion body
    b. reaction
Bassen-Kornzweig syndrome
BAT
    brightness acuity test
bathomorphic
Batten
    B. disease
    B. syndrome
Batten-Mayou
    B.-M. disease
    B.-M. syndrome
battered
    b. baby syndrome
    b. child syndrome
battle
    b. casualty injury
    B. sign
Baumgarten gland
Bausch
    B. & Lomb concentrated cleaner
    B. & Lomb manual keratometer
    B. & Lomb Moisture Eyes Protect
      Lubricant Eye Drops
    B. & Lomb Optima lens
    B. & Lomb Surgical L161U lens

bay
>junctional b.
>lacrimal b.

Baylisascaris procyonis
Baylor-Video Acuity Tester (BVAT)
bayonet forceps
BC
>base curve

BCBC
>bulbar conjunctival blood column

BCC
>basal cell carcinoma

B-cell proliferative response
BD
>base-down
>Becton Dickinson
>>BD K-3000 microkeratome
>>BD needle
>>BD prism
>>BD safety knife
>>BD Xstar blade

BDMP
>birth defect monitoring program

BDR
>background diabetic retinopathy

bead
>glass b.

beading
>retinal venous b.
>venous b.

beaked forceps
Béal
>B. conjunctivitis
>B. syndrome

beam
>aiming b.
>collimated b.
>convergent b.
>divergent b.
>gaussian b.
>helium-neon b.
>HeNe b.
>probe b.
>proton b.
>returning light b.
>b. scatter
>b. splitter
>The Summit HeNe aiming b.
>Visx Star Reticule aiming b.

Beard-Cutler operation
bear tracks
beaten
>b. bronze appearance

>b. copper appearance
>b. metal appearance

Beaupre cilia forceps
beaver
>B. cataract cryoextractor
>B. clear cornea incision system
>B. Dam Eye Study
>B. discission blade
>B. eye blade
>B. goniotomy needle knife
>B. handle
>B. keratome
>B. scleral Lundsgaard blade
>B. Xstar knife

BEB
>benign essential blepharospasm

Bechert
>B. lens-holding forceps
>B. 7-mm lens
>B. nucleus rotator

Bechert-McPherson angled tying forceps
Bechterew, Bekhterev
>B. nystagmus
>B. reflex
>B. sign

Becker
>B. corneal section spatulated
>scissors
>B. gonioscopic prism
>B. phenomenon
>B. sign

Becton Dickinson (BD)
bed
>capillary b.
>corneal stromal b.
>recipient b.
>retinal capillary b.
>stromal b.
>tissue b.

bedewing
>corneal b.
>epithelial b.

Beebe
>B. lens
>B. loupe

Beehler irrigating pupil expander
beer
>B. blade
>B. canaliculus knife
>B. cataract knife
>B. law
>B. operation

before meals (a.c.)

NOTES

behavior
> eye movement b.
> visual b.

Behçet
> B. disease
> B. skin puncture test
> B. syndrome
> B. uveitis

Behler
> B. LASIK enhancement hook
> B. LASIK retreatment hook

Behr
> B. disease
> B. optic atrophy
> B. pupil
> B. syndrome

Behren rule
Bekhterev (*var. of* Bechterew)
Belin double-ended needle holder
Belix Oral
bell
> B. palsy
> B. phenomenon
> B. reflex
> B. sign

belladonna alkaloid
Bellows cryoextractor
bell-shaped curve
belly
> muscle b.
> b. of pterygium

Belz lacrimal sac rongeur
Benadryl Oral
Benazol
Bence Jones test
bench
> optical b.

bendazac
bender
> Watt stave b.

bending power
Benedikt syndrome
beneficial effect
bengal
> rose b.

benign
> b. anisocoria
> b. concentric anular macular dystrophy
> b. dyskeratosis
> b. essential blepharospasm (BEB)
> b. lesion
> b. mucosal pemphigoid
> b. paroxysmal positional vertigo (BPPV)
> b. reactive lymphoid hyperplasia
> b. retinal vasculitis
> b. tumor

Bennett cilia forceps
benoxinate hydrochloride
Benson
> B. disease
> B. sign

bent
> b. blunt blade
> b. blunt needle
> b. 22-gauge needle
> b. infusion cannula

Benton Facial Recognition Test
benzalkonium chloride (BAK)
benzathine
> penicillin G b.

benzethonium chloride
benzoate
> sodium b.

benzododecinium bromide
benzyl alcohol
Béraud valve
Berens
> B. blade
> B. cataract knife
> B. 3-character test
> B. conical implant
> B. corneal dissector
> B. corneal transplant forceps
> B. corneal transplant scissors
> B. corneoscleral punch
> B. dilator
> B. electrode
> B. expressor
> B. glaucoma knife
> B. iridocapsulotomy scissors
> B. keratoplasty knife
> B. lens loupe
> B. lid everter
> B. lid retractor
> B. marking caliper
> B. muscle clamp
> B. muscle forceps
> B. orbital compressor
> B. partial keratome
> B. pinhole and dominance test
> B. prism
> B. prism bar
> B. ptosis forceps
> B. ptosis knife
> B. pyramidal implant
> B. refractor
> B. scleral hook
> B. sclerectomy operation
> B. spatula
> B. speculum
> B. suturing forceps
> B. test object
> B. tonometer

Berens-Rosa scleral implant

Berens-Smith
>B.-S. cul-de-sac restoration
>B.-S. operation

Berens-Tolman ocular hypertension indicator

Berger
>B. sign
>B. space

Bergmeister papilla

Berke
>B. approach
>B. clamp
>B. operation
>B. ptosis
>B. ptosis forceps

Berke-Krönlein orbitotomy

Berkeley
>B. glare test
>The B. Orthokeratology Study

Berlin
>B. disease
>B. retinal edema

Berman foreign body locator

Bernard-Horner syndrome

Bernard syndrome

Bernell tangent screen

Bernoulli law

berry aneurysm

besiclometer

best
>b. corrected vision
>b. corrected visual acuity
>B. disease
>b. ophthalmic correction
>b. spectacle-corrected visual acuity (BSCVA)
>b. uncorrected visual acuity
>B. vitelliform macular dystrophy

beta
>b. carotene
>b. crystallin
>b. radiation
>b. therapy eye applicator

beta-1a
>interferon b.-1a

beta-adrenergic antagonist

beta-blocker

Betadine

Betagan
>B. Liquifilm
>B. R

betamethasone
>postoperative b.
>b. sodium phosphate eye drops

Betaseron

BetaSite

betaxolol
>b. HCl
>b. hydrochloride

Betaxon

Betimol
>B. beta-blocker solution
>B. Ophthalmic

Betoptic
>B. S
>B. S Ophthalmic

better
>b. seeing eye
>b. visual response

bevacizumab

beveled-edge lens

beveled trocar

Beverly Douglas procedure

Bextra

Bezold-Brücke phenomenon

BFVW
>blood flow velocity waveform

BI
>base in
>BI prism

Bianchi valve

bias
>nonius b.

Biaxin

Biber-Haab-Dimmer
>B.-H.-D. corneal dystrophy
>B.-H.-D. degeneration

bicanalicular tubing

bicarbonate
>potassium b.
>sodium b.

bicentric
>b. grinding
>b. spectacle lens

Bick procedure

bicolor
>iris b.

biconcave contact lens

biconvex
>b. lens
>b. optic

bicoronal scalp flap

bicurve contact lens

bicylindrical lens

NOTES

bidimensional image
Bidwell ghost
Bielschowsky
    B. disease
    B. head-tilt phenomenon
    B. operation
    B. sign
    B. 3-step head-tilt test
    B. strabismus
Bielschowsky-Jansky
    B.-J. disease
    B.-J. syndrome
Bielschowsky-Lutz-Cogan syndrome
Bielschowsky-Parks head-tilt 3-step test
Biemond syndrome
Bietti
    B. corneal retinal dystrophy
    B. crystalline corneoretinal
      dystrophy
    B. crystalline retinopathy
    B. keratopathy
    B. lens
    B. syndrome
    B. tapetoretinal degeneration
bifermentans
    Clostridium b.
bifixation
bifocal, pl. **bifocals**
    cement b.
    b. contact lens
    curved-top b.
    Emerson 1-piece segment b.
    executive b.
    b. fixation
    flat-top b.
    Franklin b.
    Ful-Vue b.
    b. glasses
    high-add b.
    b. intracorneal lens
    invisible b.
    Kryptok b.
    Morck cement b.
    occupational b.
    Panoptic b.
    1-piece b.
    plastic b.
    progressive-add b.
    round top b.
    b. segment
    b. spectacle lens
    b. spectacles
    straight-line b.
    Ultex b.
    Univis b.
bifoveal
    b. fixation
    b. fusion
bifurcation

big
    b. blind spot syndrome
    b. bubble technique
BIGH3 gene mutation
biguanide
    polyaminopropyl b.
    polyhexamethylene b.
    tropical polyhexamethylene b.
bilaminar membrane
bilateral
    b. altitudinal field defect
    b. anterior ischemic optic
      neuropathy
    b. homonymous altitudinal defect
    b. homonymous hemianopsia
    b. hypotony
    b. juxtafoveal telangiectasis (BJT)
    b. keratoconjunctivitis
    b. occipital lobe lesion
    b. ptosis
    b. simultaneous laser in situ
      keratomileusis
    b. simultaneous LASIK
    b. sporadic retinoblastoma
    b. strabismus
    b. uveal effusion syndrome
    b. uveitis
    b. visual field defect
biliaire
    masque b.
biloba
    ginkgo b.
bilobalide
Biltricide
bimanual
    b. delamination
    b. irrigation/aspiration
    b. microincision phacoemulsification
    b. phaco chop
    b. technique
bimatoprost ophthalmic solution
bimedial recession
binasal
    b. field defect
    b. hemianopia
    b. hemianopsia
    b. quadrant field
bind
    vitronectin b.
binding
    bacterial corneal b.
Binkhorst
    B. collar stud lens implant
    B. equation
    B. formula
    B. intraocular lens
    B. iridocapsular lens
    B. irrigating cannula
    B. 2-loop intraocular lens implant

B. 4-loop iris-fixated implant
B. 4-loop iris-fixated lens
B. 2-loop lens
B. tip
binocular
  b. accommodation
  b. accommodative facility
  b. amplitude
  b. aphakia
  b. bandage
  b. coordination
  b. depth perception
  b. diplopia
  b. disparity
  b. eye patch
  b. field
  b. fixation
  b. fixation forceps
  b. function
  b. fusion
  b. hemianopsia
  b. heterochromia
  b. imbalance
  b. indirect ophthalmomicroscope
    (BIOM)
  b. indirect ophthalmoscope
  b. indirect ophthalmoscopy
  b. internuclear ophthalmoplegia
  b. loupe
  b. luster
  b. microscope
  b. parallax
  b. perimetry
  b. polyopia
  b. rivalry
  b. single vision (BSV)
  b. strabismus
  b. vision
  b. visual acuity
  b. visual acuity test
binocularity maintenance
binophthalmoscope
binoscope
bioceramic implant
biochrome test
biocompatible artificial cornea
biodendrimer adhesive
Bio-Eye ocular implant
biofilm
Biogel Sensor surgical glove
Biohist-LA
BioLon solution

BIOM
  binocular indirect ophthalmomicroscope
  BIOM lens
  BIOM noncontact panoramic
  viewing system
  BIOM noncontact wide-angle
  viewing system
BioMask
biomatrix ocular implant
Biomedics contact lens
biometric ruler
biometry
  B-scan b.
  b. test
biomicroscope
  Haag-Streit slitlamp b.
  high-frequency ultrasound b.
  Nikon FS-3 photo slitlamp b.
  slitlamp b.
  ultrasonic b. (UBM)
  ultrasound b. (UBM)
biomicroscopic
  b. examination
  b. indirect lens
biomicroscopy
  confocal b.
  contact lens b.
  laser b.
  slitlamp b.
  ultrasonographic b.
  ultrasound b. (UBM)
biomydrin
Bion
  B. Tears
  B. Tears eye drops
  B. Tears Solution
bionic
  b. eye
  B. eye microdetector subretinal
  implant
Bio-Optics
  B.-O. Bambi cell analysis system
  B.-O. Bambi fixed-frame method
  B.-O. Bambi image analysis system
  B.-O. camera
  B.-O. specular microscope
  B.-O. telescope system
biophotometer
Biophysic
  B. Medical YAG laser
  B. Ophthascan S instrument
Biopore membrane

B

NOTES

biopsy
    corneal b.
    greater superficial temporal artery b.
    temporal artery b.
    vitreous aspiration b.
biopter test
bioptic amorphic lens system
bioptics
biorbital angle
biperiden
biphasic curve
biphosphate
    sodium b.
bipolar
    b. cable
    b. cautery
    b. cone
    b. diathermy adapter clip
    b. electrode position
    b. forceps
    b. horizontal interaction
    b. radiofrequency capsulotomy
    b. retinal cell
    b. rod
biprism applanation tonometer
Birbeck granule
Birch-Hirschfeld
    B.-H. entropion operation
    B.-H. lamp
birdshot
    b. chorioretinitis
    b. chorioretinopathy
    b. choroiditis
    b. lesion
    b. retinochoroiditis
    b. retinochoroidopathy
    b. retinopathy
    b. spot
birefractive
birefringence
    corneal b.
birefringent
birth
    b. defect monitoring program (BDMP)
    b. ocular trauma
    poor vision from b.
    premature b.
    trauma at b.
    b. weight
Bishop-Harman
    B.-H. anterior chamber cannula
    B.-H. anterior chamber irrigator
    B.-H. crisscross forceps
    B.-H. foreign body forceps
    B.-H. irrigating/aspirating unit
    B.-H. knife
    B.-H. tissue forceps

Bishop tendon tucker
Bi-Soft lens
Bisolvon
bispherical lens
bisulfite
    sodium b.
bitartrate
    epinephrine b.
bitemporal
    b. disparity
    b. field defect
    b. fugax hemianopsia
    b. hemianopia
    b. hemianopic scotoma
16-bite nylon suture
biting rongeur
bitoric
    b. contact lens
    b. LASIK
Bitot
    B. patch
    B. spot
Bitumi monobjective microscope
bivariate
    b. analysis
    b. normal ellipse
bizygomatic
Bjerrum
    B. area
    B. scope
    B. scotoma
    B. scotometer
    B. screen
    B. sign
BJT
    bilateral juxtafoveal telangiectasis
BK virus
black
    b. ball hyphema
    b. braided nylon suture
    b. braided silk suture
    b. cataract
    b. cornea
    b. dot sign
    b. eye
    b. iris diaphragm
    b. patch psychosis
    b. reflex
    b. silk bridle suture
    b. silk sling suture
    b. sunburst
    b. sunburst sign
blackout
    visual b.
black/white occluder
blade
    #15 b.
    Accutome black diamond b.

Alfonso diamond corneal transplant b.
Bard-Parker b.
BD Xstar b.
Beaver discission b.
Beaver eye b.
Beaver scleral Lundsgaard b.
Beer b.
bent blunt b.
Berens b.
broken razor b.
Castroviejo razor b.
circular b.
clear cornea b.
ClearCut dual-bevel b.
crescent b.
Curdy b.
Curdy-Hebra b.
3D angled stainless phaco trapezoid b.
diamond crescent b.
diamond-dusted knife b.
dull-sided diamond b.
Duotrak b.
EpiVision b.
fine b.
Fugo b.
b. gauge
Gill b.
Grieshaber b.
b. holder
Katena double-edged sapphire b.
b. knife
Lange b.
Lieberman-type speculum, reversible thin solid b.
Lieberman-type speculum with Kratz open wire b.
Lieberman wire aspirating speculum with V-shape b.
Mastel trifaceted diamond b.
M4-400 freedom b.
Micra double-edged diamond b.
Micro-Sharp b.
microvitreoretinal b.
miniature b.
multiincision 10-facet diamond b.
MVR b.
myringotomy b.
ophthalmic b.
Optimum b.
orbit b.
oscillating b.

Personna steel b.
plasma b.
Prizm keratome b.
razor b.
rectangular b.
replaceable b.
retractable b.
Rhein 3D trapezoid diamond b.
Scheie b.
scleral b.
Sharpoint spoon b.
Sharpoint V-lance b.
b. size
slimcut b.
snub-nose diamond b.
spoon b.
Sputnik Russian razor b.
stab incision angled b.
Stealth DBO diamond b.
Surgistar ophthalmic b.
Thornton arcuate b.
Thornton tri-square b.
trapezoid b.
trephine b.
trifacet b.
ultra-thin surgical b.
V-lance b.
Wheeler b.
Ziegler b.

bladebreaker
blade/knife
    V-lance b./k.
bladeless alternative
Blairex
    B. Hard Contact Lens Cleaner
    B. sterile preserved saline solution
    B. sterile saline
    B. system
Blair retractor
blanching of sclera
Bland-Altman plot
bland ophthalmic ointment
blank
    blocking of lens b.
    contact lens b.
    lens b.
    semifinished b.
    b. spot
Blaskovics
    B. canthoplasty operation
    B. dacryostomy operation
    B. flap
    B. inversion of tarsus operation

NOTES

Blaskovics *(continued)*
 B. lid operation
 B. tarsectomy
blastoma
 pineal b.
Blastomyces dermatitidis
blastomycosis
Blaydes
 B. corneal forceps
 B. lens-holding forceps
BLD
 basal laminar deposit
blear eye
bleary eye
bleb
 b. appearance
 b. classification
 conjunctival b.
 b. cup
 cystic b.
 b. disorder of cornea
 encapsulated b.
 endothelial b.
 epithelial b.
 b. failure
 filtering b.
 b. filtering
 flat filtration b.
 b. grading approach
 b. grading system
 b. height
 ischemic b.
 leaking b.
 leaking glaucoma filtering b.
 b. migration
 mixed morphology b.
 b. needling
 nonleaking b.
 b. outcome
 postcataract b.
 retinal b.
 b. revision
 b. size
 thin b.
 b. vascularity
bleb-associated endophthalmitis
blebitis
bleb-related complication
bleed
 subarachnoid b.
 vitreal b.
bleeding
 intraoperative b.
 intraretinal b.
 limbal b.
Blefcon
blended artificial tears

Blenderm
 B. tape
 B. tape dressing
blennophthalmia
blennorrhagica
 keratoderma b.
blennorrhea
 inclusion b.
 neonatal inclusion b.
 b. neonatorum
blennorrheal conjunctivitis
Bleph-10
 B.-10 Liquifilm
 B.-10 Ophthalmic
 B.-10 SOP
Blephamide
 B. Ophthalmic
 B. SOP
blepharadenitis
blepharal
blepharectomy
blepharedema
blepharelosis
blepharism
blepharitis
 b. acarica
 allergic b.
 angular b.
 b. angularis
 bacterial b.
 chlamydial b.
 chronic b. (CB)
 b. ciliaris
 ciliary b.
 clostridial b.
 b. conjunctivitis
 contact b.
 demodectic b.
 diplobacillary b.
 eczematoid b.
 b. follicularis
 fungal b.
 herpes simplex b.
 marginal b.
 b. marginalis
 meibomian b.
 nonulcerative b.
 b. oleosa
 parasitic b.
 b. parasitica
 pediculous b.
 b. phthiriatica
 posterior b.
 pustular b.
 rickettsial b.
 b. rosacea
 seborrheic b.
 b. sicca
 b. squamosa

squamous seborrheic b.
staphylococcal b.
streptococcal b.
b. ulcerosa
viral b.
blepharoadenitis
blepharoadenoma
blepharoatheroma
blepharochalasis
b. forceps
b. repair
blepharochromidrosis
blepharoclonus
blepharocoloboma
blepharoconjunctivitis
acne rosacea b.
allergic b.
angular b.
bacterial b.
chronic b.
herpes simplex b.
b. rosacea
staphylococcal b.
b. vaccinia
blepharodiastasis
blepharokeratoconjunctivitis
blepharomelasma
blepharoncus
blepharopachynsis
blepharophimosis ptosis syndrome
blepharophyma
blepharoplast
blepharoplastic
blepharoplasty
Ammon b.
conservative b.
laser b.
transconjunctival b. (TCB)
transconjunctival lower eyelid b.
upper b.
blepharoplegia
blepharoptosis, blepharoptosia
b. adiposa
false b.
involutional b.
progressive myopathic upper
eyelid b.
b. repair
blepharoptosis-related blindness
blepharopyorrhea
blepharorrhaphy
Elschnig b.

blepharospasm, blepharospasmus
benign essential b. (BEB)
essential b.
hemifacial b.
nonorganic b.
ocular b.
primary infantile glaucoma b.
reflex b.
secondary b.
symptomatic b.
blepharospasm-oromandibular
b.-o. dystonia
b.-o. dystonia syndrome
blepharosphincterectomy
blepharostat
Goldman scleral fixation ring
and b.
McNeill-Goldman b.
blepharostenosis
blepharosynechia
blepharotomy
Blessig
B. cyst
B. groove
B. lacunae
B. space
blind
b. child
color b.
b. infant
legally b.
b. painful eye
b. spot
b. spot enlargement
b. spot of Mariotte
b. spot reflex
b. spot syndrome
blinding
b. eye disease
b. glare
b. keratoconjunctivitis
blindness
amnesic color b.
blepharoptosis-related b.
blue b.
bright b.
cerebral b.
change b.
color b.
concussion b.
congenital color b.
congenital stationary night b.
corneal b.

B

NOTES

blindness *(continued)*
    cortical psychic b.
    day b.
    deuton color b.
    eclipse b.
    electric light b.
    epidemic b.
    factitious b.
    flash b.
    flight b.
    functional b.
    glaucoma-related b.
    green b.
    hysterical b.
    Ishihara test for color b.
    legal b.
    letter b.
    mind b.
    miner's b.
    monocular b.
    moon b.
    National Institute of Neurologic
      Diseases and B. (NINDB)
    night b.
    note b.
    nutritional b.
    object b.
    postoperative b.
    protan color b.
    psychic b.
    red b.
    red-green b.
    retinal b.
    river b.
    Schubert-Bornschein congenital
      stationary night b.
    self-inflicted b.
    severe visual impairment and b.
      (SVI/BL)
    snow b.
    solar b.
    soul b.
    stationary night b.
    syllabic b.
    b. test
    text b.
    total b.
    transient b.
    twilight b.
    word b.
    X-linked congenital night b.
    yellow b.
blindsight
blink
    b. adequacy
    b. inadequacy
    b. out lagophthalmia
    b. reflex
Blinkeze external lid weight

blink-free period
blinking disorder
Blink-N-Clean
blink-related microtrauma
BLL
    brow, lids, lashes
Bloch-Stauffer syndrome
Bloch-Sulzberger syndrome
block
    aphakic pupillary b.
    Atkin lid b.
    Atkinson b.
    ciliary b.
    ciliolenticular b.
    ciliovitreal b.
    cocaine b.
    corneal b.
    facial b.
    b. glaucoma
    lid b.
    modified Van Lint b.
    Nadbath facial b.
    b. nerve
    nerve b.
    O'Brien lid b.
    paraffin b.
    phakic pupillary b.
    posterior peribulbar b.
    primary pupillary b.
    punch b.
    pupil b.
    pupillary b.
    regional b.
    retrobulbar lid b.
    reverse pupillary b.
    Smith modification of Van Lint
      lid b.
    Stahl caliper b.
    sun b.
    Tanne corneal cutting b.
    Teflon b.
    Van Lint b.
    vitreous b.
blockade
    nasolacrimal b.
    pharmacological b.
blockage nystagmus
blocked fluorescence
blocker
    H1 b.
    ultraviolet b.
blocking of lens blank
blond fundus
blood
    b. barrier
    b. cyst
    extravasated b.
    b. flow velocity waveform
      (BFVW)

b. loss
b. oxygenation level-dependent (BOLD)
b. oxygenation level-dependent effect
retinal b.
b. staining
b. staining of cornea
subhyaloid b.
subretinal b.
vitreous b.
blood-and-thunder retinopathy
blood-aqueous
 b.-a. barrier (BAB)
 b.-a. barrier breakdown
blood-eye barrier
blood-influx phenomenon
blood-ocular barrier
blood-optic nerve barrier
blood-retinal barrier (BRB)
blood-retinal-barrier breakdown
bloodshot
blood-streaked hypopyon
blood-vitreous barrier
bloody tears
Bloomberg
 B. SuperNumb anesthetic ring
 B. trabeculotome set
blooming
 b. of lens
 b. spectacle lens
blot
 b. hemorrhage
 Western b.
blot-and-dot hemorrhage
blotchy positive staining
blow-in fracture
blown pupil
blowout
 b. fracture
 b. fracture of orbit
 b. fracture of orbital floor
blue
 b. blindness
 b. cataract
 b. cone
 b. cone monochromasy
 b. cone monochromatism
 B. core PMMA
 b. field entoptic phenomenon
 b. field stimulation technique
 b. filtering lens
 b. filtration hydrophobic IOL

b. flash stimulus
b. light-absorbing intraocular lens
b. light filter
b. limbus
b. line
B. Mountain Eye Study
b. nevus
b. opaque Herrick lacrimal plug
b. rubber bleb nevus syndrome
b. sclera
b. spike
b. spot
trypan b.
b. vision
B. Vista
blue-blocking lens
blue-dot cataract
blue-filtering IOL
blue-green
 b.-g. argon laser
 b.-g. photic phototoxicity
blue-yellow perimetry
Blumenthal
 B. anterior chamber maintainer
 B. conjunctival dissector
 B. nucleus delivery technique
 B. push-pull irrigating cystotome
blunt
 b. needle
 b. trauma
blunted
 b. red reflex
 b. retinoscopic reflex
blunt-tipped Vannas scissors
blur
 b. anatomy point source of light
 astigmatic image b.
 b. circle
 b. and clear exercise
 b. detection
 b. discrimination
 interocular differential b.
 optical b.
 b. pattern
 b. perception
 b. point
 b. sensitivity
 spectacle b.
 b. spot
 symmetrical image b.
 b. zone
blur-buffering mechanism
blurred vision

NOTES

blurring
    considerable b.
    mild b.
    b. of vision
BM
    basement membrane
B-mode handpiece
BO
    base out
boat hook
bobbing
    converse b.
    inverse ocular b.
    ocular b.
    reverse b.
Boberg-Ans
    B.-A. lens
    B.-A. lens implant
Bochdalek valve
Bodian
    B. lacrimal pigtail probe
    B. mini lacrimal probe
Bodkin thread holder
body, pl. **bodies**
    adipose b.
    amyloid b.
    asteroid b.
    Barr b.
    basal lamina of ciliary b.
    basophilic intranuclear inclusion b.
    cellular inclusion b.
    ciliary b.
    colloid b.
    conjunctival foreign b.
    copper foreign b.
    corneal foreign b.
    Cowdry type A intranuclear
      inclusion b.
    cystoid b.
    cytoid b.
    cytoplasmic b.
    Dutcher b.
    electromagnetic removal of
      foreign b.
    Elschnig b.
    embryonal medulloepithelioma of
      ciliary b.
    embryonal tumor of ciliary b.
    eosinophilic intranuclear
      inclusion b.
    external geniculate b.
    foreign b. (FB)
    geniculate b.
    Guarnieri inclusion b.
    Halberstaedter-Prowazek inclusion b.
    Hassall b.
    Hassall-Henle b.
    Henderson-Patterson inclusion b.
    Henle b.

    Hensen b.
    hyaline b.
    hyaloid b.
    inclusion b.
    intracytoplasmic inclusion b.
    intranuclear eosinophilic
      inclusion b.
    intraocular foreign b. (IOFB)
    intraorbital foreign b.
    ischemic necrosis of ciliary b.
    lateral geniculate b. (LGB)
    Leishman-Donovan b.
    lenticular fossa of vitreous b.
    Lewy b.
    Lipschütz inclusion b.
    multivesicular b.
    nigroid b.
    occult anular ciliary b.
    pigmented layer of ciliary b.
    pituitary b.
    Prowazek-Greeff b.
    Prowazek-Halberstaedter b.
    Prowazek inclusion b.
    psammoma b.
    racquet b.
    radiopaque intraocular foreign b.
    refractile b.
    removal of foreign b.
    retained foreign b. (RFB)
    retained intraorbital metallic
      foreign b.
    Rosenmüller b.
    Rucker b.
    Russell b.
    Schaumann inclusion b.
    sclerotomy removal of foreign b.
    subconjunctival foreign b.
    suprachoroidal foreign b.
    synaptic b.
    trachoma b.
    vitreous foreign b.
    wartlike b.
    Weibel-Palade b.
body-referenced stimulus
Boeck sarcoid
boggy edema
Böhm operation
Bohr model
Boil-n-Soak
BOLD
    blood oxygenation level-dependent
      BOLD effect
bolus dressing
bombé
    b. configuration
    iris b.
Bonaccolto
    B. fragment forceps
    B. jeweler forceps

B

B. magnet tip forceps
B. utility and splinter forceps
Bondek suture
bone

coffin b.
b. cutter
ethmoid b.
foramen of sphenoid b.
frontal b.
glandular fossa of frontal b.
b. graft
lacrimal sulcus of lacrimal b.
b. marrow-derived progenitor cell
maxillary b.
orbital arch of frontal b.
orbital border of sphenoid b.
orbital plate of ethmoid b.
orbital plate of frontal b.
orbital sulcus of frontal b.
orbital wing of sphenoid b.
palatine b.
petrous b.
b. punch
b. removal orbital decompression
b. rongeur
sphenoid b.
b. spicule
supraorbital arch of frontal b.
supraorbital margin of frontal b.
temporal b.
b. trephine
uncinate process of lacrimal b.
zygomatic b.
bone-biting

b.-b. forceps
b.-b. punch
b.-b. trephine
Bonferroni test
Bonn

B. iris forceps
B. iris scissors
B. microiris hook
B. suturing forceps
Bonnet

B. capsule
B. enucleation operation
B. sign
B. syndrome
Bonnet-Dechaume-Blanc syndrome
Bonnier syndrome
bony

b. cataract

b. orbit
b. orbit of eye
boomerang-shaped lesion
borate

epinephrine b.
epinephryl b.
potassium b.
sodium b.
border

brushfire b.
corneoscleral b.
rolled-up epithelium with wavy b.
scalloped b.
b. tissue of Jacoby
Bordetella pertussis
Bores

B. axis marker
B. optic zone marker
B. radial marker
B. twist fixation ring
boric

b. acid
b. acid solution
boring pain
Borrelia

B. burgdorferi
B. burgdorferi infection
B. recurrentis
borreliosis

ocular Lyme b.
Borsch

B. bandage
B. dressing
Borthen iridotasis operation
Boston

B. Advance cleaner
B. Advance Comfort Formula
Conditioning Solution
B. Advance reconditioning drops
B. cleaner solution
B. 7 contact lens
B. Envision contact lens
B. EO, ES contact lens
B. II, IV contact lens
B. One Step Liquid Enzymatic
Cleaner
B. Rewetting Drops
B. RXD contact lens
B. sign
B. Simplicity multi-action solution
B. Simplus

NOTES

Boston *(continued)*
>B. trephine
>B. XO contact lens

both eyes (OU)

Bothnia dystrophy

Botox

botulin toxin (BTX)

botulinum
>b. A toxin
>b. toxin A
>b. toxin A injection
>b. toxin type F

botulism
>infantile b.

botulism-induced
>b.-i. blurred vision
>b.-i. ptosis

botulismotoxin

Botvin iris forceps

bouche de tapir

boundary
>lesion b.

bound-down muscle

bounding
>b. mydriasis
>b. pupil

Bourneville
>B. phakomatosis
>B. syndrome

bouton
>b. en passant
>b. terminaux

Bovie
>B. electrocautery unit
>B. electrosurgical unit
>B. retinal detachment unit
>B. wet-field cautery

bovina
>facies b.

bovis
>*Moraxella b.*
>*Mycobacterium b.*

Bowen disease

bowl
>Ganzfeld b.
>lenticular b.

Bowman
>B. capsule
>B. cataract needle
>B. lacrimal probe
>B. lamina
>B. layer
>B. membrane
>B. muscle
>B. needle stop
>B. operation
>B. stop needle
>B. tube
>B. zone

bowstring

bow-tie
>b.-t. hypoplasia
>b.-t. knot
>b.-t. optic atrophy
>b.-t. stitch

box-and-whisker plot

boxcarring

boxing system

box measurement

Boyce needle holder

Boyd
>B. operation
>B. orbital implant

Boyden chamber technique

boydii
>*Allescheria b.*
>*Petriellidium b.*
>*Pseudallescheria b.*

Boynton needle holder

BOZR
>back optic zone radius

BPI
>bactericidal permeability-increasing
> protein

BPPV
>benign paroxysmal positional vertigo

BRA
>branch retinal artery

brachial
>b. arch syndrome
>b. plexus palsy

brachium conjunctivum

brachymetropia

brachymetropic

brachyrhynchus

brachytherapy
>b. episcleral plaque
>orbital plaque b.
>palladium 103 ophthalmic
> plaque b.
>plaque b.
>radioactive plaque b.
>radon ring b.

Bracken
>B. anterior chamber cannula
>B. effect
>B. fixation forceps
>B. iris forceps
>B. irrigating/aspirating unit

bradykinin

braided
>b. silk suture
>b. Vicryl suture

Braid strabismus

braille
>b. access
>b. writer

brailler
    Perkins b.
brain
    b. cortex
    b. damage
    b. dysfunction
    b. heart infusion broth
    b. stem
    b. tumor
    b. tumor headache
brainstem, brain stem
    b. disease
    b. dysfunction
    b. lesion
    b. motor nucleus
branch
    b. retinal artery (BRA)
    b. retinal artery occlusion (BRAO)
    b. retinal vein (BRV)
    b. retinal vein occlusion (BRVO)
    B. Vein Occlusion Study
brancher enzyme deficiency
branching
    b. dendrite
    b. filament
    b. infiltration
    b. lesion
Branhamella catarrhalis
BRAO
    branch retinal artery occlusion
brasiliensis
    Nocardia b.
brass scleral plug
Brawner orbital implant
brawny
    b. edema
    b. scleritis
    b. trachoma
Brazilian ophthalmia
BRB
    blood-retinal barrier
breadth of accommodation
break
    chevron-shaped b.
    conjunctival b.
    giant retinal b.
    iatrogenic retinal b.
    b. phenomenon
    b. point
    retinal b.
    b. in retinal integrity
    retinochoroidal b.
    sclerotomy-related retinal b.

breakdown
    blood-aqueous barrier b.
    blood-retinal-barrier b.
    optical b.
    surface b.
breakpoint
    fusion b.
breakthrough
breakup
    b. phenomenon
    premature tear b.
    tear b.
    b. time (BUT)
    b. time of tear
    b. time test
Brems astigmatism marker with level
breves
    nervi ciliares b.
Brevital
Brickner sign
bridge
    b. coloboma
    comfort b.
    keyhole b.
    B. operation
    b. pedicle flap
    b. pedicle flap operation
    saddle b.
    b. of spectacles
    b. suture
bridle suture
Brierley nucleus splitter
bright
    b. blindness
    b. empty field
    B. eye
    b. staining
bright-field
    b.-f. accommodation
    b.-f. magnifier
brightness
    b. acuity test (BAT)
    b. comparison
    b. difference threshold
bright-sense
bright-white flash stimulus
brimonidine-P
brimonidine tartrate ophthalmic solution
brinzolamide ophthalmic suspension
British N system
Britt
    B. argon/krypton laser
    B. argon pulsed laser

B

NOTES

Britt *(continued)*
  B. BL-12 laser
  B. krypton laser
brittle
  b. cornea syndrome
  b. diabetes
broad-beam ablation
broad-spectrum
  b.-s. antibiotic
  b.-s. heater (BSH)
Broca
  B. aphasia
  B. visual plane
Brockhurst technique
Broders grading
Brodmann area
broken razor blade
Brolene
Bromarest
Brombach perimeter
Brombay
bromfenac ophthalmic
bromhexine
bromide
  benzododecinium b.
  demecarium b.
  pancuronium b.
bromocriptine
bromovinyldeoxyuridine (BVDU)
Bromphen
brompheniramine
Bronson foreign body removal operation
bronze diabetes
bronzing
  nuclear b.
Brooke tumor
broth
  brain heart infusion b.
  thioglycate b.
  trypticase soy b.
brow
  b. droop
  b. fixation
  b., lids, lashes (BLL)
  b. tape
brown
  b. cataract
  B. insertion forceps
  B. interchangeable lid speculum
  B. limbal relaxing incision guide
  B. pocket starter
  B. sterile adhesive
  B. syndrome
  B. technique of nuclear flipping
  B. tendon
  B. tendon sheath syndrome
  B. vertical retraction syndrome

Brown-Grabow capsulorrhexis cystotome forceps
Brown-McLean syndrome
Brucella suis
Bruch
  B. gland
  B. layer
  B. membrane
Bruchner
  B. reflex testing
  B. test
Brücke
  B. fiber
  B. lens
  B. line
  B. muscle
  B. reagent
Brücke-Bartley phenomenon
Brueghel syndrome
Bruening forceps
Brunati sign
brunescens
  cataracta b.
brunescent cataract
Bruns nystagmus
Brunsting-Perry cicatricial pemphigoid
brush
  Alger b.
  Barraquer sable b.
  Cytobrush S b.
  5139 flexible retinal b.
  Haidinger b.
  mechanical epithelial b.
  rotating b.
  Thomas b.
Brushfield spot
Brushfield-Wyatt syndrome
brushfire border
BRV
  branch retinal vein
BRVO
  branch retinal vein occlusion
  BRVO knife
B-Salt Forte
B-scan
  B-s. biometry
  contact B-s.
  Humphrey B-s.
  B-s. ultrasonogram
  B-s. ultrasonography
  B-s. ultrasound
BSCVA
  best spectacle-corrected visual acuity
BSD
  back surface debris
BSH
  broad-spectrum heater
BSS
  balanced salt solution

BSS flow
BSS Plus
BSS Plus ophthalmic irrigating
solution
BSS sterile irrigating solution
BSV
binocular single vision
BTX
botulin toxin
BU
base up
bubble
air b.
gas b.
intraocular gas b.
bubbling
air b.
buckle
balloon b.
encircling band for scleral b.
encircling silicone b.
b. height
Miragel episcleral b.
prominent b.
scleral b. (SB)
segmental b.
temporary balloon b.
buckling
conventional scleral b.
b. procedure
b. sclera
scleral b.
budding yeast cell
Budge
ciliospinal center of B.
buffer
Tris-borate b.
buffy coat
bufilcon A
build-up implant
bulb
b. of eye
terminal b.
bulbar
b. conjunctiva
b. conjunctival blood column
(BCBC)
b. conjunctival scarring
b. fascia
b. paralysis
b. sheath
bulbi (*pl. of* bulbus)
xanthomatosis b.

bulbocapnine
bulbous atrophy
bulbus, pl. **bulbi**
atrophia bulbi
camera vitrea bulbi
capsula bulbi
cholesterosis bulbi
cyanosis bulbi
endothelium camerae anterioris
bulbi
essential phthisis bulbi
hemosiderosis bulbi
melanosis bulbi
musculi bulbi
musculus obliquus inferior bulbi
musculus obliquus superior bulbi
musculus rectus inferior bulbi
musculus rectus lateralis bulbi
musculus rectus medialis bulbi
b. oculi
phthisis bulbi
siderosis bulbi
Tenon fascia bulbi
trochlea musculi obliqui superioris
bulbi
tunica fibrosa bulbi
tunica interna bulbi
tunica sensoria bulbi
tunica vasculosa bulbi
xanthelasmatosis bulbi
xanthomatosis bulbi
bulge
vitreous b.
bulging eye
bulla, pl. **bullae**
epithelial b.
ethmoid b.
b. ethmoidalis ossis
bulldog clamp
Buller eye shield
bullosa
concha b.
epidermolysis b.
keratitis b.
recessive dystrophic
epidermolysis b.
bullosum
erythema multiforme b.
bullous
b. detachment
b. disorder
b. keratopathy

NOTES

bullous *(continued)*
> b. pemphigoid
> b. retinoschisis

bull's-eye
> b.-e. macular lesion
> b.-e. maculopathy
> b.-e. retinopathy

Bumke pupil

bundle
> arcuate nerve fiber b.
> inferior arcuate b.
> nerve fiber b.
> papillomacular nerve fiber b.
> paracentral nerve fiber b.
> superior arcuate b.

Bunge evisceration spoon

Bunker implant

Bunsen grease spot photometer

Bunsen-Roscoe law

buphthalmia, buphthalmos, buphthalmus

bupivacaine

bur, burr
> aftercataract b.
> Allport cutting b.
> corneal foreign body b.
> cutting b.
> diamond b.
> foreign body b.
> lacrimal sac b.
> Storz corneal b.

Buratto
> B. contact lens spoon and spatula
> B. flap forceps
> B. flap protector
> B. III acrylic implantation forceps
> B. LASIK Forceps
> B. LASIK irrigating cannula
> B. ophthalmic forceps
> B. technique

Burch
> B. caliper
> B. eye evisceration operation
> B. pick

Burch-Greenwood tendon tucker

burgdorferi
> *Borrelia b.*

Burian-Allen
> B.-A. bipolar contact lens electrode
> B.-A. contact lens

buried
> b. disc drusen
> b. suture

burn
> acid b.
> alkali b.
> alkaline b.
> ammonia alkali b.
> ammonium hydroxide alkali b.
> chemical b.

corneal alkali b.
> foveal b.
> laser b.
> light argon laser b.
> ocular adnexal b.
> radiation b.
> retinal b.
> solar b.
> b. spot size
> thermal b.
> ultraviolet b.

burnetii
> *Coxiella b.*

burning
> localized transient b.
> ocular b.
> b. sensation

Burns amaurosis

Burow flap operation

burr *(var. of* bur)

burst
> b. hemiflip procedure
> laser b.
> phaco b.

Burton
> B. BAR-7 autorefractor
> B. lamp

Busacca nodule

BUT
> breakup time

butacaine

Butazolidin

butterfly
> b. macular dystrophy
> b. needle
> b. needle infusion port
> b. pattern steepening of cornea
> b. test

butterfly-shaped
> b.-s. macular dystrophy
> b.-s. pigment epithelial dystrophy

button
> collar b.
> corneal b.
> corneoscleral b.
> donor b.
> Graether collar b.
> penetrating keratoplasty b.
> silicone b.

buttonhole
> conjunctival b.
> b. incision
> b. iridectomy

button-tip manipulator

butyl
> b. cyanoacrylate
> b. cyanoacrylate glue

butyrate
> cellulose acetate b. (CAB)

Buzard Diamond Barraqueratome Microkeratome System
Buzzi operation
BV100 needle
BVAT
  Baylor-Video Acuity Tester
BVDU
  bromovinyldeoxyuridine

BVP
  back vertex power
b-wave
  b-w. amplitude
  b-w. implicit time
Byron
  B. Smith ectropion operation
  B. Smith lazy-T correction

NOTES

B

C
contraction
cylinder
cylindrical lens
adjunctive mitomycin C
C loop
C measurement
mitomycin C (MMC)
C value
C wave

CA
carbonic anhydrase
carcinoma
corneal abrasion

CAB
cellulose acetate butyrate

cable
bipolar c.
c. temple

cabufocon A

CAC
central anterior curve

CA/C
convergence accommodation to convergence
CA/C ratio

CACT
computer-assisted corneal topography

cadaver eye

caddie
tip cleaner c.

Caenorhabditis elegans

caerulea
cataracta c.

caespitosus
Streptomyces c.

CAG
closed-angle glaucoma

CAI
carbonic anhydrase inhibitor

Cairns trabeculectomy

Cajal
interstitial nucleus of C.

calcareous
c. cataract
c. conjunctivitis
c. degeneration
c. degeneration of cornea
c. deposit

calcarine
c. artery
c. cortex
c. fissure
c. gyrus

calcein-AM stain

calciferol
calcific
c. band keratopathy
c. corneal degeneration
c. phacolysis

calcification
conjunctival c.
lamellar c.
optic disc drusen c.
sclerochoroidal c.
sellar c.

calcified retinoblastoma

calcinosis cutis, Raynaud phenomenon, esophageal motility disorder, sclerodactyly, and telangiectasia (CREST)

calcitriol
calcium
c. alginate swab
c. chloride dihydrate
c. deposit
c. deposition
c. hydroxide

calcium-containing opacity

calcoaceticus
Acinetobacter c.

calcofluor
c. white
c. white stain

calculating equivalent defocus
calculation
corneal power c.
IOL power c.
lens power c.
power c.

calculator
glaucoma risk c.
pediatric IOL c.

calculus, pl. **calculi**
lacrimal c.

Caldwell
C. suction trephine
C. view

Caldwell-Luc approach
Calhoun needle
calibrator
keratometer c.

caliper
Berens marking c.
Burch c.
Castroviejo c.
Jameson c.
Stahl c.
Storz c.

caliper *(continued)*
> surgical c.
> Thorpe c.

Callahan
> C. fixation forceps
> C. operation

Callender cell type classification

callipaeda
> *Thelazia c.*

callosum
> corpus c.
> splenium of corpus c.

Calmette
> C. conjunctival reaction
> C. ophthalmic reaction
> C. ophthalmoreaction

caloric
> c. irrigation test
> c. nystagmus

caloric-induced nystagmus

calotte

calvaria, pl. **calvariae**

Cambridge
> C. acuity card
> C. low-contrast grating
> C. Research Systems (CRS)

camera, pl. **camerae, cameras**
> Bio-Optics c.
> Canon CF-60U fundus c.
> Canon CF-60Z fundus c.
> Carl Zeiss Jena Retinophot fundus c.
> CCD c.
> CFA digital c.
> CF-60DSi fundus c.
> Coburn c.
> color fundus c.
> CooperVision c.
> CR6-45NMf retinal c.
> Docustar fundus c.
> Donaldson fundus c.
> 3Dx digital stereo disc c.
> Eyecor c.
> fiberoptic digital fundus c.
> fundus c.
> handheld fundus c.
> Handy video fundus c.
> Kowa PRO II retinal c.
> Kowa RC-XV fundus c.
> c. lucida
> Neitz CT-R cataract c.
> Nidek 3Dx stereodisk c.
> Nikon D100 digital c.
> Nikon Retinopan fundus c.
> NM-1000 digital non-mydriatic fundus c.
> c. oculi anterior
> c. oculi major
> c. oculi minor

> c. oculi posterior
> Olympus fundus c.
> photoscreener pediatric c.
> RC-2 fundus c.
> Reichert c.
> RetCam 120 fiberoptic fundus c.
> retinal c.
> Retinopan 45 c.
> Scheimpflug c.
> spectacle-mounted c.
> Topcon 50IA c.
> Topcon TRC-501A fundus c.
> Topcon TRC-50VT retinal c.
> Topcon TRC-50X retinal c.
> Topcon TRV-50VT fundus c.
> TRC-SS2 stereoscopic fundus c.
> Visucam nonmydriatic fundus c.
> c. vitrea bulbi
> Zeiss FF450 fundus c.
> Zeiss-Nordenson fundus c.

cAMP
> cyclic adenosine monophosphate
> > cAMP final common pathway
> > cAMP mediated mechanism

Campbell slit lamp

campimeter

campimetry

Cam vision stimulator

Canada
> C. balsam
> Fellow of the Royal College of Physicians of C. (FRCPC)

Canadian
> C. Ophthalmology Society
> C. Study of Health and Aging

canal
> ampulla of lacrimal c.
> central c.
> ciliary c.
> Cloquet c.
> collateral pulp c.
> Dorello c.
> emissary c.
> ethmoid c.
> Ferrein c.
> Fontana c.
> Gartner c.
> Hannover c.
> Hovius c.
> hyaloid c.
> infraorbital c.
> lacrimal c.
> Lauth c.
> nasal c.
> nasolacrimal c.
> optic c.
> orbital c.
> Petit c.
> ruffed c.

Schlemm c.
scleral c.
semicircular c.
Sondermann c.
c. of Stilling
supraciliary c.
supraoptic c.
supraorbital c.
tarsal c.
zygomaticofacial c.
zygomaticotemporal c.
canalicular
c. disorder
c. duct
c. laceration
c. obstruction
c. pathway
c. route
c. scissors
c. visualization aid
canaliculi (*pl. of* canaliculus)
canaliculitis
canaliculodacryocystostomy
canaliculodacryorhinostomy
canaliculorhinostomy
canaliculum
canaliculus, pl. canaliculi
ampulla of lacrimal c.
common c.
inferior c.
lacrimal c.
c. lacrimalis
lower c.
c. rod and suture
superior c.
upper c.
canalis hyaloideus
Canavan disease
cancer
periocular basal cell c.
sebaceous eyelid c.
cancer-associated retinopathy (CAR)
cancrum nasi
candela (cd)
c. laser
c. laser lithotriptor
c. videoimaging system
candela/m²
Candida
C. albicans
C. endophthalmitis
C. glabrata
C. guilliermondii

C. keratitis
C. krusei
C. parapsilosis
C. tropicalis
candidal
c. conjunctivitis
c. endophthalmitis
c. granuloma
c. keratitis
c. retinitis
c. uveitis
candle
candle-meter
candle-power
candlewax drippings
canis
Toxocara c.
canities
c. circumscripta
c. poliosis
cannula
air injection c.
Akahoshi hydrodissection c.
alpha-chymotrypsin c.
angled left/right c.
anterior chamber washout c.
ASSI air injection c.
Bailey lacrimal c.
Banaji irrigation c.
Banaji LASIK irrigating c.
Bansal LASIK c.
Barraquer c.
Barrett hydrodelineation c.
bent infusion c.
Binkhorst irrigating c.
Bishop-Harman anterior chamber c.
Bracken anterior chamber c.
Buratto LASIK irrigating c.
Castroviejo cyclodialysis c.
Chang hydrodissection c.
coaxial irrigation/aspiration c.
Cobra LASIK irrigating c.
cortical cleaving hydrodissector c.
Corydon expression c.
Corydon hydroexpression c.
cyclodialysis c.
DeCamp viscoelastic c.
Dishler irrigation c.
Dishler type LASIK irrigating c.
double irrigating/aspirating c.
Drews irrigating c.
Fasanella lacrimal c.
Feaster K7-5460 hydrodissecting c.

NOTES

C

cannula *(continued)*

Gans cyclodialysis c.
Gass cataract-aspirating c.
Gass vitreous-aspirating c.
Gills double irrigating/aspirating c.
Gills double Luer-Lok c.
Gills-Welsh aspirating c.
Gills-Welsh double-barreled irrigating/aspirating c.
Gills-Welsh irrigating/aspirating c.
Gills-Welsh olive-tip c.
Gimbel fountain c.
Girard irrigating c.
Goldstein c.
goniotomy knife c.
Grizzard subretinal fluid c.
Guell irrigation c.
Guell LASIK irrigating c.
Gulani triple function LASIK c.
Healon aspirating c.
hydrodissection c.
I/A c.
infusion c.
iris hook c.
irrigating/aspirating c.
irrigating J-hook c.
irrigation/aspiration c.
Jensen capsule polisher c.
Johnson double c.
Johnson hydrodelineation c.
Johnson hydrodissection c.
J-shaped irrigating/aspirating c.
Karickhoff double c.
Kelman cyclodialysis c.
Knolle anterior chamber irrigating c.
lacrimal irrigating c.
Landers subretinal aspiration c.
Lewicky threaded infusion c.
liquid vitreous-aspirating c.
Manche irrigation c.
Manche-type LASIK irrigating c.
Maumenee goniotomy knife c.
Maumenee knife goniotomy c.
McIntyre anterior chamber c.
McIntyre-Binkhorst irrigating c.
McIntyre coaxial c.
model 177-33 viscocanalostomy c.
Morris flexible c.
Nichamin hydrodissection c.
Nichamin LASIK irrigating c.
O'Gawa cataract-aspirating c.
O'Gawa 2-way aspirating c.
olive tip c.
Packo pars plana c.
Pautler infusion c.
PeaceKeeper c.
Pearce coaxial irrigating/aspirating c.
perfluorocarbon coaxial I/A c.
Pettigrove irrigation c.
Pettigrove LASIK irrigating c.
quad-ported LASIK irrigating c.
Rainin air injection c.
Randolph cyclodialysis c.
reel aspiration c.
Rhein aspiration c.
Rhein irrigation c.
Roper alpha-chymotrypsin c.
Rowsey fixation c.
Rubenstein LASIK C.
Rubenstein-type LASIK irrigating c.
Rycroft c.
Scheie anterior chamber c.
Scheie cataract-aspirating c.
Seibel LASIK flap irrigator and squeegee c.
self-retaining infusion c.
self-retaining irrigating c.
Shepard incision irrigating c.
Shepard radial keratotomy irrigating c.
side port c.
sidewall infusion c.
Simcoe cortex extractor aspiration c.
Simcoe II PC double c.
Simcoe reverse aperture c.
Simcoe reverse irrigating/aspirating c.
Slade formed irrigation c.
smooth c.
soft-tipped c.
Steriseal disposable c.
subretinal aspiration c.
sub-Tenon anesthesia c.
Swets goniotomy knife c.
Tenner lacrimal c.
Thomas irrigating-aspirating c.
Thurmond nucleus-irrigating c.
transzonular vitreal injection c.
Tri-Port sub-Tenon anesthesia c.
Troutman c.
TruPro lacrimal c.
Tulevech c.
Veirs c.
Vidaurri double irrigation c.
Visco expression c.
Viscoflow c.
Visitec irrigating/aspirating c.
vitreous-aspirating c.
2-way cataract-aspirating c.
Weil lacrimal c.
Welsh cortex stripper c.
Welsh flat olive-tip double c.
West lacrimal c.
Yamagishi viscocanalostomy c.

Canny
- C. edge algorithm
- C. edge detection program

Canon
- C. Auto Keratometer K-1
- C. auto refraction keratometer
- C. auto refractometer
- C. CF-60U fundus camera
- C. CF-60Z fundus camera
- C. perimeter
- C. R-5+ Auto Ref-Keratometer
- C. R-50+ autorefractor
- C. refractor
- C. RO-4000 slit lamp
- C. RO-5000 slit lamp
- C. SLO scanning laser ophthalmoscope

can-opener anterior capsulotomy
Cantelli sign
canthal
- c. hypertelorism
- c. keratinization
- c. ligament
- c. raphe
- c. recess
- c. tendon

canthaxanthin retinopathy
canthectomy
canthi (*var. of* canthus) (*pl. of* canthus)
canthitis
cantholysis
canthomeatal
canthopexy
canthoplasty
- Agnew c.
- Ammon c.

canthorrhaphy
canthorum
- dystopia c.

canthotomy
- external c.
- lateral c.

canthus, canthi, pl. **canthi**
- basal cell carcinoma of medial c.
- inner c.
- c. inversus
- lateral c.
- medial c.
- nasal c.
- outer c.
- temporal c.

CAP
- contoured ablation pattern

cap
- compliance c.
- corneal c.
- donor c.
- Gelfilm c.

capability
- erosion c.
- extra-wide field c.
- fade-to-clear c.
- self-sealing c.

capacity
- infusion c.

capillaritis
- retinal c.

capillary
- c. bed
- choroidal c.
- c. closure
- filigree-like c.
- c. hemangioma
- c. hemangioma of eyelid
- c. leakage
- c. lumen
- c. microaneurysm
- nonfenestrated c.
- c. nonperfusion
- c. perfusion
- c. plexus
- c. scaffolding
- c. tube plasma viscosimeter

capillary-free zone
capitis
- dolor c.

caplet
- Triptone C.'s

Caprogel
capsitis
capsomere
capsula, pl. **capsulae**
- c. bulbi
- c. lentis

capsular
- c. advancement
- c. bag
- c. bag complex
- c. bag distention syndrome
- c. bag opacification
- c. cataract
- c. debris
- c. delamination
- c. exfoliation syndrome

NOTES

69

capsular *(continued)*
    c. fixation
    c. fornix
    c. glaucoma
    c. opacity
    c. phimosis
    c. plug
    c. retraction device
    c. support
    c. tension ring
    c. tension segment
capsular-zonular
capsulatum
    Histoplasma c.
capsule
    anterior lens c.
    Bonnet c.
    Bowman c.
    ciliary neurotrophic factor c.
    c. contraction syndrome
    crystalline c.
    CTNF c.
    curling of c.
    exfoliation of lens c.
    fibrotic c.
    c. forceps technique
    c. fragment forceps
    c. fragment spatula
    leaves of c.
    c. of lens
    lens c.
    ocular c.
    c. polisher
    c. polishing
    pseudoexfoliation of lens c.
    residual c.
    c. retractor
    Tenon c.
capsulectomy
    anterior c.
    pars plana posterior c.
    vitrector-cut anterior c.
capsulitis
capsulolenticular cataract
capsuloplasty
capsulorrhexis
    anterior c.
    c. capsulotomy
    circular tear c.
    continuous circular c.
    continuous curvilinear c. (CCC)
    dye-assisted anterior c.
    c. forceps
    minicircular c.
capsulotome
capsulotomy
    anterior c.
    automated c.
    bipolar radiofrequency c.

    can-opener anterior c.
    capsulorrhexis c.
    circular tear c.
    continuous tear anterior c.
    Fugo plasma blade anterior c.
    large c.
    laser c.
    manual anterior c.
    modified anterior c.
    multipuncture c.
    posterior c.
    c. scissors
    triangular c.
    Vannas c.
    YAG laser c.
    YAG posterior c.
CAPT
    Complications of Age-Related Macular Degeneration Prevention Trial
capture
    iris c.
    optic c.
    pupillary c.
caput medusae
CAR
    cancer-associated retinopathy
    CAR syndrome
carbachol
    Isopto C.
Carbastat Ophthalmic
carbenicillin
carbinoxamine and pseudoephedrine
Carbiset Tablet
Carbiset-TR Tablet
Carbocaine
carbocholine
Carbodec
    C. Syrup
    C. TR Tablet
carbohydrate sulfotransferase gene mutation
carbomycin
carbon
    c. arc lamp
    c. dioxide (CO_2)
    c. dioxide laser
    c. monoxide retinopathy
carbonate
    sodium c.
carbonic
    c. anhydrase (CA)
    c. anhydrase inhibitor (CAI)
    c. anhydrase tomography
carboplatin
Carbopol
Carboptic Ophthalmic
carboxymethylcellulose sodium
Carcholin

carcinoid tumor
carcinoma (CA)
    adenoid cystic c.
    basal cell c. (BCC)
    embryonal c.
    epidermoid c.
    c. of eyelid
    lacrimal gland adenoid cystic c.
    linear basal cell c.
    meibomian gland c.
    metastatic c.
    mucoepidermoid c.
    radiation-induced c.
    sebaceous cell c.
    sebaceous gland c.
    signet-ring c.
    squamous cell c.
carcinomatosis
    meningeal c.
carcinomatous meningitis
card
    Allen preschool c.
    Cambridge acuity c.
    digital acuity c.
    flash picture c.
    Glasgow c.
    Howell phoria c.
    illuminated near c. (INC)
    Jaeger acuity c.
    Keeler and Teller c.
    microendoscopic test c.
    MIM c.
    reading c.
    reduced Snellen c.
    Rosenbaum c.
    Sherman c.
    SKILL c.
    Sloan reading c.
    Smith-Kettlewell Institute low
      luminance c.
    Snellen near-vision c.
    Snellen reading c.
    standard near c.
    stigmatometric test c.
    Teller acuity c.
    test c.
    VSG 2/3F graphic c.
Cardec-S Syrup
cardinal
    c. diagnostic position of gaze
    c. direction of gaze
    c. field test
    c. ocular movement

    c. point
    c. position
    c. suture
Cardiobacterium hominis
Cardona threading forceps
Cardrase
care
    AoSept Clear C.
    cataract primary c.
    cataract secondary c.
    cataract tertiary c.
    low vision c.
    monitored anesthesia c. (MAC)
carinii
    Pneumocystis c.
Carl
    C. Zeiss instrument
    C. Zeiss Jena Retinophot fundus
      camera
    C. Zeiss lens
    C. Zeiss lensometer
    C. Zeiss tonometer
    C. Zeiss YAG laser
carnitine deficiency
Carones
    C. LASEK pump
    C. LASEK spatula
carotene
    beta c.
carotid
    c. aneurysm
    c. angiography
    c. arteriogram
    c. artery
    c. artery dissection
    c. artery occlusion
    c. artery stenosis
    c. artery thrombosis
    c. cavernous sinus fistula
    c. ischemia
    c. obstruction
    c. occlusive disease retinopathy
Carpel trabeculectomy punch
Carpenter syndrome
Carpine
    E C.
    Isopto C.
    PV C.
Carriazo-Barraquer
    C.-B. instrument set
    C.-B. microkeratome
    C.-B. principle
Carriazo-Pendular microkeratome

C

NOTES

carrier
>Barraquer needle c.
>minus c.
>obligate c.

carteolol
>c. HCl
>c. hydrochloride

Carter
>C. operation
>C. sphere
>C. sphere introducer

cartilage
>central c.
>ciliary c.
>palpebral c.
>posterior scleral c.
>tarsal c.

Cartman lens insertion forceps
cartridge
>Monarch C c.

Cartrol Oral
caruncle
>lacrimal c.

caruncula, pl. **carunculae**
>c. lacrimalis
>trichosis carunculae

caruncular papilloma
CAS
>congenital anterior staphyloma

Casanellas lacrimal operation
cascade
>angiogenic c.
>inflammatory c.
>phototransduction c.

cascade-induced angiogenesis
case
>eyeglass c.
>jeweled eye c.
>trial c.

caseating tubercle
Casebeer capsulorrhexis forceps
caseosa
>rhinitis c.

caseous necrosis
caspofungin
cast
>c. molding
>c. resin lens

castellanii
>*Acanthamoeba c.*

Castroviejo
>C. acrylic implant
>C. angled keratome
>C. anterior synechia scissors
>C. blade holder
>C. caliper
>C. capsule forceps
>C. clip-applying forceps
>C. compressor

C. corneal dissector
C. corneal-holding forceps
C. corneal scissors with inside stop
C. corneal section scissors
C. corneal transplant marker
C. corneal transplant scissors
C. corneal transplant trephine
C. corneoscleral forceps
C. corneoscleral punch
C. cyclodialysis cannula
C. cyclodialysis spatula
C. discission knife
C. double-ended spatula
C. electro keratome
C. electrokeratotome
C. enucleation snare
C. fixation forceps
C. improved trephine
C. iridectomy
C. iridocapsulotomy scissors
C. keratectomy
C. keratoplasty scissors
C. lacrimal dilator
C. lacrimal sac probe
C. lens loupe
C. lens spoon
C. lid clamp
C. lid forceps
C. lid retractor
C. mini-keratoplasty
C. mucotome
C. needle holder
C. needle holder clamp
C. orbital aspirator
C. radial iridotomy
C. razor blade
C. refractor
C. scleral fold forceps
C. scleral marker
C. scleral shortening clip
C. snare enucleator
C. speculum
C. suture forceps
C. suturing forceps
C. synechia scissors
C. synechia spatula
C. twin knife
C. tying forceps
C. vitreous aspirating needle
C. wide grip handle forceps

Castroviejo-Barraquer needle holder
Castroviejo-Colibri forceps
Castroviejo-Kalt needle holder
casualty
>ocular c.

catadioptric
Catalano
>C. corneoscleral forceps

C. intubation set
C. muscle hook
C. tying forceps
catalase
Catalin
cataphoria
    mature c.
cataplexy
Catapres
cataract
    acquired c.
    aculeiform c.
    adherent c.
    adolescent c.
    adult-onset c.
    age-related c.
    aminoaciduria c.
    anterior axial developmental c.
    anterior axial embryonal c.
    anterior axonal embryonal c.
    anterior polar c.
    anterior pyramidal c.
    anterior subcapsular c. (ASC)
    anular c.
    arborescent c.
    c. aspiration
    atopic c.
    autosomal dominant congenital c.
    (ADCC)
    autosomal dominant congenital c.
    (ADCC)
    axial embryonal c.
    axial fusiform developmental c.
    axial partial childhood c.
    black c.
    blue c.
    blue-dot c.
    bony c.
    brown c.
    brunescent c.
    calcareous c.
    capsular c.
    capsulolenticular c.
    central c.
    cerulean c.
    c. characteristic
    cheesy c.
    childhood c.
    choroidal c.
    Christmas tree c.
    complete c.
    complete congenital c.
    complicated c.

concussion c.
congenital c.
c. conservative management
contusion c.
copper c.
Coppock c.
coralliform c.
coronary c.
cortical spokes c.
corticosteroid-induced c.
crystalline c.
cuneiform c.
cupuliform c.
cystic c.
degenerative c.
delayed onset c.
dendritic c.
dermatogenic c.
developmental c.
diabetic c.
diabetic-osmotic c.
diffuse c.
dilacerated c.
disc-shaped c.
drug-induced c.
dry-shelled c.
dumbbell-shaped c.
dye-enhanced c.
early mature c.
electric shock c.
embryonal nuclear c.
embryonic c.
embryopathic c.
c. etiology
evolutional c.
extracapsular c. (ECC)
extracapsular extraction of c.
c. extraction (CE)
extraction of intracapsular c.
c. extraction operation
c. extraction plateau
c. extraction with intraocular lens
    (CE/IOL)
fetal nuclear c.
fibrinous c.
fibroid c.
flap operation c.
floriform c.
fluid c.
c. fragment
furnacemen's c.
fusiform c.
galactose c.

NOTES

cataract *(continued)*
    galactosemia c.
    general c.
    glassblower's c.
    c. glasses
    glassworker's c.
    glaucomatous c.
    global c.
    gray c.
    green c.
    hard c.
    heat-generated c.
    heat-ray c.
    hedger c.
    hereditary c.
    heterochromic c.
    hook-shaped c.
    hypermature c.
    hypocalcemic c.
    hypoglycemic c.
    iatrogenic c.
    immature c.
    c. incidence
    incipient c.
    infantile c.
    infrared c.
    intracapsular extraction of c.
    intumescent c.
    irradiation c.
    isolated hereditary c.
    juvenile developmental c.
    c. knife
    c. knife guard
    lacteal c.
    lamellar developmental c.
    lamellar zonular perinuclear c.
    c. lens
    lenticular c.
    life-belt c.
    lightning c.
    light perception c.
    Marner c.
    c. mask ring
    c. mask shield
    mature c.
    membranous c.
    metabolic syndrome c.
    milk-bag c.
    milky c.
    mixed c.
    Morgagni c.
    morgagnian c.
    c. morphology
    myotonic dystrophy c.
    c. needle
    NS c.
    nuclear developmental c.
    nuclear sclerotic c.
    nutritional deficiency c.

oil droplet c.
onion ring-like posterior polar c.
osmotic c.
overripe c.
partial c.
pear c.
pediatric c.
c. pencil
perinuclear c.
peripheral c.
pisciform c.
poikiloderma atrophicans and c.
poisoning degenerative c.
polar c.
polymorphic c.
posterior polar c.
posterior subcapsular c. (PSC)
postinflammatory c.
postvitrectomy c.
C. PPO project
c. of prematurity
presenile c.
c. prevalence
primary c.
c. primary care
probe c.
progressive c.
puddler's c.
pulverulent c.
punctate c.
pyramidal c.
radiation c.
reduplicated c.
ring-form congenital c.
ring-shaped c.
ripe c.
rubella c.
sanguineous c.
saucer-shaped c.
sclerotic c.
secondary c.
c. secondary care
sector cortical c.
sedimentary c.
senescent cortical degenerative c.
senescent nuclear degenerative c.
senile nuclear sclerotic c.
c. senilis
shaped c.
siderotic c.
siliculose c.
c. simulator
snowflake c.
snowstorm c.
Soemmerring ring c.
soft c.
spear developmental c.
c. spectacles
c. spindle

spindle c.
spoke-like sutural c.
c. spoon
spurious c.
stationary c.
stellate c.
steroid-induced c.
subcapsular c.
sugar c.
sugar-induced c.
sunflower c.
supranuclear c.
c. surgery
c. surgery and clear lens extraction
sutural developmental c.
syndermatotic c.
syphilitic c.
c. tertiary care
tetany c.
thermal c.
total c.
toxic c.
traumatic degenerative c.
tremulous c.
umbilicated c.
uniocular c.
vascular c.
visually significant c.
Vogt c.
Volkmann c.
white pediatric c.
c. with Down syndrome
X-linked congenital c.
x-ray-induced c.
zonular nuclear c.
zonular pulverulent c.
zonular sutural c.
cataracta
    c. adiposa
    c. brunescens
    c. caerulea
    c. centralis pulverulenta
    c. cerulea
    c. dermatogenes
    c. electrica
    c. fibrosa
    c. nigra
cataract-aspirating needle
cataractogenesis
cataractogenic drug
cataractous
catarrh
    sinus c.

spring c.
vernal c.
catarrhal
    c. conjunctivitis
    c. corneal ulcer
    c. ophthalmia
catarrhalis
    Branhamella c.
    Moraxella c.
catastrophic
    c. operative complication
    c. ophthalmic sequelae
catatonic pupil
catatropic image
caterpillar-hair ophthalmia
Catford visual acuity test
catgut suture
catheter
    C-flex c.
    French c.
    LacriCATH balloon c.
    LacriCATH lacrimal duct c.
    lacrimal balloon c.
    Lincoff balloon c.
    red rubber c.
    Teflon injection c.
catheterization
    c. of lacrimal duct
    c. of lacrimonasal duct
catoptric
catscratch disease neuroretinitis
cat's-eye
    c.-e. amaurosis
    c.-e. effect
    c.-e. pupil
    c.-e. reflex
    c.-e. syndrome
CAU
    chronic anterior uveitis
caudate hemorrhage
Cauer chalazion forceps
causative organism
cauterization
    tunnel c.
cautery
    Alcon hand c.
    bipolar c.
    Bovie wet-field c.
    Codman wet-field c.
    Colorado c.
    Concept disposable c.
    Concept handheld c.
    disposable c.

C

NOTES

cautery *(continued)*
    Eraser c.
    Geiger c.
    Hildreth c.
    Mentor wet-field c.
    Mira c.
    Mueller c.
    c. operation
    ophthalmic c.
    Op-Temp disposable c.
    pencil c.
    phacoemulsification c.
    Prince c.
    punctal c.
    Scheie ophthalmic c.
    scleral c. (SC)
    thermal c.
    Todd c.
    von Graefe c.
    Wadsworth-Todd c.
    wet-field c.
    Ziegler c.
cave
    myopic c.
cavern
    Schnabel c.
cavernoma
    orbital c.
cavernous
    c. angioma
    c. optic atrophy
    c. orbital hemangioma
    c. portion of oculomotor nerve
    c. sinus
    c. sinus aneurysm
    c. sinus fistula
    c. sinus/superior orbital fissure syndrome
    c. sinus syndrome
    c. sinus thrombosis
caviae
    Nocardia c.
cavitary uveal melanoma
cavitation
Cavitron
    C. aspirator
    C. I/A handpiece
    C. irrigation/aspiration system
Cavitron-Kelman irrigation/aspiration system
cavity
    laser c.
    opening of orbital c.
    optic papilla c.
    orbital c.
    schisis c.
    vitreous c.
CB
    chronic blepharitis

CBS
    Charles Bonnet syndrome
cc
    with correction
CCA
    central choroidal apposition
C-CAP
    custom-contoured ablation pattern
CCC
    continuous curvilinear capsulorrhexis
CCD
    choriocapillaris degeneration
        CCD camera
CCF
    critical corresponding frequency
c̄cl
    with contact lenses
CCT
    central corneal thickness
CCTS
    Collaborative Corneal Transplantation Studies
C/D
    cup-to-disc ratio
cd
    candela
CD-5 needle
CD8 cell
CDC
    Centers for Disease Control
CDCR
    conjunctivodacryocystorhinostomy
CDR
    cup-to-disc ratio
CDS
    Cornea Donor Study
CE
    cataract extraction
Ceclor
cecocentral
    c. depression
    c. scotoma
cecum, pl. **ceca**
    punctum c.
CeeNU
CeeOn
    C. Edge
    C. Edge foldable IOL
    C. heparin surface-modified lens
    C. Model 920 foldable intraocular lens
cefaclor
cefadroxil
cefamandole sodium
cefazaflur
cefazolin
    aminoglycoside with c.
cefixime
cefmenoxime

cefoperazone
ceforanide
cefotaxime
cefsulodin
ceftazidime
Ceftin
ceftizoxime
ceftriaxone
cefuroxime
CE/IOL
    cataract extraction with intraocular lens
      CE/IOL implant
Celestone
Celita
    C. elite knife
    C. sapphire knife
cell
    c. adhesion
    air c.
    allogeneic retinal epithelial c.
    amacrine c.
    amniotic c.
    antigen-presenting c.
    B c.
    basal c.
    basaloid c.
    bipolar retinal c.
    bone marrow-derived progenitor c.
    budding yeast c.
    CD8 c.
    chick lens c.
    circulating tumor c.
    clump c.
    cluster of retinoblastoma c.'s
    collagen c.
    cone c.
    conjunctival epithelial c.
    conjunctival goblet c.
    corneal c.
    c. cycle
    cytoxic T c.
    c. debris
    c. density
    downgaze paralysis, ataxia/athetosis
      and foam c. (DAF)
    E c.
    endoneural c.
    endothelial c.
    eosin-Y c.
    epithelial c.
    epithelioid c.
    fat c.
    fetal c.

fiber c.
c. and flare
foam c.
foreign body c.
ganglion c.
ghost c.
giant epithelial c.
goblet c.
granulomatous inflammatory c.
helper/inducer T c.
heterogeneous c.
horizontal c.
inflammatory c.
interplexiform c.
killer c.
koniocellular retinal ganglion c.
Leber c.
lens epithelial c. (LEC)
leukemic c.
limbal stem c.
lipid c.
c. lysis
M c.
magnocellular c.
mast c.
melanin-containing c.
membrane lipid c.
meningeal c.
mesangial c.
metaplastic epithelial c.
c. migration
Mueller c.
Müller c.
multinucleated giant epithelial c.
mural c.
myoepithelial c.
myoid visual c.
necrotic lymphomatous c.
nests and strands of c.'s
neural crest c.
neural ganglionic c.
nevus c.
nonneural ganglionic c.
occult tumor c.
off-center bipolar c.
on-center bipolar c.
Onodi c.
paracentral c.
parvocellular c.
perineural c.
perivascular stromal c.
photoreceptor c.
phytohemagglutinin c.

NOTES

C

cell *(continued)*
 pigment c.
 pigmented trabecular meshwork c.
 plasma c.
 polygonal pigmented c.
 polyhedral c.
 posterior lens c.
 Reed-Sternberg c.
 reticulum c.
 retinal glial c.
 retinal visual c.
 retinoblastoma c.
 rod c.
 satellite ganglionic c.
 Schwann c.
 sebaceous c.
 secretory epithelial c.
 somatic c.
 spillover c.
 spindle c.
 spindle-shaped c.
 squamous c.
 stem c. (SC)
 suppressor T c.
 Touton giant c.
 tumor c.
 vascular endothelial c.
 visual c.
 vitreous c.
 water c.
 wet c.
 white c.
 wing c.
 X c.
 Y c.
cell-mediated immunity
cellophane
 crinkled c.
 c. macular reflex
 c. maculopathy
 c. retinopathy
cellophane-like band
CellPlant stent
Cell-Tak autologous fibrin
Cellufluor
Cellufresh Formula
cellular
 c. aggregate
 c. atypia
 c. debris
 c. disorganization
 c. inclusion body
cellularity
cellulite
 orbital c.
cellulitis
 amyloid c.
 herpes simplex c.
 orbital c.

 pediatric orbital c.
 periorbital c.
 preseptal c.
celluloid frame
cellulose
 c. acetate
 c. acetate butyrate (CAB)
 c. acetate butyrate contact lens
 c. acetate frame
 hydroxyethyl c.
 hydroxypropyl c.
 c. nitrate
 c. nitrate frame
 oxidized c.
 c. surgical sponge
Celluvisc
cement
 c. bifocal
 Morck c.
center
 C.'s for Disease Control (CDC)
 distance between c.'s (DBC)
 Dutch Ophthalmic Research C. (DORC)
 foveal c.
 gaze c.
 geometric c.
 horizontal gaze c.
 C.'s for Medicare & Medicaid Services
 optic c.
 optical c.
 pontine gaze c. (PGC)
 pupillary c.
 c. of rotation
 c. of rotation distance
 supranuclear gaze c.
 vertical gaze c.
centering ring
centrad
centrage
central
 c. abrasion
 c. achromatopsia
 c. amaurosis
 c. angiospastic retinitis
 c. angiospastic retinopathy
 c. anisocoria
 c. anterior curve (CAC)
 c. areolar choroidal atrophy
 c. areolar choroidal dystrophy
 c. areolar choroidal sclerosis
 c. areolar pigment epithelial dystrophy
 c. astigmatism
 c. canal
 c. cartilage
 c. cataract
 c. chorioretinitis

c. choroidal apposition (CCA)
c. choroiditis
c. cloudy corneal dystrophy
c. cloudy corneal dystrophy of François
c. cloudy parenchymatous dystrophy
c. corneal thickness (CCT)
c. corneal ulcer
c. crystalline corneal dystrophy of Schnyder
c. crystalline dystrophy
c. defect
c. discoid corneal dystrophy
c. disc-shaped retinopathy
c. dissecting tip
c. dyslexia
c. edema
c. edema of cornea
c. endothelial photography
c. field loss (CFL)
c. fovea
c. fovea of retina
c. fusion
c. gyrate atrophy
c. illumination
c. iridectomy
c. island
c. island of vision
c. keyhole of vision
c. lesion
c. light
c. nervous system (CNS)
c. pigmentary retinal dystrophy
c. posterior curve (CPC)
c. posterior curve of contact lens
c. reflex stripe
c. retinal artery (CRA)
c. retinal artery occlusion (CRAO)
c. retinal degeneration
c. retinal detachment
c. retinal lens
c. retinal vein (CRV)
c. retinal vein occlusion (CRVO)
c. retinal vein occlusion knife
c. scotoma
c. scotoma syndrome
c. serous chorioretinopathy (CSC, CSCR)
c. serous choroidopathy
c. serous retinitis
c. serous retinochoroidopathy
c. serous retinopathy (CSR)
c. speckled corneal dystrophy

c., steady and maintained (CSM)
c., steady and maintained fixation
c. steep zone
c. stellate laceration
c. striate keratopathy
c. stromal infiltrate
c. suppression
c. thickness of contact lens
c. unilateral lens opacity
C. Vein Occlusion Study (CVOS)
c. vestibular imbalance
c. vestibular nystagmus
c. visual acuity
c. visual field (CVF)
c. yellow point
centralis
amaurosis c.
area c.
fovea c.
centrally fixing eye
centration
optical zone c.
centraxonial
centrifugal
c. incision
c. separation
centripetal
c. incision
c. movement
c. nystagmus
centrocecal
c. defect
c. scotoma
centronuclear myopathy
centrophose
Centurion SES microkeratome
CEOS
Congenital Esotropia Observational Study
cepacia
Pseudomonas c.
cephalexin
cephalgia
cephalic
cephalosporin
cephalothin
Ceralas I laser
Ceralink slit lamp laser adapter
ceramic effect
ceratectomy
cerclage
c. operation
c. pupilloplasty
cerclage-type fashion

NOTES

cerebellar
    c. artery
    c. astrocytoma tumor
    c. ataxia
    c. ataxia-cone dystrophy
    c. cortex
    c. dysfunction
    c. eye sign
    c. flocculus
    c. hemisphere
    c. hemorrhage
    c. lesion
    c. notch
    c. tonsil
    c. vermis
cerebellomedullary
cerebellopontine
    c. angle (CPA)
    c. angle lesion
    c. angle mass
    c. angle tumor
cerebelloretinal
cerebellospinal
cerebellotegmental
cerebellothalamic
cerebellum
cerebra (*pl. of* cerebrum)
cerebral
    c. abscess
    c. achromatopsia
    c. akinetopsia
    c. amaurosis
    c. amyloid angiopathy
    c. arteriography
    c. arteriosclerosis
    c. artery
    c. artery aneurysm
    c. atrophy
    c. blindness
    c. cortex
    c. cortex reflex
    c. diplopia
    c. dyschromatopsia
    c. edema
    c. fluid shunt
    c. giantism
    c. hemisphere lesion
    c. heterotopia
    c. infarction
    c. layer of retina
    c. metamorphopsia
    c. micropsia
    c. palsy
    c. phycomycosis
    c. polyopia
    c. ptosis
    c. radionuclide angiography
    c. stratum of retina

    c. tunnel vision
    c. venous drainage
    c. ventricle
cerebri
    idiopathic pseudotumor c.
    pseudotumor c. (PTC)
cerebritis
cerebrohepatorenal syndrome
cerebroocular
cerebropupillary reflex
cerebroretinal angiomatosis
cerebrospinal fluid (CSF)
cerebrotendinous xanthomatosis
cerebrum, pl. **cerebra, cerebrums**
cereus
    Bacillus c.
ceroid
    c. lipofuscinosis
certified
    c. ophthalmic medical technologist (COMT)
    c. ophthalmic technologist (COT)
    c. orthoptist (CO)
    c. paraoptometric assistant (CPOA)
    c. paraoptometric technician (CPOT)
    c. registered nurse in ophthalmology (CRNO)
cerulea
    cataracta c.
ceruleae
    maculae c.
cerulean cataract
cervical
    c. ganglion
    c. lesion
    c. nystagmus
cervicoocular reflex (COR)
cervicooculoacoustic syndrome
Cestan
    C. sign
    C. syndrome
Cestan-Chenais syndrome
Cestan-Raymond syndrome
Cetamide
    Isopto C.
    C. Ophthalmic
Cetapred
    Isopto C.
    C. ophthalmic
Cetazol
cetylpyridinium chloride
CF
    counting fingers
C3F8
    perfluoropropane
    C3F8 gas
CF-60DSi fundus camera

CFA
    color filter array
      CFA digital camera
CFEOM
    congenital fibrosis of extraocular muscles
CFF
    critical flicker frequency
    critical flicker fusion
CFL
    central field loss
C-flex catheter
CFTD
    congenital fiber-type disproportion
cGMP
    cyclic guanosine monophosphate
chafing
      iris c.
chain
      collagen alpha c.
      fenestrated c.
      gamma light c.
      kappa light c.
      sialylated c.
chalazion, chalaza, pl. **chalazia**
      acute c.
      c. clamp
      collar-stud c.
      c. curette
      c. forceps
      c. trephine
chalcosis lentis
challenge
      perceptual c.
      visual c.
Challenger digital applanation tonometer
chamber
      air c.
      c. angle
      angle of anterior c.
      anterior c. (AC)
      aqueous c.
      artificial anterior c.
      axial c.
      Barron disposable artificial
        anterior c.
      choroidal c.
      closed c.
      c. collapse
      depth of c.
      eye c.
      flat anterior c.
      hydrometric c.
      MoistAir humidifying c.

      moisture c.
      multicorneal perfusion c.
      optical zone c.
      parallel-plate flow c.
      peripheral anterior c.
      phakic posterior c.
      post c.
      posterior c. (PC)
      postoperative flat anterior c.
      pump c.
      quiet c.
      reformation of c.
      shallow anterior c.
      shallowing of c.
      c. stability
      vitreous c.
chamber-deepening glaucoma
CHAMPS
    Controlled High Risk Avonex Multiple
    Sclerosis Prevention Study
chancre
      c. of conjunctiva
      primary conjunctival c.
      primary eyelid c.
chancroid
Chandler
      C. iridectomy
      C. iris forceps
      C. syndrome
      C. vitreous operation
Chang
      C. combination phaco chopper
      C. combo chopper
      C. hydrodissection cannula
change
      arterial occlusive c.
      c. blindness
      contact lens power c.
      contralateral disc c.
      cortical c.
      crossing c.
      disease-related c.
      fatty c.
      c. of fixation
      Keith-Wagener retinal c.
      multifocal electroretinographic c.
      nuclear c.
      optic disc c.
      pigment c.
      saccadic c.
      senile choroidal c.
      skin c.
      surgically induced refractive c.

C

NOTES

change *(continued)*
> trophic c.
> UV c.
> visual field c.

changer
> Galilean magnification c.
> Littmann Galilean magnification c.

channel
> c. dissector
> lamellar c.
> scleral c.
> vascular c.

2-channel Badal optical system

character
> Ishihara c.

characteristic
> cataract c.
> high-risk c.

3-character test

charcoal
> Amies transport medium with c.
> Amies transport medium without c.

Charcot
> C. sign
> C. triad

CHARGE
> coloboma, heart defects, atresia choanae,
> retarded growth, genital hypoplasia, and
> ear anomalies
> CHARGE association
> CHARGE syndrome

Charleaux
> C. oil droplet reflex
> C. oil droplet sign

Charles
> C. anterior segment sleeve
> C. Bonnet syndrome (CBS)
> C. flute needle
> C. handheld infusion lens
> C. infusion sleeve
> C. intraocular lens
> C. irrigating/aspirating unit
> C. irrigating contact lens
> C. lensectomy
> C. vacuuming needle

Charlin syndrome

chart
> aberrated acuity c.
> Amsler c.
> astigmatic dial c.
> Aurora luminous acuity c.
> Bailey-Lovie logMar c.
> Bailey-Lovie test c.
> Bailey-Lovie visual acuity c.
> color c.
> contemporary nearpoint c.
> cross-Polaroid projection c.
> Donders c.
> E c.

> Early Treatment of Diabetic
> Retinopathy Study visual
> acuity c.
> eye c.
> illiterate E c.
> illiterate eye c.
> kindergarten eye c.
> Konig bar c.
> Landolt C acuity c.
> Lebensohn reading c.
> Lebensohn visual acuity c.
> Lighthouse ET-DRS acuity c.
> logMAR c.
> Low-Contrast Sloan Letter C.
> (LCSLC)
> pedigree c.
> Pelli-Robson contrast sensitivity c.
> Pelli-Robson letter c.
> picture c.
> pseudoisochromatic c.
> Randot c.
> reading c.
> Regan low-contrast acuity c.
> Reuss color c.
> Snellen c.
> sunburst dial c.
> symbol c.
> unaberrated c.
> University of Waterloo c.
> vectograph c.
> Vistech wall c.

charting
> EyeSys c.

chatter line

Chayet type corneal LASIK marker

ChBFlow
> choroidal blood flow

ChBVol
> choroidal blood volume

checkerboard
> c. hemianopsia
> c. visual field

check ligament

Chédiak-Higashi
> C.-H. anomaly
> C.-H. syndrome

Chédiak-Steinbrinck-Higashi anomaly

cheek
> c. clamp
> c. flap

cheese wire

cheesewiring of sutures

cheesy cataract

chelation
> EDTA c.

chelator
> copper c.

chelonae
> *Mycobacterium c.*

chemical
    c. burn
    c. conjunctivitis
    c. diabetes
    c. injury
    c. procedure
    c. vapor deposition (CVD)
chemically treated spectacle lens
chemiluminescence assay
chemofluorescent dye
chemoreduction
chemosis
    conjunctival c.
chemotherapy
    c. drops
    intraarterial cytoreductive c.
    subconjunctival c.
chemotic
cherry-red
    c.-r. spot
    c.-r. spot in macula
    c.-r. spot myoclonus syndrome
chevron incision
chevron-shaped
    c.-s. break
    c.-s. defect
Cheyne nystagmus
chi
Chiari malformation
chiaroscuro
chiasm
    glioma of optic c.
    optic c.
chiasma
    c. opticum
chiasmal
    c. aplasia
    c. arachnoiditis
    c. compression
    c. disease
    c. dysplasia
    c. glioma
    c. hypoplasia
    c. lesion
    c. metastasis
    c. sulcus
    c. syndrome
    c. tumor
    c. visual field loss
chiasmapexy
chiasmatic
    c. cisterna

    c. field defect
    c. syndrome
chiasmometer
Chiba eye needle
Chibroxin
chickenpox
chick lens cell
chief fiber
Chievitz
    fiber layer of C.
    transient layer of C.
child, pl. **children**
    An Evaluation of Treatment of
      Amblyopia in Children 7-18
    blind c.
    Fisher-Price polycarbonate lens for
      children
    c. glasses
    c. lens
    oculodermal melanosis in children
    partially sighted c.
    Refractive Error Study in Children
    tearing c.
    visually impaired c.
child-friendly VDS test
childhood
    c. blindness pattern
    c. cataract
    c. episcleritis
    ocular tumor of c.
    oculomotor apraxia of c.
    c. uveitis
    c. vision screening
children (*pl. of* child)
chilled balanced salt solution
chiller
    Geggel PRK c.
chip-and-flip phacoemulsification
    technique
Chiroflex C11UB lens
Chiron
    C. ACS microkeratome
    C. automated corneal shaper
    C. Hansatome
    C. Hansatome microkeratome
chiroscope
chirped-pulse amplification system
chisel
    cornea c.
    Freer c.
    lacrimal sac c.
    West lacrimal sac c.
chi-squared test

NOTES

Chlamydia
- C. conjunctivitis
- C. *psittaci*
- C. *trachomatis*

chlamydial
- c. blepharitis
- c. inclusion conjunctivitis
- c. infection

Chlo-Amine
Chloracol
chlorambucil
chloramphenicol
- c., polymyxin B, and hydrocortisone
- c. and prednisolone

chlorate
chlordecone
chlordiazepoxide
chlorhexidine
chloride
- acetylcholine c.
- aluminum c.
- benzalkonium c. (BAK)
- benzethonium c.
- cetylpyridinium c.
- edrophonium c.
- hexamethonium c.
- methacholine c.
- potassium c. (KOH)
- quaternary ammonium c.
- sodium c. (NaCl)
- tetraethylammonium c.

chlorisondamine
chloroacetophenone
chlorobutanol
Chlorofair
chloroform
chlorolabe
chloroma
chlorophane
chloropia
chloroprocaine
chloropsia
Chloroptic
- C. Ophthalmic
- C. SOP

Chloroptic-P Ophthalmic
chloroquine
- c. keratopathy
- c. retinopathy
- c. toxicity

chloroquine/hydroxychloroquine
- c. maculopathy
- c. retinopathy
- c. toxicity

Chlorphed
chlorpheniramine maleate
chlorphentermine
Chlor-Pro

chlorpromazine
chlorpropamide
chlorprothixene
chlortetracycline
chlorthalidone
Chlor-Trimeton
chocolate agar
choked
- c. optic disc
- c. reflex

cholesterinosis
cholesterol
- c. embolus of retina
- c. granuloma
- c. plaque

cholesterolosis
cholesterosis bulbi
cholinergic
- c. drug
- c. mechanism
- c. neuron
- c. pupil

cholinesterase
chondrodystrophic myotonia
chondroitin
- hyaluronate sodium with c.
- c. sulfate
- c. sulfate medium

chondroitinase
choo-choo chop and flip phacoemulsification
chop
- bimanual phaco c.

chopper
- Agarwal irrigating phaco c.
- Chang combination phaco c.
- Chang combo c.
- combination phaco c.
- Dodick-Kammann bimanual c.
- Dodick nucleus irrigating c.
- dull-tipped horizontal c.
- Fine irrigating reverse actuating splitting c.
- Fine-Nagahara phaco c.
- Fine sideport actuating quick c.
- Fukasaku snap & split tip irrigating c.
- 19-gauge irrigating c.
- Inamura race c.
- Katena MicroFinger tip irrigating c.
- Koch-Minami c.
- Lane quick c.
- Langerman bi-directional phaco c.
- Minardi phaco c.
- Miyoshi c.
- Nagahara karate c.
- Nagahara phaco c.
- Nagahara quick c.

Nichamin I and II nucleus
quick c.
Nichamin triple c.
Nichamin vertical c.
Olson phaco c.
Olson quick c.
Seibel nucleus c.
Seibel vertical safety quick c.
Shepherd tomahawk c.
Steinert double-ended claw c.
Steinert II claw c.
Sung reverse nucleus c.
Tsuneoka irrigating c.

chopper/manipulator
Universal phaco c./m.

chord length

chordoma
clivus c.

choriocapillaris
c. atrophy
c. compression
c. degeneration (CCD)
c. fenestrae
lamina c.
membrana c.
c. vascular network

choriocapillary layer

choriocele

chorioid
ischemic necrosis of c.
lymphatic sinusoid c.

chorioidea

chorionic vesicle

choriopathy

chorioretinal (C/R)
c. adhesion
c. atrophic spot
c. atrophy
c. coloboma
c. degeneration
c. fold
c. granuloma
c. inflammatory disease
c. lesion
c. scar
c. venous anastomosis

chorioretinitis
birdshot c.
central c.
cryptococcal c.
Histoplasma c.
luetic c.
miliary tuberculosis c.

peripheral multifocal c. (PMC)
salt-and-pepper c.
sclerosing panencephalitis c.
c. sclopetaria
senile c.
septic c.
syphilitic c.
Toxoplasma c.
toxoplasmosis c.
vitiliginous c.

chorioretinopathy
birdshot c.
central serous c. (CSC, CSCR)
disciform c.
idiopathic central serous c. (ICSC)
c. and pituitary dysfunction (CPD)
serous c.

choriovaginal vein

choristoma
epibulbar limbal dermoid c.
epibulbar osseous c.
episcleral osteocartilaginous c.
limbal c.
osseous c.
phakomatous c.
c. tumor

choroid
basal lamina of c.
basement membrane of c.
coloboma of c.
contusion of c.
crescent c.
c. fissure
knuckle of c.
malignant melanoma of c.
peripapillary c.
reattachment of c.
vascular lamina of c.
c. vein

choroidal
c. abscess
c. amelanotic melanoma
c. blood flow (ChBFlow)
c. blood volume (ChBVol)
c. capillary
c. cataract
c. chamber
c. coloboma
c. detachment
c. dystrophy
c. edema
c. effusion
c. epithelial atrophy

C

NOTES

choroidal *(continued)*
- c. filling
- c. flush
- c. fold
- c. granuloma
- c. gyrate atrophy
- c. hemangioma
- c. hemorrhage
- c. hyperfluorescence
- c. infarct
- c. infiltration
- c. ischemia
- c. lesion
- c. mass
- c. melanocytic tumor
- c. metastasis
- c. myopic atrophy
- c. neoplasm
- c. neovascularization (CNV)
- c. neovascular membrane (CNVM)
- c. nevus
- c. osteoma
- c. primary sclerosis
- c. pulse
- c. ring
- c. rupture
- c. scan
- c. secondary atrophy
- c. tap
- c. thinning
- c. vascular atrophy
- c. vascular occlusion
- c. vasculature
- c. vessel
- c. watershed zone

choroideae
- lamina vasculosa c.

choroidectomy
choroideremia
choroiditis
- acute diffuse serous c.
- anterior c.
- areolar central c.
- birdshot c.
- central c.
- diffuse c.
- disseminated c.
- Doyne familial honeycomb c.
- exudative c.
- focal c.
- Förster c.
- geographic peripapillary c.
- c. guttata senilis
- histoplasmic c.
- Holthouse-Batten superficial c.
- Hutchinson-Tays central guttate c.
- Jensen juxtapapillary c.
- juxtapupillary c.
- macular c.

- metastatic c.
- multifocal c. (MFC)
- c. myopia
- nongranulomatous c.
- posterior c.
- proliferative c.
- punctate inner c.
- recurrent c.
- senescent macular exudative c.
- senile macular exudative c.
- serpiginous c.
- suppurative c.
- syphilitic c.
- Tay c.
- toxoplasmic c.
- traumatic c.
- unifocal helioid c.
- vitiliginous c.

choroidocapillaris
- lamina c.

choroidocyclitis
choroidoiritis
choroidopathy
- areolar c.
- central serous c.
- Doyne honeycomb c.
- geographic c.
- geographic helicoid peripapillary c.
- guttate c.
- helicoid c.
- inner punctate c.
- myopic c.
- peripapillary central serous c.
- *Pneumocystis carinii* c.
- punctate inner c. (PIC)
- senile guttate c.
- serpiginous c.
- systemic lupus erythematosus c.

choroidoretinal dystrophy
choroidoretinitis
choroidosis
choroidovitreal neovascularization
Choyce
- C. intraocular lens
- C. lens-inserting forceps
- C. Mark VIII implant
- C. Mark VIII lens

Christmas tree cataract
chromatic
- c. aberration
- c. asymmetry
- c. contrast threshold
- c. dispersion
- c. induction effect
- c. lens aberration
- c. perimetry
- c. spectrum
- c. vision

chromaticity
   complementary c.
chromatism
chromatometer
chromatopsia
chromatoptometer
chromatoptometry
chromic
   c. catgut suture
   c. collagen suture
   c. gut suture
chromodacryorrhea
chromogranin antibody
chromometer
chromophane
chromophobe adenoma
chromophore
chromoscope
chromoscopy
chromostereopsis
chronic
   c. actinic keratopathy
   c. anterior uveitis (CAU)
   c. blepharitis (CB)
   c. blepharoconjunctivitis
   c. catarrhal conjunctivitis
   c. catarrhal rhinitis
   c. cicatrizing conjunctivitis
   c. cyclitis
   c. dacryocystitis
   c. demyelinating optic neuritis
   c. dry eye
   c. dry eye syndrome
   c. endophthalmitis
   c. follicular conjunctivitis
   c. immunogenic conjunctivitis
   c. myopia
   c. narrow-angle glaucoma
   c. open-angle glaucoma (COAG)
   c. optic disc swelling
   c. optic nerve compression
   c. papilledema
   c. paroxysmal hemicrania
   c. prephthisical ocular hypotony
   c. primary angle-closure glaucoma
      (C-PACG)
   c. progressive external
      ophthalmoplegia (CPEO)
   c. red eye
   c. serpiginous ulcer
   c. simple glaucoma
   c. smoldering toxicity syndrome
   c. superficial keratitis

CHRPE
   congenital hypertrophy of retinal pigment
      epithelium
chrysiasis
chrysocyanosis
chrysoderma
Chrysosporium parvum
Chu Foldable Lens Cutter
Churg-Strauss syndrome
Chvostek sign
Chymar
   Alpha C.
chymotrypsin
CI
   complete iridectomy
   convergence insufficiency
Ciaccio gland
Cianca syndrome
Ciba
   C. TearSaver punctual gauging
      system
   C. Vision Cleaner
   C. Vision Daily Cleanser
   C. Vision lens drops
   C. Vision Saline
CibaSoft Visitint contact lens
cibisotome
cicatricial
   c. adhesion
   c. conjunctivitis
   c. ectropion
   c. entropion
   c. mass
   c. pemphigoid
   c. pterygium
   c. retinopathy of prematurity
   c. retrolental fibroplasia
   c. shortening
   c. strabismus
cicatrix, pl. **cicatrices**
   cystoid c.
   filtering c.
cicatrization
cicatrizing
   c. conjunctivitis
   c. trachoma
CICE
   combined intracapsular cataract
      extraction
CID
   cytomegalic inclusion disease

C

NOTES

cidofovir
    c. eye drops
    c. therapy
CIF4 needle
CIGTS
    Collaborative Initial Glaucoma Treatment
    Study
Cilco
    C. argon laser
    C. Frigitronics
    C. Frigitronics laser
    C. krypton laser
    C. lens forceps
    C. YAG laser
cilia (*pl. of* cilium)
    cilia base
    cilia ectopia
    cilia follicle
    cilia forceps
ciliare
    corpus c.
ciliares
    plicae c.
    processus c.
ciliaris
    acne c.
    anulus c.
    blepharitis c.
    corona c.
    musculus c.
    pars plana corporis c.
    pars plicata corporis c.
    plica c.
    radix oculomotoria ganglii c.
    radix sympathica ganglii c.
    striae c.
    tylosis c.
    zona c.
    zonula c.
ciliariscope
ciliarotomy
ciliary
    c. apparatus
    c. artery
    c. blepharitis
    c. block
    c. block glaucoma
    c. body
    c. body band
    c. body coloboma
    c. body contraction
    c. body edema
    c. body inflammation
    c. body melanoma
    c. body melanoma with extrascleral
      extension
    c. body muscle
    c. canal
    c. cartilage

    c. crown
    c. disc
    c. epithelium
    c. flush
    c. fold
    c. ganglion
    c. ganglionectomy
    c. ganglionic plexus
    c. gland
    c. hyperemia
    c. injection
    c. ligament
    c. margin
    c. margin of iris
    c. nerve
    c. neurotrophic factor (CTNF)
    c. neurotrophic factor capsule
    c. neurotrophic factor capsule
      protein eye implant
    c. part of retina
    c. poliosis
    c. procedure
    c. process
    c. reflex
    c. region
    c. ring
    c. spasm
    c. staphyloma
    c. sulcus
    c. vein
    c. vessel
    c. wreath
    c. zone
    c. zonule
ciliate
ciliectomy
ciliochoroidal
    c. detachment
    c. effusion
    c. melanoma
ciliodestructive surgery
cilioequatorial fiber
ciliogenesis
ciliolenticular block
cilioposterocapsular fiber
cilioretinal
    c. artery
    c. artery occlusion
    c. collateral
    c. vein
cilioscleral
ciliospinal
    c. center of Budge
    c. reflex
ciliotomy
ciliovitreal block
cilium, pl. **cilia**
    intraocular cilia
cillosis, cillo

Ciloxan Ophthalmic
CIN
    conjunctival intraepithelial neoplasia
cinching operation
cinema eye
cine-magnetic resonance imaging
Cine-Microscope
Cionni capsular tension ring
Cipro
ciprofloxacin
    c. hydrochloride
    postoperative c.
circadian
    c. heterotropia
    c. pattern of IOP
    c. tonometric curve
    c. variation of intraocular pressure
circinata
    retinitis c.
circinate
    c. exudate
    c. retinitis
    c. retinopathy
circle
    arterial c.
    blur c.
    c. diffusion
    c. of dispersion
    c. dissipation
    episcleral arterial c.
    c. of greater iris
    c. of Haller
    Hovius c.
    c. of least confusion
    least confusion c.
    least diffusion c.
    c. of lesser iris
    Minsky c.
    Randot c.
    Vieth-Müller c.
    c. of Willis
    Wort c.
    c. of Zinn
    Zinn-Haller arterial c.
circlet
    Zinn c.
circline magnifier
circling band
circular
    c. blade
    c. ciliary muscle
    c. ciliary muscle fiber
    c. dichroism

    c. nystagmus
    c. synechia
    c. tear
    c. tear capsulorrhexis
    c. tear capsulotomy
    c. vection
circulating
    c. antipericyte autoantibody
    c. immune complex
    c. tumor cell
circulation
    conjunctival c.
    episcleral c.
    foveolar choroidal c.
    perilimbic c.
    retinal venous c.
    sludging of c.
circulus, pl. circuli
    c. arteriosus iridis major
    c. arteriosus iridis minor
    c. vasculosus nervi optici
circumbulbar
circumciliary flush
circumcorneal injection
circumduction
    c. of the eye
    c. hyperphoria
circumferential vascular plexus of limbus
circumlental space
circumocular
circumorbital
circumpapillary
    c. light reflex
    c. measurement
    c. telangiectatic microangiopathy
circumscribed
    c. episcleritis
    c. posterior keratoconus
    c. retinal edema
circumscripta
    canities c.
cirsoid aneurysm
cirsophthalmia
cisterna
    chiasmatic c.
cisternography
CIT
    corneal impression test
Citelli rongeur
citrate
    potassium c.

NOTES

citrate *(continued)*
     Reynold lead c.
     sodium c.
CK
     conductive keratoplasty
     CK conventional pressure technique
CL
     contact lens
Cladosporium
cladribine
Claforan
CLAMP
     Contact Lens and Myopia Progression
     CLAMP study
clamp
     Backhaus c.
     Barraquer needle holder c.
     Berens muscle c.
     Berke c.
     bulldog c.
     Castroviejo lid c.
     Castroviejo needle holder c.
     chalazion c.
     cheek c.
     cross-action towel c.
     curved mosquito c.
     Desmarres lid c.
     Downes lid c.
     Halsted curved mosquito c.
     Halsted straight mosquito c.
     Jones towel c.
     Kalt needle holder c.
     King c.
     lid c.
     mosquito c.
     muscle c.
     needle holder c.
     Prince muscle c.
     Putterman levator resection c.
     Putterman ptosis c.
     recession c.
     Robin chalazion c.
     Schaedel cross-action towel c.
     Schnidt c.
     serrefine c.
     straight mosquito c.
CLAO
     Contact Lens Association of
     Ophthalmologists
CLARE
     contact lens-induced acute red eye
Clariflex
     C. foldable silicone intraocular lens
     C. OptiEdge foldable intraocular
     lens
Clarine
Claris
     C. Cleaning and Soaking Solution
     C. Rewetting Drops

clarithromycin
Claritin
clarity
     corneal c.
     lens c.
     optical c.
     vitreous c.
clariVit
     c. central mag lens
     c. central magnification vitrectomy
     lens
     c. wide angle vitrectomy lens
Clark
     C. capsule fragment forceps
     C. probe
     C. speculum
Clark-type polarographic electrode
classic
     c. choroidal neovascularization
     c. dendritic keratitis
     c. flower petal pattern
     c. migraine
classical congenital esophoria
classification
     Ann Arbor Hodgkin disease
      staging c.
     bleb c.
     Callender cell type c.
     Duane c.
     Gass macular hole c.
     Keith-Wagener-Barker c.
     Knapp c.
     KWB c.
     Leishman c.
     MacCallan c.
     Nelson c.
     Reese-Ellsworth c.
     Retina Society c.
     Roper-Hall c.
     Scheie c.
     Shaffer anterior angle c.
     Shaffer-Weiss c.
     Spaeth c.
     tear secretion c.
     Tessier c.
Claude-Lhermitte syndrome
clavulanate
Clayman
     C. guide
     C. intraocular lens
     C. lens-holding forceps
     C. lens implant forceps
     C. lens-inserting forceps
     C. posterior chamber lens
Clayman-Knolle irrigating lens loop
CLBF-100 blood flowmeter
CLE
     clear lens extraction

cleaner
Allergan Enzymatic C.
Barnes Hind Gas Permeable Daily C.
Bausch & Lomb concentrated c.
Blairex Hard Contact Lens C.
Boston Advance c.
Boston One Step Liquid Enzymatic C.
Ciba Vision C.
ComfortCare GP Dual Action Daily C.
Complete Weekly Enzymatic C.
enzymatic c.
enzyme c.
gas-permeable daily c.
LC-65 Daily Contact Lens C.
lens c.
Lens Plus daily c.
MiraFlow Daily C.
Opti-Free Daily C.
Opti-Free Enzymatic C.
Optimum extra-strength c.
Optimum by Lobob Daily C.
Opti-Soak Daily C.
Opti-Zyme enzymatic c.
ProConcept Contact Lens C.
ProFree/GP weekly enzymatic c.
ReNu Effervescent enzymatic c.
ReNu 1 Step Enzymatic C.
ReNu Thermal enzymatic c.
Sensitive Eyes daily c.
Sensitive Eyes Enzymatic C.
Sereine c.
SofLens enzymatic contact lens c.
Soft Mate Enzyme Plus c.
Soft Mate Hands Off daily c.
sterile preserved daily c.
Ultrazyme enzymatic c.
Unizyme enzymatic c.
Vision Care enzymatic c.
Cleaner/Rinse
Pure Eyes C./R.
cleaning cloth
cleanser
Ciba Vision Daily C.
Hibiclens antiseptic/antimicrobial skin c.
OCuSoft eyelid c.
cleanup
cortical c.
phaco c.

clear
c. cornea angled CVD diamond knife
c. cornea blade
c. corneal phacoemulsification
c. corneal step incision
c. corneal tunnel incision
c. crystalline lens
deep and c. (D&C)
C. Eyes
C. Eyes ACR
c. keratin sleeve
Lens C.
c. lensectomy
c. lens extraction (CLE)
c. lid vesicle
Swim'n C.
C. View hydrophilic shield
c. window
clearance
apical c.
fluorescein tear c.
tear fluorescein c.
ClearChart digital acuity system
ClearCut
C. dual-bevel blade
C. dual-bevel line knife
C. ophthalmic dual bevel knife
C. SatinSlit knife
clearing
media c.
Clearpath corneal diamond knife
ClearView contact lens
Cleasby
C. iridectomy operation
C. spatula
C. spatulated needle
cleavage syndrome
cleaver
Haefliger c.
CLEERE
Collaborative Longitudinal Evaluation in Ethnicity and Refractive Error
CLEERE study
cleft
corneal c.
cortical c.
cyclodialysis c.
excessive cyclodialysis c.
facial c.
sonolucent c.
c. syndrome

C

NOTES

clefting
> cortical c.
> Tessier c.

CLEK
> Collaborative Longitudinal Evaluation of Keratoconus
> CLEK Study

clemastine

clerical spectacles

Clerz
> C. 2
> C. 2 artificial tears
> C. 2 Lubricating and Rewetting Drops
> C. Plus lens drops

click phenomenon

climatic
> c. droplet keratopathy
> c. proteoglycan stromal keratopathy

clindamycin

clinical
> c. applications of aberrometry
> c. conference
> c. severity
> C. Trial of Eye Prophylaxis in the Newborn

clinically viable methods maximum optimization of visual performance

clinicopathologic finding

clinometer

clinoscope

clioquinol

clip
> AGV pars plana c.
> Backhaus towel c.
> bipolar diathermy adapter c.
> Castroviejo scleral shortening c.
> double tantalum c.
> Duraclose scleral c.
> Federov 4-loop iris c.
> Friedman tantalum c.
> Halberg trial c.
> holding c.
> Janelli c.
> lens c.
> Opticaid spring c.
> Platina c.
> scleral shortening c.
> tantalum c.
> trial c.
> 2-way towel c.

clip-applying forceps

clip-on/tie-on occluder

clivus, pl. **clivi**
> c. chordoma

clobetasol propionate

clock
> astigmatic c.
> c. dial
> lens c.

clock-mechanism esotropia

clofazimine

clonidine

C-loop
> C-l. intraocular lens
> C-l. IOL
> C-l. posterior chamber lens

Cloquet canal

closed
> c. chamber
> eyelids sutured c.
> c. globe injury
> c. loop
> c. road driving performance
> c. surgery on eye

closed-angle glaucoma (CAG)

closed-dissection technique

closed-eye surgery

closed-funnel vitreoretinopathy

closed-loop infrared video tracking system

closed-system pars plana vitrectomy

clostridial
> c. blepharitis
> c. panophthalmitis

Clostridium
> *C. bifermentans*
> *C. difficile*
> *C. histolyticum*
> *C. perfringens*
> *C. subterminale*
> *C. tetani*
> *C. welchii*

closure
> capillary c.
> crow-foot c.
> endovascular c.
> forced eye c.
> hallucination with eye c.
> insufficiency of eyelid c.
> miotic-induced angle c.
> synechial c.
> watertight c.
> wound c.

cloth
> cleaning c.
> microfiber cleaning c.

clotrimazole

cloud
> photon c.
> plasma c.

clouding
> corneal c.
> feathery c.
> hyaloid c.
> retinal c.
> vitreous c.

cloudy natural cornea
clove-hitch suture
cloxacillin
CLPU
    contact lens-induced peripheral ulcer
cLSO
    confocal laser scanning ophthalmoscopy
clump
    c. cell
    vortex-like c.
clumped
    c. pigmentation
    c. retinal pigment
clumping
    pigment c.
    pigmentary rarefaction and c.
cluster
    c. headache
    macular c.
    c. of pigmented spots
    c. of retinoblastoma cells
CMAP
    compound muscle action potential
CMD
    cystoid macular degeneration
CME
    cystoid macular edema
CMID
    cytomegalic inclusion disease
CMV
    cytomegalovirus
    macular CMV
    CMV retinitis
    CMV retinopathy
CN
    cranial nerve
    CN III
    CN IV
    CN V
    CN VI
    CN VII
CNS
    central nervous system
CNTGS
    Collaborative Normal Tension Glaucoma
      Study
CNV
    choroidal neovascularization
CNVM
    choroidal neovascular membrane
CO
    certified orthoptist
    corneal opacity

CO_2
    carbon dioxide
    CO_2 Sharplan laser
COAG
    chronic open-angle glaucoma
coagulating electrode
coagulation
    c. cascade protease
    disseminated intravascular c.
    endodiathermy c.
    endolaser c.
    light c.
    Meyer-Schwickerath light c.
coagulator
    argon laser c.
    ASSI Polar-Mate c.
    Grieshaber micro-bipolar c.
    Laserflex c.
    Meyer-Schwickerath c.
    Walker c.
coagulopathy
coalescent mass
coal-mining lensectomy
coaptation bipolar forceps
coarctate retina
coarse
    c. punctate staining
    c. stereopsis
    c. vascular pattern
COAS
    Complete Ophthalmic Analysis System
coast erosion
coat
    buffy c.
    sclerotic c.
    uveal c.
coated Vicryl suture
coater
    Polaron sputter c.
coating
    antireflection c.
    color c.
    edge c.
    c. material
    mirror c.
    nondeposited tear c.
    proteinaceous c.
    c. for spectacle lens
Coats
    C. disease
    C. retinitis
    C. syndrome
    C. white ring

NOTES

C

coaxial
    c. illumination
    c. irrigation/aspiration cannula
    c. microincision surgery
    c. microphacoemulsification
    C. Multicolor LIO
coaxially sighted corneal reflex
cobalt
    c. blue filter
    c. blue light
    c. therapy
cobalt-60 eye plaque
cobblestone
    c. appearance
    c. conjunctivitis
    c. papilla
    c. retinal degeneration
Cobra LASIK irrigating cannula
Coburn
    C. camera
    C. intraocular lens
    C. irrigation/aspiration system
    C. irrigation/aspiration unit
    C. lensometer
    C. refractor
    C. tonometer
cocaine
    c. block
    crack c.
    c. hydrochloride
    c. methylphenidate
    c. test
cocamidopropylamine oxide
cocamidopropyl hydroxysultaine
cocci (*pl. of* coccus)
Coccidioides immitis
coccidioidomycosis
    c. immitis
    intraocular c.
coccus, pl. **cocci**
    Gram-positive cocci
Cochet-Bonnet esthesiometer
cochleopupillary reflex
Cochran-Mantel-Haenszel analysis
Cockayne syndrome
co-contraction syndrome
codeine
    acetaminophen with c.
Codman wet-field cautery
CoEase viscoelastic
coefficient
    c. of facility of outflow
    Spearman correlation c.
    c. of variation
    Zernike c.
coffin bone
Coffin-Lowry syndrome
Cogan
    C. congenital oculomotor apraxia

    C. disease
    C. interstitial keratitis
    C. lid twitch
    C. lid-twitch sign
    C. microcystic dystrophy
    C. microcystic dystrophy of corneal
      epithelium
    C. patch
    C. syndrome
Cogan-Reese syndrome
cogwheel
    c. ocular movement
    c. pupil
Cohan-Vannas iris scissors
Cohan-Westcott scissors
Cohen
    C. corneal forceps
    C. needle holder
    C. syndrome
coherent
    C. 920 argon/dye laser
    C. 900, 920 argon laser
    C. dye laser
    C. krypton laser
    C. 7910 laser
    C. LaserLink slit lamp
    c. light
    C. Medical YAG laser
    C. Novus Omni multiwavelength
      laser
    C. photocoagulator
    C. radiation argon/krypton laser
    C. radiation argon model 800 laser
    C. radiation Fluorotron
    C. Schwind Keraton 2 laser
    C. Selecta 7000 laser
cohesiveness
cohort study
coil
    basal c.
    electromagnetic scleral search c.
    scleral search c.
colchicine
cold compress
cold-opposite, warm-same (COWS)
Coleman retractor
colforsin
coli
    Escherichia c.
Colibri
    C. forceps
    C. microforceps
coliform organism
colistin
collaborative
    C. Corneal Transplantation Studies
      (CCTS)
    C. Initial Glaucoma Treatment
      Study (CIGTS)

C. Longitudinal Evaluation in Ethnicity and Refractive Error (CLEERE)
C. Longitudinal Evaluation of Keratoconus (CLEK)
C. Longitudinal Evaluation of Keratoconus Study
C. Normal Tension Glaucoma Study (CNTGS)
C. Ocular Melanoma Study (COMS)

collagen
  c. alpha chain
  c. bandage lens
  c. cell
  c. fiber
  c. fibril
  c. fibril interweaving
  c. implant
  c. lamella
  native vitreous c.
  c. plug
  c. and rheumatoid-related disease
  c. shield
  thermally altered c.
  c. tissue
  c. vascular disease
  c. wick procedure

collagenase
  bacterial c.

collagenolysis

collagenolytic trabecular ring

collagenous trabecular ring

Collamer
  C. 1-piece intraocular lens
  C. 3-piece intraocular lens
  C. 3-piece IOL

collapse
  chamber c.

collar button

collarette
  iris c.

collar-stud chalazion

collateral
  cilioretinal c.
  c. pulp canal
  c. vessel

colliculus
  superior c.

Collier
  tucked lid of C.
  C. tucked lid sign

collimated beam

Collin-Beard operation

collision tumor

collodion dressing

colloid
  c. body
  c. cyst
  c. deposit

collyr.
  eyewash

collyrium
  c. eye drops
  C. Fresh Ophthalmic

colmascope

coloboma, pl. **colobomata**
  c. anomaly
  atypical c.
  bridge c.
  chorioretinal c.
  c. of choroid
  choroidal c.
  ciliary body c.
  complete c.
  congenital eyelid c.
  congenital optic nerve c.
  dysplastic c.
  eyelid c.
  fissure c.
  Fuchs inferior c.
  Fuchs spot c.
  c. of fundus
  c., heart defects, atresia choanae, retarded growth, genital hypoplasia, and ear anomalies (CHARGE)
  c. iridis
  iris c.
  c. of iris
  c. of lens
  c. lentis
  c. lobuli
  macular c.
  ocular c.
  optic nerve c.
  c. of optic nerve
  c. palpebrale
  peripapillary c.
  c. of retina
  retinochoroidal c.
  typical c.
  uveal c.
  vitreous c.
  c. of vitreous

C

NOTES

colobomatous
  c. cyst
  c. microphthalmia
  c. optic disc
colomba
  optic disc c.
color
  c. aberration
  c. adaptation
  c. adaptometer
  c. agnosia
  c. amblyopia
  c. anomia
  c. bar Schirmer strip
  c. bar Schirmer tear test
  c. blind
  c. blindness
  c. chart
  c. coating
  c. comparison
  c. comparison test
  complementary c.'s
  confusion c.
  c. confusion
  c. confusion index
  c. constancy
  c. contrast
  deviant c.
  c. disc
  c. discrimination
  c. Doppler imaging
  end-point c.
  eye c.
  c. filter array (CFA)
  c. fundus camera
  c. fundus photograph
  c. fusion
  incidental c.
  c. match
  metameric c.
  c. mixing
  Munsell c.
  c. naming
  c. neglect
  opponent c.
  c. perception
  c. perimetry
  primary c.
  pure c.
  reflected c.
  saturated c.
  c. saturation
  c. scotoma
  C. Screening Inventory
  c. sense
  simple c.
  solid c.
  c. spectrum
  c. theory

  c. triangle
  c. vision (CV)
  c. vision abnormality
  c. vision defect
  c. vision test
  c. vision testing device
  C. Vision Testing Made Easy test
    (CVTMET)
  c. washout
Colorado
  C. cautery
  C. needle
colorblindness
  total c.
ColorChecker
  Macbeth C.
color-coded corneal topography
color-contrast
  c.-c. sensitivity measurement
  c.-c. threshold
colored
  c. contact lens
  c. vision
colorimeter
colossal agenesis
column
  bulbar conjunctival blood c.
    (BCBC)
  ocular dominance c.
columnar layer
Colvard handheld infrared pupillometer
Coly-Mycin S
COMA
  congenital ocular motor apraxia
coma
  c. aberration
  eyes-open c.
  metabolic c.
Comberg
  C. contact lens
  C. foreign body operation
  C. localization
Combiline system
combination
  c. phaco chopper
  c. therapy
combined
  c. cataract/trabeculectomy surgery
  c. cilioretinal artery and central
    retinal vein occlusions
  c. dystrophy of Fuchs
  c. exfoliation
  c. fracture
  c. glaucoma
  c. intracapsular cataract extraction
    (CICE)
  c. phacoemulsification and
    nonpenetrating deep sclerotomy
  c. trabeculotomy-trabeculectomy

combined-mechanism glaucoma
comedo pattern
COMET
Correction of Myopia Evaluation Trial
comet scotoma
comfort
c. bridge
C. eye drops
C. Ophthalmic
subjective ocular c.
C. Tears
C. Tears Solution
ComfortCare
C. GP Dual Action Daily Cleaner
C. GP One Step
C. GP Wetting and Soaking
Solution
ComfortKone lens
comitance
comitant
c. esotropia
c. exodeviation
c. exophoria
c. exotropia
c. heterotropia
c. squint
c. strabismus
c. vertical deviation
commercial segmentation algorithm
comminuted orbital fracture
commissura, pl. **commissurae**
c. palpebrarum lateralis
c. palpebrarum medialis
commissure
arcuate c.
c. of Gudden
interthalamic c.
Meynert c.
nucleus of posterior c.
optic c.
palpebral c.
posterior chiasmatic c.
supraoptic c.
common
c. canaliculus
c. migraine
c. subtype
c. tendinous ring
c. tendinous ring of extraocular
muscle
commotio retinae

communicating
c. artery aneurysm
internal carotid-posterior c. (IC-PC)
communication
aqueous c.
arteriole c.
arteriovenous c.
communis
anulus tendineus c.
community-acquired corneal ulcer
company
American Surgical Instrument C.
(ASICO)
Neitz Instruments C.
comparative genomic hybridization
comparison
brightness c.
color c.
c. eyepiece
compass
Mastel diamond c.
compensated
c. glaucoma
c. segment
compensating eyepiece
compensation
cornea-lens c.
compensator
GDx-variable corneal c.
compensatory head tilt
complaint
debilitating visual c.
migrainous visual c.
night vision c.
complement
c. component
c. fixation test
c. system
complementary
c. afterimage
c. chromaticity
c. colors
complement-fixing antibody
complete
c. achromatopsia
C. Blink-N-Clean Lens Drops
c. blood count
c. but pupil-sparing oculomotor
nerve paresis
c. cataract
c. coloboma
C. Comfort Plus multi-purpose
solution

NOTES

complete *(continued)*
  c. congenital cataract
  c. hemianopia
  c. hemianopsia
  c. iridectomy (CI)
  c. iridoplegia
  C. Lubricating and Rewetting Drops
  C. Moisture Plus Multi-Purpose Solution No Rub
  C. Ophthalmic Analysis System (COAS)
  c. palsy
  c. vitrectomy
  C. Weekly Enzymatic Cleaner
completer
  Akahoshi nucleus c.
complex
  AIDS-related c. (ARC)
  c. astigmatism
  capsular bag c.
  circulating immune c.
  c. ectropion
  Golgi c.
  immune c.
  c. laceration
  major histocompatibility c. (MHC)
  c. microphthalmia
  c. motion tomography
  c. retinal detachment
  triple symptom c.
  tuberous sclerosis c. (TSC)
  c. visual process
compliance
  c. cap
  patient c.
complicated
  c. cataract
  c. migraine
complication
  C.'s of Age-Related Macular Degeneration Prevention Trial (CAPT)
  bleb-related c.
  catastrophic operative c.
  contact lens c.
  devastating ocular c.
  incision-related c.
  intraoperative c.
  perioperative c.
  postoperative c.
  serious corneal c.
  sight-threatening contact lens c.
  vision-limiting c.
  vision-threatening c.
component
  amyloid P c.
  complement c.
  quick left/right c.

composite
  Multiple Sclerosis Functional C. (MSFC)
composition
  altered tear c.
  c. of spectacle lens
compound
  c. eye
  Hurler-Scheie c.
  c. hyperopic astigmatism
  intraocular pressure-lowering docosanoid c.
  c. lens
  c. muscle action potential (CMAP)
  c. myopic astigmatism
  c. nevus
  quaternary ammonium c.
  silver c.
  skin cancer c.
  c. spectacles
  c. vesicle
compress
  cold c.
  warm c.
compression
  chiasmal c.
  choriocapillaris c.
  chronic optic nerve c.
  c. cyanosis
  c. dressing
  c. gonioscopy
  limbal c.
  c. molding
  optic tract c.
  prechiasmal c.
  c. retinopathy
  c. suture
compressive
  c. nystagmus
  c. optic nerve defect
  c. optic nerve tumor
  c. optic neuropathy
compressor
  Anthony orbital c.
  Berens orbital c.
  Castroviejo c.
  orbital enucleation c.
compromise
  immune c.
compulsive eye opening
computed
  C. Anatomy Corneal Modeling System
  c. perimetry
  c. tomographic angiography
  c. tomography (CT)
  c. tomography scan
computer
  C. Eye Drops

c. simulation
c. vision syndrome (CVS)
computer-assisted
c.-a. corneal topography (CACT)
c.-a. videokeratography
c.-a. videokeratoscope
computerized
c. corneal topography
c. corneal videokeratography
c. photokeratoscope
c. static perimetry
c. tomography scan
computer-related eye irritation
COMS
Collaborative Ocular Melanoma Study
Cooperative Ocular Melanoma Study
COMT
certified ophthalmic medical technologist
concave
c. cylinder
double c. (DCC)
c. mirror
c. reflecting surface
c. spectacle lens
concavity
iris c.
concavoconcave lens
concavoconvex lens
concentration
aqueous protein c.
c. deficit
immunoreactive adrenomedullin c.
steroid c.
concentric
c. constriction
c. fold
c. lesion
c. sclerosis of Balo
c. stria
concentrica
encephalitis periaxialis c.
concentrically
Concentrix dual aspiration pump system
concept
C. disposable cautery
C. handheld cautery
lover's eye c.
concha bullosa
conclination
concomitance
concomitant
c. exophoria

c. heterotropia
c. injury
c. strabismus
concretion
conjunctival c.
concussion
c. blindness
c. cataract
c. injury
c. of retina
condensation
demisting c.
vitreoretinal c.
vitreous c.
condenser
dark-field c.
condensing lens
condition
abnormal ocular c.
aggravating c.
allergic c.
conjunctival cell c.
mesopic c.
normal viewing c.
null c.
predisposing c.
steroid-responsive inflammatory
  ocular c.
test c.
conditioning film
conductive keratoplasty (CK)
cone
c. achromatopsia
apical c.
bipolar c.
blue c.
c. b-wave amplitude
c. b-wave implicit time
  electroretinogram
c. cell
c. degeneration
distraction c.
c. dysfunction
c. dystrophy
c. dystrophy-cerebellar ataxia
c. fiber
c. function
c. granule
layer of rods and c.'s
McIntyre truncated c.
c. monochromat
monochromatic c.
c. monochromatism

NOTES

cone *(continued)*
>   muscle c.
>   ocular c.
>   c. opsin
>   pedicle c.
>   c. photopigment
>   c. response
>   retinal c.
>   28-ring Placido c.
>   c. and rod amplitude
>   rods and c.'s
>   triad of retinal c.
>   twin c.
>   c. vision
>   visual c.
>   X-linked c.

cone-rod
>   c.-r. degeneration
>   c.-r. dystrophy (CRD)
>   c.-r. retinal dystrophy

conference
>   clinical c.

confidence interval

configuration
>   bombé c.
>   double pentagon c.
>   plateau iris c.
>   vacuolar c.
>   whorl-like c.

confluent
>   c. defect
>   c. drusen
>   c. lipid wall

confocal
>   c. biomicroscopy
>   c. laser scanning microscope
>   c. laser scanning ophthalmoscope
>   c. laser scanning ophthalmoscopy
>   (cLSO)
>   c. laser scanning topography
>   c. microscopy
>   c. microscopy identification of
>   *Acanthamoeba* keratitis
>   c. optics
>   c. scanning laser (CSL)
>   c. scanning laser Doppler
>   flowmetry
>   c. scanning laser ophthalmoscopy
>   c. scanning laser polarimeter
>   c. scanning laser polarimetry
>   c. scanning laser tomography

conformer
>   eye implant c.
>   silicone c.
>   Universal c.

ConfoScan
>   C. 3 microscope
>   C. 2.0 slit corneal confocal
>   microscope

confrontation
>   c. field defect
>   full to c. (FTC)
>   c. method
>   c. visual field
>   c. visual field test
>   c. visual field testing

confusion
>   circle of least c.
>   color c.
>   c. color
>   congenital c.
>   visual c.

congenita
>   dyskeratosis c.
>   ectopia pupillae c.
>   myotonia c.
>   paramyotonia c.

congenital
>   c. abducens facial paralysis
>   c. abducens nerve lesion
>   c. abducens nerve palsy
>   c. abduction paralysis
>   c. abnormality
>   c. absence of abduction
>   c. adduction palsy with synergistic
>   divergence
>   c. adherence syndrome
>   c. amaurosis
>   c. anomaly
>   c. anophthalmos
>   c. anterior staphyloma (CAS)
>   c. anterior synechia
>   c. astigmatism
>   c. brain malformation
>   c. bulbar paralysis
>   c. cataract
>   c. cleft of iris
>   c. color blindness
>   c. confusion
>   c. conus
>   c. crescent
>   c. cupping
>   c. dacryocele
>   c. dacryocystitis
>   c. dermoid of limbus
>   c. developmental cyst
>   c. dichromatism
>   c. dyschromatopsia
>   c. dyskeratosis
>   c. dystrophic ptosis
>   c. dysversion
>   c. ectropion
>   c. entropion
>   c. esophoria
>   c. esotropia
>   C. Esotropia Observational Study
>   (CEOS)
>   c. eyelid coloboma

c. facial diplegia
c. fiber-type disproportion (CFTD)
c. fibrosis
c. fibrosis of extraocular muscles (CFEOM)
c. fibrosis syndrome
c. glaucoma
c. grouped pigmentation of retina
c. hemianopsia
c. hereditary endothelial corneal dystrophy
c. Horner syndrome
c. hypertrophy of retinal pigment epithelium (CHRPE)
c. hypophosphatasia
c. ichthyosis
c. III nerve lesion
c. impatency
c. iris heterochromia
c. juxtafoveolar syndrome
c. lens dislocation
c. lens opacity
c. leukopathia
c. limbal corneal dermoid
c. limbal corneal dermoid tumor
c. macular degeneration
c. medullated optic nerve fiber
c. melanosis oculi
c. miosis
c. muscular dystrophy
c. mydriasis
c. myopathic eyelid retraction
c. myopathic ptosis
c. myopathy
c. myotonic dystrophy
c. nasolacrimal duct obstruction
c. nasolacrimal obstruction
c. nystagmus
c. ocular melanocytosis
c. ocular motor apraxia (COMA)
c. oculodermal melanocytosis
c. oculofacial paralysis
c. oculomotor nerve palsy
c. oculopalpebral synkinesia
c. optic atrophy
c. optic disc elevation
c. optic disc pigmentation
c. optic nerve coloboma
c. optic nerve defect
c. optic nerve pit
c. paradoxic gustolacrimal reflex
c. pit of optic disc
c. prepapillary vascular loop

c. pterygium
c. ptosis oculus sinister
c. punctal agenesis
c. retinal fold
c. retinal macrovessel
c. retinoschisis
c. rubella
c. rubella syndrome
c. sporadic aniridia
c. stationary night blindness
c. subluxated crystalline lens
c. superior oblique underaction
c. syphilis
c. syphilitic conjunctivitis
c. tent-shaped retinal detachment
c. third nerve palsy
c. tilted disc syndrome
c. toxoplasmosis

congenitale
  poikiloderma c.
congenitum
  corestenoma c.
congested vessel
congestion
  c. of conjunctiva
  deep c.
  orbital venous c.
  superficial c.
  transient c.
  vascular c.
  venous c.
congestive
  c. glaucoma
  c. orbitopathy
congruent point
congruity
congruous
  c. field defect
  c. hemianopia
  c. hemianopsia
  c. homonymous hemianopic scotoma
  c. homonymous horizontal sectoranopia
  c. homonymous quadruple sectoranopia
coni (*pl. of* conus)
conical
  c. cornea
  c. implant
  c. protrusion
conjugate
  c. deviation of eyes

C

NOTES

conjugate *(continued)*
 c. disparity
 c. focus
 c. gaze
 c. gaze palsy
 c. horizontal deviation
 c. horizontal eye movement
 c. movement of eyes
 c. nystagmus
 c. ocular movement
 c. paralysis
 c. point
conjugately
conjunctiva, pl. **conjunctivae**
 anulus of c.
 bulbar c.
 chancre of c.
 congestion of c.
 c. dryness
 emphysema of c.
 epitheliosis desquamativa
  conjunctivae
 c. forceps
 fornical c.
 fornix c.
 Förster c.
 glandulae mucosae conjunctivae
 leptotrichosis conjunctivae
 limbal c.
 lithiasis conjunctivae
 marginal c.
 ocular c.
 orbital c.
 pale c.
 pallor of c.
 palpebral c.
 plica semilunaris conjunctivae
 c. retractor
 saccus conjunctivae
 scleral c.
 sebaceous gland of c.
 semilunar fold of c.
 c. sensitivity
 siderosis conjunctivae
 c. spreader
 supertemporal bulbar c.
 c. swelling
 tarsal c.
 temporal bulbar c.
 tunica c.
 upper palpebral c.
 upper tarsal c.
 xerosis conjunctivae
conjunctiva-associated lymphoid tissue
conjunctivae
 lithiasis c.
 tyloma c.
conjunctival
 c. abrasion

 c. advancement
 c. advancement technique
 c. allergen
 c. amyloidosis
 c. angioma
 c. artery
 c. autograft
 c. bleb
 c. break
 c. buttonhole
 c. calcification
 c. cell condition
 c. chemosis
 c. ciliary injection
 c. circulation
 c. concretion
 c. contusion
 c. crystal
 c. cul-de-sac
 c. cyst
 c. deposit
 c. dermoid
 c. dermolipoma
 c. discharge
 c. dysplasia
 c. edema
 c. epithelial cell
 c. epithelium
 c. exudate
 c. fixation
 c. flap
 c. flap hemorrhage
 c. follicle
 c. foreign body
 c. gland
 c. goblet cell
 c. goblet cell density
 c. granuloma
 c. hemangioma
 c. hyperemia
 c. impression cytology
 c. incision
 c. infiltration
 c. intraepithelial neoplasia (CIN)
 c. laceration
 c. limbal graft
 c. limbus
 c. lipodermoid
 c. lithiasis
 c. lymphangioma
 c. lymphoid proliferation
 c. lymphoid tumor
 c. MALT lymphoma
 c. melanoma
 c. melanotic lesion
 c. membrane
 c. mucosa-associated lymphoid
  tissue
 c. necrosis

c. nodule
c. papilla
c. papilloma
c. patch graft
c. perforation
c. perimetry
c. phlyctenule
c. phlyctenulosis
c. pigmented nevus
c. pseudomembrane
c. pterygium
c. reaction
c. recession
c. reflex
c. resection
c. rhinosporidiosis
c. ring
c. rotation autografting
c. sac
c. scarring
c. scissors
c. scraping
c. semilunar fold
c. slough
c. smear
c. sporotrichosis
c. squamous cell neoplasia
c. squamous metaplasia
c. staining
c. tear
c. ulcer
c. varix
c. vascular engorgement
c. vascularization
c. vein
c. vessel
c. xerosis

conjunctivalis
saccus c.

conjunctival-limbal autograft
conjunctiviplasty (*var. of*
conjunctivoplasty)
conjunctivitis
acne rosacea c.
actinic c.
acute atopic c.
acute catarrhal c.
acute congestive c.
acute contagious c.
acute epidemic c.
acute follicular c.
acute hemorrhagic c.
acute viral c.

adenoviral c.
adenovirus c.
adult inclusion c.
allergic c.
anaphylactic c.
angular c.
Apollo c.
arc-flash c.
c. arida
atopic c.
atropine c.
Axenfeld follicular c.
bacterial c.
Béal c.
blennorrheal c.
blepharitis c.
calcareous c.
candidal c.
catarrhal c.
chemical c.
Chlamydia c.
chlamydial inclusion c.
chronic catarrhal c.
chronic cicatrizing c.
chronic follicular c.
chronic immunogenic c.
cicatricial c.
cicatrizing c.
cobblestone c.
congenital syphilitic c.
contact c.
contagious granular c.
croupous c.
diphtheritic c.
diplobacillary c.
drug-induced cicatrizing c.
eczematous c.
Egyptian c.
Elschnig c.
epidemic c.
erythema multiforme major c.
exanthematous c.
factitious c.
follicular c.
giant papillary c. (GPC)
gonococcal c.
gonorrheal c.
granular c.
hay fever c.
hemorrhagic c.
herpes simplex c.
herpes zoster c.
herpetic c.

C

NOTES

conjunctivitis *(continued)*
    hyperacute purulent c.
    immunological c.
    inclusion c.
    infantile purulent c.
    infectious c.
    Koch-Weeks c.
    lacrimal c.
    lagophthalmia c.
    larval c.
    ligneous c.
    limbal c.
    lithiasis c.
    Lymphogranuloma venereum c.
    c. medicamentosa
    meibomian c.
    membranous c.
    meningococcus c.
    molluscum c.
    Morax-Axenfeld c.
    Moraxella c.
    mucopurulent c.
    c. necroticans infectiosus
    necrotic infectious c.
    neisserial c.
    neonatal inclusion c.
    c. of newborn
    newborn c.
    c. nodosa
    nodular c.
    nonatopic allergic c.
    ocular vaccinial c.
    oculoglandular c.
    papillary c.
    Parinaud oculoglandular c.
    Pascheff c.
    c. petrificans
    phlegmatous c.
    phlyctenular c.
    pinkeye c.
    pneumococcal c.
    prairie c.
    pseudomembranous c.
    pseudovernal c.
    purulent c.
    Reiter c.
    rubeola c.
    Samoan c.
    scrofulous c.
    seasonal allergic c.
    shipyard c.
    simple acute c.
    Singapore epidemic c.
    snow c.
    spring c.
    springtime c.
    squirrel plague c.
    staphylococcal c.
    superior tarsal papillary c.
    swimming pool c.
    Thygeson chronic follicular c.
    toxic follicular c.
    toxicogenic c.
    trachoma-inclusion c. (TRIC)
    trachomatous c.
    tuberculosis c.
    tularemic c.
    c. tularensis
    unilateral c.
    uratic c.
    vernal c.
    viral c.
    Wegener granulomatosus c.
    welder's c.
    Widmark c.
    c. xeroderma pigmentosum

conjunctivochalasis
conjunctivodacryocystorhinostomy
    (CDCR)
conjunctivodacryocystostomy
conjunctivoma
conjunctivoplasty, conjunctiviplasty
conjunctivorhinostomy
conjunctivum
    brachium c.
connection
    Luer c.
    supranuclear c.
    synaptic c.
connective
    c. tissue
    c. tissue membrane
connector
    McIntyre nylon cannula c.
Connor
    C. angled wand
    C. capsulorrhexis peeler forceps
    C. curved wand
    C. straight irrigating wand
    C. straight nonirrigating wand
Conn syndrome
conoid
    c. lens
    Sturm c.
    c. of Sturm
conomyoidin
conophthalmus
conotruncal anomalies face syndrome
Conradi syndrome
Conrad orbital blowout fracture
    operation
consecutive
    c. anophthalmia
    c. diplopia
    c. esotropia
    c. exotropia
    c. optic atrophy

consensual
    c. light reflex
    c. light response
    c. pupillary reflex
    c. pupillary response
    c. reaction
consent
    informed c.
conservative blepharoplasty
considerable blurring
consistency
    jelly-like c.
constancy
    color c.
constant
    c. esotropia
    c. exophoria
    c. exotropia
    c. hypertropia
    c. hypotropia
    c. monocular tropia
    c. nystagmus
    c. strabismus
constricted pupil
constriction
    concentric c.
    focal c.
    vessel c.
constructional
    c. ability contact lens
    c. apraxia
consummatum
    glaucoma c.
ContaClair multi-purpose contact lens solution
contact
    c. angle
    arc of c.
    c. A-scan
    c. bandage lens
    c. blepharitis
    c. B-scan
    c. B-scan ultrasonography
    c. burns of globe
    c. conjunctivitis
    c. dermatitis
    c. dermatoconjunctivitis
    eye c.
    c. glasses
    haptic c.
    c. illumination
    iridociliary process c.
    iridolenticular c.

    iridozonular c.
    c. lens (CL)
    C. Lens Association of Ophthalmologists (CLAO)
    c. lens biomicroscopy
    c. lens blank
    c. lens chord diameter
    c. lens complication
    c. lens curve
    c. lens fitting technique
    c. lens height
    c. lens-induced acute red eye (CLARE)
    c. lens-induced keratopathy
    c. lens-induced peripheral ulcer (CLPU)
    c. lens-induced warpage
    c. lens insertion
    C. Lens and Myopia Progression (CLAMP)
    C. Lens and Myopia Progression study
    c. lens noncompliance
    c. lens overwear syndrome
    c. lens power change
    c. lens prescriber
    c. lens-related microbial keratitis
    c. lens removal
    c. lens thickness
    c. lens training mirror
    c. lens vertex power
    c. lens wearer
    c. low-vacuum lens
    c. method
    c. side field lens
contact lens (CL) *(See also* lens)
contactology
contactoscope
contagiosa
    impetigo c.
contagiosum
    ecthyma c.
    molluscum c.
contagious granular conjunctivitis
contaminant
    wind-blown c.
contaminated orbit
contamination
    bacterial c.
    culture-proven c.
    lens c.
    silicone c.
contemporary nearpoint chart

NOTES

content
    orbital c.
    water c.
contiguous
    c. fibers
    c. pattern
continua
    hemicrania c.
continuous
    c. ambient lighting
    c. circular capsulorrhexis
    c. curvilinear capsulorrhexis (CCC)
    c. fiber
    c. laser
    c. tear anterior capsulotomy
    c. wave (CW)
continuous-wave
    c.-w. argon laser
    c.-w. diode laser
    c.-w. photocoagulator
contour
    c. contact lens
    convex iris c.
    corneal c.
    edge c.
    eyelid c.
    c. interaction
    iris c.
    scalloped c.
    c. stereo test
contoured ablation pattern (CAP)
contracted socket
contraction (C)
    anisocoria c.
    ciliary body c.
    c. of cyclitic membrane
    c. and liquefaction
    orbicularis c.
    c. of pupil
    pupillary sphincter c.
    vermiform c.
    vitreous c.
contracture
    socket c.
    spastic paretic facial c.
contraindication
contralateral
    c. antagonist
    c. disc change
    c. eye
contrapulsion
    saccadic c.
contrast
    c. acuity
    color c.
    c. detection
    c. discrimination
    gallium citrate c.
    long-scale c.

low c.
    c. material
    c. medium
    retinal-image c.
    c. sensitivity
    c. sensitivity reduction
    c. sensitivity test (CST)
    c. sensitivity testing
    short-scale c.
    simultaneous color c.
    successive c.
    c. threshold for motion perception (CTMP)
    c. visualization
contrast-enhancing mass
contrecoup injury
control
    astigmatic c.
    Centers for Disease C. (CDC)
    corneal hydration c.
    inflammation c.
    intraocular pressure c.
    IOP c.
    pain c.
    supranuclear c.
Controlled High Risk Avonex Multiple Sclerosis Prevention Study (CHAMPS)
controller
    Siepser endocapsular c.
    viscous fluid c. (VFC)
contusion
    c. angle glaucoma
    c. cataract
    c. of choroid
    conjunctival c.
    corneal c.
    c. of eye
    c. of globe
    ocular c.
    c. of orbit
    vitreoretinal c.
conular
conus, pl. **coni**
    congenital c.
    distraction c.
    inferior c.
    lateral oblique c.
    myopic c.
    c. of optic disc
    c. shell-type eye implant
    supertraction c.
    c. supertraction
    underlying c.
conventional
    c. outflow
    c. pars plana vitrectomy
    c. perimetry

c. scleral buckling
c. shell implant

converge

convergence

c. accommodation
accommodative c. (AC)
c. amplitude
amplitude of c.
angle of c.
c. angle
barrel card c.
convergence accommodation to c. (CA/C)
c. excess
c. excess esotropia
far point of c.
fusional c.
c. insufficiency (CI)
c. insufficiency exotropia
near point of c. (NPC)
negative c.
c. paralysis
c. paresis
point of c.
c. point
point of basal c. (PBC, PcB)
c. position
positive c.
proximal c.
punctum proximum of c. (PP)
range of c.
relative c.
c. retraction
c. spasm
string c.
tonic c.
unit of ocular c.
voluntary c.

convergence-accommodation

accommodative c.-a. (AC/A)
c.-a. ratio

convergence-accommodative micropsia

convergence-evoked nystagmus

convergence-retraction nystagmus

convergency

c. reflex
voluntary c.

convergent

c. beam
c. deviation
c. exercise
c. lens
c. light
c. misalignment
c. ray
c. squint
c. strabismus
c. wavefront

convergent-divergent pendular oscillation

converging

c. meniscus
c. meniscus lens
c. ray

convergiometer

converse

c. bobbing
C. double-ended alar retractor

convex

double c. (DCx)
high c.
c. iris approach
c. iris contour
low c.
c. mirror
c. plano lens
c. reflecting surface
c. spectacle lens

convexity

convexoconcave lens

convexoconvex lens

convolution product

Conway lid retractor

Cook speculum

Cool Touch laser

Cooper

C. aspirator
C. blade fragment
C. Clear DW contact lens
C. I&A unit
C. implant
C. irrigating/aspirating unit
C. 2000, 2500 laser
C. Laser Sonics laser
C. operation
C. Toric contact lens

Cooperative Ocular Melanoma Study (COMS)

CooperVision

C. argon laser
C. balanced salt solution
C. camera
C. Diagnostic Imaging refractor
C. Fragmatome
C. I/A machine
C. imaging perimeter
C. irrigating/aspirating unit

C

NOTES

CooperVision *(continued)*
    C. irrigating needle
    C. irrigation/aspiration unit
    C. microscope
    C. ocutome
    C. PMMA-ACL Flex lens
    C. refractive surgery
      photokeratoscope
    C. spatulated needle
    C. ultrasonography
    C. ultrasound
    C. vitrector
    C. YAG laser
coordination
    binocular c.
    head-eye c.
Copaxone
Copeland
    C. implant
    C. radial panchamber intraocular
      lens
    C. radial panchamber UV lens
    C. retinoscopy
    C. streak retinoscope
Cophene-B
copiopia
copper
    c. cataract
    c. chelator
    c. deposition
    c. foreign body
    c. wiring
copper-wire
    c.-w. arteriole
    c.-w. artery
    c.-w. effect
    c.-w. reflex
Coppock cataract
coquille plano lens
COR
    cervicoocular reflex
Coracin
coralliform cataract
Corboy
    C. hemostat
    C. needle holder
Cordarone
**cordless monocular indirect
ophthalmoscope**
cord of Schwann
core
    nerve c.
    c. vitrectomy
    c. vitreous
corecleisis, coreclisis
corectasia, corectasis
corectome
corectomedialysis
corectomy

corectopia
    midbrain c.
coredialysis
corediastasis
corelysis
coremorphosis
corenclisis
coreometer
coreometry
coreoplasty
corepraxy
    laser c.
    mechanical c.
corestenoma congenitum
coretomedialysis
coretomy
corkscrew
    c. artery
    c. visual field defect
cornea
    c. abnormality
    c. abrader
    abrasion of c.
    alkali burn of c.
    AlphaCor artificial c.
    AlphaCor hydrogel synthetic c.
    c. anesthesia
    anterior corneal epithelium of c.
    anterior limiting lamina of c.
    anterior limiting layer of c.
    anterior surface of c.
    apical zone of c.
    artificial c.
    aspheric c.
    axial c.
    c. barrier function
    biocompatible artificial c.
    black c.
    bleb disorder of c.
    blood staining of c.
    butterfly pattern steepening of c.
    calcareous degeneration of c.
    central edema of c.
    c. chisel
    cloudy natural c.
    conical c.
    degeneration of c.
    deturgescence of c.
    diameter of c.
    donor c.
    C. Donor Study (CDS)
    dystrophy of c.
    ectatic marginal degeneration of c.
    edema of c.
    endothelial cell surface of c.
    c. farinata
    fistula of c.
    flat c.
    fleck dystrophy of c.

floury c.
c. globosa
gutter dystrophy of c.
c. herpes zoster virus
host c.
indolent ulceration of c.
inferior c.
infiltrate in c.
keratoconus c.
keratoglobus c.
lash abrasion of c.
lattice dystrophy of c.
lead incrustation of c.
limbus of c.
marginal degeneration of c.
marginal ring ulcer of c.
meridian of c.
metaherpetic ulceration of c.
nasal-hinged flap c.
natural c.
c. opaca
opalescent c.
oval c.
pigmented line of c.
c. plana
posterior conical c.
posterior epithelium of c.
recurrent erosion of c.
ring ulcer of c.
rust ring of c.
serpent ulcer of c.
c. specialist
spherical c.
superficial line of c.
superior c.
superior-hinged flap c.
thick c.
thin c.
tissue-engineered c.
transparent ulcer of c.
transplantation of c.
transplanted c.
trepanation of c.
trophic ulceration of c.
c. tunnel incision
ulceration of c.
underlying c.
c. urica
c. verticillata
c. vesicle
Vogt c.
white ring of c.
xerosis of c.

corneae
anterior epithelium c.
dystrophia adiposa c.
dystrophia endothelialis c.
dystrophia epithelialis c.
epithelium anterius c.
epithelium posterius c.
facies anterior c.
facies posterior c.
herpes corneae
ichthyosis c.
lamina limitans anterior c.
lamina limitans posterior c.
leukoma c.
lipoidosis corneae
liquor c.
maculae corneae
substantia propria c.
ulcus serpens corneae
cornea-holding forceps
corneal
c. ablation plumes
c. abrasion (CA)
c. abscess
c. abscission
c. alkali burn
c. amyloidosis
c. apex
c. astigmatism
c. avulsion
c. barrier function
c. bedewing
c. biopsy
c. birefringence
c. blindness
c. block
c. button
c. cap
c. cell
c. clarity
c. cleft
c. clouding
c. conjunctival intraepithelial
   neoplasia
c. contact lens
c. contact lens electrode
c. contour
c. contusion
c. corpuscle
c. cross-linking
c. crystal
c. curette
c. curvature (K)

NOTES

corneal *(continued)*
 c. cylinder
 c. cyst
 c. damage
 c. débrider
 c. decompensation
 c. deep opacity
 c. dehydration
 c. dellen
 c. dendrite
 c. denervation
 c. deposit
 c. desiccation
 c. deturgescence
 c. diameter
 c. distortion
 c. dysgenesis
 c. dysplasia
 c. dystrophy of Waardenburg-
  Jonkers
 c. ectasia
 c. edema
 c. elevation
 c. endothelial decompensation
  etiology
 c. endothelial guttate dystrophy
 c. endothelial pigmentary dispersion
 c. endothelial polymorphism
 c. endothelial touch
 c. endothelium
 c. enlargement
 c. epithelial barrier function
 c. epithelial integrity
 c. epithelial permeability
 c. epithelial scrape
 c. epithelial scraping
 c. epithelium
 c. erosion
 c. facet
 c. fascia lata spatula
 c. filament
 c. fissure
 c. fistula
 c. fixation forceps
 c. flap by rotation
 c. fleck dystrophy
 c. fluorescein staining
 c. foreign body
 c. foreign body bur
 c. furrow degeneration
 c. graft
 c. graft operation
 c. graft rejection
 c. graft spatula
 c. graft step
 c. guttata
 c. guttate dystrophy
 c. guttering
 c. haze

 c. hook
 c. hydration control
 c. hydrops
 c. hypoesthesia
 c. hysteresis
 c. implant
 c. impression test (CIT)
 c. inferior limbus
 c. infiltrative event
 c. inlay
 c. intercept
 c. iron line
 c. iron ring
 c. irregularity
 c. keratitis
 c. keratometric map
 c. knife
 c. knife dissector
 c. laceration
 c. lamella
 c. lamellar groove
 c. lathing
 c. leakage
 c. lens aberration
 c. leukoma
 c. light reflex
 c. light shield
 c. luster
 c. margin
 c. marginal furrow
 c. melt
 c. melting
 c. meridian
 c. microincision
 c. microscope
 C. Modeling System
 c. mushroom
 c. nebula
 c. needle
 c. neovascularization
 c. nerve density
 c. nerve inflammation
 c. nociceptor
 c. opacification
 c. opacity (CO)
 c. optical density
 c. oxygenation
 c. pachometer
 c. pachymeter
 c. pachymetry
 c. pannus
 c. paracentesis track
 c. pellucid
 c. penetration
 c. perforation
 c. phlyctenule
 c. phlyctenulosis
 c. pocket
 c. polarization axis (CPA)

c. power calculation
c. prosthesis forceps
c. prosthesis trephine
c. protrusion
c. punch
c. punctate infiltrate
c. punctate lesion
c. punctate staining
c. reflection
c. reflection pupillometer (CRP)
c. relaxing incision
c. ring segment
c. scar
c. scarring
c. scleral limbus
c. section spatulated scissors
c. sensation
c. sensitivity
C. Shaper microkeratome
c. splinter forceps
c. spot
c. staining test
c. staphyloma
c. steepening
c. storage medium
c. stria
c. stroma
c. stromal bed
c. stromal blood staining
c. stromal disease
c. stromal dystrophy
c. stromal neovascularization
c. stromal remodeling
c. stroma tissue
c. subbasal nerve
c. substance
c. superinfection
c. surface disease
c. surgery
c. swelling
c. tattooing
c. thickness
c. thinning
c. topographic analysis
c. topography
c. topography system (CTS)
c. toxicity
c. transparency
c. transplant
c. transplantation
c. transplant centering ring
c. transplant marker
c. transplant rejection

c. trauma
c. trepanation
c. tube
c. ulcer
c. vascularization
c. velum
c. vesicle
c. vortex dystrophy
c. warpage
c. whorling
c. xerosis
cornea-lens
   c.-l. compensation
   preexisting well-balanced c.-l.
cornealis
   arcus c.
   rima c.
Corneascope 9-ring photokeratoscope
CorneaSparing LTK system
corneitis
Cornelia de Lange syndrome
corneoblepharon
corneoiritis
corneolenticular
corneolimbal ring graft
corneomandibular reflex
corneomental reflex
corneopterygoid reflex
corneoscleral
   c. border
   c. button
   c. forceps
   c. groove
   c. incision
   c. junction
   c. laceration
   c. lamella
   c. limbus
   c. melt
   c. punch
   c. right/left hand scissors
   c. rim
   c. spur
   c. sulcus
   c. trabecula
corneoscleralis
   pars c.
corneum
   Nosema c.
cornpicker's pupil
corona
   c. ciliaris

NOTES

111

corona *(continued)*
    c. radiata
    Zinn c.
coronal
    c. CT scan
    c. view
coronaria
coronary cataract
coroparelcysis
coroplasty
coroscopy
Cor-Oticin
corotomy
corpus
    c. adiposum orbitae
    c. callosum
    c. callosum lesion
    c. ciliare
    c. vitreum
corpuscle
    corneal c.
    hyaloid c.
    Leber c.
    Toynbee c.
    Virchow c.
Correct-a-Prizm
Correct-a-Prizmbar
corrected
    c. FCT
    c. pattern standard deviation
    (CPSD)
    c. spectacle lens
    c. SVST
    c. visual acuity (Va_{cc})
correction
    aphakic c.
    astigmatism c.
    best ophthalmic c.
    Byron Smith lazy-T c.
    dioptric c.
    distance c.
    epicanthal c.
    habitual c.
    c. of hyperopia
    hyperopic c.
    multistage c.
    C. of Myopia Evaluation Trial
    (COMET)
    optical c.
    prism c.
    refractive c.
    spectacle c.
    spectacle-free refractive c.
    vision c.
    with c. (cc)
    without c. (s̄c)
    Yates c.

corrective
    c. movement
    c. procedure
correlation
    test-retest c.
correspondence
    abnormal harmonious retinal c.
    abnormal unharmonious retinal c.
    anomalous retinal c. (ARC)
    dysharmonious retinal c.
    harmonious abnormal retinal c.
    Hering law of motor c.
    normal retinal c. (NRC)
    c. point
    retinal c.
    sensory c.
corresponding retinal point
corridor incision
corrodens
    Eikenella c.
corrugated retinal detachment
corrugator muscle
Cort-Dome
cortex, pl. **cortices**
    aspiration of c.
    brain c.
    calcarine c.
    cerebellar c.
    cerebral c.
    c. of hair shaft
    c. of lens
    c. lentis
    occipital c.
    peristriate visual c.
    primary visual c.
    proliferated c.
    c. proliferation
    residual c.
    striate visual c.
    vestibular c.
    visual c.
cortical
    c. change
    c. cleanup
    c. cleaving hydrodissection
    c. cleaving hydrodissector
    c. cleaving hydrodissector cannula
    c. cleft
    c. clefting
    c. oculomotor area
    c. opacification
    c. opacity
    c. psychic blindness
    c. ptosis
    c. spokes cataract
    c. stripping
    c. substance of lens
    c. vacuole
    c. visual impairment

c. visual insufficiency
c. vitreous
cortication
cortices (*pl. of* cortex)
corticonuclear fiber
corticooculocephalogyric area
corticopupillary reflex
corticosteroid
c. drops
ophthalmic c.
postoperative c.
systemic c.
c. therapy
c. treatment
corticosteroid-induced
c.-i. cataract
c.-i. glaucoma
corticosteroid-responsive
corticosteroid-sparing
c.-s. agent
c.-s. regimen
corticotropin
cortisol
cortisone acetate
Cortisporin
C. Ophthalmic Ointment
C. Ophthalmic Suspension
Cortone Acetate
coruscation
Corydon
C. expression cannula
C. hydroexpression cannula
corymbifera
Absidia c.
Corynebacterium
C. diphtheriae
C. keratitis
C. pseudodiphtheriticum
C. xerosis
cosegregation
Cosmegen
cosmesis
cosmetic
c. contact shell implant
c. defect
c. iris
c. oculoplastic surgery
c. outcome
c. shell contact lens
Cosopt ophthalmic solution
cost-effective analysis
cost-ineffective current screening technique

COT
certified ophthalmic technologist
cotransmission of disease
cotton
C. effect
c. pledget
c. thread tear test
cottonoid
cotton-tipped applicator
cotton-wool
c.-w. exudate
c.-w. patch
c.-w. spot (CWS)
couching needle
Coulter counter method
counseling
genetic c.
sight c.
count
complete blood c.
endothelial cell c.
finger c.
optic nerve axon c.
counterrolling
countertorsion
static c.
counting
down to finger c.
c. fingers (CF)
c. fingers vision
coup injury
coupling
c. of aberration
c. agent
c. of progressive power lens
course
arcuate c.
extramedullary c.
cover
Eye-Pak II c.
prism and c. (P&C)
c. test
cover-uncover test
Cowdry type A intranuclear inclusion body
Cowen sign
cow face
cowhitch knot
COWS
cold-opposite, warm-same
COX
cyclooxygenase
COX pathway

C

NOTES

Cox
    C. II ocular laser shield
    C. rapid dry heat transfer sterilizer
Coxiella burnetii
Cozean-McPherson tying forceps
CPA
    cerebellopontine angle
    corneal polarization axis
    CPA lesion
C-PACG
    chronic primary angle-closure glaucoma
CPC
    central posterior curve
CPD
    chorioretinopathy and pituitary
      dysfunction
      CPD syndrome
CPEO
    chronic progressive external
      ophthalmoplegia
CPOA
    certified paraoptometric assistant
CPOT
    certified paraoptometric technician
CPSD
    corrected pattern standard deviation
CR
    cycloplegic refraction
      CR IV
C/R
    chorioretinal
CR-39 lens
CR6-45NMf retinal camera
CRA
    central retinal artery
crack
    c. cocaine
    lacquer c.
crack-and-flip phacoemulsification
  technique
cracked windshield stromal lesion
cracker
    Dodick nucleus c.
    Ernest nucleus c.
    nucleus c.
cranial
    c. arteritis
    c. foramen
    c. nerve (CN)
    c. nerve abnormality
    c. nerve palsy
    c. nerve testing
    c. stenosis syndrome
craniectomy
    suboccipital c.
craniocervical junction
craniofacial
    c. anomaly

    c. defect
    c. fibroosseous tumor
    c. syndrome
cranioorbital surgery
craniopharyngioma
craniostenosis, pl. **craniostenoses**
craniosynostosis
craniotabes
craniotomy
    frontal c.
CRAO
    central retinal artery occlusion
crassus
    pannus c.
crater depression
Crawford
    C. fascial stripper
    C. forceps
    C. hook
    C. lacrimal intubation set
    C. method
    C. needle
    C. sling operation
    C. technique
    C. tube
    C. tubing intubation
CRD
    cone-rod dystrophy
C-reactive protein
cream
    Drysol c.
crease
    eyelid c.
    lid c.
    superior eyelid c.
creation
    femtosecond laser channel c.
Credé
    C. method
    C. prophylaxis
crepe bandage dressing
crepitation in eyelid
crescent
    c. blade
    c. choroid
    congenital c.
    c. corneal graft
    c. CVD diamond knife
    gray c.
    homonymous c.
    monocular temporal c.
    c. myopia
    myopic c.
    c. operation
    scleral c.
    c. scleral tunneler
    temporal c.
crescentic circumpapillary light reflex

CREST
calcinosis cutis, Raynaud phenomenon, esophageal motility disorder, sclerodactyly, and telangiectasia
CREST syndrome
crest
lacrimal anterior c.
lacrimal posterior c.
neural c.
orbital c.
cretinism
Creutzfeldt-Jakob disease
cribra orbitalia
cribriform
c. field
c. ligament
c. spot
cribrosa
lamina c.
scleral lamina c.
cri du chat syndrome
Crigler massage
Crile needle holder
crinkled cellophane
crisis, pl. **crises**
glaucomatocyclitic c.
myasthenic c.
ocular c.
oculogyric c.
Pel c.
Pel-Ebstein c.
cristallinus
criterion, pl. **criteria**
Dandy criteria
Hodapp-Parrish-Anderson grading criteria
modified dandy criteria
c. shift
visual field criteria
criterion-free measurement
critical
c. angle
c. corresponding frequency (CCF)
c. flicker frequency (CFF)
c. flicker fusion (CFF)
c. flicker fusion frequency
c. flicker fusion test
c. illumination
c. period
CRNO
certified registered nurse in ophthalmology

crocodile
c. lens
c. shagreen
c. tears
c. tears syndrome
crofilcon A
Crolom ophthalmic solution
cromoglycate
disodium c.
sodium c.
cromolyn
c. sodium
c. sodium ophthalmic solution
Crookes
C. glass
C. lens
cross
c. cover test
c. cylinder
optical c.
C. retinoscopy
cross-action
c.-a. capsule forceps
c.-a. towel clamp
cross-cylinder
c.-c. ablation
c.-c. technique
crossed
c. amblyopia
c. binasal quadrantanopia
c. bitemporal quadrantanopia
c. cylinder
c. diplopia
c. eyes
c. fixation
c. hemianopia
c. hemianopsia
c. lens
c. parallax
c. reflex
cross-eye
cross-eyed
cross-fixation
crossing
AV c.
c. change
c. eyes
cross-linking
corneal c.-l.
cross-polarization photography
cross-Polaroid projection chart
cross-section
optical retinal c.-s.

C

NOTES

cross-validation
cross-vector A-scan
croupous
    c. conjunctivitis
    c. rhinitis
Crouzon
    C. disease
    C. syndrome
crowding phenomenon
crow-foot closure
crown
    ciliary c.
    c. glass
    c. glass lens
    spectacle c.
CRP
    corneal reflection pupillometer
CRRT
    Cytomegalovirus Retinitis Retreatment
    Trial
CRS
    Cambridge Research Systems
    CRS Color Vision Test
CRS-Master software program
cruciate incision
crusting
    eyelid c.
    lid c.
crust removal
crusty eyelid
crutch glasses
CRV
    central retinal vein
CRVO
    central retinal vein occlusion
    CRVO knife
    nonischemic CRVO
CRVRS
    Cytomegalovirus Retinitis and Viral
    Resistance Study
cryoablation
cryoanalgesia
cryoapplication
cryocoagulation
cryoenucleator
cryoextraction
    open-sky c.
    c. operation
cryoextractor
    Alcon c.
    Beaver cataract c.
    Bellows c.
    Kelman c.
    Thomas c.
cryolathe
Cryomedical Sciences AccuProbe 450 system
cryopencil
    Mira endovitreal c.

cryopexy
    double freeze-thaw c.
    c. probe
    retinal c.
    transconjunctival c.
    transscleral c.
cryophake
    Alcon c.
cryopreservation
cryopreserved amniotic membrane
cryoprobe
    Thomas c.
cryoptor
    Thomas c.
cryoretinopexy
CRYO-ROP
    Cryotherapy for Retinopathy of
    Prematurity
    CRYO-ROP Cooperative Group
CryoSeal FS System
cryostat
cryosurgery
cryosurgical unit
cryotherapy
    double freeze-thaw c.
    freeze-thaw c.
    c. operation
    c. probe
    retinal c.
    C. for Retinopathy of Prematurity
    (CRYO-ROP)
    C. for Retinopathy of Prematurity
    Cooperative Group
    transscleral c.
crypt
    Fuchs c.
    c. of Henle
    c. of iris
    iris c.
cryptochrome
cryptococcal
    c. chorioretinitis
    c. meningitis
cryptococcosis
Cryptococcus
    C. laurentii
    C. laurentii keratitis
    C. neoformans
cryptoglioma
cryptophthalmus, cryptophthalmia, cryptophthalmos
crystal
    c. clear vision
    conjunctival c.
    corneal c.
    cystine c.
    refractile c.
    retinal c.

Crystalens
C. IOL
C. model AT-45 implant
crystallin
alpha c.
beta c.
gamma c.
crystallina
lens c.
crystalline
c. capsule
c. cataract
c. corneal dystrophy
c. deposit
c. humor
c. infiltrate
c. keratopathy
c. lens
c. lens aberration
c. lens capsule staining
c. lens equator
c. opacity
c. protein
c. protein mutation
c. retinopathy
crystallizable
fragment c. (Fc)
CSC
central serous chorioretinopathy
C-Scan
C-S. color-ellipsoid topometer
C-S. corneal topography system
Technomed C-S.
CSCR
central serous chorioretinopathy
CSF
cerebrospinal fluid
CSI toric contact lens
CSL
confocal scanning laser
CSL tomography
CSM
central, steady and maintained
CSM fixation
CSR
central serous retinopathy
CST
contrast sensitivity test
CT
computed tomography
CT 200 corneal topographer
CT scan of orbit

CTMP
contrast threshold for motion perception
CTNF
ciliary neurotrophic factor
CTNF capsule
CTNF capsule protein eye implant
CTS
corneal topography system
Cuban epidemic optic neuropathy
cube
tumbling E c.
cuboidal
cue
monocular c.
cuff
fibrous tissue c.
Honan c.
opacified c.
subretinal fluid c.
Cuignet method
cul-de-sac
conjunctival c.-d.-s.
glaucomatous c.-d.-s.
c.-d.-s. irrigation T-tube
c.-d.-s. irrigator
ocular c.-d.-s.
ophthalmic c.-d.-s.
optic c.-d.-s.
Culler
C. fixation forceps
C. iris spatula
C. lens spoon
C. muscle hook
C. speculum
culture
bacterial c.
c. medium
organ c.
vitreous c.
culture-proven contamination
culturette
Mini-tip c.
Cummings folding forceps
cuneate-shaped scotoma
cuneiform cataract
cup
AoSept Lens Holder and C.
bleb c.
eye c.
flat c.
c. forceps
Galin bleb c.
glaucomatous c.

NOTES

cup *(continued)*
    large physiologic c.
    ocular c.
    ophthalmic c.
    optic c.
    perilimbal suction c.
    physiologic c.
    slitlamp c.
cupped disc
Cüppers method of pleoptics
cupping
    congenital c.
    glaucomatous c.
    optic disc c.
    c. of optic disc
    optic nerve c.
    c. of optic nerve
    pathologic c.
    physiologic optic nerve c.
cup-to-disc ratio (C/D, CDR)
cupuliform cataract
cupulolithiasis
curb tenotomy
Curdy
    C. blade
    C. sclerotome
Curdy-Hebra blade
curette, curet
    Alvis c.
    chalazion c.
    corneal c.
    Gills-Welsh c.
    Heath chalazion c.
    Hebra c.
    Kraff capsule polisher c.
    Meyhoefer chalazion c.
    Skeele c.
    Spratt mastoid c.
    Visitec capsule polisher c.
curlback shell implant
curling of capsule
curl temple
Curran knife needle
current
    eddy c.
    c. symptoms questionnaire
curvature
    c. aberration
    c. ametropia
    anterior corneal c.
    corneal c. (K)
    c. hyperopia
    c. of lens
    c. myopia
    posterior corneal c.
    radius of c.
curve
    anterior central c. (ACC)
    anterior peripheral c.

    base c. (BC)
    bell-shaped c.
    biphasic c.
    central anterior c. (CAC)
    central posterior c. (CPC)
    circadian tonometric c.
    contact lens c.
    intermediate posterior c. (IPC)
    IOP c.
    luminosity c.
    posterior central c.
    posterior intermediate c.
    posterior peripheral c. (PPC)
    c. response
    c. of spectacle lens
    visibility c.
    c. width
curved
    c. Connor wand
    c. iris forceps
    c. iris scissors
    c. laser probe
    c. mosquito clamp
    c. needle eye spud
    c. reflecting surface
    c. retinal probe
    c. scleral-limbal incision of
      Flieringa
    c. tenotomy scissors
    c. tying forceps
curved-top bifocal
Curvularia lunata
cushingoid appearance
Cushing syndrome
Custodis
    C. nondraining procedure
    C. operation
custom-contoured
    c.-c. ablation pattern (C-CAP)
    c.-c. ablation pattern method
CustomCornea
    C. wavefront-guided LASIK
    C. wavefront measurement system
customized
    c. ablation treatment
    c. hyperopic ablation
CustomVue LASIK procedure
cut
    field c.
    sector c.
cutaneomucouveal syndrome
cutaneous
    c. horn
    c. melanoma
    c. myiasis
    c. pupillary reflex
    c. tissue
cutdown incision
Cuterebra ophthalmomyiasis

cuticular
c. drusen
c. layer
c. stitch
cutis laxa
Cutler
C. implant
C. lens spoon
C. operation
Cutler-Beard
C.-B. bridge flap
C.-B. operation
cutter
Alcon Accurus vitrectomy c.
bone c.
Chu Foldable Lens C.
electronic vitreous c.
guillotine-type c.
high-speed c.
infusion suction cutter vitreous c.
Katena soft IOL c.
Koo foldable intraocular lens c.
Koo foldable IOL c.
Machemer vitreous c.
Maguire-Harvey vitreous c.
membrane peeler-c. (MPC)
Millennium vitreous c.
rotating-type c.
soft IOL c.
Tolentino vitreous c.
Utrata foldable lens c.
vitreoretinal infusion c.
vitreous infusion suction c. (VISC)
cutting bur
CV
color vision
CV232 square-round-edge IOL
CVD
chemical vapor deposition
CVD black diamond keratome line
CVD diamond knife
CVF
central visual field
CVOS
Central Vein Occlusion Study
CVS
computer vision syndrome
CVTMET
Color Vision Testing Made Easy test
CW
continuous wave
CWS
cotton-wool spot

cyanoacrylate
butyl c.
ethyl c.
c. retinopexy
c. tissue adhesive
c. tissue adhesive augmented tenoplasty
c. tissue glue
cyanographic contrast material
cyanolabe
cyanopsia, cyanopia
cyanopsin
cyanosis
c. bulbi
compression c.
c. retinae
cycle
cell c.
micropulse duty c.
pump c.
variable duty c.
visual c.
cyclectomy
cyclic
c. adenosine monophosphate (cAMP)
c. esotropia
c. guanidine monophosphate
c. guanosine monophosphate (cGMP)
c. ocular motor spasm
c. oculomotor palsy
c. oculomotor paresis
c. strabismus
cyclicotomy
cyclitic membrane
cyclitis
chronic c.
Fuchs heterochromic c. (FHC)
heterochromic Fuchs c.
c. in pars planitis
plastic c.
pure c.
purulent c.
serous c.
cycloablation
endoscopic laser c.
cycloceratitis
cyclochoroiditis
cyclocoagulation
cyclocongestive glaucoma
cyclocryopexy

C

NOTES

cyclocryotherapy
    YAG c.
cyclodamia
cyclodestruction
cyclodestructive procedure
cyclodeviation
cyclodextrin
cyclodialysis
    Allen c.
    c. cannula
    c. cleft
    Heine c.
    c. spatula
cyclodiathermy
    c. electrode
    c. operation
cyclodiplopia
cycloduction
cycloelectrolysis
cyclofilcon A
Cyclogyl
cyclokeratitis
Cyclomydril Ophthalmic
cyclooxygenase (COX)
cyclopea
cyclopean eye
cyclopentolate hydrochloride
cyclophoria
    accommodative c.
    minus c.
    plus c.
    position c.
    c. positive
cyclophorometer
cyclophosphamide
cyclophotocoagulation
    endoscopic c. (ECP)
    laser transscleral c.
    Nd:YAG laser c.
    transpupillary c.
    transscleral laser c.
    c. vitreoretinal surgery
    YAG laser c.
cyclopia
cyclopian
cycloplegia
cycloplegic
    c. refraction (CR)
    topical c.
cyclorotary muscle
cyclorotation
cyclorotational registration
cycloscope
cycloscopy
cycloserine
cyclospasm
cyclosporin A

cyclosporine
    efficacy of c.
    safety of c.
cyclotherapy
    laser c.
cyclotome
cyclotomy
cyclotorsion
cyclotorsional registration
cyclotropia
cyclovergence
cycloversion
cyclovertical
    c. muscle
    c. muscle palsy
cyl, cyl.
    cylinder
Cylate
cylinder (C, cyl, cyl.)
    anterior c.
    c. axis
    concave c.
    corneal c.
    cross c.
    crossed c.
    diopter c.
    Jackson cross c.
    minus c.
    3-month postoperative refractive c.
    c. retinoscopy
    c. spectacle lens
cylindric
    c. lens
    c. refraction
cylindrical lens (C, cyl.)
Cylindrocarpon
cylindroma
CYP1B1 gene
cyproheptadine
cyst
    Acanthamoeba c.
    aneurysmal bone c.
    arachnoidal c.
    Blessig c.
    blood c.
    colloid c.
    colobomatous c.
    congenital developmental c.
    conjunctival c.
    corneal c.
    c. degeneration
    dermoid c.
    Echinococcus c.
    epibulbar dermoid c.
    epidermal inclusion c.
    epidermoid c.
    epithelial implantation c.
    epithelial inclusion c.
    foveal c.

Gartner c.
hematic c.
inclusion c.
infundibular c.
intracorneal c.
intraepithelial c.
iris c.
lacrimal ductal c.
lacrimal gland c.
meibomian c.
Naegleria c.
orbital c.
pearl c.
proteinaceous c.
pupillary iris c.
Rathke cleft c.
retinal c.
scleral c.
sebaceous inclusion c.
serous c.
spontaneous congenital iris c.
subconjunctival c.
subretinal hydatid c.
sudoriferous c.
tarsal c.
traumatic corneal c.
traumatic scleral c.
Vahlkampfia c.
vitrectomy for subretinal c.

cystadenoma
Moll gland c.

cysteamine HCl

cystic
c. amelanotic nevus
c. bleb
c. cataract
c. eye
c. fibrosis
c. hydrocystoma tumor
c. maculopathy
c. microphthalmia
c. retinal tuft

cysticerci (*pl. of* cysticercus)

cysticercoid

cysticercosis

cysticercus, pl. **cysticerci**
intraocular c.

cysticum
epithelioma adenoides c.

cystine crystal

cystinosis
nephropathic c.

cystoid
c. body
c. cicatrix
c. cicatrix of limbus
intraretinal c.
c. macular degeneration (CMD)
c. macular dystrophy
c. macular edema (CME)
c. macular hole
c. maculopathy
c. retinal degeneration

cystotome, cystitome
air c.
Atkinson 25-G short curved c.
Azar curved c.
Blumenthal push-pull irrigating c.
double-cutting sharp c.
Drews angled c.
Graefe c.
irrigating c.
Kelman air c.
kibisitome c.
Knolle-Kelman cannulated c.
Kratz angled c.
Lewicky formed c.
Lieppman c.
Look c.
McIntyre reverse c.
Mendez c.
Nevyas double sharp c.
Visitec double-cutting c.
von Graefe c.
Wheeler c.
Wilder c.

cytarabine

Cytobrush S brush

CytoFluor II fluorometer

cytogenetic
c. abnormality
c. test

cytoid body

cytokeratin 7, 20 antibody

cytokine therapy

cytologic examination

cytology
conjunctival impression c.
impression c.

cytomegalic
c. inclusion disease (CID, CMID)
c. inclusion virus

cytomegalovirus (CMV)
AIDS-related c.
c. disease

NOTES

cytomegalovirus *(continued)*
    macular c.
    c. retinitis
    C. Retinitis Retreatment Trial
    (CRRT)
    C. Retinitis and Viral Resistance
    Study (CRVRS)
    c. retinopathy
cytophotocoagulation
cytoplasm
    intracellular c.
cytoplasmic body

cytoskeletal agent
cytotoxic antibody
Cytovene
Cytoxan
    C. Injection
    C. Oral
cytoxic T cell
Czapski microscope
Czermak
    C. keratome
    C. pterygium operation

D
> dexter
> diopter
>> D chromosome ring syndrome
>> hypervitaminosis D
>> D trisomy syndrome
>> D wave

3D
> 3-dimensional
>> 3D angled stainless phaco trapezoid blade
>> 3D i-Scan ophthalmic ultrasound
>> 3D i-Scan ultrasound tomography
>> 3D stainless steel knife

D-15 Hue Desaturated Panel test
3Dx digital stereo disc camera
d
> day

daclizumab
Dacroise irrigating eye solution
Dacron suture
dacryadenalgia
dacryadenitis
dacryadenoscirrhus
dacryagogatresia
dacryagogic
dacryagogue
dacrycystalgia
dacrycystitis
dacryelcosis
dacryoadenalgia
dacryoadenectomy operation
dacryoadenitis
> bacterial d.
> infectious d.
> inflammatory d.

dacryoblennorrhea
dacryocanaliculitis
dacryocele
> congenital d.

dacryocyst
dacryocystalgia
dacryocystectasia
dacryocystectomy operation
dacryocystitis
> acute d.
> chronic d.
> congenital d.
> phlegmonous d.
> silent d.
> syphilitic d.
> trachomatous d.
> tuberculous d.

dacryocystoblennorrhea
dacryocystocele

dacryocystoethmoidostomy
dacryocystogram
dacryocystography (DCG)
dacryocystoptosis, dacryocystoptosia
dacryocystorhinostenosis
dacryocystorhinostomy (DCR)
> endonasal d.
> endonasal laser d. (ENL-DCR)
> endoscopic laser d.
> endoscopic laser-assisted d.
> external d. (EXT-DCR)
> intranasal endoscopic d.
> therapeutic d.

dacryocystostenosis
dacryocystotome
dacryocystotomy
> Ammon d.

dacryogenic
dacryogram
dacryohelcosis
dacryohemorrhea
dacryolin
dacryolith
> Desmarres d.
> Nocardia d.

dacryolithiasis
dacryoma
dacryon
dacryoplasty
> balloon d.

dacryops
dacryopyorrhea
dacryopyosis
dacryorhinocystotomy
dacryorrhea
dacryoscintigraphy
dacryosinusitis
dacryosolenitis
dacryostenosis
dacryostomy
> Arroyo d.
> Arruga d.
> Dupuy-Dutemps d.
> Kuhnt d.

dacryosyrinx
dactinomycin
DAF
> downgaze paralysis, ataxia/athetosis and foam cell
> DAF syndrome

Dailies contact lens
daily
> D. cataract needle
> d. wear contact lens (DWCL)

Daisy irrigation/aspiration instrument

Dakrina Ophthalmic Solution
Dalalone
Dalcaine
Dalen-Fuchs nodule
Dallas lens-inserting forceps
Dalrymple
    D. disease
    D. sign
daltonian
daltonism
damage
    brain d.
    corneal d.
    dorsal rostral d.
    endothelial cell d.
    glaucoma d.
    glaucomatous optic nerve d.
    (GOND)
    optic nerve d.
    optic tract d.
    oxidative d.
    pressure-related d.
    solar d.
    sun d.
    UV d.
    UV-mediated ocular d.
    visual field d.
    zonular d.
dammini
    Ixodes d.
Dan chalazion forceps
dancing eye
Dandy criteria
dantrolene sodium
dapiprazole
    d. HCl
    d. hydrochloride
DAPS
    dark-adapted pupil size
dapsone
Daranide
Daraprim
Dardenne nucleus forceps
dark
    d. adaptation
    d. adaptometry
    d. disc
    d. empty field
    d. event
    d. retinoscopy
dark-adapted
    d.-a. eye
    d.-a. pupil size (DAPS)
dark-field
    d.-f. accommodation
    d.-f. condenser
    d.-f. examination
    d.-f. illumination
dark-ground illumination

darkly pigmented nodular mass
dark-room
    d.-r. gonioscopy
    d.-r. test
    d.-r. testing
darting eye movement
Dartmouth Eye Institute
data
    d. handling
    d. selection
database
    autopsy eye d.
datum line
Daubenton plane
daunorubicin
Daviel
    D. lens spoon
    D. operation
    D. scoop
Davis
    D. forceps
    D. knife needle
    D. spud
    D. trephine
day (d)
    d. blindness
    d. sight
    d. vision
90-day glaucoma
Dazamide
dazzle
    monocular d.
    d. reflex
dazzling glare
DBC
    distance between centers
DBL
    distance between lenses
DC
    dermatochalasis
D&C
    deep and clear
DCC
    double concave
DCG
    dacryocystography
DCR
    dacryocystorhinostomy
DCx
    double convex
DD
    disc diameter
    disc diffusion
dd
    disc diameter
DDHT
    dissociated double hypertropia
DDLS
    disc damage likelihood scale

DDMS
    diamond-dusted membrane scraper
    Synergetics DDMS
DDT
    dye disappearance test
de
    de Grandmont operation
    de Grouchy syndrome
    de Juan ophthalmic pick forceps
    de Lange syndrome
    de Morsier-Gauthier syndrome
    de Morsier syndrome
    de Wecker iris scissors
deaf-blindness
deafness
    diabetes insipidus, diabetes mellitus, optic atrophy, d. (DIDMOAD)
    lentigines, electrocardiogram abnormalities, ocular hypertelorism, pulmonary stenosis, abnormal genitalia, retardation of growth, and d. (LEOPARD)
Dean
    D. iris knife
    D. knife holder
    D. knife needle
death-to-preservation time
debilitating visual complaint
debrancher enzyme deficiency
débridement
    epithelial d.
    impression d.
    surgical d.
    wipe d.
débrider
    corneal d.
    Sauer corneal d.
debris
    back surface d. (BSD)
    capsular d.
    cell d.
    cellular d.
    desquamated epithelial d.
    epithelial d.
    phagocytosed cellular d.
    d. removal
    seborrheic d.
    tear film d.
debris-laden tear film
decalvans
    keratosis follicularis spinulosa d.
DeCamp viscoelastic cannula
decenter

decentered
    d. ablation
    d. lens
    d. spectacles
decentration
    d. of contact lens
    intraocular lens d.
    IOL d.
    lens d.
decision-making
    therapeutic d.-m.
declination
decolorize
decompensated
    d. accommodative esotropia
    d. phoria
decompensation
    corneal d.
    endothelial d.
decomposition
    Zernike d.
decompression
    bone removal orbital d.
    extracranial optic nerve d.
    fat removal orbital d. (FROD)
    intracranial optic nerve d.
    lateral orbital d.
    microvascular d.
    Naffziger orbital d.
    optic canal d.
    optic nerve sheath d. (ONSD)
    orbital d.
    d. of orbit operation
    posterior fossa nerve d.
    d. surgery
    surgical d.
    transantral orbital d.
    3-wall d.
decompressive surgery
decongestant
    ocular d.
decrease
    visual acuity d.
decreased corneal sensation
decreasing vision
decrement
    age-related d.
decussation
    oculomotor d.
    optic d.
deep
    d. blunt rake retractor
    d. and clear (D&C)

D

NOTES

deep *(continued)*
  d. congestion
  d. corneal stromal opacity
  d. dyslexia
  d. filiform dystrophy
  d. lamellar endothelial keratoplasty
    (DLEK)
  d. lamellar keratectomy
  d. lamellar keratoplasty (DLK,
    DLKP)
  d. parenchymatous dystrophy
  d. punctate keratitis
  d. pustular keratitis
  d. and quiet (D&Q)
  d. retina
  d. scleritis
  d. sclerotomy
  d. socket

DeepLight glaucoma treatment system
defect
  acquired color d.
  afferent pupillary d. (APD)
  altitudinal visual field d.
  arcuate field d.
  arteriovenous crossing d.
  AV crossing d.
  bilateral altitudinal field d.
  bilateral homonymous altitudinal d.
  bilateral visual field d.
  binasal field d.
  bitemporal field d.
  central d.
  centrocecal d.
  chevron-shaped d.
  chiasmatic field d.
  color vision d.
  compressive optic nerve d.
  confluent d.
  confrontation field d.
  congenital optic nerve d.
  congruous field d.
  corkscrew visual field d.
  cosmetic d.
  craniofacial d.
  directional d.
  enzyme d.
  epithelial d. (ED)
  field d.
  functional d.
  glaucoma field d.
  gun-barrel field d.
  homonymous field d.
  hyperfluorescent window d.
  hysterical visual field d.
  incongruous field d.
  inferior altitudinal d.
  IOFB-caused d.
  iris transillumination d. (ITD)
  levator aponeurosis d.

  Marcus Gunn relative afferent d.
  monocular field d.
  nasal step d.
  nerve fiber bundle d.
  paracentral d.
  parietal lobe field d.
  patchy window d.
  persistent epithelial d.
  pie-in-the-sky d.
  pie-on-the-floor d.
  posterior corneal d.
  preexisting posterior capsule d.
  punctate corneal epithelial d.
  quadrantic d.
  radial transillumination d.
  relative afferent pupillary d.
    (RAPD)
  retinal pigment epithelial d.
  retrochiasmal visual field d.
  sector d.
  sector-shaped d.
  superior homonymous quadrantic d.
  temporal lobe field d.
  trophic d.
  vascular filling d.
  visual corkscrew d.
  visual field d.
  window d.
defective
  d. accommodation
  d. zonule
deficiency
  acetylcholine receptor d.
  acetylcholinesterase d.
  acid maltase d.
  aqueous tear d. (ATD)
  brancher enzyme d.
  carnitine d.
  debrancher enzyme d.
  familial lecithin-cholesterol
    acyltransferase d.
  familial lipoprotein d.
  folic acid d.
  galactokinase d.
  iatrogenic limbal stem cell d.
  lecithin-cholesterol acyltransferase d.
  limbal stem cell d.
  nutritional d.
  partial limbal stem cell d.
  primary acetylcholine receptor d.
  supranuclear d.
  vitamin A d.
deficit
  abduction d.
  amplitude d.
  concentration d.
  hemisensory d.
  horizontal gaze d.
  latency d.

neurologic d.
permanent d.

definition
area of critical d.

Definity contact lens

defocus
calculating equivalent d.

defocus-induced ametropia

deformans
osteitis d.

deformation
eye d.
eyeball d.
globe d.

deformity
d. angle
scleral d.
S-shaped d.

degeneration
aberrant d.
advanced pellucid marginal d.
age-related disciform macular d.
age-related macular d. (AMD, ARMD)
amyloid corneal d.
anterograde d.
atrophic age-related macular d.
balloon d.
Biber-Haab-Dimmer d.
Bietti tapetoretinal d.
calcareous d.
calcific corneal d.
central retinal d.
choriocapillaris d. (CCD)
chorioretinal d.
cobblestone retinal d.
cone d.
cone-rod d.
congenital macular d.
d. of cornea
corneal furrow d.
cyst d.
cystoid macular d. (CMD)
cystoid retinal d.
diabetic macular d.
disciform macular d.
Doyne familial colloid d.
Doyne honeycomb d.
dry senile macular d.
ectatic marginal d.
elastoid d.
end-stage age-related macular d.
equatorial d.

exudative age-related macular d.
familial colloid d.
familial pseudoinflammatory macular d.
fine fibrillar vitreal d.
furrow d.
hepatolenticular d.
hereditary d.
heredomacular d.
hyaline d.
hyaloideoretinal d.
hydropic d.
juvenile macular d.
keratinoid d.
Kuhnt-Junius macular d.
lattice retinal d.
lenticular d.
lipid d.
macular disciform d.
marginal corneal d.
marginal furrow d.
myopic retinal d.
nodular corneal d.
nonneovascular age-related macular d.
opticocochleodentate d.
paraneoplastic cerebellar d.
paving-stone d.
pellucid corneal marginal d. (PCMD)
pellucid marginal corneal d.
pellucid marginal retinal d.
peripheral cystoid d.
peripheral disciform d.
peripheral tapetochoroidal d.
photoreceptor d.
pigmentary perivenous chorioretinal d.
primary pigmentary d.
primary retinal d.
progressive cone d.
progressive myopic d.
prophylactic treatment of age-related macular d. (PTAMD)
red cone d.
reticular cystoid d.
retinal lattice d.
retrograde transsynaptic d.
rod-cone d.
Salzmann nodular corneal d.
scleral d.
secondary retinal d.
senescent disciform macular d.

D

NOTES

degeneration *(continued)*
 senile disciform macular d.
 senile exudative macular d.
 senile furrow d.
 snail track d.
 Sorsby pseudoinflammatory
  macular d.
 spheroid d.
 spheroidal d.
 spinocerebellar d.
 striatal nigral d.
 tapetochoroidal d.
 tapetoretinal d.
 Terrien marginal d.
 tractional retinal d.
 transneuronal d.
 transsynaptic d.
 trophic retinal d.
 vitelliform macular d.
 vitelline macular d.
 vitelliruptive d.
 vitreoretinal d.
 Vogt d.
 Wagner hereditary vitreoretinal d.
 Wagner hyaloid retinal d.
 wallerian d.
 wet form of age-related macular d.
 Wilson d.
 xerotic d.
degenerative
 d. cataract
 d. cerebellar disease
 d. myopia
 d. ocular disease
 d. pannus
 d. retinal disease
 d. retinoschisis
degenerativus
 pannus d.
Degos syndrome
degradation
 image d.
degraded image artifact
degree
 prism d.
45-degree
 45-d. bent reform implant
 45-d. scissor with membrane pick
dehiscence
 iris d.
 levator muscle d.
 retinal d.
 traumatic wound d.
 wound d.
 Zuckerkandl d.
dehiscent
dehiscing

dehydration
 corneal d.
 d. injury
Dehydrex
dehydrogenase
 glucose 6-phosphate d.
 lactate d.
dehydroretinol
deinsertion
Deiter operation
Deitz
 D. incision depth gauge
 D. ophthalmic gauge
Dejean syndrome
Deknatel silk suture
delacrimation
delamination
 bimanual d.
 capsular d.
delayed
 d. massive suprachoroidal
  hemorrhage
 d. mucous plaque
 d. onset cataract
 d. postoperative opacification
 d. rectifier
 d. visual maturation
deletion mapping
delicate
 d. grasping forceps
 d. serrated straight dressing forceps
delimiting keratotomy
delivery system
Dell
 D. astigmatism marker
 D. fixation ring
dellen
 corneal d.
 d. of Fuchs
Deltasone
DEM
 developmental eye movement
 DEM test
demarcated detachment
demarcation line of retina
demecarium bromide
demeclocycline
Demerol
demisting condensation
demodectic blepharitis
Demodex folliculorum
demodicosis
demonstration
 d. eyepiece
 d. ophthalmoscope
demonstrator
 halo d.
Demours membrane

demyelinating
    d. disease
    d. optic neuritis
    d. optic neuropathy
    d. plaque
demyelination
    autoimmune d.
    nystagmus with d.
    viral-induced d.
demyelinization
dendriform
    d. corneal lesion
    d. keratitis
    d. ulcer
dendrite
    branching d.
    corneal d.
    epithelial d.
    fragmented d.
    herpetic d.
    d. keratitis
    VZV d.
dendritic
    d. cataract
    d. epithelial lesion
    d. epitheliopathy
    d. ghost
    d. herpes simplex corneal ulcer
    d. herpes zoster keratitis
    d. keratopathy
    d. line
dendritiform appearance
denervate
denervation
    corneal d.
    d. supersensitivity test
    trigeminal d.
Dennie-Morgan fold
densa
    lamina d.
dense
    d. brunescent nucleus
    d. core granule
    d. hemorrhage
    d. opacity
    d. vitreitis
densitometer
density
    arciform d.
    average lens d. (ALD)
    cell d.
    conjunctival goblet cell d.
    corneal nerve d.

    corneal optical d.
    endothelial cell d. (ECD)
    Fas receptor d.
    hemorrhage d.
    macular pigment d.
denudation
denuded corneal epithelium
deorsumduction
deorsumvergence
    left d.
    right d.
deorsumversion
dependent
    steroid d.
depigmentation
    periocular d.
depigmented spot
deposit
    adrenochrome d.
    amorphous corneal d.
    amyloid d.
    basal laminar d. (BLD)
    calcareous d.
    calcium d.
    colloid d.
    conjunctival d.
    corneal d.
    crystalline d.
    discrete micro gel d.
    fibrillogranular d.
    intraretinal lipid d.
    iron d.
    jelly bump lipid d.
    lipid d.
    mutton-fat d.
    optic d.
    pigment d.
    posterior corneal d. (PCD)
    protein d.
    refractile d.
    subretinal d.
    superficial retinal refractile d.
    tear protein d.
deposition
    calcium d.
    chemical vapor d. (CVD)
    copper d.
    epithelial adrenochrome d.
    iron d.
    pigment d.
depressed fracture
depression
    cecocentral d.

D

NOTES

depression *(continued)*
    crater d.
    foveal d.
    d. of orbital floor
    posterior corneal d.
    scleral d.
depressor
    muscle d.
    O'Connor d.
    orbital d.
    Schepens scleral d.
    Schepens thimble d.
    Schocket scleral d.
    scleral d.
    Simcoe scleral d.
    Wilder scleral d.
deprimens oculi
deprivation
    d. amblyopia
    stimulus d.
depth
    anterior chamber d.
    d. of chamber
    d. of field
    focal d.
    d. of focus
    d. gauge
    d. perception
    d. plate
    sagittal d.
derangement
    pigment d.
Derf needle holder
derivative
    imidazole d.
    propionic acid d.
    pyrazolone d.
Derma-K laser
dermal
    d. amyloid infiltration
    d. nevus
Dermalon suture
dermatan sulfate
dermatitidis
    Blastomyces d.
dermatitis, pl. **dermatitides**
    contact d.
    herpes simplex d.
    hyperkeratotic d.
    trigeminal herpes zoster d.
dermatoblepharitis
dermatochalasis (DC)
    eyelid d.
dermatoconjunctivitis
    contact d.
dermatogenes
    cataracta d.
dermatogenic cataract
dermatolysis palpebrarum

dermatome
    Hall d.
dermatomyositis
dermatosis
    acute febrile neutrophilic d.
    papillopruritic d.
dermis
    acellular d.
    d. fat graft
    d. patch graft
dermochondral corneal dystrophy of François
dermoid
    congenital limbal corneal d.
    conjunctival d.
    d. cyst
    limbal d.
    d. of orbit
    orbital d.
    pedunculated congenital corneal d.
    d. tumor
dermolipoma
    conjunctival d.
Dermostat implant
DES
    dry eye syndrome
desaturation
    red d.
Descartes law
Descemet
    D. fold
    D. membrane
    D. membrane detachment
    D. membrane punch
    D. plane
descemetitis
descemetocele
    surgical d.
    d. ulcer
Descemet-stripping automated endothelial keratoplasty (DSAEK)
desflurane
desiccant
desiccate
desiccation
    corneal d.
    d. keratitis
design
    aspheric optic d.
    double pentagon slight d.
    gripflex d.
    prism ballast d.
    single-loop sling d.
    sling d.
Desmarres
    D. chalazion forceps
    D. corneal dissector
    D. dacryolith
    D. eyelid retractor

D. fixation pick
D. knife
D. lamellar dissector
D. lid clamp
D. lid elevator
desmopressin
desmosomal cellular attachment
desmosome
desquamated epithelial debris
destroyed globe
DET
dry eye test
DET fluorescein strip
detached
d. iris
d. retina
d. vitreous
detachment
aphakic d.
bullous d.
central retinal d.
choroidal d.
ciliochoroidal d.
complex retinal d.
congenital tent-shaped retinal d.
corrugated retinal d.
demarcated d.
Descemet membrane d.
disciform retinal d.
extrafoveal retinal d.
exudative retinal d. (ERD)
exudative serous retinal d.
fibrovascular pigment epithelium d.
foveal retinal d.
foveolar retinal d.
funnel-shaped retinal d.
hemorrhagic choroidal d.
hyaloid membrane d.
d. infusion
late phase d.
macula-off rhegmatogenous
retinal d.
macula-on rhegmatogenous
retinal d.
macular retinal d.
macular traction d.
morning glory retinal d.
myopic macular hole d.
neurosensory retinal d.
nonrhegmatogenous retinal d.
open-funnel d.
perifoveal posterior vitreous d.
(PPVD)

pigment epithelial d. (PED)
d. pocket
posterior vitreous d. (PVD)
pseudophakic d.
d. of retina
retinal d. (RD)
retinal pigment epithelium
serous d.
rhegmatogenous retinal d. (RRD)
schisis-related d.
sensory d.
serous choroidal d.
serous macular d.
serous pigment epithelial d.
serous retinal pigment
epithelium d.
shallow d.
tear-induced retinal d.
total exudative d.
tractional retinal d. (TRD)
traction macular d.
traction retinal d.
vitreous d.
detectability
ophthalmoscopic d.
detectable focus
detection
d. acuity
blur d.
contrast d.
glaucoma d.
mosaic retinal dysfunction d.
progression d.
detector
thermoluminescence d. (TLD)
deterenol HCl
deturgescence
d. of cornea
corneal d.
deturgescent state
deuteranomalopia
deuteranomalous
deuteranomaly
deuteranope
deuteranopia, deuteranopsia
deuteranopic
deuton color blindness
devascularization
devastating
d. ocular adnexal injury
d. ocular complication

NOTES

development
- National Institute of Child Health and Human D. (NICHHD)
- ocular d.
- visual d.

developmental
- d. anomaly
- d. anterior segment abnormality
- d. cataract
- d. eye movement (DEM)
- d. eye movement test
- d. glaucoma
- d. optometry
- d. prosopagnosia
- d. ptosis
- d. vision therapy

deviant color

deviating eye

deviation
- angle of d.
- comitant vertical d.
- conjugate horizontal d.
- convergent d.
- corrected pattern standard d. (CPSD)
- dissociated horizontal d.
- dissociated vertical d. (DVD)
- divergent d.
- downward d.
- esotropic d.
- forced downward d.
- frequency doubling technology mean d. (FDT-MD)
- frequency doubling technology pattern standard d. (FDT-PSD)
- global d. (GD)
- Hering-Hellebrand d.
- heterotropic d.
- high-pass resolution perimetry global d. (HRP-GD)
- high-pass resolution perimetry local d. (HRP-LD)
- horizontal d.
- incomitant vertical d.
- intermittent d.
- latent d.
- local d. (LD)
- manifest d.
- mean d. (MD)
- minimum d.
- pattern standard d. (PSD)
- periodic alternating gaze d.
- primary d.
- right d.
- secondary d.
- skew d.
- squint d.
- standard d. (SD)
- strabismal d.

- supranuclear d.
- tonic downward d.
- tonic upward d.
- torsional d.
- tropia d.
- tropic d.
- vertical comitant d.

deviational nystagmus

Devic disease

device
- Ahmed d.
- AquaFlow collagen glaucoma drainage d.
- AquaLase liquefaction d.
- capsular retraction d.
- color vision testing d.
- DisCoVisc ophthalmic viscosurgical d.
- doubling d.
- Envision TD ophthalmic drug delivery d.
- explosive d.
- glaucoma drainage d. (GDD)
- improvised explosive d.
- Joseph d.
- Krupin d.
- laser-argon d.
- laser-ruby d.
- liquefaction d.
- Look micropuncture d.
- measuring d.
- Microjet-based cutting and debriding d.
- MTI photoscreener vision screening d.
- myReader low-vision auto-reading d.
- Novus 3000 photocoagulation d.
- oblique prism d.
- Ocusert d.
- OptiMed d.
- Panoramic200 Ultra-Widefield Ophthalmic Imaging D.
- PerfectCapsule irrigation d.
- Perfect Pupil expansion d.
- Pocket Starter d.
- portable d.
- retrieval d.
- sealed capsule irrigation d.
- seton drainage d.
- spectacle-borne d.
- Stratus OCT d.
- subjective d.
- SureSight vision screening d.
- Venturi aspiration vitrectomy d.
- viscosurgical d.
- Welch 4-drop d.

deviometer

devitalized epithelium

Dexacidin
Dexacine ointment
Dexair
dexamethasone
    d. acetate
    neomycin, polymyxin B, and d.
    d. sodium phosphate
    d. solution
    tobramycin and d.
Dexasol
Dexasone L.A.
Dexasporin
Dexcaine
Dexchlor
dexchlorpheniramine
Dexedrine
Dexone LA
Dexon suture
Dexsol
Dexsone
dexter (D)
    oculus d. (right eye)
dextran medium
dextroclination
dextrocular
dextrocularity
dextrocycloduction
dextrodepression
dextroduction
dextrogyration
dextrose
dextrotorsion
dextroversion
DFP
    diisopropyl fluorophosphate
DGH
    DGH 2000 AP ultrasonic
    pachymeter
    DGH 5000 A-scan
DGI
    disability glare index
DHPG
    dihydrophenylethylene glycol
DHQ
    driving habits questionnaire
D-15 Hue Desaturated Panel test
D&I
    dilation and irrigation
diabetes
    alloxan d.
    artificial d.
    brittle d.
    bronze d.

    chemical d.
    D. Control and Complications Trial
    experimental d.
    gestational d.
    gouty d.
    growth-onset d.
    d. innocens
    d. insipidus
    d. insipidus, diabetes mellitus, optic
      atrophy, deafness (DIDMOAD)
    insulin-deficient d.
    juvenile d.
    ketosis-prone d.
    ketosis-resistant d.
    Lancereaux d.
    latent d.
    lipoatrophic d.
    lipoplethoric d.
    lipuric d.
    masked d.
    maturity-onset d.
    d. mellitus (DM)
    Mosler d.
    overflow d.
    overt d.
    pancreatic d.
    phlorhizin d.
    phosphate d.
    poorly controlled d.
    puncture d.
    renal d.
    skin d.
    steroid d.
    steroidogenic d.
    subclinical d.
    temporary d.
    toxic d.
    type 1, 2 d.
diabetic
    d. amaurosis
    d. Argyll Robertson pupil
    d. cataract
    d. diffuse macular edema
    d. iritis
    d. keratoepitheliopathy
    d. macular degeneration
    d. macular edema (DME)
    d. macular heterotopia
    d. maculopathy
    d. melanosis
    d. membrane
    d. optic atrophy
    d. papilledema

D

NOTES

diabetic *(continued)*
    d. papillitis
    d. papillopathy
    d. patient
    d. retinitis
    d. retinopathy (DR)
    D. Retinopathy Clinical Research (DRCR)
    D. Retinopathy Clinical Research Network
    D. Retinopathy Vitrectomy Study (DRVS)
    d. traction
diabetica
    rubeosis iridis d.
diabetic-osmotic cataract
diabeticus
    fundus d.
diagnosis, pl. **diagnoses**
    differential d.
    neuroophthalmologic d.
    nonorganic disorder d.
    preimplantation genetic d.
    prenatal d.
    presumptive d.
diagnostic
    d. contact lens
    d. fiberoptic lens
    d. fitting set
    d. position of gaze
    d. probing
    d. program
    d. testing
dial
    astigmatic d.
    clock d.
    Mendez astigmatism d.
    Regan-Lancaster d.
    sunburst d.
dialer
    angled iris hook and IOL d.
    intraocular lens d.
    Lester lens d.
    Spadafora MemoryLens d.
    Visitec intraocular lens d.
dialysis
    large nasal zonular d.
    retinal d.
    zonular d.
Diamatrix trapezoidal diamond knife
diameter
    anterior optic zone d.
    contact lens chord d.
    d. of cornea
    corneal d.
    disc d. (DD, dd)
    effective d. (ED)
    iris d.
    large pupil d.

    minimal effective d. (MED)
    optical zone d.
    overall d. (OAD)
    pupillary d.
    visible iris d. (VID)
3,4-diaminopyridine
diamond
    d. blade knife
    d. bur
    d. crescent blade
    D. Dye
    d. laser knife
    d. micrometer
    d. phaco knife
    d. wound separator
diamond-bur polishing
diamond-dusted
    d.-d. knife
    d.-d. knife blade
    d.-d. membrane eraser
    d.-d. membrane scraper (DDMS)
    d.-d. scraper
Diamontek knife
Diamox Sequels
diaphanoscopy
diaphragm
    black iris d.
    iris-lens d.
    lens-iris d.
    Potter-Bucky d.
diaphragma sellae
diapositive
diaschisis
diastasis
    iris d.
diathermy
    d. application
    d. electrode
    Mira d.
    d. operation
    d. point
    d. puncture
    d. tip
    transscleral d.
    d. unit
    wet-field d.
Diatracin
dibromopropamidine isethionate
dichlorphenamide
dichoptic separation
dichroic
dichroism
    circular d.
dichromasy
dichromat
dichromatic
    d. light
    d. vision

dichromatism
    congenital d.
dichromatopsia
dichromic
Dickinson
    Becton D. (BD)
diclofenac
    postoperative d.
    d. sodium
dicloxacillin
Dicon
    D. CT 200 corneal topographer
    D. ocular blood flow analyzer
dicoria
dictyoma
didanosine
DIDMOAD
    diabetes insipidus, diabetes mellitus, optic atrophy, deafness
    DIDMOAD syndrome
Dieffenbach
    D. operation
    D. serrefine
diencephalic
    d. lesion
    d. syndrome
diencephalon
difference
    frame d.
    interocular axial length d. (IALD)
    light d.
differential diagnosis
differentiation
    stem cell d.
difficile
    Clostridium d.
Diff-Quik stain
diffraction
    Fraunhofer d.
diffraction-limited pupil
diffractive multifocal lens
diffusa
    encephalitis periaxialis d.
diffuse
    d. angiokeratoma
    d. anterior scleritis
    d. atherosclerosis
    d. cataract
    d. choroidal sclerosis
    d. choroiditis
    d. deep keratitis
    d. drusen
    d. endotheliitis

    d. granuloma
    d. illumination
    d. inflammatory eyelid atrophy
    d. lamellar keratitis
    d. Lewy body disease
    d. neonatal hemangiomatosis
    d. retina pigment epitheliopathy
    d. unilateral subacute neuroretinitis (DUSN)
diffusion
    circle d.
    disc d. (DD)
diffusion-weighted imaging/magnetic resonance imaging (DWI/MRI)
diffusum
    angiokeratoma corporis d.
Diflucan
difumarate
    emedastine d.
DiGeorge syndrome
digestion
    enzymatic d.
Digilab tonometer
digital
    d. acuity card
    3Dx d. stereo disc camera
    d. fitting measurement
    D. fundus imager
    d. image analysis
    d. nonmydriatic fundus imaging
    d. pressure
    D. slit-lamp imager
    d. subtraction indocyanine green angiography (DS-ICGA)
    d. subtraction photokeratoscopy
    d. tonometry
Digitalis purpurea
digitized video fundus image
digitoocular sign
digitoxin
digoxin
dihydrate
    calcium chloride d.
    sodium citrate d.
dihydrophenylethylene glycol (DHPG)
diisopropyl fluorophosphate (DFP)
dilacerated cataract
dilaceration
Dilantin
Dilatair
dilatation
    balloon catheter d.
    vascular d.

D

NOTES

dilate
dilated
    d. episcleral vessel
    d. pupil
    d. retinal examination
    d. stereoscopic fundus examination
dilating drop
dilation
    balloon catheter d.
    ectatic d.
    d. and irrigation (D&I)
    d. lag
    pharmacological d.
    d. of punctum
    d. of punctum operation
    pupil d.
    saccular d.
    transient unilateral d.
dilator
    Berens d.
    Castroviejo lacrimal d.
    French lacrimal d.
    Galezowski lacrimal d.
    Heyner d.
    Hosford lacrimal d.
    House lacrimal d.
    iris d.
    Keuch pupil d.
    lacrimal d.
    Muldoon lacrimal d.
    d. muscle
    d. muscle of pupil
    Nettleship-Wilder d.
    Perfect Pupil d.
    polyurethane d.
    punctal d.
    punctum d.
    pupil d.
    Ruedemann lacrimal d.
    Sisler punctum d.
    Wilder lacrimal d.
    Ziegler lacrimal d.
dilution
    pigmentary d.
dimefilcon A
dimenhydrinate
dimension
    orbital d.
3-dimensional (3D)
    3-d. conformal fractionated radiation
    therapy
    3-d. retinal image
Dimetabs Oral
Dimetane Extentabs
dimethylaminoethanol
dimethylpolysiloxane
dimethyl sulfate
diminazene aceturate
Dimmer nummular keratitis

dimness of vision
dimple
    Fuchs d.
    d. veil
dimpling
    d. of eyeball
    foveal d.
diode
    d. endolaser
    d. endophotocoagulation
    d. laser
    d. laser therapy
    d. laser trabeculoplasty (DLT)
    light-emitting d. (LED)
    d. microlaser
diode-pumped
    d.-p. solid-state (DPSS)
    d.-p. solid-state photocoagulation
    laser
diolamine
    sulfisoxazole d.
diolipin antibody
diopsimeter
diopter, dioptre (D)
    d. cylinder
    d. prism
    prism d. (PD, p.d.)
    d. sphere (DS)
4-diopter base-out prism testing
66-diopter iridectomy laser lens
dioptometer, dioptrometer
dioptometry, dioptrometry
dioptoscope, dioptroscope
dioptoscopy, dioptroscopy
dioptre (*var. of* diopter)
dioptric
    d. aberration
    d. apparatus
    d. correction
    d. medium
    d. power
    d. system
dioptrics
dioptrometer (*var. of* dioptometer)
dioptrometry (*var. of* dioptometry)
Dioptron
    D. Nova
    D. Ultima
dioptroscope (*var. of* dioptoscope)
dioptroscopy (*var. of* dioptoscopy)
dioptry
dioxide
    carbon d. (CO_2)
Diphenhist
diphenhydramine hydrochloride
diphtheriae
    Corynebacterium d.
diphtheritic conjunctivitis
diphtheroid

dipivalyl epinephrine
dipivefrin HCl
diplegia
    congenital facial d.
diplexia
diplobacillary
    d. blepharitis
    d. conjunctivitis
diplocoria
diplopia
    binocular d.
    cerebral d.
    consecutive d.
    crossed d.
    direct d.
    heteronymous d.
    homonymous d.
    horizontal d.
    monocular d.
    paradoxical d.
    peribulbar anesthesia-related d.
    simple d.
    stereoscopic d.
    torsional d.
    uncrossed d.
    vertical d.
diplopiometer
diploscope
dipping
    ocular d.
    reverse d.
Diprivan
diquafosol tetrasodium
direct
    d. astigmatism
    d. carotid cavernous fistula
    d. chlamydial immunofluorescence
      test
    d. diplopia
    d. fluorescent antibody stain
    d. glare
    d. gonioscopic lens
    d. illumination
    d. image
    d. measurement
    d. method
    d. ophthalmoscope
    d. ophthalmoscopy
    d. parallax
    d. pupillary light reaction
    d. pupillary reflex
    d. pupillary response
    d. vision

direction
    angle of d.
    line of d.
    principal line of d.
    principal visual d.
    rotational d.
    visual d.
directional
    d. defect
    d. preponderance
direct-light
    d.-l. reflex
    d.-l. refraction
    d.-l. response
director
    grooved d.
Dirofilaria repens
disability
    auditory perceptual d.
    d. glare
    glare d. (GD)
    d. glare index (DGI)
    motor-output d.
    visual d.
disc, disk
    Airy d.
    angioid d.
    anomalous d.
    aperture d.
    choked optic d.
    ciliary d.
    colobomatous optic d.
    color d.
    congenital pit of optic d.
    conus of optic d.
    cupped d.
    cupping of optic d.
    d. damage likelihood scale (DDLS)
    dark d.
    d. diameter (DD, dd)
    d. diffusion (DD)
    donor d.
    doubling of optic d.
    dragged d.
    d. drusen
    d. drusen hemorrhage
    d. edema
    edema of optic d.
    d. elevation
    excavation of optic d.
    d. forceps
    gelatin d.
    glass d.

D

NOTES

disc *(continued)*
    hypoplastic d.
    d. intraocular lens
    d. IOL
    ischemic d.
    Krill d.
    Krupin eye d.
    leukemic infiltration of optic d.
    micrometer d.
    morning glory d.
    nasal border of optic d.
    d. neovascularization
    neovascularization of d. (NVD)
    d. neurovascular vessel
    Newton d.
    optic d.
    pale optic d.
    d. pallor
    pinhole d.
    pinkeye d.
    Placido da Costa d.
    planoconvex-shaped d.
    posterior lamellar d.
    Rekoss d.
    stenopeic d.
    stroboscopic d.
    d. stroma
    swelling of d.
    tilted d.
    d. vasculature
    Whipple d.
disc-fovea distance
discharge
    conjunctival d.
    mucoid d.
    mucous d.
    purulent d.
    serous d.
    socket d.
    watery d.
disci (*pl. of* discus)
DisCide disinfecting towelette
disciform
    d. chorioretinopathy
    d. degeneration of retina
    d. endotheliitis
    d. herpes simplex keratitis
    d. macular degeneration
    d. macular scar
    d. opacity
    d. process
    d. retinal detachment
    d. scar
disciformis
    keratitis d.
discission
    d. hook
    d. knife
    d. of lens operation

    d. needle
    posterior d.
discitis
disclination
discoloration
    lens d.
    d. of pigment
discomfort
    morning d.
    visual d.
disconjugate
    d. gaze
    d. movement of eyes
    d. nystagmus
    d. roving eye movement
discontinuity
    zone of d.
DisCoVisc ophthalmic viscosurgical device
discrete
    d. colliquative keratopathy
    d. granuloma
    d. micro gel deposit
discrimination
    blur d.
    color d.
    contrast d.
    light d.
    2-light d.
    light-dark d. (LDD)
    spatial d.
    visual d.
disc-shaped cataract
discus, pl. **disci**
    excavatio disci
    d. nervi optici
    d. opticus
discussion pallor
disease
    age-related eye d.
    AIDS-related eye d.
    Åland Island eye d.
    Albers-Schönberg d.
    Albright d.
    allergic eye d.
    allergic ocular d.
    Alström d.
    angio-Behçet d.
    Apollo d.
    Arlt d.
    arterial occlusive d.
    Ballet d.
    basal ganglia d.
    Basedow d.
    Batten d.
    Batten-Mayou d.
    Behçet d.
    Behr d.
    Benson d.

Berlin d.
Best d.
Bielschowsky d.
Bielschowsky-Jansky d.
blinding eye d.
Bowen d.
brainstem d.
Canavan d.
chiasmal d.
chorioretinal inflammatory d.
Coats d.
Cogan d.
collagen and rheumatoid-related d.
collagen vascular d.
corneal stromal d.
corneal surface d.
cotransmission of d.
Creutzfeldt-Jakob d.
Crouzon d.
cytomegalic inclusion d. (CID, CMID)
cytomegalovirus d.
Dalrymple d.
degenerative cerebellar d.
degenerative ocular d.
degenerative retinal d.
demyelinating d.
Devic d.
diffuse Lewy body d.
dry eye ocular surface d.
Dyggve d.
Eales d.
end-stage d.
epithelial basement membrane d.
epithelial herpetic d.
Erdheim-Chester d.
exogenous d.
extraorbital d.
eyelid margin d.
Fabry d.
Farber d.
Flajani d.
Flatau-Schilder d.
flecked retina d.
Förster d.
Franceschetti d.
Gaucher d.
Gerstmann-Straussler-Scheinker d.
Goldflam d.
Goldflam-Erb d.
Goldmann-Favre d.
Gorham d.
Graefe d.

graft versus host d.
Graves d.
Hand-Schüller-Christian d.
Harada d.
Heerfordt d.
helminthic d.
herpetic ocular d.
Hippel d.
HIV-related eye d.
HSV ocular d.
HSV stromal d.
Hurler d.
idiopathic inflammatory d.
infantile Refsum d.
infectious d.
inflammatory meibomian gland d.
interpalpebral stromal d.
Jansky-Bielschowsky d.
Jensen d.
Kawasaki d.
Kikuchi-Fujimoto d.
Kimmelstiel-Wilson d.
Kjer d.
Krabbe d.
Krill d.
Kuhnt-Junius d.
Kyrle d.
Lauber d.
Leber d.
Leigh d.
Lindau-von Hippel d.
Lyme d.
lysosomal storage d.
Machado-Joseph d.
macular d.
Marfan d.
Marsh d.
medullary cystic d.
medullary optic d.
meibomian gland d.
midbrain d.
Mikulicz d.
miner's d.
mitochondrial d.
Möbius d.
multicore d.
multifactorial d.
multifocal Best d.
multifocal chorioretinal d.
muscle-eye-brain d.
mycobacterial d.
neonatal onset multisystem inflammatory d. (NOMID)

D

NOTES

139

disease *(continued)*
  neuro-Behçet d.
  neuroophthalmologic d.
  neuropathic d.
  Niemann-Pick d. type A, B
  Norrie d.
  occlusive vascular d.
  ocular Lyme d.
  ocular surface d. (OSD)
  ocular syphilitic d.
  oculoglandular d.
  Oguchi d.
  ophthalmic Graves d.
  optic nerve d.
  orbital inflammatory d.
  pancreatic d.
  Parry d.
  plus d.
  prethreshold d.
  primary demyelinating d.
  primary ocular d.
  prion-mediated d.
  pulseless d.
  Purtscher d.
  Refsum d.
  Reis-Bücklers d.
  Reiter d.
  retinal d.
  Rosai-Dorfman d.
  Sanders d.
  Schilder d.
  d. severity
  shipyard d.
  Sichel d.
  sickle cell d.
  Sjögren d.
  Sneddon-Wilkinson d.
  Spielmeyer-Sjögren d.
  Spielmeyer-Stock d.
  Spielmeyer-Vogt d.
  Stargardt and Best d.
  Steele-Richardson-Olszewski d.
  Steinert d.
  Strachan d.
  stromal d.
  Sturge-Weber d.
  syphilitic ocular d.
  systemic autoimmune d.
  Tangier d.
  Tay d.
  Tay-Sachs d.
  threshold d.
  Thygeson d.
  thyroid eye d.
  toxic-nutritional d.
  van der Hoeve d.
  vanishing bone d.
  vascular cerebellar d.
  vascular occlusive d.
  venous occlusive d.
  viral ocular d.
  visual pathway d.
  Vogt d.
  Vogt-Koyanagi-Harada d.
  Vogt-Spielmeyer d.
  von Gierke d.
  von Hippel d.
  von Hippel-Lindau d.
  von Recklinghausen d.
  Wagner d.
  Weil d.
  Werdnig-Hoffmann d.
  Westphal-Strümpell d.
  Whipple d.
  Wilson d.
  zone 1 d.
disease-causing gene
diseased
  d. endothelium
  d. eye
disease-modifying therapy
disease-related change
disequilibrium
Dishler
  D. Excimer Laser System for
    LASIK
  D. irrigation cannula
  D. type LASIK irrigating cannula
disinfectant
  AoSept D.
disinfecting solution
disinfection
disinserted
  d. muscle
  d. retina
disinsertion
  levator aponeurosis d.
  d. of retina
disjugate
  d. movement
  d. movement of eyes
disjunctive
  d. movement
  d. nystagmus
disk *(var. of* disc)
dislocated
  d. crystalline lens
  d. intraocular lens
  d. intraocular lens fixation
  ocular circulation d.
dislocation
  congenital lens d.
  intraocular lens d.
  lens d.
  posterior d.
dislocator
  Kirby lens d.

dismutase
    manganese superoxide d.
disodium
    d. cromoglycate
    edetate d.
    d. hydrogen phosphate
disorder
    accommodation d.
    adrenal d.
    autonomic nervous system d.
    basement membrane d.
    blinking d.
    bullous d.
    canalicular d.
    epithelial bleb d.
    extraocular muscle d.
    d. of eye
    eyelid d.
    eye movement d.
    gaze d.
    hemorrhagic d.
    histiocytic d.
    hyperkeratotic d.
    infranuclear d.
    lacrimation d.
    motion perception d.
    myelin d.
    myopathic d.
    neurologic d.
    neuromuscular d.
    ocular motility d.
    ocular surface d.
    oculodermal d.
    oculomotor d.
    ophthalmic d.
    optic nerve d.
    outflow d.
    parathyroid d.
    peroxisomal d.
    postsynaptic congenital myasthenic d.
    prechiasmal d.
    presynaptic congenital myasthenic d.
    pupil d.
    pupillary d.
    pursuit d.
    retinal artery d.
    retinal vein d.
    saccadic d.
    Sanders d.
    seasonal affective d. (SAD)
    sensorimotor d.
    single gene d.
    spatial perception d.
    supranuclear d.
    tear film d.
    thyroid gland d.
    vascular d.
    vestibular d.
    visuospatial d.
    vitreoretinal d.
disorganization
    cellular d.
disorganized globe
disorientation
    topographic d.
disparate retinal point
disparity, pl. **disparities**
    d. angle
    binocular d.
    bitemporal d.
    conjugate d.
    fixation d.
    horizontal retinal d.
    retinal d.
    subjective fixation d.
disparometer
    Sheedy d.
dispensary
    optical d.
dispenser
    optical d.
dispersing lens
dispersion
    chromatic d.
    circle of d.
    corneal endothelial pigmentary d.
    peripheral retinal pigment d.
    pigment d.
    point of d.
    d. prism
    d. syndrome
dispersiveness
displacement
    eye d.
    globe d.
    image d.
    macular d.
    object d.
    d. threshold
display
    point-of-purchase d.
    virtual reality head-mounted d.
    Virtual Retinal D. (VRD)
    Yorktown-style designer series d.

NOTES

disposable
8.4 BC d. lens
d. cautery
d. contact lens
d. Keratoplast tip
d. ocutome
d. separator
d. trephine

disproportion
congenital fiber-type d. (CFTD)

disruption
posterior capsular zonular d.
YAG laser d.
zonular d.

dissecting
d. scissors
d. tip

dissection
arterial d.
carotid artery d.
open-sky d.
pre-descemetic d.
tunnel d.

dissector
Barraquer corneal d.
Berens corneal d.
Blumenthal conjunctival d.
Castroviejo corneal d.
channel d.
corneal knife d.
Desmarres corneal d.
Desmarres lamellar d.
d. knife
LASEK bow d.
Martinez d.
Troutman corneal d.
Troutman nonincisional lamellar d.
Wagner epiretinal membrane d.

disseminated
d. asymptomatic unilateral
   neovascularization
d. choroiditis
d. intravascular coagulation
d. nonosteolytic myelomatosis

dissimilar
d. image test
d. segment
d. target test

dissipation
circle d.

dissociated
d. alkaloid
d. double hypertropia (DDHT)
d. horizontal deviation
d. hyperdeviation
d. position
d. vertical deviation (DVD)
d. vertical divergence (DVD)
d. vertical nystagmus

dissociation
light-near d.
perception d.
pupillary light-near d.
d. of visual perception

distal
d. optic nerve syndrome
d. optic neuropathy

distance
angular d.
d. between centers (DBC)
d. between lenses (DBL)
center of rotation d.
d. correction
disc-fovea d.
egocentric fixation d.
equivalent d.
focal d. (FD)
frame papillary d.
geometric center d. (GCD)
infinite d.
intercanthal d. (ICD)
interpupillary d. (IPD)
intraocular d.
marginal reflex d. (MRD)
d. and near
object d.
pupillary d. (PD)
test d.
vertex of d.
d. vision
d. visual acuity (DVA)
d. visual performance

distant
d. direct ophthalmoscopy
d. gaze

distantial aberration

distichiasis
acquired d.

distinct flicker

distometer
Haag-Streit d.

distortion
d. aberration
barrel d.
corneal d.
d. of lens
pincushion d.
d. of vision
xeroscope grid d.

distraction
d. cone
d. conus

distribution
altered tear d.
gaussian d.
normal d.

districhiasis

disturbance
    equilibrium d.
    psychological d.
    sensation d.
    tear-film d.
    visual d.
diuretic
diurnal
    d. fluctuation
    d. intraocular pressure measurement
    d. variation
divergence
    d. amplitude
    congenital adduction palsy with
      synergistic d.
    dissociated vertical d. (DVD)
    d. excess
    d. excess exotropia
    fusional d.
    d. insufficiency
    d. insufficiency exotropia
    negative vertical d.
    d. nystagmus
    d. paralysis
    d. paresis
    point of d.
    positive vertical d.
    relative d.
    d. reserve
    strabismus d.
    synergistic d.
    vertical d.
divergent
    d. beam
    d. cut angle
    d. deviation
    d. lens
    d. light
    d. ray
    d. squint
    d. strabismus
diverging
    d. meniscus
    d. meniscus lens
divers' spectacles
diverticulum, pl. **diverticula**
    lacrimal sac d.
divide-and-conquer
    d.-a.-c. method
    d.-a.-c. technique
divided spectacles
Dix foreign body spud
Dix-Hallpike test

Dixon Mann sign
Dk
    oxygen permeability
    Dk IOL insertion forceps
    Dk value
Dk/L
    oxygen transmissibility
DLEK
    deep lamellar endothelial keratoplasty
DLK
    deep lamellar keratoplasty
DLKP
    deep lamellar keratoplasty
DLT
    diode laser trabeculoplasty
DM
    diabetes mellitus
DME
    diabetic macular edema
D/N
    at distance and at near
dobutamine
doctor-patient relationship
Docustar fundus camera
Dodick
    D. laser cataract surgery
    D. laser photolysis system
    D. lens-holding forceps
    D. nucleus cracker
    D. nucleus irrigating chopper
    D. photolysis
    D. photolysis probe
Dodick-Kammann bimanual chopper
Doherty
    D. sphere
    D. sphere implant
Dohlman keratoprosthesis
dolasetron
dolichoectasia
dolichoectatic anterior cerebral artery
Döllinger tendinous ring
doll's
    d. eye
    d. eye reflex
    d. eye response
    d. eye sign
    d. head phenomenon
dolor capitis
dolorosa
    atrophia d.
D'Ombrain operation
Domeboro solution
dome receptacle

D

NOTES

dominance
> ocular d.

dominant
> d. action plan
> d. cystoid macular dystrophy
> d. eye
> d. gene
> d. optic atrophy
> d. optic neuropathy
> d. progressive foveal dystrophy
> d. slowly progressive macular dystrophy
> d. strategy

Donaldson
> D. eye patch
> D. fundus camera
> D. stereoviewer

Donders
> D. chart
> D. glaucoma
> D. law
> D. ring

donor
> d. button
> d. cap
> d. cornea
> d. disc
> d. eye
> d. graft
> d. lamella
> d. material
> d. punch
> d. tissue

donut-cut flap
donut-shaped flap
dopamine
Doppler
> D. flowmetry measure
> Hadeco intraoperative D.
> Siemens Quantum 2000 Color D.
> transcranial D. (TCD)
> D. ultrasonogram
> D. ultrasonography
> D. ultrasound
> D. velocimeter

DORC
> Dutch Ophthalmic Research Center
> DORC backflush instrument
> DORC fast freeze cryosurgical system
> DORC handle
> DORC Hexon Illumination System 1266 XII
> DORC illuminated diamond knife
> DORC microforceps and microscissors
> DORC subretinal instrument set

Dorello canal

dorsal
> d. midbrain syndrome
> d. rostral damage
> d. vermis

dorsalis
> tabes d.

dorzolamide
> d. hydrochloride
> d. hydrochloride ophthalmic solution
> d. hydrochloride-timolol maleate ophthalmic solution

dot
> d. dystrophy
> granular hyperfluorescent d.
> Gunn d.
> d. hemorrhage
> Horner-Trantas d.
> lamina d.
> Marcus Gunn d.
> d. method
> Mittendorf d.
> Trantas d.
> white d.

4-dot
> 4-d. test
> Worth 4-d. (W4D)

dot-and-blot hemorrhage
dot-and-fleck retinopathy
dot-like lens
double
> d. arcuate scotoma
> d. concave (DCC)
> d. concave lens
> d. convex (DCx)
> d. convex lens
> d. dissociated hypertropia
> d. elevator palsy
> d. eversion of eyelid
> d. freeze-thaw cryopexy
> d. freeze-thaw cryotherapy
> d. graft
> d. homonymous hemianopsia
> d. irrigating/aspirating cannula
> d. K method
> d. lid eversion
> d. lower lid fold
> d. Maddox rod
> d. Maddox rod test
> d. pentagon configuration
> d. pentagon slight design
> d. pentagon technique
> d. refraction
> d. ring sign
> d. slab-off contact lens
> d. spatula
> d. tantalum clip
> d. vision (DV)

double-armed suture

double-barreled injector-aspirator
double-blind study
double-contrast visualization
double-cutting sharp cystotome
double-headed pterygium
double-pronged forceps
double-quadrant testing
double-row diathermy barrage
double-running penetrating keratoplasty
  suture
doublet
  achromatic d.
  Wollaston d.
doubling
  d. device
  frequency d.
  d. of optic disc
Dougherty
  D. irrigating/aspirating unit
  D. irrigator
Douglas cilia forceps
douloureux
  tic d.
Douvas rotoextractor
down
  base d.
  endothelial cell side d.
  d. to finger counting
  D. syndrome
downbeat nystagmus
Downes lid clamp
downgaze
  d. paralysis, ataxia/athetosis and
    foam cell (DAF)
  d. saccade
downgrowth
  epithelial d.
  stromal d.
down-regulated gene
downward
  d. deviation
  d. gaze
  d. squint
doxycycline
Doyne
  D. familial colloid degeneration
  D. familial honeycomb choroiditis
  D. guttate iritis
  D. honeycomb choroidopathy
  D. honeycomb degeneration
  D. honeycomb dystrophy
  D. syndrome

DPSS
  diode-pumped solid-state
D&Q
  deep and quiet
DR
  diabetic retinopathy
Draeger
  D. forceps
  D. modified keratome
  D. tonometer
dragged
  d. disc
  d. macula
  d. retina
dragging
  macular d.
  optic disc d.
  retinal d.
drain
  Mentor precut d.
drainage
  d. angle
  aqueous humor d.
  cerebral venous d.
  d. implant surgery
  indirect argon laser d.
  lacrimal d.
  d. of lacrimal gland
  d. of lacrimal gland operation
  d. of lacrimal sac
  d. of lacrimal sac operation
  lymphatic d.
  quadrantic sclerectomy with
    internal d.
  sclerotomy with d.
  subretinal fluid d.
  tear d.
Drance hemorrhage
drape
  1021 d.
  Alcon disposable d.
  Barrier d.
  Eye-Pak II d.
  Hough d.
  LASIK eyelid d.
  miniophthalmic d.
  3M Steri-Drape d.
  Opraflex d.
  Steri-Drape d.
  Surgikos disposable d.
  Visi-Drape Elite ophthalmic d.
  Visi-Drape mini aperture d.

D

NOTES

drape *(continued)*
    Visi-Drape mini incise d.
    Visiflex d.
DRCR
    Diabetic Retinopathy Clinical Research
    DRCR Network
dressing
    AmnioGraft wound d.
    Blenderm tape d.
    bolus d.
    Borsch d.
    collodion d.
    compression d.
    crepe bandage d.
    Elastoplast d.
    eye pad d.
    fluff d.
    fluffed gauze d.
    d. forceps
    Harman eye d.
    lens d.
    moistened fine mesh gauze d.
    monocular d.
    pressure patch d.
    ribbon gauze d.
    saline-saturated wool d.
    sterile adhesive bubble d.
    Telfa plastic film d.
    tulle gras d.
    wet d.
    wool saturated in saline d.
Drews
    D. angled cystotome
    D. capsule polisher
    D. cataract needle
    D. cilia forceps
    D. inclined prism
    D. irrigating/aspirating unit
    D. irrigating cannula
    D. lens
    D. syndrome
Drews-Knolle reverse irrigating vectis
drift
    d. movement
    postsaccadic d.
drifting-text method
drill
    ophthalmic d.
drippings
    candlewax d.
drive
    safe to d.
    unsafe to d.
driver
    visually impaired d.
driving
    d. assessment
    d. habits questionnaire (DHQ)
    d. maneuver

droop
    brow d.
    lid d.
drooping of eyelid
droopy lid
drop
    AC eye d.'s
    Acular d.'s
    Akwa Tears lubricant eye d.'s
    Allerest eye d.'s
    Alomide d.'s
    antibiotic eye d.'s
    Aquify long-lasting comfort d.'s
    autologous serum eye d.'s
    Bausch & Lomb Moisture Eyes
      Protect Lubricant D.'s
    betamethasone sodium phosphate
      eye d.'s
    Bion Tears eye d.'s
    Boston Advance reconditioning d.'s
    Boston Rewetting D.'s
    chemotherapy d.'s
    Ciba Vision lens d.'s
    cidofovir eye d.'s
    Claris Rewetting D.'s
    Clerz 2 Lubricating and
      Rewetting D.'s
    Clerz Plus lens d.'s
    collyrium eye d.'s
    Comfort eye d.'s
    Complete Blink-N-Clean Lens D.'s
    Complete Lubricating and
      Rewetting D.'s
    Computer Eye D.'s
    corticosteroid d.'s
    dilating d.
    drop by d. (guttat.)
    Dry Eyes lubricant eye d.'s
    Enuclene eye d.'s
    eye d.'s
    20/20 eye d.'s
    Focus Lens D.'s
    GenTeal Mild lubricant eye d.'s
    hypertonic d.'s
    HypoTears Select lubricant eye d.'s
    d. instillation
    Lens Drops lubricating and
      rewetting d.'s
    Lens Plus rewetting d.'s
    lubricating d.'s
    Mallazine eye d.'s
    Moisture Eyes liquid gel lubricant
      eye d.'s
    Moisture Eyes liquid gel
      preservative-free eye d.'s
    Moisture ophthalmic d.'s
    Neosporin d.'s
    Opcon Maximum Strength
      Allergy D.'s

Opti-Free Rewetting D.'s
Optimum by Lobob wetting and
   rewetting d.'s
Opti-One Rewetting D.'s
Optique 1 Eye D.'s
OptiZen lubricating eye d.'s
placebo eye d.'s
Prefrin Liquifilm D.'s
Refresh contact lens comfort d.'s
Refresh Endura d.'s
Refresh Liquigel eye d.'s
Refresh Plus lubricant eye d.'s
Refresh Tears eye d.'s
ReNu Rewetting D.'s
Rondec D.'s
Sensitive Eyes d.'s
Similasan eye d.'s
Soothe emollient eye d.'s
sympathomimetic eye d.'s
Systane lubricant eye d.'s
Teargen II lubricant eye d.'s
Tears Again eye d.'s
Tears Again gel d.'s
Tears Again preservative-free d.'s
Tears Naturale Free lubricant
   eye d.'s
Tears Naturale II lubricant
   eye d.'s
Tears Naturale II Polyquad
   eye d.'s
Tears Naturale PM lubricant
   eye d.'s
Tears Natural Forte lubricant
   eye d.'s
Tears Plus lubricant eye d.'s
TheraTears lubricant eye d.'s
topical anesthetic eye d.'s
trifluridine eye d.'s
Viva-Drops eye d.'s
droperidol
dropout
   acinar d.
   nerve fiber layer d.
   pigmentary d.
   retinal pigment epithelium d.
dropped-socket appearance
dropper
   eye d.
droxifilcon A
drug
   d. abuse retinopathy
   adrenergic d.
   amphiphilic d.

antiadrenergic d.
anticataract d.
anticholinergic d.
antimalarial d.
antimicrobial d.
antirejection d.
cataractogenic d.
cholinergic d.
immunosuppressive d.
d. interaction
investigational new d. (IND)
IOP-lowering d.
light-activated d.
neuromuscular blocking d.
neuromuscular disorder-causing d.
neuroprotective antiglaucoma d.
nonsteroidal antiinflammatory d.
   (NSAID)
ophthalmic d.
orphan d.
parasympatholytic d.
parasympathomimetic d.
photosensitizing d.
d. reflux
steroid anti-infective ophthalmic
   combination d.
sulfa d.
sympatholytic d.
systemic d.
therapeutic neuroprotective
   antiglaucoma d.
topical d.
drug-dosing schedule
drug-induced
   d.-i. cataract
   d.-i. cicatrizing conjunctivitis
   d.-i. glaucoma
   d.-i. nystagmus
   d.-i. ptosis
drum
   optokinetic d.
drusen
   autosomal dominant d.
   basal laminar d.
   basal linear d.
   buried disc d.
   confluent d.
   cuticular d.
   diffuse d.
   disc d.
   equatorial d.
   exudative d.
   familial d.

D

NOTES

147

drusen *(continued)*
- giant d.
- hard d.
- intrapapillary d.
- d. of macula
- macular d.
- nerve head d.
- optic disc d.
- optic nerve head d. (ONHD)
- d. of optic nerve head
- d. of optic papilla
- radial d.
- retinal d.
- soft d.
- typical d.
- visible d.

DRVS
Diabetic Retinopathy Vitrectomy Study

dry
- d. ARMD
- d. eye algorithm
- d. eye goggles
- d. eye ocular surface disease
- d. eye prevalence
- d. eye questionnaire
- D. Eyes
- D. Eyes lubricant eye drops
- D. Eyes lubricant ointment
- d. eye state
- d. eye syndrome (DES)
- d. eye test (DET)
- d. eye therapy
- D. Eye Therapy Solution
- d. fold
- d. senile degenerative maculopathy
- d. senile macular degeneration
- d. spot

dryness
- conjunctiva d.

Drysdale nucleus manipulator
dry-shelled cataract
Drysol cream
DS
diopter sphere

DSAEK
Descemet-stripping automated endothelial keratoplasty

D-shaped keratometric reflection
DS-ICGA
digital subtraction indocyanine green angiography

dual
- d. eye shield
- d. lens
- d. mechanism lens

Dual-Wet
Duane
- D. classification

D. classification of squint
D. retraction syndrome

duboisii
Histoplasma d.

Duchenne
- D. dystrophy
- D. paralysis

Duchenne-Erb paralysis
Ducournau fine gripping forceps
duct
- ampulla of lacrimal d.
- canalicular d.
- catheterization of lacrimal d.
- catheterization of lacrimonasal d.
- excretory d.
- Gartner d.
- lacrimal d.
- lacrimonasal d.
- meibomian d.
- nasal d.
- nasolacrimal d. (NLD)
- probing lacrimonasal d.
- tear d.

ductal orifice obliteration
duction
- forced d.
- full versions and d.'s
- ocular d.
- passive d.
- d. test
- d.'s and versions (D&V)
- vertical d.

ductional
ductus
- d. lacrimales
- d. nasolacrimalis

Duddell membrane
Duet system
Duke-Elder
- D.-E. lamp
- D.-E. operation

Dulaney
- D. LASIK marker
- D. lens

dull-sided diamond blade
dull-tipped horizontal chopper
dumbbell opening
dumbbell-shaped cataract
duochrome test
Duolube
Duotrak blade
Duovisc
- D. solution
- D. viscoelastic system

duplex scan
duplicity theory of vision
Dupuy-Dutemps
- D.-D. dacryocystorhinostomy dye test

D.-D. dacryostomy
D.-D. operation
Duraclose scleral clip
dural
d. arteriovenous malformation
d. carotid cavernous fistula
d. cavernous sinus fistula
d. sheath
d. shunt
d. shunt syndrome
Duralone
Duralube
Duramist Plus
Duranest
D. HCl
D. HCl with epinephrine
Durasoft
D. 2 ColorBlends lens
D. 3 Optifit Toric ColorBlends contact lens
D. 2 Optifit Toric for light eyes contact lens
Duratears Naturale
duration
hemorrhage d.
Dura-T lens
Durazyme
Duredge knife
Durette external laser shield
Durham tonometer
Duricef
DUSN
diffuse unilateral subacute neuroretinitis
dusting
fibrin d.
iris pigment d.
dust-like opacity
Dutcher body
Dutch Ophthalmic Research Center (DORC)
DV
double vision
D&V
ductions and versions
DVA
distance visual acuity
DVD
dissociated vertical deviation
dissociated vertical divergence
DWCL
daily wear contact lens

DWI/MRI
diffusion-weighted imaging/magnetic resonance imaging
dyclonine
dye
alizarin red S d.
chemofluorescent d.
Diamond D.
d. disappearance test (DDT)
fluorescein d.
indocyanine green d.
materials primary d.
ophthalmic d.
pooling of d.
tricarbocyanine d.
vital d.
d. yellow laser
dye-assisted anterior capsulorrhexis
dye-enhanced
d.-e. cataract
d.-e. cataract surgery
d.-e. feeder vessel treatment
d.-e. photocoagulation
Dyer
D. nomogram system of lens ordering
D. nomogram system of ordering contact lens
Dyggve disease
Dymadon
Dynacin
dynamic
d. accommodation insufficiency
d. refraction
d. scanning laser ophthalmoscopy
d. stabilization
d. strabismus
d. visual acuity
dynamics
fluid d.
Dyonics syringe injector
dysacusia
dysadaptation
dysaptation, dysadaptation
dysautonomia
familial autonomic d.
dyscephalic
d. syndrome
d. syndrome of François
dyschromasia
dyschromatopsia
acquired d.

D

NOTES

dyschromatopsia *(continued)*
    cerebral d.
    congenital d.
dysconjugate gaze
dyscoria
dyscrasia
    retinopathy of blood d.
dysesthesia
    glaucoma filtering bleb d.
dysfunction
    anterior visual pathway d.
    brain d.
    brainstem d.
    cerebellar d.
    chorioretinopathy and pituitary d.
      (CPD)
    cone d.
    familial autonomic d.
    foveal outer retinal d.
    intraorbital nerve d.
    iris d.
    isolated oculomotor nerve d.
    meibomian gland d. (MGD)
    meshwork d.
    minimal brain d.
    mosaic pattern of d.
    mosaic retinal d.
    neurologic d.
    oblique muscle d.
    oculosympathetic d.
    optic nerve d.
    photoreceptor d.
    pontomesencephalic d.
    primary cone d.
    rod-cone d.
    visual d.
dysfunctional tear syndrome
dysgenesis
    anterior segment d.
    corneal d.
    iridocorneal mesenchymal d.
    iridocorneal mesodermal d.
    mesenchymal d.
    mesodermal d.
    posterior amorphous corneal d.
dysharmonious retinal correspondence
dysjunctive nystagmus
dyskeratosis
    benign d.
    d. congenita
    congenital d.
    hereditary benign intraepithelial d.
    intraepithelial d.
    malignant d.
dyslexia
    attentional d.
    central d.
    deep d.
    endogenous d.

    hemianopic d.
    mixed d.
    neglect d.
    surface d.
dysmegalopsia
dysmetria
    flutter d.
    ocular d.
    saccadic d.
dysmetropsia
dysmorphopsia
dysmotility
    ocular d.
dysoric retinopathy
dysphotopsia
    negative d.
    phakic d.
    positive d.
    pseudophakic d.
dysplasia
    chiasmal d.
    conjunctival d.
    corneal d.
    encephalo-ophthalmic d.
    fibromuscular d.
    fibrous d.
    forebrain d.
    hereditary renal-retinal d.
    macular d.
    OAV d.
    oculoauricular d.
    oculoauriculovertebral d.
    oculodentodigital d.
    oculovertebral d.
    ODD d.
    ophthalmomandibulomelic d.
    optic disc d.
    optic nerve d.
    orodigitofacial d.
    retinal d.
    septooptic d.
    vitreoretinal d.
dysplastic
    d. coloboma
    d. retina
Dysport
dysproteinemic retinopathy
dysthyroid
    d. myopathy
    d. ophthalmopathy
    d. optic neuropathy
    d. orbitopathy
dysthyroidism
dystonia
    blepharospasm-oromandibular d.
    focal d.
dystopia
    d. canthorum

foveal d.
orbital d.
dystrophia
d. adiposa corneae
d. endothelialis corneae
d. epithelialis corneae
dystrophica
elastosis d.
dystrophy
adult foveomacular retinal d.
adult-onset foveomacular d.
(AOFMD)
adult-onset vitelliform macular d.
adult vitelliform macular d.
amorphous corneal d.
anterior basement membrane d.
(ABMD)
anterior corneal d.
anular macular d.
Avellino d.
basement membrane d.
benign concentric anular macular d.
Best vitelliform macular d.
Biber-Haab-Dimmer corneal d.
Bietti corneal retinal d.
Bietti crystalline corneoretinal d.
Bothnia d.
butterfly macular d.
butterfly-shaped macular d.
butterfly-shaped pigment
epithelial d.
central areolar choroidal d.
central areolar pigment epithelial d.
central cloudy corneal d.
central cloudy parenchymatous d.
central crystalline d.
central discoid corneal d.
central pigmentary retinal d.
central speckled corneal d.
cerebellar ataxia-cone d.
choroidal d.
choroidoretinal d.
Cogan microcystic d.
cone d.
cone-rod d. (CRD)
cone-rod retinal d.
congenital hereditary endothelial
corneal d.
congenital muscular d.
congenital myotonic d.
d. of cornea
corneal endothelial guttate d.
corneal fleck d.

corneal guttate d.
corneal stromal d.
corneal vortex d.
crystalline corneal d.
cystoid macular d.
deep filiform d.
deep parenchymatous d.
dominant cystoid macular d.
dominant progressive foveal d.
dominant slowly progressive
macular d.
dot d.
Doyne honeycomb d.
Duchenne d.
ectatic corneal d.
endothelial cell d.
endothelial corneal d. (ECD)
epithelial basement membrane d.
Favre d.
Fehr macular d.
fenestrated sheen macular d.
filiform d.
fingerprint corneal d.
flecked corneal d.
Fleischer d.
foveomacular vitelliform d.
Franceschetti d.
François d.
François-Neetens d.
Fuchs combined corneal d.
Fuchs endothelial corneal d.
Fuchs epithelial corneal d.
Fuchs epithelial-endothelial d.
furrow d.
gelatino-lattice corneal d.
gelatinous droplike corneal d.
Goldmann-Favre d.
granular corneal d.
Groenouw corneal d.
Groenouw type I, II d.
gutter d.
hereditary anterior membrane d.
hereditary epithelial corneal d.
hereditary hemorrhagic macular d.
hereditary vitelliform d.
honeycomb d.
infantile neuroaxonal d. (INAD)
juvenile corneal epithelial d.
keratoconus d.
lattice corneal d.
lattice corneal d. type I
lattice corneal d. type IIIA
(LCDIIIA)

D

NOTES

dystrophy *(continued)*
Lisch corneal d.
macroreticular d.
macular corneal d.
macular retinal d.
map d.
map-dot corneal d.
map-dot-fingerprint corneal
  epithelial d.
marginal crystalline d.
MDF corneal d.
Meesmann epithelial corneal d.
Meesmann juvenile epithelial d.
microcystic corneal d.
microcystic epithelial d.
multifocal pattern d.
muscular d.
myotonic d.
North Carolina macular d.
ocular pharyngeal d.
oculocerebrorenal d.
oculopharyngeal d.
ophthalmoplegic muscular d.
parenchymatous corneal d.
pattern retinal d.
pericentral rod-cone d.
pigment epithelial d.
Pillat d.
polymorphous d.
posterior amorphous corneal d.
posterior polymorphic d. (of
  cornea) (PPMD)
posterior polymorphous corneal d.
pre-Descemet corneal d.
progressive cone d.
progressive cone-rod d.
progressive foveal d.
progressive macular d.

progressive tapetochoroidal d.
pseudoendothelial d.
pseudoinflammatory macular d.
Reis-Bücklers ring-shaped d.
Reis-Bücklers superficial corneal d.
reticular d.
retinal-choroidal d.
retinal cone d.
retinal pigmentary d.
ringlike corneal d.
ring-shaped d.
rod-cone d.
Salzmann nodular corneal d.
Schlichting d.
Schnyder crystalline corneal d.
sheen d.
Sjögren reticular d.
Sorsby fundus d.
Sorsby pseudoinflammatory
  macular d.
speckled corneal d.
Stargardt d.
Stocker-Holt d.
Stocker-Holt-Schneider d.
stromal corneal d.
tapetochoroidal d.
Thiel-Behnke corneal d.
unilateral corneal lattice d.
vitelliform macular d.
vitelliform retinal d.
vitelliruptive macular d.
vitreotapetoretinal d.
vortex corneal d.
d. of Waardenburg-Jonkers
Wagner vitreoretinal d.
X-linked cone d.

dysversion
congenital d.

E
- E Carpine
- E cell
- E chart
- E Clips computer eyewear
- E Clips prescription computer lens
- E game
- E syndrome
- E test

E′
- esophoria
- apolipoprotein E′
- illiterate E′

E¹
- esophoria at near

Eagle FlexPlug
EaglePlug tapered-shaft punctum plug
EagleVision Freeman punctum plug
Eales disease
early
- e. antigen
- e. bleb failure
- e. lens opacity
- e. lesion
- E. Manifest Glaucoma Trial (EMGT)
- e. mature cataract
- e. postoperative suture adjustment (EPSA)
- e. receptor potential
- e. receptor potential mottling
- E. Treatment Diabetic Retinopathy Study (ETDRS)
- E. Treatment of Diabetic Retinopathy Study visual acuity chart
- E. Treatment of Retinopathy of Prematurity (ETROP)
- E. Treatment for Retinopathy of Prematurity study

early-onset myopia
early-phase reaction
EAS-1000 anterior eye segment analysis system
easily everted upper eyelid
Easyloupes
- Oculus E.

Eaton-Lambert syndrome
EBAA
- Eye Bank Association of America

Eber needle-holder forceps
EBV
- Epstein-Barr virus
- EBV nuclear antigen

EBV-associated antigen

EC-5000 excimer laser
ecabet sodium
ECC
- extracapsular cataract

ECCE
- extracapsular cataract extraction

eccentric
- e. ablation
- e. fixation
- e. gaze
- e. gaze-holding
- e. limitation
- e. photorefraction
- e. vision

eccentricity
- angle of e.
- retinal e.

ecchymosis
- e. of eyelid
- periocular e.

ECD
- endothelial cell density
- endothelial corneal dystrophy

ECF
- epicanthic fold

Echinococcus
- *E.* cyst
- *E. granulosus*

echinophthalmia
echo
- e. ophthalmogram
- e. ophthalmography

Echodide
echogram
- intraoperative B-scan e.

echography
- kinetic e.
- ocular e.
- orbital e.
- quantitative e.
- topographic e.

echothiophate
- e. iodide
- e. phospholine

Eckardt
- E. ILM microforceps
- E. temporary keratoprosthesis

eclamptic hypertensive retinopathy
eclipse
- e. amblyopia
- e. blindness
- e. retinopathy
- e. scotoma

ECM
- extracellular matrix

E

Econochlor
Econopred
    E. Ophthalmic
    E. Plus
ECP
    endoscopic cyclophotocoagulation
    eosinophil cationic protein
ectasia, ectasis
    corneal e.
    iris e.
    post-LASIK e.
    e. of sclera
    scleral e.
    stromal e.
ectatic
    e. corneal dystrophy
    e. dilation
    e. marginal degeneration
    e. marginal degeneration of cornea
ecthyma
    e. contagiosum
    e. gangrenosum
ectiris
ectochoroidea
ectocornea
ectopia
    cilia e.
    e. lentis
    e. maculae
    macular e.
    posterior pituitary e.
    e. pupillae congenita
ectopic
    e. eyelash
    e. tissue
ectropion, ectropium
    Adams operation for e.
    atonic e.
    cicatricial e.
    complex e.
    congenital e.
    eyelid e.
    flaccid e.
    inflammatory e.
    involutional senile e.
    e. iridis
    lid e.
    e. luxurians
    mechanical e.
    medial e.
    paralytic e.
    pigment layer e.
    punctal e.
    e. sarcomatosum
    senescent e.
    senile e.
    spastic e.
    e. spasticum

    tarsal e.
    e. uveae
ectropionize
eczematoid blepharitis
eczematosa
    ophthalmia e.
eczematosus
    pannus e.
eczematous
    e. conjunctivitis
    e. pannus
ED
    effective diameter
    epithelial defect
eddy current
edema
    acute disc e.
    aphakic cystoid macular e.
    autosomal dominant cystoid
     macular e.
    Berlin retinal e.
    boggy e.
    brawny e.
    central e.
    cerebral e.
    choroidal e.
    ciliary body e.
    circumscribed retinal e.
    conjunctival e.
    e. of cornea
    corneal e.
    cystoid macular e. (CME)
    diabetic diffuse macular e.
    diabetic macular e. (DME)
    disc e.
    endothelial cell e.
    epithelial e.
    experimentally nduced retinal e.
    eyelid e.
    focal vasogenic e.
    foveal e.
    graft e.
    hereditary corneal e.
    high altitude cerebral e. (HACE)
    ischemic e.
    lid e.
    macular e.
    microcystic e.
    mucinous e.
    e. of optic disc
    optic disc e.
    perifoveal e.
    periorbital e.
    periretinal e.
    phakic cystoid macular e.
    progressive orbital e.
    prolonged eyelid e.
    pseudocystoid macular e.
    pseudophakic cystoid macular e.

recalcitrant diabetic macular e.
retinal e.
sight-threatening diabetic macular e.
Stellwag brawny e.
stromal e.
subconjunctival e.
tractional diabetic macular e. (TDME)
transient optic disc e.
widespread diffuse corneal e.

edetate disodium
edge
CeeOn E.
e. coating
e. contour
epithelial rolled e.
fimbriated e.
flap e.
e. glare
E. III hydrogel contact lens
optic e.
ragged wound e.
e. stand-off
wound e.

EdgeAhead
E. crescent knife
E. microsurgical knife
E. phaco slit knife

edge-light pupil cycle time
edger
edging of spectacle lens
Edinger-Westphal nucleus
edrophonium
e. chloride
e. chloride test

EDSS
Expanded Disability Status Scale
EDTA
ethylene diamine tetraacetic acid
EDTA chelation
Edwards syndrome
EEG
electroencephalogram
electroencephalography
EFEMP1 gene
effect
autokinetic e.
beneficial e.
blood oxygenation level-dependent e.
BOLD e.
Bracken e.
cat's-eye e.

ceramic e.
chromatic induction e.
copper-wire e.
Cotton e.
experimental secondary e.
Faden e.
fatigue e.
flash-lag e.
histopathologic e.
hyperchromic e.
immunosuppressive e.
lens flexure e.
E.'s of Light Reduction on Retinopathy of Prematurity
McCollough e.
muscarinic cholinergic side e.
myotonic dystrophy e.
neuromuscular e.
ocular motility e.
optical side e.
pantoscopic e.
prismatic e.
Pulfrich e.
pupillary e.
Purkinje e.
radiation e.
Raman e.
silver wire e.
Stiles-Crawford e.
sunburst e.
telephoto e.
thermal e.
threshold e.
Tyndall e.
Venturi e.
visual side e.
Zeeman e.

effective
e. diameter (ED)
e. refractory period (ERP)
efferent
e. fiber
e. nerve
efficacy of cyclosporine
efficiency
phaco e.
visual e. (VE)
effusion
choroidal e.
ciliochoroidal e.
e. light pipe
serous choroidal e. (SCE)
uveal e.

NOTES

Eflone
Efricel
EGb 761
Egger line
Egna-Neumarkt study
egocentric fixation distance
EGPS
European Glaucoma Prevention Study
Egyptian
E. conjunctivitis
E. ophthalmia
Ehlers-Danlos syndrome
Ehrhardt lid forceps
Ehrlich-Türk line
Ehrmann test
eidoptometry
eighth cranial nerve
Eikenella corrodens
eikonometer
Eisenmenger syndrome
EKC
epidemic keratoconjunctivitis
EKV
erythrokeratodermia variabilis
E-LASIK
epithelial laser-assisted intrastromal
keratomileusis
elasticity
elastic pseudoxanthoma
elasticum
pseudoxanthoma e. (PXE)
xanthoma e.
elastodysplasia
elastodystrophy
elastoid degeneration
Elastoplast
E. bandage
E. dressing
E. eye occlusor
elastorrhexis
elastosis
e. dystrophica
senescent e.
senile e.
elastotic band keratopathy
Elavil
El Bayadi-Kajiura lens
Eldridge-Green lamp
electric
e. light blindness
e. retinopathy
e. shock cataract
electrica
cataracta e.
ophthalmia e.
electrocauterizer
electrocautery
Geiger e.
Hildreth e.

Mentor wet-field e.
Mira e.
Mueller e.
ophthalmic e.
Op-Temp disposable e.
Rommel e.
Scheie e.
Todd e.
Valilab e.
von Graefe e.
wet-field e.
Ziegler e.
electrocoagulation
electrode
Berens e.
Burian-Allen bipolar contact lens e.
Clark-type polarographic e.
coagulating e.
corneal contact lens e.
cyclodiathermy e.
diathermy e.
gold disc Grass e.
Grass e.
Walker e.
electrodiaphake
electroencephalogram (EEG)
electroencephalography (EEG)
electroepilation
electrokeratotome
Castroviejo e.
electromagnetic
e. energy
e. interference (EMI)
e. radiation
e. removal of foreign body
e. scleral search coil
e. spectrum
electron
e. interferometer
e. interferometry
e. microscope
e. microscopy
electron-dense meshwork
electronegative
electroneurography (ENG)
electronic
e. tonometer
e. vitreous cutter
electronystagmogram (ENG)
electronystagmograph (ENG)
electronystagmography (ENG)
electrooculogram (EOG)
monocular e.
electrooculograph (EOG)
electrooculography (EOG)
electroolfactogram (EOG)
electroolfactography (EOG)
electroparacentesis
electroperimeter

electrophysiology
> visual e.

electroretinogram (ERG)
> cone b-wave implicit time e.
> flash e. (fERG)
> flicker e.
> e. flicker response
> focal e.
> full-field e.
> mosaic retinal dysfunction detection using multifocal e.
> multifocal e. (mfERG)
> pattern e.
> pattern-evoked e. (PERG)
> peak latencies of pattern e.
> rod e.
> standard full-field e.
> topographical e.

electroretinograph (ERG)
> Ganzfeld e.

electroretinographic monitoring

electroretinography (ERG)
> foveal cone e.
> multifocal e. (MFE)
> topographic e.

electrostatic interaction

elegans
> Caenorhabditis e.

element
> encircling e.
> imaging e.
> Kollmorgen e.
> Mira encircling e.
> retinal e.

Elestat ophthalmic solution

elevated glutamine level

elevation
> e. angle
> congenital optic disc e.
> corneal e.
> disc e.
> immediate e.
> parafoveal serous retinal e.
> sensory e.
> e. topography
> e. topography map
> Z-axis e.

elevator
> Desmarres lid e.
> Freer periosteal e.
> Joseph periosteal e.
> e. muscle
> e. palsy

> Sayre e.
> Tenzel e.

Elimite

Eliprodil

ELISA
> enzyme-linked immunosorbent assay
> ELISA antibody

ELK
> endothelial lamellar keratoplasty

Ellingson syndrome

Elliot
> E. corneal trephine
> E. operation
> E. sign
> E. trephine handle

ellipse
> bivariate normal e.
> superimposed e.

ellipsoid

ellipsoidal back surface

ellipsometer
> neovascularization of new vessel e.
> retinal e.

elliptic
> e. pupil

elliptical
> e. nystagmus
> e. trephination

Ellis
> E. astigmatism marker
> E. foreign body needle
> E. foreign body spud
> E. foreign body spud needle probe
> E. needle holder

Elschnig
> E. blepharorrhaphy
> E. body
> E. capsule forceps
> E. cataract knife
> E. central iridectomy
> E. conjunctivitis
> E. corneal knife
> E. cyclodialysis spatula
> E. extrusion needle
> E. fixation forceps
> E. keratoplasty
> E. pearl
> E. pterygium knife
> E. refractor
> E. retractor
> E. spoon
> E. spot

E

NOTES

Elschnig *(continued)*
 E. syndrome
 E. trephine
Elschnig-O'Brien forceps
Elschnig-O'Connor fixation forceps
Elschnig-Weber loupe
elsewhere
 neovascularization e. (NVE)
EM-1000 specular microscope
EMA
 epithelial membrane antigen
Emadine
embedded suture knot
embolic retinopathy
embolism
 retinal e.
embolus
 retinal e.
embryonal
 e. carcinoma
 e. epithelial cyst of iris
 e. medulloepithelioma
 e. medulloepithelioma of ciliary
  body
 e. nuclear cataract
 e. tumor of ciliary body
embryonic
 e. cataract
 e. fixation syndrome
 e. lens
 e. plate
embryopathic cataract
embryotoxon
 anterior e.
 posterior e.
EMDR
 eye movement desensitization and
  reprocessing
emedastine
 e. difumarate
 e. difurmarate ophthalmic solution
emergence
 angle of e.
emergency light reflex
emergent
 e. ray
 e. ray of light
Emerson 1-piece segment bifocal
EMGT
 Early Manifest Glaucoma Trial
EMI
 electromagnetic interference
 EMI digital imaging system
emissary canal
emittance
 radiant e.
emmetropia
emmetropic eye

emmetropization
 active e.
 e. process
EMP
 epiretinal membrane proliferation
emphysema
 e. of conjunctiva
 e. of orbit
 orbital e.
 subconjunctival e.
Empire needle
empirical
 e. horopter
 e. steroid treatment
empowerment
 Adolescent and Child Health
  Initiative to Encourage Vision E.
  (ACHIEVE)
empty
 optically e.
 e. sella
 e. sella syndrome
Emsley reduced eye
emulsification
 endocapsular vortex e.
emulsifier
 Pulsatome cataract e.
E-Mycin
en
 en bloc excision
 en bloc removal
encapsulated bleb
encephalitis
 e. periaxialis concentrica
 e. periaxialis diffusa
 Schilder e.
Encephalitozoon hellem
encephalocele
 basal e.
 orbital e.
 transsphenoidal e.
encephalofacial
 e. angiomatosis
 e. cavernous hemangiomatosis
encephalomyelitis
encephalomyelopathy
 subacute necrotizing e.
encephalomyopathy
encephalo-ophthalmic dysplasia
encephalopathy
 hypertensive e.
 lead e.
 Leigh e.
 Wernicke e.
encephalotrigeminal angiomatosis
encircling
 e. band
 e. band for scleral buckle
 e. element

e. explant
e. of globe operation
e. implant
e. polyethylene tube
e. procedure
e. of scleral buckle operation
e. silicone buckle
enclavation needle
Encore monthly disposable contact lens
endarteritis obliterans
end-gaze nystagmus
end-gripping forceps with standard jaw
end-labeling
in situ DNA nick e.-l.
endocapsular
e. balloon
e. balloon implantation
e. equator ring
e. phacoemulsification
e. vortex emulsification
endocrine
e. exophthalmos
e. lid retraction
e. myopathy
e. ophthalmopathy
endocrine-inactive adenoma
endocryopexy
endocryoretinopexy
endocyclophotocoagulation
endodiathermy coagulation
endogenous
e. bacterial endophthalmitis
e. dyslexia
e. fungal endophthalmitis
e. surface organism
e. uveitis
endoillumination
xenon e.
endoilluminator
Grieshaber e.
endolaser
e. coagulation
diode e.
e. probe tip
endolenticular phacoemulsification
endonasal
e. dacryocystorhinostomy
e. laser dacryocystorhinostomy
(ENL-DCR)
endoneural cell
endophlebitis of retinal vein

endophotocoagulation
argon laser e.
diode e.
endophthalmitis
Acanthamoeba e.
acute-onset e.
aseptic e.
bacterial e.
bleb-associated e.
Candida e.
candidal e.
chronic e.
endogenous bacterial e.
endogenous fungal e.
exogenous e.
fungal e.
granulomatous e.
infectious e.
Klebsiella e.
latent e.
metastatic e.
nocardial e.
e. ophthalmia nodosa
phacoanaphylactic e.
phacoantigenic e.
pneumococcal e.
postcataract e.
postinjection infectious e.
postinjection sterile e.
postoperative e.
posttraumatic e.
Propionibacterium acnes e.
recalcitrant anaerobic e.
sterile e.
systemic bacterial e.
toxocariasis e.
traumatic e.
E. Vitrectomy Study (EVS)
endophthalmodonesis
endophytum
glioma e.
endoplasmic reticulum
EndoProbe handpiece
endoresection
endoretinal
endoscope
MicroProbe integrated laser e.
ophthalmic e.
endoscopic
e. cyclophotocoagulation (ECP)
e. lacrimal surgery
e. laser-assisted
dacryocystorhinostomy

E

NOTES

endoscopic *(continued)*
    e. laser cycloablation
    e. laser dacryocystorhinostomy
    e. PEELS
    e. pigment epithelial endoscopic laser surgery
    e. raking
Endosol Extra
endothelial
    e. bleb
    e. cell
    e. cell activation
    e. cell analysis
    e. cell basement membrane
    e. cell count
    e. cell damage
    e. cell density (ECD)
    e. cell dystrophy
    e. cell edema
    e. cell loss
    e. cell morphometry
    e. cell side down
    e. cell surface of cornea
    e. cell transplantation
    e. corneal dystrophy (ECD)
    e. decompensation
    e. exudate
    iridocorneal e. (ICE)
    e. lamellar keratoplasty (ELK)
    e. permeability
    e. photograph
    e. plaque
    e. rejection line
    vesiculosus linear e.
endothelialitis
endotheliitis
    diffuse e.
    disciform e.
    HSV e.
    linear e.
    peripheral e.
endotheliopathy
    autoimmune corneal e.
    idiopathic corneal e.
    progressive herpetic corneal e.
endothelium
    e. camerae anterioris bulbi
    corneal e.
    diseased e.
    monolayered e.
Endotine TransBleph implant
endotracheal
    e. anesthesia
    e. intubation
    e. tube
endovascular closure
EndoView sapphire lens
end-piece

end-point
    e.-p. color
    e.-p. nystagmus
end-position nystagmus
Endrate
endrysone
end-stage
    e.-s. age-related macular degeneration
    e.-s. disease
Endura
energetic pulse
energy
    electromagnetic e.
    radiant e.
    radiofrequency e.
enflurane
enfolding
ENG
    electroneurography
    electronystagmogram
    electronystagmograph
    electronystagmography
engorgement
    conjunctival vascular e.
    episcleral vascular e.
    venous e.
enhancement
    astigmatic keratotomy e.
    LASIK e.
enlarged globe
enlargement
    blind spot e.
    corneal e.
    optical zone e.
    orbital e.
    tunnel e.
ENL-DCR
    endonasal laser dacryocystorhinostomy
enolase
    neuron-specific e. (NSE)
enophthalmia
enophthalmos, enophthalmus
    e. of fellow eye
    senescent e.
    e. wedge implant
enoxacin
Enroth sign
enstrophe
Enterobacter aerogenes
Enterococcus faecalis
enteropathica
    acrodermatitis e.
entochoroidea
entocornea
entophthalmia
entopic foveal avascular zone measurement

entoptic
 e. phenomenon
entoptoscope
entoptoscopy
entoretina
entrance pupil
entrapment
 extraocular muscle e.
 pupillary e.
entropion, entropium
 acquired e.
 acute spastic e.
 atonic e.
 cicatricial e.
 congenital e.
 eyelid e.
 e. forceps
 involutional e.
 involutional lower eyelid e.
 involutional senile e.
 marginal e.
 noncicatricial e.
 senescent e.
 senile e.
 spastic e.
 e. spasticum
 e. uveae
 uveal e.
entropionize
entry
 eyelid e.
 implant e.
entry-site alignment (ESA)
enucleate
enucleated
enucleation
 e. of eyeball operation
 e. scissors
 e. scoop
 e. spoon
 whole-globe e.
 e. wire snare
enucleator
 Castroviejo snare e.
 Foster snare e.
 snare e.
Enuclene eye drops
env **gene**
environment
 low-humidity e.
 telepresence e.
environmental risk factor

envision
 E. TD implant with fluocinolone
 E. TD intravitreal implant
 E. TD ophthalmic drug delivery
 device
enzymatic
 e. cleaner
 e. cleaner for extended wear
 e. digestion
 e. galactosemia
 e. glaucoma
 e. sclerostomy
 e. zonulolysis
enzyme
 antioxidant e.
 autologous plasmin e.
 e. cleaner
 e. defect
 e. glaucoma
 mitochondrial e.
 proteolytic e.
 surgical e.
**enzyme-linked immunosorbent assay
 (ELISA)**
EOG
 electrooculogram
 electrooculograph
 electrooculography
 electroolfactogram
 electroolfactography
EOM
 extraocular movement
 extraocular muscle
EOMI
 extraocular movement intact
eosinophil cationic protein (ECP)
eosinophilic
 e. globule
 e. granuloma
 e. intranuclear inclusion body
 e. reaction
 e. response
eosin-Y cell
ependymoma tumor
ephaptic transmission
epiblepharon
epibulbar
 e. dermoid cyst
 e. Fordyce nodule
 e. lesion
 e. limbal dermoid choristoma
 e. osseous choristoma
 e. tissue

E

NOTES

epicanthal
  e. correction
  e. inversus
  e. skin fold
epicanthic fold (ECF)
epicanthus
  e. inversus
  e. palpebralis
  e. supraciliaris
  e. tarsalis
epicapsular lens star
epicauma
epicenter
epiciliary proliferative tissue
epicorneascleritis
epidemic
  e. blindness
  e. conjunctivitis
  e. keratoconjunctivitis (EKC)
  e. typhus
epidermal
  e. growth factor
  e. inclusion cyst
epidermidis
  Staphylococcus e.
epidermoid
  e. carcinoma
  e. cyst
epidermolysis
  e. bullosa
  e. bullosa acquisita
  e. bullosa simplex
epidialysis
epidiascope
Epifrin
epikeratome
  Amadeus e.
  Norwood EyeCare e.
epikeratophakia
epikeratophakic keratoplasty
epikeratoplasty
  e. lenticule
  tectonic e.
epikeratoprosthesis
Epi-K microkeratome
epi-LASIK
  e.-LASIK procedure
  e.-LASIK surgery
epilation
epilator
epileptic nystagmus
EpiLift epikeratome system
E-Pilo
epimacular
  e. membrane
  e. proliferation
epimysium

epinastine
  E. HCl
  E. HCl ophthalmic solution
epinephrine
  e. bitartrate
  e. borate
  dipivalyl e.
  Duranest HCl with e.
  e. HCl
  lidocaine with e.
  Lidoject-1 with e.
  Marcaine HCl with e.
  e. and pilocarpine
  pilocarpine and e.
  Sensorcaine with e.
  Xylocaine with e.
epinephryl borate
epinucleus
epipapillary membrane
Epi-Peeler
  Sloane E.-P.
epiphora
  atonic e.
  episodic e.
  late-onset e.
epiretinal
  e. macular membrane
  e. membrane (ERM)
  e. membrane formation
  e. membrane proliferation (EMP)
  e. membrane traction
  e. pathology
episclera
episcleral
  e. angioma
  e. arterial circle
  e. artery
  e. blood vessel
  e. circulation
  e. explant
  e. eye plaque
  e. fibrosis
  e. hemangioma
  e. injection
  e. lamina
  e. nevus
  e. osteocartilaginous choristoma
  e. rheumatic nodule
  e. scarring
  e. space
  e. sponge
  e. tissue
  e. vascular engorgement
  e. vein
  e. venous pressure (EVP)
  e. vessel
episclerale
  spatium e.

episcleritis, episclerotitis
  childhood e.
  circumscribed e.
  gouty e.
  e. multinodularis
  nodular e.
  e. partialis fugax
  e. periodica fugax
  simple e.
  syphilitic e.
episode
  ischemic e.
  microembolic e.
  stroke-like e.
  thromboembolic e.
episodic
  e. epiphora
  e. unilateral mydriasis
episphaeria
  Fusarium e.
epitarsus pterygium
epithelia (*pl. of* epithelium)
epithelial
  e. adrenochrome deposition
  e. barrier
  e. basement layer
  e. basement membrane
  e. basement membrane disease
  e. basement membrane dystrophy
  e. bedewing
  e. bleb
  e. bleb disorder
  e. bulla
  e. cell
  e. congenital melanosis
  e. débridement
  e. debris
  e. defect (ED)
  e. dendrite
  e. diffuse keratitis
  e. downgrowth
  e. dystrophy of Fuchs
  e. edema
  e. erosion
  e. flap
  e. herpetic disease
  e. hyperplasia
  e. hypertrophy
  e. implantation cyst
  e. inclusion
  e. inclusion cyst
  e. infectious crystalline keratopathy
  e. ingrowth

  e. integrity
  e. invasion
  e. iron line
  e. laser-assisted intrastromal
    keratomileusis (E-LASIK)
  e. LASIK
  e. membrane antigen (EMA)
  e. microcyst
  e. migration
  e. mitosis
  e. nerve plexus
  e. nevus
  e. orientation
  e. plug
  e. punctate haze
  e. punctate keratitis
  e. rolled edge
  e. scrape
  e. scraper
  e. scraping
  e. separator
  e. slide
  e. transplantation
  e. trephine
  e. tumor
  e. turnover
  e. wrinkling
epithelialization
epitheliitis
  e. focal retinal pigment
  pigment e.
  retinal pigment e.
epitheliocapsularis
  fibrillopathia e.
epithelioid
  e. cell
  e. hemangioma
epithelioma, pl. epitheliomata
  e. adenoides cysticum
  intraepithelial e.
  Malherbe calcifying e.
  malignant ciliary e.
epitheliopathy
  acute multifocal placoid pigment e.
  acute multifocal posterior placoid
    pigment e. (AMPPPE)
  advancing wave-like e. (AWE)
  dendritic e.
  diffuse retina pigment e.
  lid wiper e.
  multifocal posterior pigment e.
  pigment e.
  placoid pigment e.

NOTES

E

epitheliopathy *(continued)*
  posterior pigment e.
  retinal pigment e.
epitheliosis desquamativa conjunctivae
epithelium, pl. **epithelia**
  e. anterius corneae
  basement membrane of corneal e.
  ciliary e.
  Cogan microcystic dystrophy of
    corneal e.
  congenital hypertrophy of retinal
    pigment e. (CHRPE)
  conjunctival e.
  corneal e.
  denuded corneal e.
  devitalized e.
  graft e.
  iris pigment e. (IPE)
  lens e.
  e. lentis
  migrating e.
  nonpigmented ciliary e.
  pigment e. (PE)
  e. pigmentosum iridis
  placoid pigmentation of e.
  e. posterius corneae
  retinal pigment e. (RPE)
  serous pigment e.
  stratified squamous e.
  subcapsular e.
  syngeneic e.
**epithelium-deprived orthotopic corneal
  allograft**
EpiVision blade
epizootic keratoconjunctivitis
Eppendorf tube
Eppy/N
EPS
  exophthalmos-producing substance
EPSA
  early postoperative suture adjustment
Epson 3200 Perfect Scanner
Epstein
  E. collar stud acrylic implant
  E. collar stud acrylic lens
  E. sign
  E. symptom
Epstein-Barr virus (EBV)
ePTFE
  expanded polytetrafluoroethylene
equal
  pupils round, regular, and e.
    (PRRE)
equation
  Baker e.
  Binkhorst e.
  Holladay-Binkhorst e.
  Rayleigh e.

equator
  anatomic e.
  e. bulbi oculi
  crystalline lens e.
  e. of crystalline lens
  eyeball e.
  geometric e.
  lens e.
  e. lentis
equatorial
  e. degeneration
  e. drusen
  e. meridian
  e. ring scotoma
  e. staphyloma
equilateral hemianopsia
equilibrating operation
equilibrium disturbance
equipment
  laser e.
  Volk Plus noncontact adapter cap
    and e.
equivalence
  therapeutic e.
equivalent
  e. distance
  mean spherical e. (MSE)
  migraine e.
  e. oxygen percentage value
  e. power
  e. refracting plane
  Snellen e.
  spherical e.
Er
  erbium
eraser
  E. cautery
  diamond-dusted membrane e.
  Mentor curved e.
  Mentor wet-field e.
  PeaceKeeper extrusion aspiration
    cannula e.
  Tano e.
Erb-Duchenne paralysis
erbium (Er)
  e. laser
**erbium:yttrium-aluminum-garnet
  (Er:YAG)**
Erb paralysis
ERD
  exudative retinal detachment
Erdheim-Chester disease
erect illumination
ERG
  electroretinogram
  electroretinograph
  electroretinography
  photopic ERG
ERG-Jet disposable contact lens

ergograph
ergonomics
    visual e.
ergonovine
ergot alkaloid
Erhardt lid forceps
erisophake
ERM
    epiretinal membrane
Ernest-McDonald soft intraocular lens-folding forceps
Ernest nucleus cracker
erosion
    e. capability
    coast e.
    corneal e.
    epithelial e.
    punctate epithelial e.
    recurrent corneal e.
    recurrent epithelial e.
    scleral e.
    sphincter e.
erosive vitreoretinopathy
ERP
    effective refractory period
erroneous projection
error
    astigmatic refractive e.
    asymmetric refractive e.
    Collaborative Longitudinal Evaluation in Ethnicity and Refractive E. (CLEERE)
    field of view e.
    hyperopic e.
    inborn e.
    myopic e.
    position e.
    refractive e.
    residual refractive e.
    retinal e.
    spherical refractive e.
    velocity e.
    wavefront e.
eruptive keratoacanthoma
Er:YAG
    erbium:yttrium-aluminum-garnet
    Er:YAG laser
    Er:YAG laser phacoemulsification
    Er:YAG phacolase
erythema
    e. chronicum migrans
    localized e.
    e. multiforme

    e. multiforme bullosum
    e. multiforme exudativum
    e. multiforme major
    e. multiforme major conjunctivitis
    ocular e.
erythematous
    e. pouting
    e. pouting of punctum
Erythrocin
erythroclastic glaucoma
erythrocyte
    ghost e.
erythroderma
    neonatal e.
erythrokeratodermia variabilis (EKV)
erythrolabe
erythrometer
erythrometry
erythromycin
erythrophagocytosis
erythropsia, erythropia
ESA
    entry-site alignment
    ESA system
escape
    e. phenomenon
    pupillary e.
Eschenbach
    E. low vision rehabilitation guide
    E. monocular telescope
    E. Optik lens
Escherichia coli
eserine
    Isopto E.
    e. sulfate
esocataphoria
esodeviation
    e. accommodation
    accommodative e.
    incomitant e.
    nonaccommodative e.
esophoria (E′)
    accommodative e.
    e. at near (E^1)
    A Trial of Bifocals in Myopic Children with E.
    classical congenital e.
    congenital e.
    near-point e.
    nonaccommodative e.
esophoric
esotropia (ET, ST)
    A e.

NOTES

E

esotropia *(continued)*
    e. accommodation
    accommodative e.
    acquired e.
    acute acquired comitant e. (AACE)
    alternate day e.
    alternating e.
    A-pattern e.
    basic e.
    clock-mechanism e.
    comitant e.
    congenital e.
    consecutive e.
    constant e.
    convergence excess e.
    cyclic e.
    decompensated accommodative e.
    essential infantile e.
    idiopathic congenital e.
    infantile e.
    intermittent e. (E(T))
    large-angle infantile e.
    late-onset e.
    left e.
    mixed e.
    near e. (ET′)
    nonaccommodative e.
    nonrefractive accommodative e.
    partial accommodative e.
    periodic e.
    refractive accommodative e.
    right e.
    sensory deprivation e.
    V-pattern e.
    X-pattern e.
esotropic
    e. amblyopia
    e. deviation
Espaillat-Deblasio nucleus rotator
essential
    e. anisocoria
    e. blepharospasm
    e. hypertension
    e. hypotony
    e. infantile esotropia
    e. iris atrophy
    e. phthisis
    e. phthisis bulbi
    e. progressive atrophy of iris
    e. telangiectasia
Esser inlay operation
ester
    unoprostone isopropyl e.
Esterman scale
esthesiometer, aesthesiometer
    Cochet-Bonnet e.
    noncontact corneal e. (NCCA)
    noncontact pneumatic e.
esthesioneuroblastoma

esthetics
    facial e.
Estivin II Ophthalmic
estropia
ET
    esotropia
ET′
    near esotropia
E(T)
    intermittent esotropia
etabonate
    loteprednol e.
etafilcon A lens
ETDRS
    Early Treatment Diabetic Retinopathy Study
        ETDRS laser photocoagulation
        ETDRS protocol
ethambutol
ether
    e. guard
    e. theory of light
Ethicon
    E. BV-75-3 needle
    E. micropoint suture
    E. Sabreloc suture
Ethicon-Atraloc suture
ethidium homodimer stain
ethmoid
    e. bone
    e. bulla
    e. canal
    e. exenteration
    e. sinus
ethmoidal
    e. artery
    e. incisure
    e. region
    e. sinus
ethmoidalis
    lamina orbitalis ossis e.
ethmoidal-lacrimal fistula
ethmoiditis
ethmoidolacrimalis
    sutura e.
ethmoidomaxillaris
    sutura e.
ethoxyzolamide
ethyl
    e. alcohol amblyopia
    e. cyanoacrylate
    e. cyanoacrylate glue
ethylene
    e. diamine tetraacetic acid (EDTA)
    e. glycol
ethylenediamine
    naphthyl e.
etidocaine

etiology
    cataract e.
    corneal endothelial
      decompensation e.
etiopurpurin
    tin ethyl e. (SnET2)
ETROP
    Early Treatment of Retinopathy of
      Prematurity
      ETROP study
EUA
    exam under anesthesia
eucatropine
euchromatopsy
European
    E. Contact Lens Society of
      Ophthalmologists
    E. Glaucoma Prevention Study
      (EGPS)
euryblepharon
euryopia
euryopic
euthyphoria
euthyscope
euthyscopy
evagination
    optic e.
evaluation
    An E. of Treatment of Amblyopia
      in Children 7-18
    genetic e.
    Low Vision Functional Status E.
      (LVFSE)
    reproducibility of e.
    scan e.
    Statpac-like Analysis for
      Glaucoma E. (SAGE)
    Structure And Function E. (SAFE)
    telemedical e.
    visual function e.
evaporation
    excess tear e.
    tear e.
evasion
    macular e.
evasive action
event
    adverse e.
    corneal infiltrative e.
    dark e.
    independent e.
Eversbusch operation

eversion
    double lid e.
    e. of eyelid
    lid e.
    e. of punctum
    single lid e.
everted
    e. eyelid
    e. punctum
everter
    Berens lid e.
    lid e.
    Roveda lid e.
    Schachne-Desmarres lid e.
    Struble lid e.
    Walker lid e.
everting suture
evisceration
    e. of eyeball
    e. operation
    e. spoon
evisceroneurotomy
Evizon
evoked
    e. nystagmus gaze
    e. potential
evolutional cataract
EVP
    episcleral venous pressure
EVS
    Endophthalmitis Vitrectomy Study
evulsion
Ewald law
EWCL
    extended wear contact lens
Ewing sarcoma
exam
    mandatory eye e.
    e. under anesthesia (EUA)
examination
    anterior segment e.
    biomicroscopic e.
    cytologic e.
    dark-field e.
    dilated retinal e.
    dilated stereoscopic fundus e.
    e. of eye
    flashlight e.
    frozen section e.
    fundus e.
    funduscopic e.
    glaucoma e.
    meibomian gland e.

E

NOTES

examination *(continued)*
 neurologic e.
 neuroophthalmologic e.
 ophthalmic e.
 ophthalmoscopic e.
 pediatric eye e.
 penlight e.
 slitlamp e. (SLE)
 Wood light e.
exanthematous conjunctivitis
excavated optic disc anomaly
excavatio disci
excavation
 atrophic e.
 glaucomatous e.
 e. of optic disc
 physiologic e.
 retinal e.
excess
 convergence e.
 divergence e.
 e. tear evaporation
excessive
 e. accommodation
 e. cyclodialysis cleft
 e. lacrimation
 e. rebound uveitis
exchange
 air-fluid e.
 fluid-air e.
 fluid-gas e.
 gas-fluid e. (GFE)
 intraocular lens e.
 IOL e.
 lens e.
 presbyopic lens e.
 refractive lens e. (RLE)
 tear e.
ExciMed
 E. UV200 excimer laser
 E. UV200LA laser
excimer
 e. laser
 e. laser, 193193-nm
 e. laser photorefractive keratectomy
 e. laser phototherapeutic
  keratectomy
 e. laser subepithelial ablation
 e. laser surgical technique
 e. laser system
 e. laser transepithelial photoablation
 e. laser trephination
 193-nm e. laser
excised eye
excision
 bare sclera e.
 en bloc e.
 eye e.
 e. of lacrimal gland operation

 e. of lacrimal sac operation
 pentagonal block e.
 primary e.
excitation
 l-cone e.
 M cone e.
 paradoxic levator e.
 s-cone e.
exciting eye
exclusion of pupil
excretory duct
excycloduction
excyclophoria
excyclorotation
excyclotorsion
excyclotropia
excyclovergence
excysting organism
exduction
executive
 American Academy of
  Ophthalmic E.'s (AAOE)
 e. bifocal
 e. spectacle lens
 e. trifocal
exenteration
 ethmoid e.
 eyelid-splitting orbital e.
 orbital e.
 e. of orbital contents operation
 subtotal orbital e.
exercise
 antisuppression e.
 blur and clear e.
 convergent e.
 eye tracking e.
 optometric visual e.
 pleoptic e.
exertional amblyopia
Exeter ophthalmoscope
exfoliation
 combined e.
 e. of lens
 e. of lens capsule
 e. syndrome (XFS)
 true e.
exfoliative
 e. glaucoma
 e. keratitis
 e. material
exit
 orbital e.
 e. pupil
exocataphoria
exodeviation
 comitant e.
exogenous
 e. disease

e. endophthalmitis
e. ochronosis
exophoria (X, XP)
alternating e.
comitant e.
concomitant e.
constant e.
near-point e.
exophoric
exophthalmic
e. goiter
e. ophthalmoplegia
exophthalmogenic
exophthalmometer
Hertel e.
Luedde e.
Marco prism e.
exophthalmometric
exophthalmometry
Hertel e.
Krahn e.
exophthalmos, exophthalmus
e. due to pressure
e. due to tower skull
endocrine e.
malignant e.
ophthalmoplegic e.
postural e.
pulsating e.
recurrent e.
e. reduction
substance e.
thyroid e.
thyrotoxic e.
thyrotropic e.
transient early e.
exophthalmos-producing substance (EPS)
exophytic
e. papillary capillary hemangioma
e. retinoblastoma
exoplant
Miragel e.
scleral e.
exorbitism
exotropia (XT)
A e.
alternating e.
A-pattern e.
basic e.
comitant e.
consecutive e.
constant e.
convergence insufficiency e.

divergence excess e.
divergence insufficiency e.
flick e.
intermittent e. (X(T))
large-angle e.
late-onset e.
left e.
paralytic pontine e.
periodic e.
right e.
secondary e.
sensory deprivation e.
V e.
V-pattern e.
X-pattern e.
exotropic
expanded
E. Disability Status Scale (EDSS)
e. polytetrafluoroethylene (ePTFE)
e. polytetrafluoroethylene SoftForm facial implant
expander
Beehler irrigating pupil e.
field e.
Graether pupil e.
irrigating pupil e.
scleral e.
expansion
normalized Zernike e.
expedition
Surgical Eye E.'s (SEE)
experience
microbiologic e.
experiment
Mariotte e.
Scheiner e.
experimental
e. apparatus
e. diabetes
e. secondary effect
experimentally induced retinal edema
explant
encircling e.
episcleral e.
Molteno episcleral e.
posterior e.
scleral e.
segmental e.
silicone sponge e.
sponge e.
trypsin-digested e.
explantation
IOL e.

NOTES

E

exploration
>sclerotomy with e.

explosive
>e. device
>e. globe rupture

exposure
>accumulated lead e.
>ambient light e.
>e. keratitis
>e. keratopathy
>ultraviolet radiation e.
>UV e.

expression
>e. of chemokine receptor
>nuclear e.
>transgene e.

expressivity

Ex-PRESS mini glaucoma shunt

expressor
>Arruga e.
>Berens e.
>hook e.
>e. hook
>Kirby hook e.
>Kirby intracapsular lens e.
>lens e.
>e. loop
>meibomian gland e.
>nucleus e.
>ring lens e.
>Rizzuti lens e.
>Verhoeff lens e.

expulsive hemorrhage

EXT-DCR
>external dacryocystorhinostomy

extend
>E. absorbable synthetic punctal implant
>E. punctal plug

extended
>e. range keratometry
>e. round needle
>e. wear contact lens (EWCL)
>e. wear hydrogel
>e. wear infection

extender
>Ahmed tube e.

extension
>ciliary body melanoma with extrascleral e.
>finger-like e.
>orbital e.

Extentabs
>Dimetane E.

externa
>axis oculi e.
>membrana limitans e.
>ophthalmoplegia e.

external
>e. ankyloblepharon
>e. axis of eye
>e. beam radiation
>e. beam radiation therapy
>e. beam radiation treatment
>e. canthotomy
>e. dacryocystorhinostomy (EXT-DCR)
>e. exudative retinopathy
>e. geniculate body
>e. hordeolum
>e. limiting membrane
>e. limiting membrane of retina
>e. ophthalmopathy
>e. ophthalmoplegia
>e. orbital fracture
>e. palsy
>e. pterygoid levator synkinesis
>e. rectus muscle
>e. route
>e. scar
>e. squint
>e. strabismus
>e. trabeculectomy

externo
>ab e.

externum
>hordeolum e.

externus
>axis bulbi e.

extinction
>e. phenomenon
>visual e.

extirpation

extorsion

extra
>AMO Endosol E.
>Endosol E.
>Ocuvite E.

extracanthic

extracapsular
>e. aphakia
>e. cataract (ECC)
>e. cataract extraction (ECCE)
>e. cataract extraction operation
>e. extraction of cataract
>e. phacoemulsification

extracellular matrix (ECM)

extraciliary fiber

extraconal fat reticulum

extracranial optic nerve decompression

extractable nuclear antigen

extraction
>Arruga cataract e.
>cataract e. (CE)
>cataract surgery and clear lens e.
>clear lens e. (CLE)

combined intracapsular cataract e.
(CICE)
extracapsular cataract e. (ECCE)
e. flap
foreign body e.
intracapsular cataract e. (ICCE)
e. of intracapsular cataract
intraocular cataract e.
lens e. (LE)
magnetic e.
planned extracapsular cataract e.

extractor
irrigating C-hook e.
irrigating cortex e.
Look cortex e.
Visitec cortex e.
Welsh cortex e.

extrafoveal retinal detachment
extramacular binocular vision
extramedullary
e. course
e. segment

extraocular
e. irrigating solution
e. motility
e. movement (EOM)
e. movement intact (EOMI)
e. muscle (EOM)
e. muscle disorder
e. muscle entrapment
e. muscle fibrosis
e. muscle palsy
e. muscles of Tillaux
e. muscle surgery
e. muscle testing

extraorbital disease
extrapyramidal
e. syndrome
e. system

extrarectus
extraretinal
e. fibrovascular proliferation
e. neovascularization

extrascleral outgrowth
Extra-Strength
MiraFlow E.-S.

extrastriate cortex lesion
extravasated blood
extravisual zone
extra-wide field capability
extrinsic muscle
extrusion
implant e.

e. needle
pellet e.

exudate
circinate e.
conjunctival e.
cotton-wool e.
endothelial e.
fatty e.
fibrin e.
fibrinous e.
foaming e.
hard lipid e.
lipid e.
macular e.
retinal e.
soft e.
waxy e.

exudation
proteinaceous aqueous e.

exudativa
retinitis e.

exudative
e. age-related macular degeneration
e. AMD
e. choroiditis
e. drusen
e. eye
e. idiopathic polypoidal choroidal
vasculopathy
e. retinal detachment (ERD)
e. retinitis
e. retinopathy
e. senile maculopathy
e. serous retinal detachment
e. vitreoretinopathy

exudativum
erythema multiforme e.

eye
aberrated e.
accessory organ of e.
accommodation of e.
acute red e. (ARE)
alkali burn to e.
amaurotic cat's e.
amblyopic e.
anterior pole of e.
anterior segment of e.
aphakic e.
appendage of e.
aqueous humor e.
artificial e.
asymmetric folds of e.'s
axial length of e.

E

NOTES

eye *(continued)*
    e. axial length
    bagginess of e.
    e. bank
    E. Bank Association of America
      (EBAA)
    e. banking risk factor
    better seeing e.
    bionic e.
    black e.
    blear e.
    bleary e.
    blind painful e.
    bony orbit of e.
    both e.'s (OU)
    Bright e.
    bulb of e.
    bulging e.
    cadaver e.
    E. Cancer Network
    E. Cap Ophthalmic Image Capture
      System
    e. care professional
    centrally fixing e.
    e. chamber
    e. chart
    chronic dry e.
    chronic red e.
    cinema e.
    circumduction of the e.
    Clear E.'s
    closed surgery on e.
    e. color
    compound e.
    conjugate deviation of e.'s
    conjugate movement of e.'s
    e. contact
    contact lens-induced acute red e.
      (CLARE)
    contralateral e.
    contusion of e.
    crossed e.'s
    crossing e.'s
    e. cup
    cyclopean e.
    cystic e.
    dancing e.
    dark-adapted e.
    e. deformation
    deviating e.
    disconjugate movement of e.'s
    diseased e.
    disjugate movement of e.'s
    disorder of e.
    e. displacement
    doll's e.
    dominant e.
    donor e.
    e. dropper

e. drops
20/20 e. drops
E. Drops AC
E. Drops Regular
Dry E.'s
emmetropic e.
Emsley reduced e.
enophthalmos of fellow e.
examination of e.
excised e.
e. excision
exciting e.
external axis of e.
exudative e.
e. fatigue
fellow e.
fibrous coat of e.
fixating e.
fixing e.
focus image quality of e.
following e.
fundus of e.
gas-filled e.
glaucomatous e.'s
e. globe
gritty e.
Gullstrand schematic e.
hare's e.
heavy e.
Helmholtz schematic e.
high myopia e.
e. holder
e. implant conformer
e. infarction
e. infirmary
inflammatory target site of e.
e. injury
internal axis of e.
iris e.
e. irrigating solution
itchy e.
jumping e.
e. knife guard
laser-treated e.
lateral angle of e.
lazy e.
left e. (LE, OS)
e. lens
light-adapted e.
Listing reduced e.
e. magnet
master e.
master-dominant e.
medial angle of e.
micromovement of e.
model e.
Moisture E.'s
Moisture E.'s PM
monochromatic e.

e. movement
e. movement behavior
e. movement desensitization and reprocessing (EMDR)
e. movement disorder
muscle of e.
e. muscle surgery
naked e.
near-emmetropic e.
nondominant e.
normal e.
e. occluder
old e.
orbicular muscle of e.
oval e.
e. pad
e. padding
e. pad dressing
painful e.
parietal e.
patch e.
phakic e.
photopic e.
phthisical e.
pineal e.
e. plaque
e. plaque surgery
e. point
Pontocaine E.
porcine e.
posterior pole of e.
posterior segment of e.
Preflex for Sensitive E.'s
Preservative-Free Moisture E.'s
e. pressing
primary e.
e. protector
protruding e.'s
pseudophakic e.
quiescent e.
raccoon e.'s
red e.
reduced e.
e. reflex
e. removed in toto
e. restored to normotensive pressure
right e. (OD)
rolling of e.'s
e. rotated inferiorly
e. rotation
e. rubbing
rudimentary e.

saccadic movement of e.
sagittal axis of e.
sandy e.
E. Scan corneal analyzer
schematic e.
scotopic e.
secondary e.
Sensitive E.'s
e. shape
e. shield
shipyard e.
e. size
Snellen reform e.
Soft Mate Comfort Drops for Sensitive E.'s
Soft Mate Saline for Sensitive E.'s
Soothe e.
e. spear
e. speculum
sphincter of e.
e. spot
e. spud
squinting e.
stony-hard e.
e. strain
E. Stream sterile eye irrigating solution
suspensory ligament of e.
e. suture scissors
e. swab
e. sweep
sympathizing e.
tension of e.
test e.
The E. Cancer Network
e. tissue
e. topography
e. tracking exercise
translocated e.
e. trauma
traumatized e.
tumor of interior of e.
vertical axis of e.
vision, each e. (VOU)
vitreous chamber of e.
e. wall
E. Wash
E. Wash solution
e. was quiet
watery e.
web e.
wet e.
white of e.

E

NOTES

eye *(continued)*
    wobbly e.
    worse e.
EyeArmor safety glasses
eyeball
    anterior chamber of e.
    anterior pole of e.
    anterior segment of e.
    e. compression reflex
    e. deformation
    dimpling of e.
    e. equator
    evisceration of e.
    fibrous tunic of e.
    luxation of e.
    meridian of e.
    pigmented layer of e.
    posterior pole of e.
    rectus muscle of e.
    e. sheath
    vascular coat of e.
eyeball-heart reflex
eyebrow
    e. fixation
    high e.
    e. laceration
    ptotic e.
eyecare
    e. practitioner
    Society for Excellence in E. (SEE)
EyeClose
    E. Adhesive strip
    E. external eyelid weight
eye-closure
    e.-c. pupil reaction
    e.-c. reflex
Eyecor camera
Eye-Cort
Eyecuity wireless visual acuity test
eyecup
eye/ear plane
Eye-Gene
eyeglass
    e. case
    e. frame
    e. repair kit
    e. retainer
eyeglobe
eyegrounds
eye-head
    e.-h. movement
    e.-h. shift
eyelash
    e. abnormality
    ectopic e.
    e. loss
    e. parallelism
    piebald e.

    e. ptosis
    e. tint
eyelash-induced leak
eyelid
    e. abnormality
    angular junction of e.
    e. apraxia
    e. architecture
    avulsion of e.
    baggy e.
    basal cell carcinoma of e.
    capillary hemangioma of e.
    carcinoma of e.
    e. coloboma
    e. contour
    e. crease
    e. crease incision
    crepitation in e.
    e. crusting
    crusty e.
    e. dermatochalasis
    e. disorder
    double eversion of e.
    drooping of e.
    easily everted upper e.
    ecchymosis of e.
    e. ectropion
    e. edema
    e. entropion
    e. entry
    eversion of e.
    everted e.
    e. fissure
    floppy e.
    e. flora
    e. flutter
    e. fold
    e. forceps
    free margin of e.
    e. fusion
    gland of e.
    gray line of e.
    e. hygiene
    e. imbrication
    incision into e.
    inelastic e.
    inflammation of e.
    e. injury
    e. innervation
    insufficiency of e.
    e. keratosis
    e. laceration
    e. landmark
    lateral commissure of e.
    e. lesion
    levator muscle of upper e.
    e. lichenification
    lower e.
    e. lymphangioma

e. malignancy
e. malposition
e. margin
e. margin disease
e. massage
medial commissure of e.
melanoma of e.
e. milia
e. molluscum contagiosum infection
e. muscle
e. myokymia
e. neurilemoma
e. neurofibroma
e. nevus
e. nystagmus
orbital portion of e.
e. papilloma
paradoxical movement of e.
e. plaque
plastic repair of e.
e. position
pseudobaggy e.
e. ptosis
e. puncture
reconstruction of e.
e. retraction
e. retractor
e. rhytide
e. sag
sign of edema of lower e.
sluggish movements of eyes and
   e.'s
e. spacer
e. spasm
e. speculum
squamous cell carcinoma of e.
1-stage reconstruction of eye
   socket and e.'s
e. strawberry hemangioma
e. surgery
e.'s sutured closed
suturing of e.
e. swelling
e. syringoma
e. taping
tarsal portion of e.
e. trauma
e. tuck
e. tumor
tumor of e.
e. twitch
unable to close e.
unilateral ptosis of e.

upper e.
e. vesiculation
xanthelasma around e.
eyelid-closure reflex
eyelid-sparing procedure
eyelid-splitting orbital exenteration
EyeLite photocoagulator
Eye-Lube-A Solution
EyeMap EH-290 corneal topography
   system
1-eye measurement
eye-of-the-tiger sign
Eye-Pak
   E.-P. II cover
   E.-P. II drape
   E.-P. II sheet
eyepiece
   comparison e.
   compensating e.
   demonstration e.
   Huygenian e.
   negative e.
   position e.
   positive e.
   Ramsden e.
   wide-field e.
eye-popping reflex
eye-referenced stimulus
eye-refractometer
eye-related variable
Eye-Scrub
Eye-Sed solution
eyeshot
eyesight
eyes-open coma
eyestone
eyestrain
EyeSys
   E. charting
   E. corneal analysis system
   E. 2000 corneal topographic
      mapping system
   E. corneal topography system
   E. surface topography system
   E. System 2000
   E. Technologies corneal topography
   E. videokeratograph
   E. videokeratoscope
eye-tracking system
eyewash (collyr.)
eyewear
   E Clips computer e.
   polycarbonate ballistic protective e.

E

NOTES

eyewear *(continued)*
    safety e.
    Timex TMX optical e.
    e. wardrobe

eyewire
EZ.1 multifocal contact lens
E-Z mount disinfectant kit
EZVue violet haptic intraocular lens

F
    filial generation
    focus
    visual field
FA
    fluorescein angiography
FAAO
    Fellow of the American Academy of
        Ophthalmology
    Fellow of the American Academy of
        Optometry
Fab fragment
Fabry
    F. disease
    F. syndrome
face
    anterior vitreous f.
    cow f.
    hyaloid f.
    intact anterior hyaloid f.
    f. line
    f. shield
    vitreous f.
face-down position
facet, facette
    corneal f.
facial
    f. anatomy
    f. anomaly
    f. asymmetry
    f. block
    f. cleft
    f. esthetics
    f. fracture
    f. hemangioma
    f. implant
    f. movement
    f. movement abnormality
    f. myokymia
    f. nerve
    f. nerve avulsion
    f. nerve lesion
    f. nerve misdirection
    f. nerve palsy
    f. nerve trunk
    f. neuroma
    f. nevus flammeus
    f. pain
    f. paralysis
    f. perception
    f. spasm
    f. synkinesis
    f. vein
    f. vision

facialis
    vena f.
facies, pl. **facies**
    f. anterior corneae
    f. anterior iridis
    f. anterior lentis
    f. anterior palpebrarum
    f. antonina
    f. bovina
    Hutchinson f.
    mask-like f.
    f. orbitalis alae magnae
    f. orbitalis alae majoris
    f. orbitalis ossis frontalis
    f. posterior corneae
    f. posterior iridis
    f. posterior lentis
    f. posterior palpebrarum
facility
    binocular accommodative f.
    letter chart accommodative f.
    loose lens accommodative f.
    f. of outflow
    vergence f.
facioauriculovertebral spectrum
FACS
    Fellow of the American College of
        Surgeons
FACT
    functional acuity contrast test
factitious
    f. blindness
    f. conjunctivitis
    f. mydriasis
factor
    ciliary neurotrophic f. (CTNF)
    environmental risk f.
    epidermal growth f.
    eye banking risk f.
    human antitumor necrosis f.
    independent risk f.
    lifestyle f.
    macrophage migration inhibitory f.
        (MMIF)
    modifiable risk f.
    nerve growth f.
    pigment epithelium-derived f.
        (PEDF)
    platelet-derived growth f.
    predictive f.
    preoperative risk f.
    risk f.
    surgery-related f.
    tumor necrosis f.
    unrecognized risk f.

F

factor *(continued)*
> vascular endothelial growth f. (VEGF)

factor-B
> platelet-derived growth f.-B

facultative
> f. hyperopia
> f. suppression

faculty
> fusion f.

Faden
> F. effect
> F. operation
> F. procedure
> F. suture

fade-to-clear capability
fading time
faecalis
> *Enterococcus f.*
> *Streptococcus f.*

FA/ICGA
> fluorescein angiography/indocyanine green angiography

failed
> f. graft
> f. ptosis surgery

failure
> bleb f.
> early bleb f.
> graft f.
> lacrimal pump f.
> late endothelial f.
> ocular surface f.
> primary graft f.
> progressive visual f.
> sympathetic innervation f.

faint
> f. flare
> f. hyperfluorescence

falciform
> f. fold of retina
> f. retinal fold

Falcon lens
Falls-Kertesz syndrome
false
> f. blepharoptosis
> f. image
> f. macula
> f. negative
> f. orientation
> f. positive
> f. projection
> f. ptosis
> f. scotoma
> f. vision

false-negative result
false-positive result

FAMA
> fluorescent-antibody-to-membrane antigen

famciclovir
familial
> f. arteriolar tortuosity
> f. autonomic dysautonomia
> f. autonomic dysfunction
> f. colloid degeneration
> f. drusen
> f. episodic ataxia
> f. exudative retinopathy (FER)
> f. exudative vitreoretinopathy (FEVR)
> f. fibrosis
> f. foveal retinoschisis (FFR)
> f. juvenile systemic granulomatosis
> f. lecithin-cholesterol acyltransferase deficiency
> f. lipoprotein deficiency
> f. paroxysmal ataxia
> f. periodic paralysis
> f. pseudoinflammatory macular degeneration
> f. pseudoinflammatory maculopathy
> f. retinoblastoma

Famvir
Fanconi syndrome
fantascope
far
> f. phoria
> f. point
> f. point of accommodation (FPA, p.r.)
> f. point of convergence
> f. sight

Farber disease
farinaceous epithelial keratitis
farinata
> cornea f.

Farkas-Bracken fixation forceps
Farnsworth
> F. D15 panel
> F. panel D15 test

Farnsworth-Munsell 100-hue color vision test
farsighted
farsightedness
Fas
> F. interaction
> F. liquid protein
> F. receptor density

Fasanella lacrimal cannula
Fasanella-Servat
> F.-S. procedure
> F.-S. ptosis operation
> F.-S. ptosis repair

fascia, pl. **fasciae**
> f. band

bulbar f.
f. lata sling for ptosis operation
f. lata stripper
muscular f.
orbital f.
palpebral f.

fascicle
abducens nerve f.
oculomotor nerve f.

fascicular
f. keratitis
f. ophthalmoplegia
f. ulcer

fasciculus
inferior longitudinal f.
longitudinal f.
maculary f.
medial longitudinal f. (MLF)
rostral interstitial medial
longitudinal f.

fasciitis
nodular f.
orbital f.

fashion
cerclage-type f.
in-tumbling f.
stepwise f.
X-linked f.

FasL interaction

fast
F. Grind 2200
F. Grind lens system
f. optic disc algorithm

FastPac
F. algorithm
F. 24-2 test

fat
f. adherence syndrome
f. cell
f. embolism of retina
f. graft
herniating orbital f.
mutton f.
orbital f.
f. pad
pterygopalatine f.
f. removal orbital decompression
(FROD)
f. reticulum
suborbicularis oculi f. (SOOF)

fatigable ptosis

fatigue
f. effect

eye f.
f. nystagmus
f. phenomenon

fatty
f. change
f. exudate

Faulkner
F. folder
F. lens-holding forceps

Favre dystrophy

FAZ
foveal avascular zone

FB
foreign body

Fc
fragment crystallizable
Fc fragment

fc
footcandle
foot-candle

FCI Ready-Set punctal plug

FCT
fluorescein clearance test
corrected FCT

FD
focal distance

FD2
Frisby-Davis 2
FD2 testing protocol

FDA-approved medication

FDACL
first definite apical clearance lens

FDT
frequency doubling technology
FDT perimetry

FDT-MD
frequency doubling technology mean
deviation

FDT-PSD
frequency doubling technology pattern
standard deviation

Feaster
F. adjustable eyelid speculum
F. Dualens lens
F. K7-5460 hydrodissecting cannula
F. radial keratotomy knife

feather
F. clear cornea knife
F. Touch CO_2 laser

feathery
f. appearance
f. clouding

F

NOTES

feature
> felt-like f.

Fechtner
> F. conjunctiva forceps
> F. ring forceps

Federov
> F. 4-loop iris clip
> F. 4-loop iris clip lens implant
> F. type I, II intraocular lens
> F. type I, II lens implant

feeder-frond technique
feeder vessel
feet
> f. motion at 3 f. (HM/3ft)
> Müller end f.

Fehr macular dystrophy
Feldman
> F. adaptometer
> F. buffer solution
> F. RK optical center marker

fellow
> F. of the American Academy of
> Ophthalmology (FAAO)
> F. of the American Academy of
> Optometry (FAAO)
> F. of the American College of
> Surgeons (FACS)
> f. eye
> F. of the Royal College of
> Physicians (FRCP)
> F. of the Royal College of
> Physicians of Canada (FRCPC)
> F. of the Royal College of
> Surgeons (FRCS)
> F. of the Royal College of
> Surgeons of Australia (FRCSA)

felt disc polisher
felt-like feature
femtosecond (FS)
> f. laser
> f. laser channel creation
> f. laser technique

fenestra, pl. **fenestrae**
fenestrae
> choriocapillaris f.

fenestrated
> f. chain
> f. sheen macular dystrophy

fenestration
> optic nerve sheath f. (ONSF)

fenretinide
fentanyl
Fenzel
> F. angled manipulating hook
> F. insertion hook
> F. lens-manipulating hook

FER
> familial exudative retinopathy

fERG
> flash electroretinogram

Ferguson implant
ferning
> tear mucus f.

Ferree-Rand perimeter
Ferrein canal
ferric
> f. ferrocyanide
> f. hyaluronate gel

Ferris-Smith
> F.-S. refractor
> F.-S. retractor

Ferris-Smith-Sewall
> F.-S.-S. refractor
> F.-S.-S. retractor

ferrocholinate
ferrocyanide
> ferric f.

ferrous sulfate
Ferry line
Ferry-Porter law
fetal
> f. cell
> f. fibronectin
> f. fibrovascular sheath
> f. hydantoin syndrome
> f. nuclear cataract
> f. nuclear opacity
> f. nucleus
> f. trimethadione syndrome
> f. vasculogenesis
> f. warfarin syndrome
> f. Y suture

fever
> acute pharyngoconjunctival f.
> pharyngoconjunctival f.

FEVR
> familial exudative vitreoretinopathy

fexofenadine
F&F
> fix and follow

FFF
> flicker fusion frequency

FFR
> familial foveal retinoschisis

FFSS
> Fluorouracil Filtering Surgery Study

FGCRT
> Foscarnet-Ganciclovir Cytomegalovirus
> Retinitis Trial

FHC
> Fuchs heterochromic cyclitis

fiber
> accessory f.
> auxiliary f.
> Brücke f.
> f. cell
> chief f.

cilioequatorial f.
cilioposterocapsular f.
circular ciliary muscle f.
collagen f.
cone f.
congenital medullated optic
  nerve f.
contiguous f.'s
continuous f.
corticonuclear f.
efferent f.
extraciliary f.
Gratiolet radiating f.
Henle f.
interciliary f.
intraocular myelination of retinal
  nerve f.
f. layer of axon
f. layer of Chievitz
lens f.
longitudinal f.
main f.
medullated nerve f.
meridional ciliary muscle f.
Monakow f.
Müller f.
myelinated retinal nerve f.
myoclonic epilepsy with ragged-
  red f.
nerve f.
oblique f.
optic nerve f.
orbiculoanterocapsular f.
orbiculociliary f.
orbiculoposterocapsular f.
parasympathetic f.
peripapillary retinal nerve f.
postganglionic f.
principal f.
pupilloconstrictor f.
pupillomotor f.
radial f.
ragged-red f.
Ritter f.
rod f.
Sappey f.
sensory f.
sphincter f.
sustentacular f.
trabecular f.
vitreous f.
zonular f.
Fiberlite microscope

fiberoptic
  f. diagnostic lens
  f. digital fundus camera
  f. light projector
  f. pick
  f. videoendoscope
fiberoptics
fiberscope
fiber-tracking method
fibra, pl. **fibrae**
fibril
  collagen f.
fibrillar material
fibrillin-1
fibrillogranular deposit
fibrillogranuloma
fibrillopathia epitheliocapsularis
fibrin
  Cell-Tak autologous f.
  f. dusting
  f. exudate
  f. gel
  f. glue
  f. influx
  intravitreal f.
  f. layer
  postvitrectomy f.
  f. pupillary block glaucoma
  f. sealant
  f. strand
  f. thrombus
fibrinogen glue
fibrinoid necrosis
fibrinolysis
  local intraarterial f. (LIF)
fibrinous
  f. aqueous
  f. cataract
  f. exudate
  f. iritis
  f. rhinitis
fibroblast
  Tenon f.
fibroblastic
  f. ingrowth
  f. meningioma
fibroglial membrane
fibroid cataract
fibroma
  orbital f.
fibromatosis
  orbital f.
fibromuscular dysplasia

F

NOTES

fibronectin
>fetal f.

fibroosseous tumor

fibroplasia
>cicatricial retrolental f.
>retrolental f. (RLF)

fibroproliferative membrane

fibrosa
>cataracta f.

fibrosarcoma
>orbital f.

fibrosclerosis
>multifocal f.

fibrosis
>congenital f.
>cystic f.
>episcleral f.
>extraocular muscle f.
>familial f.
>orbital eosinophilic angiocentric f.
>premacular f.
>preretinal macular f.
>subepithelial f.
>subretinal f.
>f. syndrome

fibrotic
>f. capsule
>f. PCO
>f. scar

fibrous
>f. coat of eye
>f. dysplasia
>f. frond
>f. proliferans
>f. tissue cuff
>f. tunic
>f. tunic of eyeball
>f. uveitis

fibrovascular
>f. frond
>f. membrane
>f. pannus
>f. pigment epithelium detachment
>f. proliferation
>f. scar
>f. sheath
>f. tunic

fibulin 5, 6 gene

Fick
>anteroposterior axis of F.
>F. axis
>axis of F.
>F. halo
>longitudinal axis of F.
>F. phenomenon
>sagittal axis of F.
>transverse axis of F.
>vertical axis of F.
>Z axis of F.

field
>altitudinal f.
>automated visual f.
>binasal quadrant f.
>binocular f.
>bright empty f.
>central visual f. (CVF)
>checkerboard visual f.
>confrontation visual f.
>cribriform f.
>f. cut
>dark empty f.
>f. defect
>depth of f.
>f. diaphragm setting
>f. expander
>f. of fixation
>Forel f.
>frontal eye f.
>f. of gaze
>Humphrey visual f. (HVF)
>hysterical constricted f.
>keyhole f.
>f. lens
>f. loss
>paracentral visual f.
>peripheral visual f.
>receptive f.
>remaining visual f.
>spiral f.
>star-shaped f.
>superonasal paracentral visual f.
>surplus f.
>Swiss-cheese visual f.
>temporal island of visual f.
>tubular visual f.
>tunnel f.
>f. of view
>f. of view error
>f. of vision
>visual f. (F, VF)
>wide f. (WF)

field-dependent aniseikonia

Fiessinger-Leroy-Reiter syndrome

fifth cranial nerve

figure
>Allen f.
>fortification f.
>Kanizsa f.
>Purkinje f.
>Rey-Osterreith Complex F.
>Zöllner f.

figure-of-8 suture

filament
>Ammon f.
>branching f.
>corneal f.
>f. keratitis
>myosin f.

filamentary
 f. keratitis (FK)
 f. keratome
 f. keratopathy
filamentosa
 keratitis f.
filamentous fungus
filariasis
Filatov keratoplasty
filial generation (F)
filiform dystrophy
filigree-like capillary
filler
 wrinkle f.
filling
 choroidal f.
 retinal arterial f.
film
 absorbable gelatin f.
 aqueous layer of tear f.
 conditioning f.
 debris-laden tear f.
 gelatin f.
 Gelfilm ophthalmic f.
 human tear f.
 plain f.
 postlens tear f.
 precorneal tear f.
 prelens tear f.
 preocular tear f. (POTF)
 proteinolipidic f.
 tear f.
 unstable tear f.
filmtab
 Rondec F.
filter
 blue light f.
 cobalt blue f.
 f. glasses for color testing
 interference f.
 f. management
 Millex f.
 Millipore f.
 neutral density f.
 f. paper strip
 pocket red f.
 Polaroid f.
 red f.
 red-free f.
 ultraviolet f.
 UV blocking f.
 Wratten f.

filtering
 bleb f.
 f. bleb
 f. bleb leak
 f. cicatrix
 f. implant
 f. operation
 f. procedure
 f. surgery
 f. valve
 f. wick
filtration
 f. angle
 f. surgery
 f. track
 transciliary f.
 Van Herick f.
filtrator
fimbriated
 f. edge
 f. margin
final threshold
finding
 clinicopathologic f.
 new physical f.
 physical f.
 posterior vitreous f.
 visual field f.
fine
 F. bimanual handpiece set
 f. blade
 F. crescent fixation ring
 F. dissecting forceps
 f. fibrillar vitreal degeneration
 F. gripping forceps
 F. III inserter
 f. iris process
 F. irrigating capsulorrhexis forceps
 F. irrigating reverse actuating
  splitting chopper
 F. magnetic implant
 f. punctate keratopathy
 f. retinal fold
 F. sideport actuating quick chopper
 F. sideport capsulorrhexis forceps
 F. suture scissors
 F. suture-tying forceps
Fine-Castroviejo suturing forceps
Fine-Nagahara phaco chopper
fine-needle aspiration
Fine-Thornton scleral fixation ring
fine-toothed forceps
fine-wire speculum

F

NOTES

finger
>f. count
>counting f.'s (CF)
>f. iridectomy technique
>f. mimicking
>f. tension
>f. vision

finger-counting vision
finger-like extension
fingerprint
>f. body myopathy
>f. corneal dystrophy
>f. line

finished
>f. contact lens
>f. glass

Fink-Weinstein 2-way syringe
Finnoff transilluminator
first definite apical clearance lens (FDACL)
first-degree relative
first-eye cataract surgery
first-grade fusion
Fisher
>F. exact test
>F. eye needle
>F. lid retractor
>F. spoon
>F. spud
>F. syndrome

Fisher-Arlt iris forceps
Fisher-Price
>F.-P. polycarbonate lens
>F.-P. polycarbonate lens for children

fishmouthing
fishmouth tear
fish-strike sign
Fison indirect binocular ophthalmoscope
fissura
>f. orbitalis inferior
>f. orbitalis superior

fissuratum
>acanthoma f.

fissure
>Ammon f.
>basin of inferior orbital f.
>calcarine f.
>choroid f.
>f. coloboma
>corneal f.
>eyelid f.
>inferior orbital f.
>interpalpebral f.
>lid f.
>orbital superior f.
>palpebral f.
>pterygomaxillary f.
>sphenoccipital f.

sphenoidal f.
sphenomaxillary f.
superior orbital f. (SOF)
water f.
f. zone

fistula, pl. fistulae, fistulas
>carotid cavernous sinus f.
>cavernous sinus f.
>f. of cornea
>corneal f.
>direct carotid cavernous f.
>dural carotid cavernous f.
>dural cavernous sinus f.
>ethmoidal-lacrimal f.
>internal lacrimal f.
>intraocular f.
>lacrimal f.
>f. lacrimalis
>scleral f.
>f. test

fistulizing surgery
fit
>prosthetic f.

fitting triangle
Fitz-Hugh and Curtis syndrome
Fitzpatrick sun-sensitivity scale
fix and follow (F&F)
fix-and-follow eye movement
fixate
fixating eye
fixation
>alternate f.
>anomalous f.
>f. assessment
>axis f.
>bifocal f.
>bifoveal f.
>binocular f.
>f. binocular forceps
>brow f.
>capsular f.
>central, steady and maintained f.
>change of f.
>conjunctival f.
>crossed f.
>CSM f.
>dislocated intraocular lens f.
>f. disparity
>eccentric f.
>eyebrow f.
>field of f.
>graft f.
>Guyton-Noyes f.
>f. hook
>f. instrument
>lens f.
>f. light
>line of f.
>locus of f.

f. mechanism
microplate f.
monocular f.
near f.
f. nystagmus
f. on moving object
f. pick
pigtail f.
point of f.
f. point
4-point f.
f. preference
f. reflex
f. ring
saccadic f.
split f.
sulcus f.
f. suture
f. target
transscleral suture f.

fixational ocular movement
fixed

f. dilated pupil
f. fold
f. forceps
f. mydriasis
f. point

fixing eye
fixus

strabismus f.
vertical strabismus f.

FK

filamentary keratitis

flaccid

f. canaliculus syndrome
f. ectropion

FLAIR

fluid-attenuated inversion recovery
FLAIR MRI

Flajani disease
flame

f. photometer
f. spot

flame-shaped hemorrhage
flammeus

facial nevus f.
nevus f.

flap

advancement f.
amputation of scleral f.
bicoronal scalp f.
Blaskovics f.
bridge pedicle f.

cheek f.
conjunctival f.
Cutler-Beard bridge f.
donut-cut f.
donut-shaped f.
f. edge
epithelial f.
extraction f.
fornix-based conjunctival f.
galeal f.
Gunderson conjunctival f.
hinged corneal f.
Hughes tarsoconjunctival f.
f. irregularity
limbus-based conjunctival f.
f. manipulation
modified Hughes f.
Mustarde rotational cheek f.
necrotic f.
f. operation cataract
partial conjunctival f. (PCF)
pedicle f.
pediculated f.
f. perforation
f. position
retinal f.
f. retraction
scalp f.
scleral f.
skin f.
sliding f.
f. stria
swinging lid f.
tarsoconjunctival f.
f. tear
Tenon f.
Tenzel rotational cheek f.
f. thickness
total conjunctival f. (TCF)
trabeculectomy f.
Van Lint f.

FlapMaker

F. disposable microkeratome
F. microkeratome system

flare

aqueous f.
cell and f.
faint f.
f. response
symptom f.

flared ABS tip
Flarex

F

NOTES

flash
- f. blindness
- f. electroretinogram (fERG)
- f. keratoconjunctivitis
- f.'s of light
- f. ophthalmia
- f. picture card
- f. stimulus
- f. visual-evoked potential (fVEP)

flash-lag effect

flashlamp-pumped microsecond pulse-dye laser

flashlight
- f. examination
- f. test

flask
- Primaria tissue culture f.

flat
- f. anterior chamber
- f. axis
- f. chorioretinal atrophy
- f. contact lens
- f. cornea
- f. cup
- f. demarcation line
- f. eye spud
- f. filtration bleb
- f. hook
- f. neovascularization

Flatau-Schilder disease

flat-edge lens

flattening
- keratometric f.

flat-top
- f.-t. bifocal
- f.-t. spectacles

flavimaculatus
- fundus f.

Flavobacterium
- *F. indoltheticum*
- *F. meningosepticum*

flavus
- *Aspergillus f.*

fleck
- f. dystrophy of cornea
- intraretinal f.

flecked
- f. corneal dystrophy
- f. retina
- f. retina disease
- f. retina of Kandori
- f. retina syndrome

flecken glaucoma

Fleischer
- F. dystrophy
- F. keratoconus ring
- F. vortex

Fleischer-Strümpell ring

flexible
- f. contact lens
- f. loop
- 5139 f. retinal brush
- f. translimbal iris retractor

flexible-wear contact lens

Flexlens lens

flexneri
- *Shigella f.*

Flexner-Wintersteiner rosette

FlexPlug
- Eagle F.

Flexsol

flick
- f. exotropia
- f. hypertropia
- f. movement

flicker
- f. amplitude
- distinct f.
- f. electroretinogram
- f. fusion
- f. fusion frequency (FFF)
- f. fusion frequency technique
- f. fusion frequency test
- f. fusion stimulus
- f. perception
- f. perimetry
- f. perimetry test
- f. phenomenon
- f. photometer

Flieringa
- curved scleral-limbal incision of F.
- F. scleral fixation ring

flight blindness

flint
- f. glass
- f. glass lens

flip-and-chop technique

flipping
- Brown technique of nuclear f.

flittering scotoma

floater
- f. eye model
- meniscus f.
- pigment f.
- pupillary f.
- vitreous f.

flocculus, pl. flocculi
- cerebellar f.
- f. syndrome

floor
- blowout fracture of orbital f.
- depression of orbital f.
- f. fracture
- irregular cup f.
- orbital f.

floppy
- f. eyelid

f. eyelid syndrome
f. eye syndrome
flora
    eyelid f.
    ocular f.
FloraGLO lutein
florid
    f. papillitis
    f. xanthelasma
floriform cataract
Floropryl Ophthalmic
Flouren law
floury cornea
flow
    aqueous humor f.
    axoplasmic f.
    BSS f.
    choroidal blood f. (ChBFlow)
    laminar f.
    ocular blood f. (OBF)
    retinal capillary blood f.
    reversed ophthalmic artery f.
     (ROAF)
    tear f.
    total steady-state tear f.
    uniform BSS f.
flow-based
    f.-b. phacoemulsification surgery
    f.-b. pump
flower petal pattern
flowgraphy
    laser speckle f.
flowmeter
    CLBF-100 blood f.
    Heidelberg retinal f.
    laser Doppler f.
flowmetry
    confocal scanning laser Doppler f.
Floxin
floxuridine
Floyd-Barraquer wire speculum
Flucaine
fluconazole
fluctuating vision
fluctuation
    diurnal f.
    visual field f.
flucytosine
fluff
    f. dressing
    vitreous f.
fluffed gauze dressing
fluffy appearance

Fluftex gauze roll
fluid
    amniotic f.
    aqueous f.
    f. cataract
    cerebrospinal f. (CSF)
    f. contact lens
    f. dynamics
    heavy f.
    Hylan biopolymer f.
    intraocular f.
    f. lamellar keratoplasty
    f. mechanics
    perioptic cerebrospinal f.
    petaloid accumulation of f.
    f. pulse
    f. retinopexy
    subarachnoid f.
    submacular f.
    submembrane f.
    subretinal f. (SRF)
    viscous ochre f.
    viscous xanthochromic f.
    Vitreon sterile intraocular f.
    warmed f.
    xanthochromic f.
fluid-air exchange
fluid-attenuated inversion recovery
   (FLAIR)
fluid-gas exchange
fluidic ILM separation
fluidless contact lens
fluid-ventilated lens
FluidVision implant
fluocinolone
    f. acetonide
    f. acetonide intravitreal implant
    Envision TD implant with f.
Fluoracaine
fluorescein
    f. angiogram
    f. angiogram test
    f. angiographer
    f. angiography (FA)
    f. angiography/indocyanine green
     angiography (FA/ICGA)
    f. clearance test (FCT)
    f. dilution test
    f. dye
    f. dye disappearance test
    f. dye and stain solution
    f. fundus angioscopy
    f. instillation test

F

NOTES

fluorescein *(continued)*
    intravenous f.
    f. irrigation
    f. isothiocyanate
    parafoveal f.
    f. pooling
    sodium f. (NaFl)
    f. sodium
    f. stain
    f. staining
    f. staining pattern
    f. stick
    f. strip test
    f. tear clearance
    f. tear clearance assessment
fluorescein-potentiated argon laser therapy (FPAL)
fluorescence
    blocked f.
    f. microscopy
    f. retinal photography
    UV-induced f.
fluorescent
    f. antibody test
    f. lamp
    f. treponemal antibody absorption
fluorescent-antibody-to-membrane antigen (FAMA)
Fluorescite
Fluoresoft
Fluorets fluorescein sodium strip
Fluorex 300, 500 contact lens
fluorexon
fluoride
    argon f. (ArF)
    neodymium:yttrium lithium f. (Nd:YLF)
fluorite
fluorobiprofen
fluorocarbon in contact lens
fluorometer
    CytoFluor II f.
fluorometholone (FML)
    f. acetate
    f. alcohol
    f. ophthalmic suspension
    sulfacetamide sodium and f.
fluorometholone/sulfacetamide (FML-S)
fluorometric technique
fluorometry
    noninvasive corneal redox f.
Fluor-Op
fluorophosphate
    diisopropyl f. (DFP)
fluorophotometer
    Fluorotron master f.
    slitlamp f.
fluorophotometry
    vitreous f.

Fluoroplex
fluoroquinolone antibiotic
Fluorotron
    Coherent radiation F.
    F. master fluorophotometer
5-fluorouracil (5-FU)
    topical 5-f.
Fluorouracil Filtering Surgery Study (FFSS)
Fluorox ophthalmic solution
flurbiprofen sodium
Fluress ophthalmic solution
flush
    choroidal f.
    ciliary f.
    circumciliary f.
    hemifacial f.
flute
    f. needle
    f. pipe
fluted spiral tubing
flutter
    f. dysmetria
    eyelid f.
    ocular f.
flux
    f. incident
    luminous f.
    oxygen f.
    radiant and luminous f.
    unit of luminous f.
fly
    f. test
    Titmus stereo f.
Flynn
    F. extrusion needle
    F. lens loop
    F. phenomenon
FM-500
    Kowa FM-500
FM-100 hue test
FML
    fluorometholone
    FML Forte
    FML SOP
FML-S
    fluorometholone/sulfacetamide
    FML-S Ophthalmic Suspension
foam cell
foaming exudate
focal
    f. attenuation
    f. choroiditis
    f. constriction
    f. depth
    f. distance (FD)
    f. dystonia
    f. electroretinogram
    f. granuloma

f. illumination
f. image point
f. interval
f. laser photocoagulation
f. laser treatment
f. length
f. myasthenia
f. necrotizing retinitis
f. scotoma
f. staining
f. trauma
f. vasogenic edema
foci (*pl. of* focus)
focimeter
focofilcon A
focus, pl. **foci (F)**
aplanatic f.
conjugate f.
F. Dailies Toric contact lens
depth of f.
detectable f.
f. image quality of eye
image-space f.
F. Lens Drops
F. Night & Day contact lens
object-space f.
principal f.
real f.
sustained f.
virtual f.
focusing
peripheral light f.
fogged manifest refraction
fogging
f. mechanism
f. retinoscopy
f. system of refraction
fog test
foil sheet
Foix syndrome
fold
arcuate retinal f.
asymmetric f.
chorioretinal f.
choroidal f.
ciliary f.
concentric f.
congenital retinal f.
conjunctival semilunar f.
Dennie-Morgan f.
Descemet f.
double lower lid f.
dry f.

epicanthal skin f.
epicanthic f. (ECF)
eyelid f.
falciform retinal f.
fine retinal f.
fixed f.
f. forceps
glabellar f.
Hasner f.
idiopathic choroidal f.
iridial f.
lacrimal f.
Lange f.
macular f.
meridional f.
mongolian f.
nasojugal f.
nasolabial f.
palpebral f.
palpebronasal f.
papillomacular retinal f.
primary retinal f.
retinal f.
retinal fixed f.
retrotarsal f.
semilunar f.
star f.
stiff retinal f.
foldable
f. acrylic lens
f. disc intraocular lens
f. intraocular lens surgery
f. IOP
f. iris-claw phakic IOL
f. 3-piece silicone IOL
f. plate-haptic silicone intraocular lens
f. silicone implant
folder
Faulkner f.
folding spectacles
folic
f. acid antagonist
f. acid deficiency
folinic acid
follicle
cilia f.
conjunctival f.
limbal f.
lymphoid f.
necrotic f.
follicular
f. conjunctivitis

F

NOTES

189

follicular *(continued)*
  f. hypertrophy
  f. iritis
  f. plugging
  f. trachoma
follicularis
  blepharitis f.
  keratosis f.
folliculorum
  Demodex f.
folliculosis
follow
  fix and f. (F&F)
following
  f. eye
  f. movement
Foltz valve
fomepizole
fomivirsen sodium
Fontana
  F. canal
  F. space
foot-candle, footcandle (fc)
  f.-c. meter
foot-lambert
footplate
  Müller cell f.
footprints of HSV
foramen, pl. **foramina**
  cranial f.
  inferior zygomatic f.
  infraorbital f.
  lacerate anterior f.
  lacerate middle f.
  lacerate posterior f.
  optic f.
  f. opticum
  orbitomalar f.
  rotundum f.
  f. of sclera
  Soemmerring f.
  f. sphenoidalis
  f. of sphenoid bone
  supraorbital f.
  f. supraorbitale
  zygomatic f.
  zygomaticofacial f.
  zygomaticoorbital f.
  zygomaticotemporal f.
force
  muscle f.
  shear f.
  tractional f.
forced
  f. choice preferential looking
  f. downward deviation
  f. duction
  f. duction test
  f. duction testing

  f. eye closure
  f. generation
  f. generation test
forceps
  Adson f.
  Akahoshi acrylic intraocular lens f.
  Akahoshi acrylic IOL loading f.
  Akahoshi implantation f.
  Akahoshi prechopper f.
  Alabama tying f.
  Alabama University utility f.
  Alfonso nucleus f.
  Alio capsulorrhexis f.
  Alio enclavation f.
  Alio iridectomy f.
  Alio MICS capsulorrhexis f.
  Allis f.
  Alvis fixation f.
  angled capsule f.
  Anis lens-holding f.
  Arroyo f.
  Arruga capsule f.
  Arruga-Nicetic ophthalmology f.
  Asch septal f.
  ASICO capsulorrhexis f.
  ASSI capsulorrhexis f.
  ASSI IOL inserter f.
  ASSI tubing introducer f.
  ASSI universal lens folding f.
  Azar lens-holding f.
  Bailey chalazion f.
  Baird chalazion f.
  Bangerter muscle f.
  Bansal LASIK f.
  Bard-Parker f.
  Barraquer cilia f.
  Barraquer-Colibri f.
  Barraquer conjunctival f.
  Barraquer corneal utility f.
  Barraquer hemostatic mosquito f.
  Barraquer-von Mandach capsule f.
  bayonet f.
  beaked f.
  Beaupre cilia f.
  Bechert lens-holding f.
  Bechert-McPherson angled tying f.
  Bennett cilia f.
  Berens corneal transplant f.
  Berens muscle f.
  Berens ptosis f.
  Berens suturing f.
  Berke ptosis f.
  binocular fixation f.
  bipolar f.
  Bishop-Harman crisscross f.
  Bishop-Harman foreign body f.
  Bishop-Harman tissue f.
  Blaydes corneal f.
  Blaydes lens-holding f.

blepharochalasis f.
Bonaccolto fragment f.
Bonaccolto jeweler f.
Bonaccolto magnet tip f.
Bonaccolto utility and splinter f.
bone-biting f.
Bonn iris f.
Bonn suturing f.
Botvin iris f.
Bracken fixation f.
Bracken iris f.
Brown-Grabow capsulorrhexis
  cystotome f.
Brown insertion f.
Bruening f.
Buratto flap f.
Buratto III acrylic implantation f.
Buratto LASIK F.
Buratto ophthalmic f.
Callahan fixation f.
capsule fragment f.
capsulorrhexis f.
Cardona threading f.
Cartman lens insertion f.
Casebeer capsulorrhexis f.
Castroviejo capsule f.
Castroviejo clip-applying f.
Castroviejo-Colibri f.
Castroviejo corneal-holding f.
Castroviejo corneoscleral f.
Castroviejo fixation f.
Castroviejo lid f.
Castroviejo scleral fold f.
Castroviejo suture f.
Castroviejo suturing f.
Castroviejo tying f.
Castroviejo wide grip handle f.
Catalano corneoscleral f.
Catalano tying f.
Cauer chalazion f.
chalazion f.
Chandler iris f.
Choyce lens-inserting f.
Cilco lens f.
cilia f.
Clark capsule fragment f.
Clayman lens-holding f.
Clayman lens implant f.
Clayman lens-inserting f.
clip-applying f.
coaptation bipolar f.
Cohen corneal f.
Colibri f.

conjunctiva f.
Connor capsulorrhexis peeler f.
cornea-holding f.
corneal fixation f.
corneal prosthesis f.
corneal splinter f.
corneoscleral f.
Cozean-McPherson tying f.
Crawford f.
cross-action capsule f.
Culler fixation f.
Cummings folding f.
cup f.
curved iris f.
curved tying f.
Dallas lens-inserting f.
Dan chalazion f.
Dardenne nucleus f.
Davis f.
de Juan ophthalmic pick f.
delicate grasping f.
delicate serrated straight dressing f.
Desmarres chalazion f.
disc f.
Dk IOL insertion f.
Dodick lens-holding f.
double-pronged f.
Douglas cilia f.
Draeger f.
dressing f.
Drews cilia f.
Ducournau fine gripping f.
Eber needle-holder f.
Ehrhardt lid f.
Elschnig capsule f.
Elschnig fixation f.
Elschnig-O'Brien f.
Elschnig-O'Connor fixation f.
entropion f.
Erhardt lid f.
Ernest-McDonald soft intraocular
  lens-folding f.
eyelid f.
Farkas-Bracken fixation f.
Faulkner lens-holding f.
Fechtner conjunctiva f.
Fechtner ring f.
Fine-Castroviejo suturing f.
Fine dissecting f.
Fine gripping f.
Fine irrigating capsulorrhexis f.
Fine sideport capsulorrhexis f.
Fine suture-tying f.

F

NOTES

forceps *(continued)*

fine-toothed f.
Fisher-Arlt iris f.
fixation binocular f.
fixed f.
fold f.
foreign body f.
Förster iris f.
Francis spud chalazion f.
Fuchs capsule f.
Fuchs extracapsular f.
Fuchs iris f.
Gaskin fragment f.
25-gauge intraocular f.
Gelfilm f.
Gifford fixation f.
Gifford iris f.
Gill-Arruga capsular f.
Gill-Colibri f.
Gill-Hess iris f.
Gill iris f.
Gills-Welsh capsule f.
Girard corneoscleral f.
Goldmann capsulorrhexis f.
Grabow f.
Gradle cilia f.
Graefe eye dressing f.
Graefe fixation f.
Graefe iris f.
Graefe tissue f.
grasping f.
Grayson corneal f.
Grazer blepharoplasty f.
Grieshaber diamond-coated f.
Grieshaber internal limiting
  membrane f.
Grieshaber iris f.
f. guard
Guist fixation f.
Gunderson muscle f.
Guyton-Noyes fixation f.
Halberg contact lens f.
Halsted curved mosquito
  hemostatic f.
Harman fixation f.
Harms-Colibri f.
Harms corneal f.
Harms-Tubingen tying f.
Harms tying f.
Hartmann mosquito hemostatic f.
Hasner lid f.
Heath chalazion f.
hemostatic f.
Henry cilia f.
Hersh LASIK retreatment f.
Hertel stone f.
Hess f.
Heyner f.
Hirschman lens f.

Hirschman lens-inserting f.
Holth f.
Hoskins beaked Colibri f.
Hoskins fine straight f.
Hoskins fixation f.
Hoskins miniaturized micro
  straight f.
Hoskins straight microiris f.
Hoskins suture f.
host tissue f.
House miniature f.
Hubbard corneoscleral f.
Hunt chalazion f.
Hyde corneal f.
Hyde double-curved f.
Ikeda microcapsulorrhexis f.
implantation f.
Inamura small incision
  capsulorrhexis f.
intraocular f.
Iowa State fixation f.
iris bipolar f.
Jacob capsule fragment f.
Jacobson hemostatic f.
Jaffe capsulorrhexis f.
Jaffe suturing f.
Jameson muscle f.
Jansen-Middleton septotomy f.
Jervey capsule fragment f.
Jervey iris f.
jeweler's bipolar f.
Jones f.
Judd f.
Kalt f.
Kansas fragment lens f.
Katena capsulorrhexis f.
Katzin-Barraquer f.
Kawai capsulorrhexis f.
Keeler extended round tip f.
Keeler intraocular foreign body
  grasping f.
Kelman-McPherson corneal f.
Kelman-McPherson lens-holding f.
Kelman-McPherson suturing f.
Kelman-McPherson tying f.
Kerrison f.
Kershner butterfly capsulorrhexis f.
Kershner LASIK flap f.
Kershner One-Step Micro
  capsulorrhexis f.
Kevorkian-Younge f.
Kirby capsule f.
Kirby corneoscleral f.
Kirby iris f.
Kirby tissue f.
Knapp f.
Knolle-Shepard lens-holding f.
Kraff fixation f.
Kraff intraocular utility f.

Kraff lens-holding f.
Kraff lens-inserting f.
Kraff suturing f.
Kraff tying f.
Kraff-Utrata capsulorrhexis f.
Kraff-Utrata intraocular utility f.
Kraft f.
Kratz lens-inserting f.
Kremer corneal fixation f.
Kremer 2-point fixation f.
Kuhnt fixation f.
Lalonde hook f.
Lambert chalazion f.
Lambert hook f.
Leahey chalazion f.
Lehner-Utrata capsulorrhexis f.
Leigh capsule f.
lens-holding f.
lens-threading f.
Lester fixation f.
lid f.
Lieberman lens-holding f.
Lieberman micro-ring lens f.
Lindstrom lens-insertion f.
Lister f.
Littauer cilia f.
Livernois lens-holding f.
Livernois pickup and folding f.
Lordan chalazion f.
Lucae dressing f.
Machemer diamond-dust-coated
  foreign body f.
Malis f.
Manche LASIK f.
Manhattan Eye & Ear suturing f.
marginal chalazion f.
Masket capsulorrhexis f.
matte black f.
Maumenee capsule f.
Maumenee-Colibri corneal f.
Maumenee corneal f.
Max Fine f.
McCollough suturing f.
McDonald lens-folding f.
McDonald soft IOL folding f.
McGregor conjunctival f.
McPherson angled f.
McPherson bent f.
McPherson corneal f.
McPherson irrigating f.
McPherson microiris f.
McPherson microsuture f.
McPherson suturing f.

McPherson tying iris f.
membrane peeling f.
Mendez multipurpose LASIK f.
Mermoud nonpenetrating
  glaucoma f.
micro Colibri f.
microserrated Tano asymmetrical
  peeling f.
miniature f.
Moody fixation f.
Moore lens f.
Moore lens-inserting f.
mosquito hemostatic f.
muscle f.
Nevyas lens f.
Newman collagen plug inserter f.
New Orleans Eye & Ear
  fixation f.
New York Eye & Ear Hospital
  fixation f.
Noble f.
Noyes f.
Nugent fixation f.
Nugent superior rectus f.
O'Brien fixation f.
Ochsner cartilage f.
Ochsner tissue f.
Ochsner tissue/cartilage f.
O'Connor iris f.
O'Connor lid f.
O'Connor sponge f.
O'Gawa suture-fixation f.
Ogura cartilage f.
Ogura tissue f.
Ogura tissue/cartilage f.
Osher foreign body f.
Passarelli 1-pass capsulorrhexis f.
Paton anterior chamber lens
  implant f.
Paton capsule f.
Paton corneal transplant f.
Paton suturing f.
Paton tying/stitch removal f.
Paufique suturing f.
Perone LASIK Flap F.
Peyman-Green vitreous f.
Phillips fixation f.
Pierse corneal Colibri-type f.
Pierse fixation f.
Pierse-type Colibri f.
Pley extracapsular f.
Pollock f.
pre-chopping f.

F

NOTES

forceps *(continued)*

Primbs suturing f.
Prince muscle f.
ptosis f.
Puntenney f.
pupil spreader/retractor f.
Quire mechanical finger f.
recession f.
Reese muscle f.
Reisinger lens-extracting f.
Rhein Artisan lens-holding f.
Rhein capsulorrhexis cystotome f.
Rhein fine foldable lens-insertion f.
Rhein LASIK flap f.
ring f.
ring-tip f.
Rizzuti rectus f.
Rizzuti scleral fixation f.
Rolf f.
roller f.
Russian f.
Rycroft tying f.
Sachs tissue f.
Sanders-Castroviejo suturing f.
Sandt f.
Sattler advancement f.
Sauer suture f.
Saupe cilia f.
Schaaf foreign body f.
Schepens f.
Schweigger capsule f.
Schweigger extracapsular f.
scleral twist-grip f.
Scott lens-insertion f.
series 5 f.
serrated conjunctival f.
Shaaf cilia foreign body f.
Shea f.
Sheets lens-inserting f.
Sheets-McPherson tying f.
Shepard intraocular lens f.
Shepard intraocular lens-holding f.
Shepard intraocular utility f.
Shepard lens-inserting f.
Shepard-Reinstein f.
Shepard tying f.
Shields f.
Shoemaker intraocular lens f.
silicone rod and sleeve f.
silicone sponge f.
Simcoe lens implant f.
Simcoe lens-inserting f.
Simcoe nucleus f.
Simcoe posterior chamber lens f.
Sinskey lens-holding f.
Sinskey micro-tying f.
Sinskey-Wilson foreign body f.
Skeleton fine f.
sleeve spreading f.

Smart f.
Smith-Leiske cross-action intraocular lens f.
smooth grasping f.
Snellen entropion f.
Snyder corneal spring f.
Spaleck f.
Spencer chalazion f.
Spero f.
splaytooth f.
Starr fixation f.
Stephens soft IOL-inserting f.
Stern-Castroviejo locking f.
Stern-Castroviejo suturing f.
Stevens iris f.
stitch-removal f.
Storz-Bonn suturing f.
Storz capsule f.
Storz cilia f.
Storz corneal f.
strabismus f.
straight-tip bipolar f.
straight tying f.
Strow corneal f.
superior rectus f.
suturing f.
Takahashi iris retractor f.
Tano micro serrated f.
Tennant-Colibri corneal f.
Tennant lens-inserting f.
Tennant titanium suturing f.
Tennant-Troutman superior rectus f.
Tennant tying f.
Tenner titanium suturing f.
Tenzel f.
Terson capsule f.
Terson extracapsular f.
Thomas fixation f.
Thornton fixation f.
Thorpe conjunctival f.
Thorpe corneal f.
Thorpe foreign body f.
Thrasher lens implant f.
tissue f.
titanium suturing f.
toothed f.
3-toothed f.
Troutman-Barraquer corneal fixation f.
Troutman-Barraquer corneal utility f.
Troutman-Castroviejo corneal fixation f.
Troutman-Llobera fixation f.
Troutman rectus f.
Troutman tying f.
tubing introducer f.
tying f.
tying/stitch removal f.

Universal II f.
Universal lens-folding f.
Utrata capsulorrhexis f.
Utrata-Kershner capsulorrhexis
cystotome f.
Verhoeff capsule f.
vertical f.
Vickers f.
vitreous foreign body f.
von Graefe fixation f.
von Graefe iris f.
von Graefe tissue f.
Waldeau fixation f.
Watzke f.
Weaver chalazion f.
Welsh pupil-spreader f.
Whitney superior rectus f.
Wies chalazion f.
Wilde f.
Wilkerson intraocular lens-
insertion f.
Wills Hospital utility f.
Wills utility eye f.
Wolfe f.
Worst implantation f.
Worth strabismus f.
Zaldivar iridectomy f.
Zaldivar micro acrylic lens
implantation f.
Zaldivar reverse capsulorrhexis f.
Ziegler cilia f.
Zurich suturing f.
Fordyce nodule
forebrain dysplasia
foreign
f. body (FB)
f. body bur
f. body cell
f. body extraction
f. body forceps
f. body locator
f. body needle
f. body sclerotomy
f. body sensation
f. body spud
Forel field
foreshortening
fornical f.
Forker retractor
form
F. Fit intracanalicular plug
medication f.
f. perception

f. sense
f. vision
wet f.
formalin-fixed tissue specimen
format
tagged image file f. (TIFF)
formation
atrophic scar f.
epiretinal membrane f.
macular hole f.
secondary membrane f.
symblepharon f.
form-deprivation myopia
formed image
forme fruste
FormFlex lens
formula, pl. **formulas, formulae**
Binkhorst f.
Cellufresh F.
Hoffer-Colenbrander f.
Hoffer Q f.
Holladay-Binkhorst f.
Holladay II · f.
ICaps Lutein & Zeaxanthin F.
IOL f.
lens-maker f.
MaxiVision ocular f.
MaxiVision whole body f.
Sanders-Retzlaff-Kraff f.
SRK f.
Vogel f.
formulation
algorithmic f.
fornical
f. conjunctiva
f. foreshortening
fornix, pl. **fornices**
f. approach
capsular f.
f. conjunctiva
inferior conjunctival f.
lacrimal f.
f. reformation
f. sacci lacrimalis
superior conjunctival f.
fornix-based conjunctival flap
forskolin
Forssman carotid syndrome
Förster
F. choroiditis
F. conjunctiva
F. disease
F. enucleation snare

NOTES

F

Förster *(continued)*
 F. iris forceps
 F. lacrimal sac
 F. operation
 F. photometer
 F. photoptometer
 F. sacci lacrimalis
 F. uveitis
Förster-Fuchs black spot
forte
 AK-Sulf F.
 B-Salt F.
 FML F.
 Inflamase F.
 Lipo-Tears F.
 Liquifilm F.
 Naphcon F.
 Ocu-Pred F.
 Pred F.
 Predair F.
 Prednefrin F.
 Sulfair F.
 Tears Naturale F.
fortification
 f. figure
 f. spectrum
fortified antibiotic
fortuitum
 Mycobacterium f.
forward
 f. light scatter
 f. traction test
Foscarnet-Ganciclovir Cytomegalovirus Retinitis Trial (FGCRT)
foscarnet sodium
Foscavir
fossa, pl. **fossae**
 f. glandulae lacrimalis
 hyaloid f.
 f. hyaloidea
 interpeduncular f.
 lacrimal gland f.
 lacrimal sac f.
 lenticular f.
 optical f.
 f. sacci lacrimalis
 trochlear f.
 f. trochlearis
 f. tumor
fossette
Foster
 F. Kennedy syndrome
 F. snare enucleator
 F. suture
Foucault knife-edge test
foundation
 American Macula Degeneration F. (AMDF)
 Glaucoma Research f.

Fourier
 F. algorithm
 F. harmonic analysis
Fourier-transformed vector
fourth
 f. cranial nerve
 f. nerve palsy
fovea, pl. **foveae**
 central f.
 f. centralis
 obscured f.
 trochlear f.
 f. trochlearis
foveal
 f. avascular zone (FAZ)
 f. burn
 f. center
 f. cone electroretinography
 f. cyst
 f. depression
 f. dimpling
 f. dystopia
 f. edema
 f. flicker fusion frequency
 f. image
 f. ischemia
 f. outer retinal dysfunction
 f. outer retinal function
 f. pit
 f. pseudocyst
 f. reflex
 f. retina
 f. retinal detachment
 f. sensitivity
 f. sparing
 f. splitting
 f. telangiectasia
 f. traction
 f. translocation
 f. vision
foveating saccade
foveola, pl. **foveolae**
 f. ocularis
foveolar
 f. choroidal circulation
 f. retinal detachment
foveomacular
 f. cone dysfunction syndrome
 f. retinitis
 f. retinopathy
 f. vitelliform dystrophy
foveoschisis
 myopic f.
Foville syndrome
Foville-Wilson syndrome
fowleri
 Naegleria f.
Fox
 F. aluminum shield

F. eye shield
F. irrigating/aspirating unit
F. irrigator
F. LASIK spatula
F. operation
F. speculum
F. sphere implant

FOZR
front optic zone radius

FP
fundus photo

FPA
far point of accommodation

FPAL
fluorescein-potentiated argon laser
therapy

FR3
third framework region

fraction
Snellen f.

fracture
apex f.
blow-in f.
blowout f.
combined f.
comminuted orbital f.
depressed f.
external orbital f.
facial f.
floor f.
midfacial f.
nasoorbital f.
f. of orbit
orbital blowout f.
orbital floor f.
orbital rim f.
orbital wall f.
pediatric orbital floor f.
roof f.
trap-door f.
tripod f.
white-eyed blowout f.
zygomatic f.

fragilis
Bacteroides f.

fragilitas ossium

fragmatome
CooperVision F.
F. flute syringe
Girard F.

fragment
anti-VEGF antibody f.
cataract f.

Cooper blade f.
f. crystallizable (Fc)
Fab f.
Fc f.
Hoskins razor blade f.
munitions f.

fragmentation
hydrogel exoplant f.
proportional f.

fragmentation/aspiration handpiece
fragment crystallizable (Fc)
fragmented dendrite
frame
celluloid f.
cellulose acetate f.
cellulose nitrate f.
f. difference
eyeglass f.
Lucite f.
molded f.
nylon f.
Oculus trial f.
optical f.
optyl f.
f. papillary distance
f. PD
Perspex f.
plastic f.
Plexiglas f.
polymethyl methacrylate f.
rimless f.
Scappa f.
f. scotoma
spectacle f.
Stryker f.
trial f.

frame-mounted pump
frameshift mutation
framework
scleral f.
uveal f.

Franceschetti
F. disease
F. dystrophy
F. syndrome

Franceschetti-Klein syndrome
Francis
F. spud
F. spud chalazion forceps

Francisella tularensis
François
central cloudy corneal dystrophy
of F.

F

NOTES

197

François *(continued)*
    dermochondral corneal dystrophy
      of F.
    dyscephalic syndrome of F.
    F. dystrophy
    F. syndrome
François-Neetens dystrophy
frank corneal ulceration
Frankfort horizontal plane
Franklin
    F. bifocal
    F. glasses
    F. spectacles
Franklin-style bifocal lenses
Fraser syndrome
Fraunhofer
    F. diffraction
    F. line
Frazier
    F. dura hook
    F. suction tube
FRCP
    Fellow of the Royal College of
      Physicians
FRCPC
    Fellow of the Royal College of
      Physicians of Canada
FRCS
    Fellow of the Royal College of Surgeons
FRCSA
    Fellow of the Royal College of Surgeons
      of Australia
freckle
    iris f.
Frederick sleeve spreader
free
    f. conjunctival autograft
    f. margin of eyelid
    f. operculum
    f. running mode
    f. skin autograft
    Tears Naturale F.
    f. tenotomy
Freeman
    F. punctum plug
    F. solution
Freeman-Sheldon syndrome
Freer
    F. chisel
    F. periosteal elevator
freezer
    Wallach cryosurgery f.
freeze-thaw cryotherapy
French
    F. catheter
    F. hook spatula
    F. lacrimal dilator
    F. lacrimal probe
    F. lacrimal spatula

    F. needle holder
    F. pattern spatula
**Frenkel anterior ocular traumatic
syndrome**
Frenzel
    F. goggles
    F. lens
frequency
    critical corresponding f. (CCF)
    critical flicker f. (CFF)
    critical flicker fusion f.
    f. doubling
    f. doubling illusion
    f. doubling perimetry
    f. doubling technique
    f. doubling technology (FDT)
    f. doubling technology mean
      deviation (FDT-MD)
    f. doubling technology pattern
      standard deviation (FDT-PSD)
    flicker fusion f. (FFF)
    foveal flicker fusion f.
    fusion f.
    F. 38 monthly disposable contact
      lens
    relevant spatial f.
fresh
    Lens F.
FreshLook
    F. ColorBlends lens
    F. contact lens
Fresnel
    F. lens
    F. membrane
    F. optics
    F. press-on prism
    F. principle
Frey syndrome
friable
Fridenberg
    F. stigmatometric card
    F. stigometric card test
Friedenwald
    F. funduscope
    F. law
    F. ophthalmoscope
    F. syndrome
Friedenwald-Guyton operation
Friedlander incision marker
Friedman
    F. hand-held Hruby lens
    F. Phaco/IOL manipulator
    F. tantalum clip
    F. test
Friedmann visual field analyzer
Friedreich
    F. ataxia
    F. syndrome

Frigitronics
Cilco F.
F. cryosurgical unit
F. freeze-thaw cryopexy probe
F. nitrous oxide cryosurgery apparatus
F. vitrector

frill
iris f.
plaited f.

Frin
Isopto F.

fringe
interference f.
Moiré f.

Frisby-Davis
F.-D. 2 (FD2)
F.-D. 2 distance stereoacuity test

Fritz vitreous transplant needle

FROD
fat removal orbital decompression

frond
fibrous f.
fibrovascular f.
sea f.
vascular f.
f. of vessel

front
f. build-up implant
f. optic zone radius (FOZR)
f. surface toric contact lens
f. vertex
f. vertex power

frontal
f. axis
f. bone
f. craniotomy
f. diploic vein
f. eye field
f. incisure
f. lobe
f. lobe unilateral cerebral hemisphere lesion
f. nerve
f. sinus
f. sinusitis
f. triangle
f. tuber

frontalis
facies orbitalis ossis f.
f. fascia lata suspension
incisura ethmoidalis ossis f.
margo supraorbitalis ossis f.

f. muscle
f. muscle sling
pars orbitalis ossis f.
f. sling technique
sulcus orbitales lobi f.
f. suspension surgery
vena diploica f.

frontolacrimal suture

frontoparietal bilateral cerebral hemisphere lesion

frontosphenoid suture

frontozygomatic suture

Frost
F. scissors
F. suture

frosted branch angiitis

Frostig Development Test of Visual Perception

Frost-Lang operation

frown line

frozen
f. globe
f. section examination
f. tissue

fruste
forme f.
keratoconus f.

FS
femtosecond

FS30 femtosecond laser

FTC
full to confrontation

5-FU
5-fluorouracil

Fuchs
F. adenoma
angle of F.
F. aphakic keratopathy
F. atrophy
F. black spot
F. canthorrhaphy operation
F. capsule forceps
F. combined corneal dystrophy
combined dystrophy of F.
F. crypt
dellen of F.
F. dimple
F. endothelial corneal dystrophy
F. epithelial corneal dystrophy
epithelial dystrophy of F.
F. epithelial-endothelial dystrophy
F. extracapsular forceps
F. heterochromia

NOTES

F

Fuchs *(continued)*
F. heterochromic cyclitis (FHC)
F. heterochromic iridocyclitis
F. inferior coloboma
F. iris bombe transfixation
operation
F. iris forceps
F. keratitis
lamella of F.
F. lancet-type keratome
F. retinal detachment syringe
F. spot coloboma
F. spur
F. stoma
F. syndrome
F. uveitis
F. 2-way syringe
Fuchs-Kraupa syndrome
fucidic acid gel
Fucidin gel
fugax
amaurosis f.
amaurosis partialis f.
episcleritis partialis f.
episcleritis periodica f.
keratitis periodica f.
saburral amaurosis f.
Fugo
F. blade
F. plasma blade anterior
capsulotomy
F. plasma knife
Fukala operation
Fukasaku
F. small pupil snapper hook
F. snap & split tip irrigating
chopper
F. spatula
Ful-Glo fluorescein strip
fulguration
full
f. to confrontation (FTC)
f. macular translocation
f. penetrating keratoplasty
f. versions and ductions
**full-arc depth-dependent astigmatic
keratotomy**
full-dimpled Lucite implant
Fuller silicone sponge
full-field
f.-f. electroretinogram
f.-f. system
full-thickness
f.-t. autograft
f.-t. corneal graft
f.-t. corneal laceration
f.-t. corneal wound
f.-t. keratoplasty

f.-t. macular hole
f.-t. retinal hole
fulminans
glaucoma f.
fulminant
f. abscess
f. glaucoma
f. myasthenia gravis
f. ocular toxoplasmosis
Ful-Vue
F.-V. bifocal
F.-V. ophthalmoscope
F.-V. spot retinoscope
F.-V. streak retinoscope
fumagillin
fumarate
ketotifen f.
Fumidil B
fumigatus
Aspergillus f.
function
bandpass f.
binocular f.
cone f.
cornea barrier f.
corneal epithelial barrier f.
foveal outer retinal f.
medial rectus f.
modulation transfer f.
motor f.
neural transfer f.
optical transfer f.
peripheral rod f.
point spread f. (PSF)
response f.
rod f.
spread f.
transfer f.
visual f.
wavefront aberration f.
f. of Zernike mode
functional
f. acuity contrast test (FACT)
f. amblyopia
f. blindness
f. defect
f. vision
f. visual acuity
f. visual acuity meter
f. visual loss
fundal reflex
fundectomy
fundus, pl. **fundi**
albinotic f.
albipunctate f.
f. autofluorescence
blond f.
f. camera
coloboma of f.

f. contact lens
f. diabeticus
f. examination
f. of eye
f. flavimaculatus
f. focalizing lens
f. laser lens
leopard f.
f. microscopy
mosaic f.
mottling of f.
normal f.
f. oculi
optic f.
pepper-and-salt f.
f. photo (FP)
f. photograph
prismatic f.
f. reflex
salt-and-pepper f.
sunset f.
tessellated f.
f. tigré
tigroid f.
tomato-ketchup f.
Funduscein
Funduscein-10, -25
funduscope
Friedenwald f.
funduscopic examination
funduscopy
fundusectomy
fungal
f. agent
f. blepharitis
f. corneal ulcer
f. endophthalmitis
f. eyelid infection
f. keratitis
f. uveitis
Fungizone
fungus, pl. **fungi**
filamentous f.
hyaline f.
nonfilamentous f.
saprophytic f.
funnel
Martegiani f.
muscular f.
vascular f.
funnel-shaped retinal detachment
furnacemen's cataract

furrow
corneal marginal f.
f. degeneration
f. dystrophy
f. keratitis
marginal f.
palpebral f.
scleral f.
superior palpebral f.
furrowing
Fusarium
F. episphaeria
F. moniliforme
F. oxysporum
F. solani
fuscin
fused
f. bifocal lens
f. multifocal lens
fusiform
f. aneurysm
f. cataract
fusion
amplitude of f.
f. area
bifoveal f.
binocular f.
f. breakpoint
central f.
color f.
critical flicker f. (CFF)
eyelid f.
f. faculty
first-grade f.
flicker f.
f. frequency
f. grade
motor f.
peripheral f.
f. reflex
second-grade f.
sensory f.
tenacious distance f.
tenacious proximal f.
third-grade f.
f. tube
f. with accommodation
f. with amplitude
Worth concept of f.
fusional
f. convergence
f. convergence amplitude
f. divergence

F

NOTES

fusional *(continued)*
    f. divergence amplitude
    f. movement
    f. reserve
    f. vergence

fusion-free position
Fusobacterium necrophorum
fVEP
    flash visual-evoked potential

Gaffee speculum
gag gene
Gaillard-Arlt suture
galactokinase deficiency
galactose cataract
galactosemia
  g. cataract
  enzymatic g.
Galassi pupillary phenomenon
galeal flap
Galen vein
galeropia
galeropsia
Galezowski lacrimal dilator
Galilean
  G. magnification changer
  G. microscope
  G. telescope
Galin
  G. bleb cup
  G. intraocular implant lens
gallium
  g. citrate contrast
  g. citrate contrast material
  g. scan
  g. scanning
galvanic nystagmus
game
  E g.
  paint-ball g.
  The Pointing G.
gamma
  g. angle
  g. crystallin
  g. irradiation
  g. light chain
ganciclovir
  g. cyclic phosphate
  G. Implant Study for
    Cytomegalovirus Retinitis
  g. intravitreal implant
  g. sodium
  g. therapy
Ganciclovir-Cidofovir Cytomegalovirus
  Retinitis Trial (GCCRT)
ganglia (pl. of ganglion)
ganglioglioma
ganglioma
ganglion, pl. ganglia
  basal g.
  g. cell
  g. cell layer
  cervical g.
  ciliary g.
  gasserian g.

geniculate g.
  g. layer of optic nerve
  g. layer of retina
  lenticular g.
  long root of ciliary g.
  motor root of ciliary g.
  oculomotor root of ciliary g.
  ophthalmic g.
  optic g.
  orbital g.
  pterygopalatine g.
  retinal g.
  sensory root of ciliary g.
  short root of ciliary g.
  sphenopalatine g.
  g. stratum of optic nerve
  superior cervical g.
  trigeminal sensory g.
ganglionectomy
  ciliary g.
ganglioneuroma
ganglionic
  g. layer of optic nerve
  g. layer of retina
  g. stratum of optic nerve
  g. stratum of retina
ganglionitis
ganglioside
gangliosidosis
gangraenescens
  granuloma g.
gangrenosa
  vaccinia g.
gangrenosum
  ecthyma g.
gangrenous rhinitis
Gans cyclodialysis cannula
Gantrisin
Ganzfeld
  G. bowl
  G. electroretinograph
  G. illumination
  G. sphere
  G. stimulation
gap
  nonius g.
gape
  wound g.
GAPO
  growth retardation, alopecia,
    pseudoanodontia, and optic atrophy
  GAPO syndrome
Garamycin
Garcia-Novito eye implant
Gardner syndrome

G

garter
  Goffman eye g.
Gartner
  G. canal
  G. cyst
  G. duct
  G. phenomenon
  G. tonometer
gas
  g. bubble
  C3F8 g.
  g. discharge lamp
  heavy g.
  hexafluoride g.
  inspired g.
  intraocular g.
  Ispan intraocular g.
  laughing g.
  long-acting g.
  mustard g.
  octafluoropropane g.
  perfluorocarbon g.
  perfluoropropane g.
  g. retinopexy
  SF6 g.
  sulfur g.
  sulfurhexafluoride g.
  g. tamponade
  tear g.
gas-filled eye
gas-fluid exchange (GFE)
Gaskin fragment forceps
gasoline
  jellied g.
gas-permeable
  g.-p. contact lens (GPCL)
  g.-p. daily cleaner
  rigid g.-p. (RGP)
Gass
  G. cataract-aspirating cannula
  G. corneoscleral punch
  G. dye applicator
  G. irrigating/aspirating unit
  G. macular hole classification
  G. muscle hook
  G. retinal detachment hook
  G. scleral marker
  G. scleral punch
  G. sclerotomy punch
  G. syndrome
  G. vitreous-aspirating cannula
gasserian ganglion
GAT
  Goldmann applanation tonometer
gatifloxacin ophthalmic solution
Gaucher disease
gauge
  blade g.
  Deitz incision depth g.

Deitz ophthalmic g.
depth g.
Katena depth g.
Marco radius g.
Mendez degree g.
radius g.
Reichert radius g.
Rowen white-to-white corneal g.
Shepard incision depth g.
Stahl lens g.
Steinert-Deacon incision g.
V-groove g.
Zaldivar degree g.
19-gauge
  19-g. irrigating axe
  19-g. irrigating chopper
25-gauge
  25-g. chandelier illumination system
  25-g. intraocular forceps
  25-g. sclerotomy
30-gauge needle
23-gauge sclerotomy
20-gauge straight bipolar pencil
Gault reflex
gaussian
  g. beam
  g. distribution
  g. optical system
  g. optics
gaze
  apraxia of g.
  cardinal diagnostic position of g.
  cardinal direction of g.
  g. center
  conjugate g.
  diagnostic position of g.
  disconjugate g.
  g. disorder
  distant g.
  downward g.
  dysconjugate g.
  eccentric g.
  evoked nystagmus g.
  field of g.
  horizontal g.
  lateral g.
  left g.
  midline position of g.
  g. movement
  near fixation position of g.
  g. palsy
  parallelism of g.
  paralysis of g.
  g. paretic nystagmus
  ping-pong g.
  primary position of g.
  psychic paralysis of fixation of g.
  right g.
  spasticity of conjugate g.

superior g.
supranuclear paresis of vertical g.
upward g.
vertical g.
gaze-evoked
    g.-e. amaurosis
    g.-e. nystagmus
    g.-e. tinnitus
gaze-holding
    eccentric g.-h.
G-banding
GC
    goniocurettage
GCA
    giant cell arteritis
GCAP1 protein
GCCRT
    Ganciclovir-Cidofovir Cytomegalovirus
      Retinitis Trial
GCD
    geometric center distance
GCM
    good, central, maintained
GCNM
    good, central, not maintained
GD
    glare disability
    global deviation
GDD
    glaucoma drainage device
GD-LD-208C minicamera
GDx
    GDx Access scanning laser
      polarimeter
    GDx nerve fiber analyzer
    GDx VCC scanning laser
      polarimeter
GDx-variable corneal compensator
Geggel
    G. corneal transplant marker
    G. PRK chiller
Geiger
    G. cautery
    G. electrocautery
gel
    Aquasonic 100 g.
    g. eye mask
    ferric hyaluronate g.
    fibrin g.
    fucidic acid g.
    Fucidin g.
    GenTeal lubricant eye g.
    HP Acthar G.

HP-Guar ophthalmic g.
Night & Day Tears Again sterile
  lubricant g.
ocular g.
Pilopine HS g.
pirenzepine ophthalmic g.
semisolid g.
silica g.
Tears Again Night & Day g.
TheraTears liquid g.
vitreous g.
gelatin
    g. disc
    g. film
gelatino-lattice
    g.-l. corneal dystrophy
    g.-l. corneal dystrophy analysis
gelatinous
    g. droplike corneal dystrophy
    g. mass
    g. material
    g. scleritis
gelatinous-appearing limbal hypertrophy
Gelfilm
    G. cap
    G. forceps
    G. ophthalmic film
    G. plate
    G. retinal implant
    Schepens G.
gel-fluid
    Hylan biopolymer g.-f.
Gelfoam
gellan
    timolol g.
Gemella
    G. haemolysans
    G. morbillorum
gene
    CYP1B1 g.
    disease-causing g.
    dominant g.
    down-regulated g.
    EFEMP1 g.
    env g.
    fibulin 5, 6 g.
    gag g.
    LMX1B g.
    g. locus
    master control g.
    metallothionein g.
    MHC g.
    myocilin g.

G

NOTES

gene *(continued)*
- nonpenetrant g.
- novel causative g.
- OCLM g.
- optineurin g.
- OPTN g.
- PEDF g.
- penetrant g.
- peripherin/RDS g.
- pol g.
- retinal degeneration slow g.
- retinitis pigmentosa GTPase regulator g. (RPGR)
- retinoblastoma g.
- SOD2 g.
- syntenic g.
- g. therapy
- TIGR g.
- TIMP3 g.
- g. transfer
- VMD2 g.

general
- g. anesthesia
- g. anesthetic
- g. cataract

generalized
- g. essential telangiectasia (GET)
- g. vaccinia

generating spectacle lens

generation
- filial g. (F)
- forced g.

genetic
- g. counseling
- g. evaluation
- g. eye research
- g. heterogeneity
- g. influence
- g. marker
- g. predisposition
- g. sequence
- g. variant

Geneva lens measure

Geneye Ophthalmic

geniculate
- g. body
- g. ganglion
- g. hemianopsia
- g. nucleus

geniculocalcarine
- g. radiation
- g. tract

genistein

genome synthesis

Genoptic S.O.P. ophthalmic

genotyping
- apolipoprotein E g.

Gentacidin ophthalmic

Gentafair

Gentak ophthalmic

gentamicin
- prednisolone and g.
- g. sulfate

gentamicin-induced vestibulotoxicity

Gentasol

GenTeal
- G. lubricant eye gel
- G. Mild
- G. Mild lubricant eye drops
- G. Moderate

Gentex PDQ polycarbonate lens

gentian violet marking pen

GentleLASE laser

Gentrasul

geographic
- g. choroidopathy
- g. helicoid peripapillary choroidopathy
- g. herpes simplex corneal ulcer
- g. keratitis
- g. lesion
- g. peripapillary choroiditis
- g. retinal atrophy
- g. ulceration

geometric
- g. axis
- g. center
- g. center distance (GCD)
- g. equator
- g. optics
- g. tenting

Geopen

geotropic nystagmus

geriatric population

Gerlach network

gerontopia

gerontoxon

Gerstmann-Straussler-Scheinker disease

Gerstmann syndrome

gestational
- g. age
- g. diabetes
- g. diabetes mellitus
- g. injury

GET
- generalized essential telangiectasia

Getman-Henderson-Marcus visual manipulation test

GFAP
- glial fibrillary acidic protein

GFE
- gas-fluid exchange

ghost
- Bidwell g.
- g. cell
- g. cell glaucoma
- dendritic g.
- g. erythrocyte

g. image
g. ophthalmoscope
g. scarring
g. vessel
ghosting
GHPI
Glaucoma Health Perceptions Index
GHT
glaucoma hemifield test
Gianelli sign
giant
g. aneurysm
g. axonal neuropathy
g. cell arteritis (GCA)
g. cyst of retina
g. drusen
g. epithelial cell
g. melanosome
g. papilla
g. papillary conjunctivitis (GPC)
g. papillary hypertrophy (GPH)
g. retinal break
g. retinal tear (GRT)
giantism
cerebral g.
Gibson
G. irrigating/aspirating unit
G. irrigator
G. technique
Giemsa stain
Gifford
G. delimiting keratotomy operation
G. fixation forceps
G. iris forceps
G. needle holder
G. reflex
G. sign
Gifford-Galassi reflex
Gilbert-Behçet syndrome
Gill
G. blade
G. corneal knife
G. incision spreader
G. intraocular implant lens
G. iris forceps
G. scissors
Gill-Arruga capsular forceps
Gill-Colibri forceps
Gillespie syndrome
Gill-Fine corneal knife
Gill-Hess iris forceps
Gillies scar correction operation

Gills
G. double irrigating/aspirating
cannula
G. double Luer-Lok cannula
G. pop-up arcuate diamond knife
Gills-Welsh
G.-W. aspirating cannula
G.-W. capsule forceps
G.-W. capsule polisher
G.-W. curette
G.-W. double-barreled
irrigating/aspirating cannula
G.-W. guillotine port
G.-W. irrigating/aspirating cannula
G.-W. knife
G.-W. olive-tip cannula
G.-W. scissors
G.-W. spatula
Gills-Welsh-Vannas angled micro scissors
Gimbel
G. fountain cannula
G. stabilization ring
ginkgo biloba
Ginsberg eye speculum
Girard
G. anterior chamber needle
G. cataract-aspirating needle
G. corneoscleral forceps
G. corneoscleral scissors
G. Fragmatome
G. irrigating cannula
G. irrigating tip
G. keratoprosthesis operation
G. phacofragmatome needle
G. phakofragmatome
G. procedure
G. scleral-expander ring
G. ultrasonic unit
Girard-Swan knife needle
girdle
limbal g.
limbus g.
Vogt white limbal g.
Gitelman syndrome
GL
green laser
glabella
glabellar
g. fold
g. frown line

G

NOTES

glabrata
  Candida g.
  Torulopsis g.
gland
  accessory lacrimal g.
  acinar lacrimal g.
  apocrine g.
  Baumgarten g.
  Bruch g.
  Ciaccio g.
  ciliary g.
  conjunctival g.
  drainage of lacrimal g.
  g. of eyelid
  Harder g.
  harderian g.
  Henle g.
  inferior lacrimal g.
  Krause lacrimal g.
  lacrimal g.
  meibomian sebaceous g.
  Moll g.
  nasolacrimal g.
  palpebral g.
  pineal g.
  pituitary g.
  Rosenmüller g.
  salivary g.
  sebaceous g.
  superior lacrimal g.
  tarsal g.
  tarsoconjunctival g.
  tear g.
  tear-secreting g.
  g. trachoma
  trachoma g.
  Waldeyer g.
  g. of Wolfring
  Wolfring lacrimal g.
  Zeis g.
  g. of Zeis
  zeisian g.
glandula, pl. **glandulae**
  g. lacrimalis
  g. lacrimalis inferior
  g. lacrimalis superior
glandular fossa of frontal bone
glare
  blinding g.
  dazzling g.
  direct g.
  g. disability (GD)
  disability g.
  g. disability measurement
  edge g.
  peripheral g.
  specular g.
  sun g.
  g. test

  veiling g.
  g. vision
glarometer
Glasgow card
glass
  g. bead
  Crookes g.
  crown g.
  g. disc
  finished g.
  flint g.
  High-Lite g.
  g. lens
  optical g.
  semifinished g.
  g. sphere implant
glassblower's cataract
glasses
  aphakic g.
  bifocal g.
  cataract g.
  child's g.
  contact g.
  crutch g.
  EyeArmor safety g.
  Franklin g.
  Grafco magnifying g.
  half g.
  Hallauer g.
  hemianopic g.
  hyperbolic g.
  liquid crystal g. (LCG)
  magnifying g.
  Masselon g.
  presbyopia g.
  protective g.
  reading g.
  red-green g.
  safety g.
  self-adjusted g.
  snow g.
  striated g.
  trifocal g.
  without g.
glassine strand
glass-rod
  g.-r. negative phenomenon
  g.-r. positive phenomenon
glassworker's cataract
glassy
  g. membrane
  g. sheet
glatiramer acetate
glaucoma
  absolute g.
  acute angle-closure g. (AACG)
  acute chronic g.
  acute congestive g.

acute primary angle-closure g.
(APACG)
g. agent
air-block g.
alpha-chymotrypsin-induced g.
angle-closure g. (ACG)
angle-recession g.
aphakic g.
apoplectic g.
aqueous misdirected g.
auricular g.
block g.
capsular g.
chamber-deepening g.
chronic narrow-angle g.
chronic open-angle g. (COAG)
chronic primary angle-closure g.
(C-PACG)
chronic simple g.
ciliary block g.
closed-angle g. (CAG)
combined g.
combined-mechanism g.
compensated g.
congenital g.
congestive g.
g. consummatum
contusion angle g.
corticosteroid-induced g.
cyclocongestive g.
g. damage
90-day g.
g. detection
developmental g.
Donders g.
g. drainage device (GDD)
drug-induced g.
enzymatic g.
enzyme g.
erythroclastic g.
g. examination
exfoliative g.
fibrin pupillary block g.
g. field defect
g. filtering bleb dysesthesia
g. filtering surgery
g. filtration surgery
g. filtration technique
flecken g.
G. Foundation of Australia
g. fulminans
fulminant g.
ghost cell g.

G. Health Perceptions Index
(GHPI)
g. hemifield test (GHT)
hemolytic g.
hemorrhagic g.
herpes zoster g.
high-tension g. (HTG)
hypersecretion g.
g. imminens
infantile g.
inflammatory g.
intermittent angle-closure g.
iris-block g.
juvenile g.
juvenile-onset high pressure g.
juvenile-onset open-angle g.
juvenile open-angle g. (JOAG)
laser-induced g.
G. Laser Trial (GLT)
G. Laser Trial Followup Study
(GLTFS)
latent angle-closure g.
late-onset g.
lens exfoliation g.
lens-induced secondary open-
angle g.
lens particle g.
lens protein g.
lenticular g.
low-pressure g.
low-tension g.
malignant g.
melanomalytic g.
monocular g.
mydriatic test for angle-closure g.
myocilin g.
narrow-angle g. (NAG)
neovascular angle-closure g.
noncongestive g.
normal-pressure g.
normal-tension g. (NTG)
obstructive g.
open-angle g. (OAG)
pediatric g.
g. pencil
penetrating keratoplasty and g.
(PKPG)
phacogenic g.
phacolytic g.
phacomorphic g.
phakic g.
pigmentary dispersion g.
postcataract pediatric g.

G

NOTES

glaucoma *(continued)*
  postoperative aphakic g.
  postoperative ghost cell g.
  primary angle-closure g.
  primary childhood g.
  primary congenital open-angle g.
  primary infantile g.
  primary open-angle g. (POAG)
  prodromal g.
  g. progression
  pseudoexfoliative g. (PEXG)
  pseudoexfoliative capsular g.
  pupil block g.
  pupillary block g.
  G. Research Foundation
  retrobulbar hemorrhage g.
  g. risk
  g. risk calculator
  rubeotic g.
  scleral shell g.
  secondary angle-closure g.
  secondary childhood g.
  secondary neovascular g.
  g. shunt
  simple g.
  g. simplex
  simplex g.
  g. sleep laboratory
  steroid g.
  steroid-induced g.
  g. suspect
  syndrome-associated g.
  trabeculitis g.
  transscleral neodymium:yttrium-
   aluminum-garnet
   cyclophotocoagulation for g.
  traumatic g.
  uveitic g.
  vitreociliary g.
  vitreous block g.
  wide-angle g.
glaucoma-related blindness
Glaucoma-Scope
glaucomatocyclitic crisis
glaucomatosa
  iritis g.
glaucomatous
  g. atrophy
  g. cataract
  g. cul-de-sac
  g. cup
  g. cupping
  g. damage detection by retinal
   thickness mapping
  g. excavation
  g. eyes
  g. habit
  g. halo
  g. nerve-fiber bundle scotoma

  g. optic nerve damage (GOND)
  g. optic neuropathy
  g. pannus
  g. ring
  g. visual field loss
Glaucon
glaucosis
Glaucotest
GlaucTabs
GLC1A locus
glia
glial
  g. fibrillary acidic protein (GFAP)
  g. fibrillary acidic protein antibody
  g. proliferation
  g. ring
glial-neural hamartoma
glide
  intraocular lens g.
  lens g.
  Sheets lens g.
glioblastoma multiforme
gliocyte
  retinal g.
glioma
  anterior visual pathway g.
  astrocytic g.
  chiasmal g.
  g. endophytum
  hypothalamic g.
  intracranial g.
  g. of optic chiasm
  optic nerve g.
  optic pathway g.
  orbital g.
  peripheral g.
  g. of retina
  retinal g.
  g. sarcomatosum
  telangiectatic g.
gliomatosis
gliomatous
glioneuroma
gliosarcoma
  retinal g.
gliosis
  neonatal g.
  premacular g.
  preretinal g.
  retinal g.
  traumatic g.
gliotic
  g. membrane
  g. strip
glistening opacity
Gln368Stop mutation
global
  g. cataract
  g. deviation (GD)

globe
>contact burns of g.
>contusion of g.
>g. deformation
>destroyed g.
>disorganized g.
>g. displacement
>enlarged g.
>eye g.
>frozen g.
>g. indentation
>luxation of g.
>open g.
>g. perforation
>g. puncture
>g. remnant
>ruptured g.

globosa
>cornea g.

globule
>eosinophilic g.
>Morgagni g.
>morgagnian g.
>ora g.

globus pallidus (GP)
glomerulonephritis
>membranoproliferative g. type II

gloss
>peripheral silvery g.

glove
>Biogel Sensor surgical g.

glower
>Nernst g.

GLP
>grid laser photocoagulation

GLT
>Glaucoma Laser Trial

GLTFS
>Glaucoma Laser Trial Followup Study

Glucantime
glucocorticoid
>ophthalmic g.
>systemic g.
>topical g.

glucose 6-phosphate dehydrogenase
glue
>butyl cyanoacrylate g.
>cyanoacrylate tissue g.
>ethyl cyanoacrylate g.
>fibrin g.
>fibrinogen g.
>histoacryl g.
>methyl cyanoacrylate g.

>N-butyl-2-cyanoacrylate g.
>g. patch
>g. patch leak
>self-gelling g.

glued-on hard contact lens
glutamine level
glutamyltransferase
glycerin
glycerin-preserved graft
glycerol
>anhydrase g.

glyceryl monostearate
glycocalyx matrix
glycogen granule
glycol
>dihydrophenylethylene g. (DHPG)
>ethylene g.
>polyethylene g.
>propylene g.

glycoprotein
>mucin-like g.
>transmembrane g.

glycosaminoglycan
glycosylated hemoglobin
Glyrol
GMS
>Gomori methenamine silver

goal
>intraocular pressure g.

goblet
>g. cell
>g. cell hyperplasia

Goffman eye garter
goggles
>dry eye g.
>Frenzel g.
>moisture g.
>night-vision g.
>pinhole g.
>plethysmographic g.
>sports g.
>swimmer's g.
>Zoom and Sniper sports g.

goiter
>exophthalmic g.

gold
>g. disc Grass electrode
>g. dust retinopathy
>g. eyelid load implant
>g. eye plaque
>g. microshunt implantation
>g. salt
>g. sodium thiomalate

G

NOTES

gold *(continued)*
    g. sphere implant
    g. tattoo pigment
    g. weight
    g. weight implantation
Goldenhar-Gorlin syndrome
Goldenhar syndrome (GS)
golden tapetal-like fundus reflex
Goldflam disease
Goldflam-Erb disease
Goldmann
    G. applanation tonometer (GAT)
    G. capsulorrhexis forceps
    G. Coherent radiation
    G. contact lens prism
    G. diagnostic contact lens
    G. fundus contact lens
    G. goniolens
    G. kinetic perimetry
    G. kinetic technique
    G. macular contact lens
    G. manual projection perimeter
    G. 3-mirror contact diagnostic lens
    G. 3-mirror implant
    G. 3-mirror prism
    G. multi-mirror lens
    G. serrated knife
    G. static technique
    G. tonometer
    G. visual field test
Goldmann-Favre
    G.-F. disease
    G.-F. dystrophy
    G.-F. retinoschisis
    G.-F. syndrome
Goldmann-Weekers dark adaptometer
Goldman scleral fixation ring and blepharostat
Goldstein
    G. anterior chamber syringe
    G. cannula
    G. golf-club spud
    G. lacrimal sac retractor
    G. lacrimal syringe
    G. refractor
Golgi
    G. apparatus
    G. complex
    G. I, II neuron
Goltz-Gorlin syndrome
Goltz syndrome
Gomori
    G. methenamine silver (GMS)
    G. methenamine silver stain
Gonak ophthalmic solution
GOND
    glaucomatous optic nerve damage
gondii
    Toxoplasma g.

Gonin
    G. cautery operation
    G. marker
goniocurettage (GC)
goniodysgenesis
goniogram
goniolens
    Allen-Thorpe g.
    Barkan g.
    Goldmann g.
    Koeppe g.
    g. lens
    4-mirror g.
    single-mirror g.
    Zeiss g.
goniometer
    Bailliart g.
goniophotocoagulation
goniophotography
gonioplasty
gonioprism
    Posner diagnostic g.
    Posner surgical g.
    Swan-Jacob g.
goniopuncture
gonioscope
    Sussman 4-mirror g.
    Thorpe surgical g.
    Zeiss g.
gonioscopic
    g. implant
    g. lens
    g. prism
gonioscopy
    compression g.
    dark-room g.
    indentation g.
    Koeppe g.
Goniosoft
Goniosol
goniosynechia
goniosynechialysis (GSL)
goniotomy
    g. knife
    g. knife cannula
    g. needle holder
    g. operation
    photoablative laser g. (PLG)
gonoblennorrhea
gonococcal
    g. bacillus
    g. conjunctivitis
    g. infection
    g. keratitis
    g. ophthalmia
gonorrheal
    g. conjunctivitis
    g. ophthalmia

gonorrhoeae
Neisseria g.
good
g., central, maintained (GCM)
g., central, not maintained (GCNM)
G. retractor
Gorham
G. disease
massive osteolysis of G.
Gorham-Stout syndrome
gossamer scarring
gouge
lacrimal sac g.
spud and g.
g. spud
Todd g.
West g.
Gould intraocular implant lens
gouty
g. diabetes
g. episcleritis
g. iritis
Gower sign
GP
globus pallidus
GPC
giant papillary conjunctivitis
GPCL
gas-permeable contact lens
GPH
giant papillary hypertrophy
Grabow forceps
graceful swirling rod
Gradal individual customized
progressive lens
grade
fusion g.
Gradenigo syndrome
gradient
hydrostatic g.
g. method
grading
Broders g.
lens opacities classification system
III g.
g. of retinal nerve fiber layer
Gradle
G. cilia forceps
G. corneal trephine
graduated
g. fine focus mechanism
g. side port
g. tenotomy

Graefe
G. cataract knife
G. cystotome
G. cystotome knife
G. disease
G. eye dressing forceps
G. fixation forceps
G. iris forceps
G. needle
G. operation
G. sign
G. strabismus hook
G. syndrome
G. test
G. tissue forceps
Graether
G. button hook
G. collar button
G. collar button micro iris
retractor
G. pupil expander
G. refractor
Grafco
G. eye shield
G. magnifying glasses
graft
Amsler corneal g.
anular corneal g.
autogenous dermis fat g.
bone g.
g. carrier spoon
conjunctival limbal g.
conjunctival patch g.
corneal g.
corneolimbal ring g.
crescent corneal g.
dermis fat g.
dermis patch g.
donor g.
double g.
g. edema
g. epithelium
failed g.
g. failure
fat g.
g. fixation
full-thickness corneal g.
glycerin-preserved g.
harvested g.
high-risk g.
g. infection
lamellar corneal g.
lamellar patch g.

NOTES

G

graft *(continued)*
    long-term g.
    mucous membrane g.
    mushroom corneal g.
    Mustarde g.
    patch g.
    pattern-cut corneal g.
    penetrating full-thickness corneal g.
    piggyback g.
    g. preservation solution
    ProKera amniotic membrane g.
    g. rejection
    retroauricular complex g.
    scleral patch g.
    skin g.
    snowman g.
    split-calvarial bone g.
    tarsoconjunctival composite g.
    tectonic corneal g.
    Tenon patch g.
    Tudor-Thomas g.
    uncomplicated g.
    g. versus host disease
    Wolfe g.
graft-host interface
grafting
    surgical patch g.
gramicidin
    neomycin, polymyxin B, and g.
Gram-negative
    G.-n. bacteria
    G.-n. medium
Gram-positive
    G.-p. bacteria
    G.-p. bacterial keratitis
    G.-p. cocci
    G.-p. infection
    G.-p. organism
Grandon T-incision marker
granisetron
granular
    g. appearance
    g. conjunctivitis
    g. corneal dystrophy
    g. hyperfluorescent dot
    g. lid
    g. ophthalmia
    g. trachoma
granularity
granule
    Birbeck g.
    cone g.
    dense core g.
    glycogen g.
    keratohyaline g.
    Langerhans g.
    neurosecretory g.
    pigment g.

    rod g.
    scintillating g.
granulocytic sarcoma
granuloma
    candidal g.
    cholesterol g.
    chorioretinal g.
    choroidal g.
    conjunctival g.
    diffuse g.
    discrete g.
    eosinophilic g.
    focal g.
    g. gangraenescens
    intracranial g.
    lethal midline g.
    midline g.
    noncaseating conjunctival g.
    orbital g.
    palisading orbital g.
    peripheral g.
    posterior pole g.
    pyogenic g.
    reparative giant cell g.
    sclerosing orbital g.
    zonal g.
granulomatosis
    familial juvenile systemic g.
    juvenile systemic g.
granulomatous
    g. anterior uveitis
    g. endophthalmitis
    g. inflammatory cell
    g. iridocyclitis
    g. keratic precipitate
    g. keratoconjunctivitis
    g. panuveitis
    g. vasculitis
granulosus
    Echinococcus g.
graph
    shadow g.
graphic neglect
grasping forceps
Grass electrode
grating
    g. acuity
    Arden g.
    Cambridge low-contrast g.
    g. monochromator
    sine-wave g.
    sinusoidal g.
Gratiolet radiating fiber
Graves
    G. disease
    G. hyperthyroidism
    G. ophthalmopathy
    G. optic neuropathy
    G. orbitography

G. orbitopathy
G. strabismus
gravidic
g. retinitis
g. retinopathy
gravis
fulminant myasthenia g.
myasthenia g.
Grawitz tumor
gray
g. atrophy
g. cataract
g. crescent
g. line
g. line of eyelid
G. oral reading test
G. photochromic lens
g. plaque
G. Standardized Oral Reading
Paragraphs
graying
g. of macula
macular g.
gray-line incision
gray-scale
g.-s. image
g.-s. ultrasonogram
Grayson corneal forceps
gray-white corneal scar
Grazer blepharoplasty forceps
great big barbie retractor
greater
g. ring of iris
g. superficial petrosal nerve
g. superficial temporal artery
biopsy
g. wing of sphenoid
green
g. blindness
g. cataract
indocyanine g. (ICG)
g. laser (GL)
g. laser light photocoagulator
lissamine g.
g. muscle hook
g. needle holder
532nm G. laser photocoagulator
g. strabismus hook
g. vision
Green-Kenyon corneal marker
Gregg syndrome
Greig syndrome
Greither syndrome

Grey-Hess screen
grid
Amsler g. (AG)
HirCal g.
g. laser photocoagulation (GLP)
g. method
Grieshaber
G. blade
G. calibrated trephine
G. corneal trephine
G. diamond-coated forceps
G. endoilluminator
G. flexible iris retractor
G. 2-function manipulator
G. 3-function manipulator
G. internal limiting membrane
forceps
G. iris forceps
G. keratome
G. micro-bipolar coagulator
G. needle holder
G. ophthalmic needle
G. power injector system
G. ruby knife
G. ultrasharp knife
G. ultrasharp microsurgery
instrument
G. vertical cutting scissors
G. vitreous scissors
Griess reaction
Griffith
G. scale
G. sign
grind
Fast G. 2200
grinding
bicentric g.
slab-off g.
grip
scleral g.
gripflex design
grittiness
gritty
g. eyes
g. foreign body sensation
Grizzard subretinal fluid cannula
Grocco sign
**Grocott-Gomori methenamine silver
nitrate**
Groenouw
G. corneal dystrophy
G. type I, II dystrophy
G. type II maculopathy

G

NOTES

Grönblad-Strandberg syndrome
groove
> Blessig g.
> corneal lamellar g.
> corneoscleral g.
> infraorbital g.
> lacrimal g.
> lamellar g.
> limbal g.
> nasolacrimal g.
> optic g.
> peptide-binding g.
> g. suture
> tunnel g.
> Verga lacrimal g.

grooved
> g. director
> g. incision
> G. Pegboard test
> g. silicone implant
> g. silicone sponge

Grossmann operation
Gross stereopsis
ground-glass sheet
group
> g. B streptococcus
> CRYO-ROP Cooperative G.
> Cryotherapy for Retinopathy of
> Prematurity Cooperative G.
> nonocular muscle g.
> Pediatric Eye Disease
> Investigator G. (PEDIG)

growth
> axial g.
> rate of refractive g.
> g. retardation, alopecia,
> pseudoanodontia, and optic
> atrophy (GAPO)

growth-onset diabetes
GRT
> giant retinal tear

Grunert spur
GS
> Goldenhar syndrome

GSL
> goniosynechialysis

gt.
GTS
> guided trephine system

gtt.
guard
> cataract knife g.
> ether g.
> eye knife g.
> forceps g.
> keratome g.
> knife g.
> LASIK eye g.
> scalpel g.

guarded filtration procedure
guarding ptosis
Guarnieri inclusion body
Gudden
> commissure of G.

Guell
> G. irrigation cannula
> G. LASIK irrigating cannula
> G. type LASIK speculum

guide
> Brown limbal relaxing incision g.
> Clayman g.
> Eschenbach low vision
> rehabilitation g.
> Lu-Mendez LRI g.
> vacuum-centering g.

guided trephine system (GTS)
guideline
> American Academy of
> Ophthalmology's Preferred Practice
> Pattern g.'s

Guillain-Barré syndrome
guilliermondii
> *Candida g.*

guillotine
> g. cutting tip
> g. vitrectomy instrument
> g. vitrector

guillotine-type cutter
Guimaraes
> G. flap spatula
> G. ICL manipulator
> G. implantable contact lens
> manipulator
> G. ophthalmic spatula

Guist
> G. fixation forceps
> G. speculum

Gulani
> G. globe stabilizer and flap
> restrainer
> G. triple function LASIK cannula

Gullstrand
> G. law
> G. monograph
> G. ophthalmoscope
> G. schematic eye
> G. slit lamp

gummate
gummatous meningitis
gun-barrel field defect
Gunderson
> G. conjunctival flap
> G. muscle forceps

Gunn
> G. crossing sign
> G. dot
> G. jaw-winking phenomenon
> Marcus G. (MG)

no Marcus G. (NMG)
G. pupil
G. pupillary reflex
G. syndrome
gunshot wound
gustatolacrimal reflex
gustatory lacrimation
Guthrie fixation hook
gutta, pl. **guttae**
g. amaurosis
g. serena
guttat.
guttatim
guttata
corneal g.
keratopathia g.
guttate choroidopathy
guttatim (guttat.)
gutter
g. dystrophy
g. dystrophy of cornea
guttering
corneal g.
limbal g.
limbus g.

guy suture
Guyton corneal transplant trephine
Guyton-Minkowski potential acuity meter
Guyton-Noyes
G.-N. fixation
G.-N. fixation forceps
Guyton-Park
G.-P. eye speculum
G.-P. lid speculum
GV
Healon GV
gymnastics
ocular g.
gyrata
atrophia g.
gyrate
g. atrophy
g. atrophy of choroid and retina
gyrus, pl. **gyri**
angular g.
calcarine g.

NOTES

H
- hyperopia
- hyperopic
- hyperphoria
  - H band

h
- hour

H1 blocker

HA
- headache
- hydroxyapatite

Haab
- H. knife needle
- H. magnet
- H. reflex
- H. scleral resection knife
- H. stria

Haag-Streit
- H.-S. Biomicroscope 900 slit lamp
- H.-S. distometer
- H.-S. keratometer
- H.-S. ophthalmometer
- H.-S. slitlamp biomicroscope

HAART
- highly active antiretroviral therapy

habit
- glaucomatous h.

habitual
- h. correction
- h. symptom

HACE
- high altitude cerebral edema

HACEK
- *Haemophilus, Actinobacillus actinomycetemicomitans, Cardiobacterium hominis, Eikenella corrodens, Kingella kingae*
  - HACEK group organism

Hadeco intraoperative Doppler

Haefliger cleaver

haemolysans
- *Gemella h.*

haemolyticus
- *Staphylococcus h.*

Haemophilus
- *H. aegyptius*
- *H., Actinobacillus actinomycetemicomitans, Cardiobacterium hominis, Eikenella corrodens, Kingella kingae* (HACEK)
- *H. influenzae*
- *H. parainfluenzae*
- *H. paraphrophilus*

haemorrhagica
- retinitis h.

Haenel symptom

Hagberg-Santavuori syndrome

Hague cataract lamp

Haidinger
- H. brush
- H. brush test

hair
- h. bulb incubation test
- h. follicle tumor

halation

Halberg
- H. contact lens forceps
- H. trial clip
- H. trial clip occluder

Halberstaedter-Prowazek inclusion body

Haldrone

half
- h. glasses
- h. vision

half-diopter increment

half-eye spectacles

half-field
- visual h.-f. (VHF)

half-glass spectacles

half-moon syndrome

HALK
- hyperopic automated lamellar keratoplasty

Hallauer
- H. glasses
- H. spectacles

Hall dermatome

Haller
- circle of H.
- H. layer
- H. membrane

Hallermann-Streiff-François syndrome

Hallermann-Streiff syndrome

Hallervorden-Spatz syndrome

Hallgren syndrome

Hallpike maneuver

hallucination
- hypnagogic h.
- hypnopompic h.
- irritative h.
- migrainous h.
- peduncular h.
- release h.
- visual h.
- h. with eye closure

hallucinogenic

halo
- h. around light

H

halo *(continued)*
    h. demonstrator
    Fick h.
    glaucomatous h.
    parafoveal h.
    h. phenomenon
    pigmentary h.
    h. saturninus
    senescent h.
    senile h.
    h. sheathing
    h. symptom
    h. vision
    visual h.
halogenated hydroxyquinoline
halogen ophthalmoscope
halogram
halometer
halometry
halophilic noncholera *Vibrio* **species**
haloscope
    phase difference h.
halothane
HALS
    Health and Activity Limitations Survey
Halsey needle holder
Halsted
    H. curved mosquito clamp
    H. curved mosquito hemostatic
      forceps
    H. hemostat
    H. strabismus scissors
    H. straight mosquito clamp
Haltia-Santavuori type of Batten
  syndrome
hamartoblastoma
hamartoma
    astrocytic h.
    glial-neural h.
    melanocytic h.
    orbit h.
    orbital h.
    retinal astrocytic h.
    smooth muscle h.
    uveal tract h.
    vascular h.
hamartomatosis
hamartomatous lesion
Hamilton
    H. repeating pipette dispenser
      system
    H. syringe
hammock pupil
hamular procedure
hamulus, pl. **hamuli**
    h. lacrimalis
    trochlear h.
hand
    h. magnifier

    h. motion (HM)
    h. movement
    Winter Helping H.
1-handed
    1-h. phacoemulsification
    1-h. stabilization
2-handed phacoemulsification
hand-eye coordination strategy
handheld
    h. autorefractor
    h. eye magnet
    h. fundus camera
    h. Hruby lens
    h. infusion lens
    h. keratometry
    h. magnifier
    h. magnifying reticle
    h. rotary prism
    h. trephine
handicapped
    National Association for the
      Visually H. (NAVH)
handle
    Beaver h.
    DORC h.
    Elliot trephine h.
handling
    data h.
hand-motion
    h.-m. vision (HMV)
    h.-m. visual acuity test
hand-movement visual acuity test
hand-painted lens
handpiece
    AMO Series 4 phaco h.
    Avit h.
    B-mode h.
    Cavitron I/A h.
    EndoProbe h.
    fragmentation/aspiration h.
    Kelman irrigating h.
    micro bimanual irrigating h.
    MicroSeal ophthalmic h.
    NeoSoniX h.
    Packer Wick extrusion h.
    phacoemulsification h.
    ProFinesse II ultrasonic h.
    soft-tipped extrusion h.
    Storz h.
Hand-Schüller-Christian
    H.-S.-C. disease
    H.-S.-C. syndrome
Handy video fundus camera
Hanley and McNeil method
Hanna
    H. arcitome
    H. trephine
Hannover canal

Hansatome
Chiron H.
H. microkeratome
H. 8.5-mm suction ring
haplopia
haploscope
mirror h.
haploscopic
h. test
h. vision
haptic
h. angulation
h. contact
lamellar h.
h. loop
modified L loop h.
h. plate lens
PMMA h.'s
violet h.
HAR
high altitude retinopathy
Harada
H. disease
H. syndrome
Harada-Ito procedure
hard
h. cataract
h. contact lens (HCL)
h. drusen
h. lipid exudate
hardened spectacle lens
hardening of lens
Harder gland
harderian gland
Hardesty
H. tendon hook
H. tenotomy hook
hard-finger tension
Hardy
H. lensometer
H. punch
Hardy-Rand-Ritter (HRR)
H.-R.-R. color vision plate
H.-R.-R. pseudoisochromatic plate
H.-R.-R. screening plate
H.-R.-R. test
hare's eye
Harman
H. eye dressing
H. fixation forceps
harmonious abnormal retinal correspondence

Harms
H. corneal forceps
H. trabeculotome
H. trabeculotomy probe
H. tying forceps
Harms-Colibri forceps
Harms-Tubingen tying forceps
Harrington
H. retractor
H. tonometer
Harrington-Flocks
H.-F. multiple pattern
H.-F. test
Hartmann mosquito hemostatic forceps
Hartmann-Shack (HS)
H.-S. wavefront aberrometer
H.-S. wavefront method
H.-S. wavefront sensor system
Hart pediatric 3-mirror lens
harvested graft
Hashimoto thyroiditis
Hasner
H. fold
H. lid forceps
valve of H.
H. valve
Hassall body
Hassall-Henle
H.-H. body
H.-H. wart
hay fever conjunctivitis
Hay-Wells syndrome
hazard avoidance
haze
aerial h.
corneal h.
epithelial punctate h.
interface h.
late-onset corneal h.
h. level
reticular h.
stromal h.
subepithelial corneal h.
vitreous h.
haziness
hazy vision
HBO
hyperbaric oxygen
HBR
holmium bleb reformation
HBr
hydrobromic acid
scopolamine HBr

NOTES

H

HC
    Ocutricin HC
    Tri-Thalmic HC
HCDVA
    high-contrast distance visual acuity
HCL
    hard contact lens
HCl
    hydrochloride
        antazoline phosphate and
          naphazoline HCl
        apraclonidine HCl
        azelastine HCl
        betaxolol HCl
        carteolol HCl
        cysteamine HCl
        dapiprazole HCl
        deterenol HCl
        dipivefrin HCl
        Duranest HCl
        epinastine HCl
        epinephrine HCl
        levobunolol HCl
        levocabastine HCl
        Marcaine HCl
        mepivacaine HCl
        naboctate HCl
        naphazoline HCl
        oxymetazoline HCl
        pheniramine maleate and
          naphazoline HCl
        pilocarpine HCl
        proparacaine HCl
        proxymetacaine HCl 0.5%
        valganciclovir HCl
head
    drusen of optic nerve h.
    h. injury
    Medusa h.
    h. mirror
    h. nystagmus
    optic nerve h. (ONH)
    h. posture
    h. tremor
headache (HA)
    brain tumor h.
    cluster h.
    migraine without h.
    muscle contraction h.
    postherpetic h.
    posttraumatic h.
    retroorbital h.
    sinus h.
head-eye coordination
head-mounted
    h.-m. instrument
    h.-m. video magnifier LVES
head-nodding
headrest

head-tilt test
head-turning reflex
healing
    stromal wound h.
Healon
    H. 5
    H. aspirating cannula
    H. GV
    H. solution
Health and Activity Limitations Survey (HALS)
Health-Related Quality of Life (HRQOL)
heat-causing radiofrequency wave
heater
    broad-spectrum h. (BSH)
    infrared h.
heat-generated cataract
Heath
    H. chalazion curette
    H. chalazion forceps
heat-ray cataract
heavy
    h. eye
    h. fluid
    h. gas
    h. ion irradiation
    h. ion radiation
Hebra curette
hedger cataract
HEDS1
    Herpetic Eye Disease Study I
HEDS2
    Herpetic Eye Disease Study II
Heerfordt
    H. disease
    H. syndrome
hefilcon A
Heidelberg
    H. laser tomographic scanner
    H. retina angiograph
    H. retinal flowmeter
    H. retinal tomography
    H. retina tomograph (HRT)
    H. retina tomograph II (HRT-II)
Heidenhain
    H. syndrome
    H. variant
height
    bleb h.
    buckle h.
    contact lens h.
    orbital h.
    peripapillary retinal h.
    sagittal h.
    segment h.
Heine
    H. cyclodialysis
    H. HSL 100 hand-held slit lamp

H. Lambda 100 retinometer
H. operation
H. penlight
helical computed tomography
helicoid
   h. choroidopathy
   h. peripapillary atrophy
helium-ion aiming laser
helium-neon
   h.-n. aiming laser
   h.-n. beam
hellem
   Encephalitozoon h.
Helmholtz
   H. keratometer
   H. line
   H. ophthalmoscope
   H. schematic eye
   H. theory
   H. theory of accommodation
   H. theory of color vision
helminthic disease
helper/inducer T cell
Helveston
   H. big barbie tissue retractor
   H. great big barbie retractor
   H. hook
   H. scleral marking ruler
HEMA
   hydroxyethyl methacrylate
hemagglutination
   immune adherence h. (IAH)
   Treponema pallidum h.
hemangioblastoma
   optic nerve h.
hemangioendothelioma
   orbital h.
hemangioma
   capillary h.
   cavernous orbital h.
   choroidal h.
   conjunctival h.
   episcleral h.
   epithelioid h.
   exophytic papillary capillary h.
   eyelid strawberry h.
   facial h.
   juxtapapillary endophytic
     capillary h.
   orbital cavernous h.
   osseous metaplasia over
     choroidal h.
   papillary capillary h.

periocular h.
periorbital h.
racemose h.
retinal capillary h.
retinal cavernous h.
retinal racemose h.
strawberry h.
uveal tract h.
venous h.
hemangiomatosis
   diffuse neonatal h.
   encephalofacial cavernous h.
   racemose h.
hemangiopericytoma
   lacrimal sac h.
   meningeal h.
   orbital h.
hematic cyst
hematogenous
   h. metastasis
   h. pigmentation
   h. sepsis
hematoma
   orbital h.
   subdural h.
hematopoietic metastasis
hematopsia
hemeralopia, hemeranopia
hemiachromatopsia
hemiakinesia
   pupillary h.
hemialexia
hemiamblyopia
hemianopia
   absolute h.
   altitudinal h.
   binasal h.
   bitemporal h.
   complete h.
   congruous h.
   crossed h.
   heteronymous h.
   homonymous h.
   incomplete h.
   incongruous h.
   quadrantic h.
   unilateral h.
   unilocular h.
hemianopic
   h. dyslexia
   h. glasses
   h. scotoma
   h. spectacles

NOTES

hemianopsia, hemianopia
    absolute h.
    altitudinal h.
    bilateral homonymous h.
    binasal h.
    binocular h.
    bitemporal fugax h.
    checkerboard h.
    complete h.
    congenital h.
    congruous h.
    crossed h.
    double homonymous h.
    equilateral h.
    geniculate h.
    heteronymous h.
    homonymous h.
    horizontal h.
    incomplete h.
    incongruous h.
    lateral h.
    lower h.
    nasal h.
    postgeniculate congenital
      homonymous h.
    quadrant h.
    quadrantic h.
    relative h.
    temporal h.
    true h.
    unilateral h.
    uniocular h.
    upper h.
    vertical h.
hemianoptic
hemianosmia
hemichiasma
hemichromatopsia
hemicrania
    chronic paroxysmal h.
    h. continua
hemicraniosis
hemi-CRVO
hemifacial
    h. atrophy
    h. blepharospasm
    h. flush
    h. spasm
hemifield slide phenomenon
hemihydrate
    timolol h.
hemimicropsia
hemiopalgia
hemiopia
hemiopic
    h. hypoplasia
    h. pupillary reaction
hemiplegia
    alternating oculomotor h.

hemiplegic migraine
hemiscotosis
hemi-seesaw nystagmus
hemisensory
    h. deficit
    h. loss
hemisphere
    cerebellar h.
    h. eye implant
    h. projection perimetry
    silicone h.
hemispherical
hemocytic mesenchyme
**hemodynamically significant carotid
  artery stenosis (HSCAS)**
hemoglobin
    glycosylated h.
hemolytic glaucoma
hemophilia
hemophthalmia
hemophthalmos, hemophthalmus
hemorrhage
    anterior chamber h.
    arachnoid h.
    8-ball h.
    blot h.
    blot-and-dot h.
    caudate h.
    cerebellar h.
    choroidal h.
    conjunctival flap h.
    delayed massive suprachoroidal h.
    dense h.
    h. density
    disc drusen h.
    dot h.
    dot-and-blot h.
    Drance h.
    h. duration
    expulsive h.
    flame-shaped h.
    hyperfluorescent h.
    intralenticular h.
    intraocular h.
    intraorbital h.
    intraretinal h.
    intraventricular h. (IVH)
    intravitreal h.
    kissing suprachoroidal h.
    h. and microaneurysm (h/ma)
    mild periocular h.
    nerve fiber layer h.
    nonclearing h.
    ochre h.
    orbital h.
    perihemangioma subretinal h.
    peripheral intraretinal h.
    premacular subhyaloid h.
    prepapillary h.

preretinal h.
punctate h.
retinal h.
retinopathy h.
retrobulbar h.
retrohyaloid premacular h.
round h.
splinter disc h.
spontaneous retrobulbar h.
spontaneous vitreous h.
subarachnoid h.
subchoroidal h.
subconjunctival h.
subhyaloid h.
subinternal limiting membrane h.
subretinal h.
suprachoroidal h. (SCH, SH)
vision-threatening vitreous h.
vitreal h.
vitreous h. (VH)
vitreous breakthrough h.
white-centered h.
yellow-ochre h.
hemorrhagic
　　h. choroidal detachment
　　h. choroidal neovascularization
　　h. conjunctivitis
　　h. disciform lesion
　　h. disorder
　　h. glaucoma
　　h. iritis
　　h. retinopathy
　　h. RPE
　　h. sarcoma
hemorrhagica
　　Leber lymphangiectasia h.
hemosiderosis bulbi
hemostat
　　Corboy h.
　　Halsted h.
　　Kelly h.
hemostatic
　　h. agent
　　h. forceps
Henderson-Patterson inclusion body
HeNe
　　H. beam
　　H. laser
Henle
　　H. body
　　crypt of H.
　　H. fiber
　　H. fiber layer

　　H. gland
　　H. layer of macula
　　H. membrane
　　H. wart
Hennebert sign
Henry cilia forceps
henselae
　　Bartonella h.
Hensen body
Henson CFS 2000 perimeter
heparin
　　h. surface-modified intraocular lens
　　(HSM-IOL)
　　h. surface-modified polymethyl
　　methacrylate
hepatica
　　ophthalmia h.
hepatolenticular degeneration
herbal medicine
Herbert
　　H. operation
　　H. peripheral pit
hereditaria
　　atrophia bulborum h.
hereditary
　　h. abetalipoproteinemia
　　h. anterior membrane dystrophy
　　h. benign intraepithelial dyskeratosis
　　h. benign intraepithelial dyskeratosis
　　syndrome
　　h. cataract
　　h. cerebellar ataxia
　　h. corneal edema
　　h. degeneration
　　h. epithelial corneal dystrophy
　　h. hemorrhagic macular dystrophy
　　h. hemorrhagic telangiectasia
　　h. hyperferritinemia-cataract
　　syndrome
　　h. optic atrophy
　　h. optic atrophy syndrome
　　h. optic neuropathy
　　h. progressive arthroophthalmopathy
　　h. renal-retinal dysplasia
　　h. vitelliform dystrophy
heredity maculopathy
heredodegeneration
　　macular h.
heredodegenerative
　　h. atrophy
　　h. neurologic syndrome
heredofamilial optic atrophy
heredomacular degeneration

NOTES

H

225

Hering
  H. after-image mechanism
  H. law of equal innervation
  H. law of equivalent innervation
  H. law of motor correspondence
  H. law of simultaneous innervation
  H. test
  H. theory
  H. theory of color vision
Hering-Bielschowsky after-image test
Hering-Hellebrand deviation
Hermann grid illusion
Hermansky-Pudlak syndrome
hernia
  h. of iris
  orbital h.
  vitreous h.
herniating orbital fat
herniation
  hippocampal gyrus h.
  vitreous h.
Herpchek herpes simplex virus test
herpes
  h. corneae
  h. epithelial tropic ulceration
  h. follicular keratoconjunctivitis
  ocular h.
  h. panuveitis
  h. simplex blepharitis
  h. simplex blepharoconjunctivitis
  h. simplex cellulitis
  h. simplex conjunctivitis
  h. simplex corneal ulcer
  h. simplex dermatitis
  h. simplex iridocyclitis
  h. simplex keratitis
  h. simplex keratoconjunctivitis
  h. simplex keratouveitis
  h. simplex retinitis
  h. simplex scar
  h. simplex scleritis
  h. simplex uveitis
  h. simplex virus (HSV)
  h. simplex virus type I
  h. zoster conjunctivitis
  h. zoster disciform keratitis
  h. zoster glaucoma
  h. zoster iridocyclitis
  h. zoster keratoconjunctivitis
  h. zoster ophthalmicus
  h. zoster oticus
  h. zoster virus
herpesvirus
herpete
  zoster sine h.
herpetic
  h. conjunctivitis
  h. dendrite
  H. Eye Disease Study

  H. Eye Disease Study I (HEDS1)
  H. Eye Disease Study II (HEDS2)
  h. fungal keratitis
  h. iridocyclitis
  h. keratoconjunctivitis
  h. necrotizing retinopathy
  h. ocular disease
  h. ocular infection
  h. stromal keratitis
  h. ulcer
herpetoid lesion
Herplex
  H. Liquifilm
  H. Ophthalmic
Herrick
  H. lacrimal plug
  H. silicone lacrimal implant
Herring law
Hersh
  H. LASIK retreatment forceps
  H. LASIK retreatment spatula
Hertel
  H. exophthalmometer
  H. exophthalmometry
  H. ophthalmometer
  H. stone forceps
  H. value
Hertwig-Magendie
  H.-M. phenomenon
  H.-M. syndrome
Hess
  H. diplopia screen
  H. eyelid operation
  H. forceps
  H. ptosis operation
  H. screen test
  H. spoon
Hessburg-Barron
  H.-B. disposable vacuum trephine
  H.-B. suction trephine
Hessburg lens
Hess-Lee screen
heterochromatic flicker photometry
heterochromia
  atrophic h.
  binocular h.
  congenital iris h.
  Fuchs h.
  h. iridis
  h. of iris
  iris h.
  monocular h.
  simple h.
  sympathetic h.
heterochromic
  h. cataract
  h. Fuchs cyclitis
  h. iridocyclitis
  h. uveitis

heterogeneity
    genetic h.
    optical h.
heterogeneous
    h. cell
    h. donor material
heterogenous keratoplasty
heterokeratoplasty
heterometropia
heteronymous
    h. diplopia
    h. hemianopia
    h. hemianopsia
    h. image
    h. parallax
    h. quadrantanopia
heterophoralgia
heterophoria method
heterophoric position
heterophthalmia, heterophthalmos, heterophthalmus
heteropsia
heteroptics
heteroscope
heteroscopy
heterotopia
    cerebral h.
    diabetic macular h.
    h. maculae
    macular h.
heterotopic pulley
heterotropia, heterotropy
    circadian h.
    comitant h.
    concomitant h.
    h. maculae
    noncomitant h.
    paralytic h.
heterotropic deviation
Hetrazan
Hexadrol Phosphate
hexafluoride
    h. gas
    sulfur h. (SF6)
hexagonal keratotomy
hexahydrate
    magnesium chloride h.
    trisodium phosphonoformate h.
hexametaphosphate
    sodium h.
hexamethonium chloride
hexamidine
Hexon illumination system

hex procedure
hexylcaine
Heyer-Schulte specular microscope
Heyner
    H. dilator
    H. double needle
    H. forceps
HFA
    Humphrey field analyzer
Hg
    mercury
HGM
    HGM argon green laser
    HGM intravitreal laser
    HGM ophthalmic laser
Hibiclens antiseptic/antimicrobial skin cleanser
hidden visual loss
hiding Heidi facial expressions test
hidrocystoma
    apocrine h.
high
    h. altitude cerebral edema (HACE)
    h. altitude illness
    h. altitude retinopathy (HAR)
    h. convex
    h. eyebrow
    h. hyperopia
    h. intensity illuminator
    h. magnification (HM)
    h. myopia
    h. myopia eye
    h. prevalence
    h. viscosity
    h. viscosity agent
high-add bifocal
high-contrast distance visual acuity (HCDVA)
higher
    h. order wavefront aberration
    h. visual function test
high-frequency ultrasound biomicroscope
high-gain
    h.-g. artifact
    h.-g. digital ultrasound
High-Lite glass
highly
    h. active antiretroviral therapy (HAART)
    h. oxygen permeable contact lens
high-pass
    h.-p. resolution perimetry (HRP)

NOTES

H

high-pass *(continued)*
    h.-p. resolution perimetry global deviation (HRP-GD)
    h.-p. resolution perimetry local deviation (HRP-LD)
high-power lens
high-resolution in vivo fundus autofluorescence imaging
high-risk
    h.-r. characteristic
    h.-r. graft
    h.-r. patient
high-sensitivity C-reactive protein (hs-CRP)
high-speed cutter
high-tension
    h.-t. glaucoma (HTG)
    h.-t. suturing technique
high-vacuum phacoemulsification
high-velocity projectile injury
Hildreth
    H. cautery
    H. electrocautery
hinge cord length
hinged corneal flap
Hippel
    H. disease
    internal corneal ulcer of von H.
    H. operation
Hippel-Lindau syndrome
hippocampal gyrus herniation
hippocampus
hippus
    respiratory h.
HirCal grid
Hirschberg
    H. magnet
    H. method
    H. reflex
    H. reflex assessment
    H. test
Hirschman
    H. iris hook
    H. lens forceps
    H. lens-inserting forceps
    H. microiris hook
    H. spatula
    H. speculum
Hismanal
histiocytic
    h. disorder
    h. lymphoma
    h. tumor
histoacryl
    h. glue
    h. glue patch
histologic subtype
histolyticum
    Clostridium h.

histopathologic effect
Histoplasma
    H. capsulatum
    H. chorioretinitis
    H. duboisii
histoplasmic choroiditis
histoplasmosis
    h. maculopathy
    ocular h.
    presumed ocular h.
    h. syndrome
history
    neuroophthalmologic case h.
    past ocular h. (POH)
histo spot
HIV
    human immunodeficiency virus
    HIV retinopathy
HIV-related
    HIV-r. eye disease
    HIV-r. retinochoroiditis
HIV-specific antibody
Hl
    latent hyperopia
HLA
    human leukocyte antigen
    HLA match
HLA-A29 antigen
HLA-B5 antigen
HLA-B7 antigen
HLA-B15 antigen
HLA-B27
    HLA-B27 antigen
    HLA-B27 syndrome
HLA-B27-associated uveitis
HLA-DR4 antigen
HM
    hand motion
    high magnification
Hm
    manifest hyperopia
h/ma
    hemorrhage and microaneurysm
H-magnetic resonance spectroscopy
HM/3ft
    hand motion at 3 feet
HMV
    hand-motion vision
Hoagland sign
hockey-end temple
Hodapp-Parrish-Anderson (HPA)
    H.-P.-A. grading criteria
    H.-P.-A. visual field staging system
hoe
    LASEK epithelial micro h.
    Rhein LASIK epithelial detaching h.
    Sloane micro h.
Hoffberger program

Hoffer
- H. optical center marker
- H. optic zone marker
- H. Q formula

Hoffer-Colenbrander formula
Hofmann-Thornton globe fixation ring
Hofmann T-incision marker
holder
- Arruga needle h.
- baby Barraquer needle h.
- Barraquer curved h.
- Barraquer needle h.
- Belin double-ended needle h.
- blade h.
- Bodkin thread h.
- Boyce needle h.
- Boynton needle h.
- Castroviejo-Barraquer needle h.
- Castroviejo blade h.
- Castroviejo-Kalt needle h.
- Castroviejo needle h.
- Cohen needle h.
- Corboy needle h.
- Crile needle h.
- Dean knife h.
- Derf needle h.
- Ellis needle h.
- eye h.
- French needle h.
- Gifford needle h.
- goniotomy needle h.
- green needle h.
- Grieshaber needle h.
- Halsey needle h.
- IOL cartridge h.
- Jaffe needle h.
- Kalt needle h.
- McIntyre fish-hook needle h.
- McPherson needle h.
- needle h.
- Neumann razor blade fragment h.
- Paton needle h.
- Stevens needle h.
- Troutman blade h.
- Troutman needle h.
- Vickers needle h.
- Webster needle h.

holding clip
hole
- atrophic h.
- cystoid macular h.
- full-thickness macular h.
- full-thickness retinal h.
- iatrogenic retinal h.
- idiopathic macular cyst and h.
- impending macular h.
- lamellar h.
- macular h. (MH)
- operculated retinal h.
- partial thickness macular h.
- h. in retina
- retinal h.
- senescent macular h.
- stage 0 macular h.
- unclosed macular h.

Holladay
- H. contrast acuity test
- H. Diagnostic Summary topography
- H. II formula
- H. posterior capsule polisher

Holladay-Binkhorst
- H.-B. equation
- H.-B. formula

Hollenhorst plaque
hollowing and shadowing
hollow-sphere implant
Holmes-Adie
- H.-A. pupil
- H.-A. syndrome

Holmgren
- H. color test
- H. method
- H. wool skein test

holmium
- h. bleb reformation (HBR)
- h. laser
- h. YAG laser sclerectomy

hologram
holoprosencephaly
Holth
- H. forceps
- H. iridencleisis
- H. operation
- H. scleral punch
- H. sclerectomy

Holthouse-Batten superficial choroiditis
Holt-Oram syndrome
Homatrocel
homatropine
- h. hydrobromide
- Isopto H.
- h. refraction

Homer syndrome
Homer-Wright rosette

NOTES

H

hominis
    Cardiobacterium h.
    Staphylococcus h.
homocitrullinuria
    hyperornithinemia, hyperammonemia,
      and h.
homocystinuria
homogeneous donor material
homogenous keratoplasty
homokeratoplasty
homologous penetrating central limbo keratoplasty
homonymous
    h. crescent
    h. diplopia
    h. field defect
    h. hemianopia
    h. hemianopic scotoma
    h. hemianopsia
    h. hemiopic hypoplasia
    h. image
    h. parallax
    h. quadrantanopia
homoplastic keratomileusis
homotropic antibody
Honan
    H. balloon
    H. cuff
    H. manometer
honey bee lens
honeycomb
    h. dystrophy
    h. macula
hook
    anchor h.
    angled discission h.
    ASSI fixation h.
    Azar lens-manipulating h.
    Behler LASIK enhancement h.
    Behler LASIK retreatment h.
    Berens scleral h.
    boat h.
    Bonn microiris h.
    Catalano muscle h.
    corneal h.
    Crawford h.
    Culler muscle h.
    discission h.
    h. expressor
    expressor h.
    Fenzel angled manipulating h.
    Fenzel insertion h.
    Fenzel lens-manipulating h.
    fixation h.
    flat h.
    Frazier dura h.
    Fukasaku small pupil snapper h.
    Gass muscle h.
    Gass retinal detachment h.

Graefe strabismus h.
Graether button h.
green muscle h.
green strabismus h.
Guthrie fixation h.
Hardesty tendon h.
Hardesty tenotomy h.
Helveston h.
Hirschman iris h.
Hirschman microiris h.
Hunkeler ball-point h.
iris h.
Jaffe iris h.
Jaffe lens-manipulating h.
Jaffe microiris h.
Jameson muscle h.
Katena boat h.
Kirby muscle h.
Knapp iris h.
Kratz K push-pull iris h.
Kuglen manipulating h.
Kuglen push/pull h.
Lewicky lens manipulating h.
Manson double-ended strabismus h.
Maumenee iris h.
McIntyre irrigating h.
McReynolds lid-retracting h.
muscle h.
Nugent h.
oblique muscle h.
Ochsner h.
O'Connor flat h.
O'Connor muscle h.
O'Connor sharp h.
O'Connor tenotomy h.
ophthalmic h.
Osher h.
pocketing h.
push-and-pull h.
recession ophthalmic muscle h.
Rentsch boat h.
retinal detachment h.
Russian 4-pronged fixation h.
scleral h.
Scobee oblique muscle h.
sharp h.
Shepard microiris h.
Shepard reversed iris h.
Sinskey lens h.
Sinskey lens-manipulating h.
Sinskey microiris h.
Sinskey microlens h.
skin h.
Smith expressor h.
Smith lid h.
h. spatula
spatula h.
squint h.
Stevens tenotomy h.

strabismus h.
suture pickup h.
tenotomy h.
Tomas iris h.
Tomas suture h.
twist fixation h.
Tyrell iris h.
Visitec angled lens h.
Visitec corneal suture
  manipulating h.
Visitec micro double-iris h.
Visitec microiris h.
Visitec straight lens h.
von Graefe muscle h.
von Graefe strabismus h.
Wiener corneal h.
Wiener scleral h.
Y h.

hook-shaped cataract
hook-type implant
Hooper Visual Organization Test
(HVOT)
Hopkins rod lens telescope
hordeolum
external h.
h. externum
internal h.
h. internum
h. meibomianum

horizontal
h. band pallor
h. cell
h. deviation
h. diplopia
h. gaze
h. gaze center
h. gaze deficit
h. hemianopsia
h. jerk nystagmus
h. laxity
h. mattress suture
h. meridian
h. muscle surgery
h. plane
h. prism bar
h. raphe
h. retinal disparity
h. scissors
h. strabismus
h. tropia

hormone
thyrotropin-releasing h.

horn
cutaneous h.
lateral h.
medial h.

Horner
H. law
H. muscle
H. ptosis
H. pupil
H. syndrome

Horner-Bernard syndrome
Horner-Trantas
H.-T. dot
H.-T. spot

horopter
empirical h.
Vieth-Müller h.

horopteric
horseshoe tear
Horton syndrome
Hosford
H. lacrimal dilator
H. spud

Hoskins
H. beaked Colibri forceps
H. fine straight forceps
H. fixation forceps
H. lens
H. miniaturized micro straight
  forceps
H. razor blade fragment
H. straight microiris forceps
H. suture forceps

Hoskins-Barkan goniotomy infant lens
hospital
King Khaled Eye Specialist H.
  (KKESH)
Wills Eye H.

host
h. cornea
h. incision
h. tissue forceps
h. trephination

host-graft junction
hot spot
HOTV visual acuity test
Hough drape
hour (h)
house
H. lacrimal dilator
H. miniature forceps
H. myringotomy knife

House-Bellucci alligator scissors

NOTES

H

231

housefly test
Houser
 H. cul-de-sac irrigator T-tube
 H. cul-de-sac irrigator tube
Hovius
 H. canal
 H. circle
 H. membrane
 H. plexus
Howard-Dolman apparatus
Howell phoria card
Hoya
 H. AR-570 autorefractor
 H. HDR objective refractometer
 H. MRM objective refractometer
Ho:YAG laser
HPA
 Hodapp-Parrish-Anderson
 HPA visual field staging system
HP Acthar Gel
HP-Guar ophthalmic gel
HPMC
 hydroxypropyl methylcellulose
HPMPC Peripheral Cytomegalovirus Retinitis Trial
HR
 hypertensive retinopathy
HRP
 high-pass resolution perimetry
HRP-GD
 high-pass resolution perimetry global deviation
HRP-LD
 high-pass resolution perimetry local deviation
HRQOL
 Health-Related Quality of Life
HRR
 Hardy-Rand-Ritter
 HRR plate
 HRR pseudoisochromatic test
HRT
 Heidelberg retina tomograph
HRT-II
 Heidelberg retina tomograph II
Hruby
 H. contact lens
 H. implant
HS
 Hartmann-Shack
 Pilopine HS
HSCAS
 hemodynamically significant carotid artery stenosis
hs-CRP
 high-sensitivity C-reactive protein
HSM-IOL
 heparin surface-modified intraocular lens

HSV
 herpes simplex virus
 HSV endotheliitis
 HSV epithelial keratitis
 footprints of HSV
 HSV ocular disease
 HSV stromal disease
 HSV trophic keratopathy
HT
 hypertropia
Ht
 hypermetropia, total
 total hyperopia
HTG
 high-tension glaucoma
Hubbard corneoscleral forceps
Huco diamond knife
Hudson line
Hudson-Stähli
 H.-S. line
 H.-S. line of corneal pigmentation
hue
 palpebral conjunctival h. (PCH)
Hueck ligament
28-Hue de Roth test
90-hue discrimination test
100-hue test
Hughes
 H. classification of chemical injury
 H. implant
 H. modification of Burch technique
 H. operation
 H. tarsoconjunctival flap
human
 h. allograft tissue
 h. antitumor necrosis factor
 h. immunodeficiency virus (HIV)
 h. leucocyte antigen match
 h. leukocyte antigen (HLA)
 h. tear film
 h. T-lymphotropic virus
humanized anti-Tac monoclonal antibody
Hummelsheim
 H. operation
 H. procedure
humor
 aqueous h.
 h. aquosus
 crystalline h.
 ocular h.
 plasmoid aqueous h.
 vitreous h.
 h. vitreus
humoral immunity
Humorsol Ophthalmic
Humphrey
 H. Atlas 991

H. Atlas Eclipse corneal topography system
H. automatic refractor
H. B-scan
H. field analyzer (HFA)
H. field analyzer II
H. 24-2 glaucoma hemifield test
H. Instruments vision analyzer
H. Instruments vision analyzer overrefraction system
H. lens analyzer
H. Mastervue corneal topography system
H. matrix
H. model 2000 optical coherence tomography
H. perimeter
H. retina imager
H. Systems ablation planner topography
H. ultrasonic pachometer
H. 992 videokeratographer
H. visual field (HVF)
H. visual field analyzer
Humphriss binocular balance
Hunkeler
H. ball-point hook
H. frown incision marker
H. lens
Hunt
H. chalazion forceps
H. chalazion scissors
Hunter-Hurler syndrome
Hunter syndrome
Hunt-Transley operation
Hurler
H. disease
H. syndrome
Hurler-Scheie
H.-S. compound
H.-S. syndrome
hurricane keratopathy
Huschke valve
Hutchinson
H. facies
H. patch
H. pupil
H. sign
H. Summer prurigo
H. syndrome
H. triad
Hutchinson-Tays central guttate choroiditis

HUV
hypocomplementemic urticarial vasculitis
Huygenian eyepiece
HVF
Humphrey visual field
HVOT
Hooper Visual Organization Test
Hy
hypermetropia
hyaline
h. artery
h. body
h. degeneration
h. fungus
h. mass
h. material
h. membrane
h. plaque
hyalinosis cutis et mucosae
hyalitis
h. of anterior membrane
asteroid h.
punctate h.
h. suppurativa
suppurative h.
hyalohyphomycosis
hyaloid
h. artery
h. asteroid
h. body
h. canal
h. clouding
h. corpuscle
h. face
h. fossa
h. membrane detachment
posterior h.
h. posterior membrane
h. system
hyaloidal fibrovascular proliferation
hyaloidea
fossa h.
membrana h.
stella lentis h.
hyaloideocapsular ligament
hyaloideoretinal degeneration
hyaloideus
canalis h.
hyaloiditis
hyaloidotomy
hyalomucoid
hyalonyxis

NOTES

H

hyalosis
asteroid h.
punctate h.
hyaluronate
h. sodium
h. sodium with chondroitin
hyaluronic
h. acid
h. acid solution
hyaluronidase
purified ovine h.
hybridization
comparative genomic h.
Hybriwix probe system
Hyde
H. astigmatism ruler
H. corneal forceps
H. double-curved forceps
H. irrigating/aspirating unit
H. irrigator/aspirator unit
Hydeltrasol
Hyde-Osher keratometric ruler
Hydracon contact lens
Hydrasoft contact lens
Hydrate Injection
hydration
stromal h.
hydraulic retinal reattachment
hydroa vacciniforme
hydroblepharon
hydrobromic acid (HBr)
hydrobromide
homatropine h.
hydroxyamphetamine h.
HydroBrush keratome
Hydrocare preserved saline
hydrochloric acid
hydrochloride (HCl)
apraclonidine h.
benoxinate h.
betaxolol h.
carteolol h.
ciprofloxacin h.
cocaine h.
cyclopentolate h.
dapiprazole h.
diphenhydramine h.
dorzolamide h.
hydromorphone h.
levobetaxolol h.
levobunolol h.
levocabastine h.
lidocaine h.
lignocaine h.
meperidine h.
naloxone h.
Neo-Synephrine H.
oxybuprocaine h.

oxymorphone h.
papaverine h.
phenacaine h.
phencyclidine h.
phenmetrazine h.
phenoxybenzamine h.
phenylephrine h.
phenylpropanolamine h.
piperocaine h.
procaine h.
proparacaine h.
protriptyline h.
quinacrine h.
tetracaine h.
tetrahydrozoline h.
thioridazine h.
thymoxamine h.
trifluoperazine h.
trifluperidol h.
tyramine h.
hydrochlorothiazide
hydrocodone
acetaminophen with h.
hydrocortisone
h. acetate
bacitracin, neomycin, polymyxin B, and h.
chloramphenicol, polymyxin B, and h.
neomycin, polymyxin B, and h.
oxytetracycline and h.
h. suspension
Hydrocortone Phosphate
Hydrocurve II lens
hydrodelamination
hydrodelineation
hydrodiascope
hydrodissection
h. cannula
cortical cleaving h.
Kellan h.
multiple-quadrant h.
multiquadrant h.
hydrodissector
anterior capsule h.
cortical cleaving h.
Pearce nucleus h.
hydrodissector/rotator
5195 nucleus h./r.
HydroDIURIL
HydroEye SoftGels
hydrogel
h. contact lens
h. disc intraocular lens
h. exoplant fragmentation
extended wear h.
h. intraocular lens
hydrogen peroxide

hydrolysis
Koch nucleus h.
h. of solution
hydrometric chamber
hydromorphone hydrochloride
Hydron
American H.
H. lens
Hydronol
hydrophila
Aeromonas h.
hydrophilic
h. acrylic intraocular lens
h. contact lens
h. hydrogel implant
hydrophobic contact lens
hydrophobicity
hydrophthalmia, hydrophthalmos, hydrophthalmus
anterior h.
posterior h.
total h.
hydropic degeneration
hydrops
acute h.
corneal h.
h. of iris
hydroquinone
hydrostatic gradient
Hydroview
H. foldable IOL
H. intraocular lens
hydroxide
calcium h.
potassium h.
sodium h.
hydroxocobalamin
hydroxyamphetamine
h. hydrobromide
h. and tropicamide
hydroxyapatite (HA)
h. ocular implant
h. orbital implant
h. spherical enucleation implant
hydroxychloroquine
h. retinopathy
h. sulfate
h. therapy
h. toxicity
hydroxyethyl
h. cellulose
h. methacrylate implant

hydroxymethylprogesterone
hydroxypropyl
h. cellulose
h. methylcellulose (HPMC)
hydroxyquinoline
halogenated h.
hydroxystilbamidine isethionate
hydroxysultaine
cocamidopropyl h.
hydroxyzine pamoate
Hy-Flow
Hyfrecator
hygiene
eyelid h.
hygroblepharic
hygroma
perioptic h.
Hygroton
hyicus
Staphylococcus h.
Hylan
H. biopolymer fluid
H. biopolymer gel-fluid
Hylashield
Hymenolepis nana
hyoscine
Isopto H.
scopolamine h.
hyoscyamine
hyperactive immune recovery
hyperactivity
sympathetic h.
hyperacuity
hyperacusis
hyperacute purulent conjunctivitis
hyperbaric
h. oxygen (HBO)
h. oxygen therapy
hyperbolic glasses
hyperburst mode
hypercalcemic
hyperchromic effect
hypercupremia
hyperdeviation
alternate h.
dissociated h.
hyperemia
ciliary h.
conjunctival h.
rebound conjunctival h.
hyperemic
hyperesophoria

NOTES

H

235

hyperesthesia
    optic h.
    h. optica
hypereuryopia
hyperexophoria
hyperfluorescence
    choroidal h.
    faint h.
    patchy h.
    stippled h.
hyperfluorescent
    h. hemorrhage
    h. window defect
hypergammaglobulinemia
hypergranulation tissue
hyperhomocysteinemia
hyperintense foci image
Hyperion LTK system
hyperkalemic periodic paralysis
hyperkeratotic
    h. dermatitis
    h. disorder
    h. plaque
hypermaturation
hypermature
    h. cataract
    h. lens
hypermetrope
hypermetropia (*var. of* hyperopia) **(Hy)**
    index h.
hypermetropia, total (Ht)
hypermetropic
    h. anisometrope
    h. astigmatism
hyperope
hyperophthalmopathic syndrome
hyperopia, hypermetropia (H)
    absolute h.
    acquired h.
    axial h.
    correction of h.
    curvature h.
    facultative h.
    high h.
    index h.
    h. index
    isolated high h.
    latent h. (Hl)
    manifest h. (Hm)
    refractive h.
    relative h.
    total h. (Ht)
hyperopic (H)
    h. ablation
    h. astigmatism (AsH)
    h. automated lamellar keratoplasty
    (HALK)
    h. correction
    h. error

    h. keratomileusis
    h. LASIK
    h. LASIK surgery
    h. LASIK technique
    h. shift
hyperopization
hyperornithinemia
hyperornithinemia, hyperammonemia,
    and homocitrullinuria
hyperosmotic agent
hyperosmotics
hyperphoria (H)
    circumduction h.
    left h.
    right h.
hyperplasia
    actinic h.
    benign reactive lymphoid h.
    epithelial h.
    goblet cell h.
    iris epithelial h.
    lymphoid h.
    pseudoepitheliomatous h.
    pseudosarcomatous endothelial h.
    reactive lymphoid h. (RLH)
    retinal epithelial pigment h.
hyperplastic primary vitreous
hyperpresbyopia
hyperpulse mode
hyperreflective tissue
Hypersal
hypersecretion glaucoma
hypersensitivity
    h. reaction
    staphylococcal h.
hyperteloric
hypertelorism
    canthal h.
    ocular h.
    orbital h.
hypertension
    adrenal h.
    arterial h.
    essential h.
    idiopathic intracranial h. (IIH)
    intracranial h.
    malignant h.
    ocular h. (OHT)
    h. period
    systemic arterial h.
hypertensive
    h. encephalopathy
    h. iridocyclitis
    h. neuroretinopathy
    h. oculopathy
    h. optic neuropathy
    h. retinitis
    h. retinopathy (HR)

hyperthermia
    malignant h.
    microwave h.
hyperthyroidism
    Graves h.
    ophthalmic h.
hyperthyroid stare
hypertonic
    h. drops
    h. osmotherapy
    h. saline
    h. solution
hypertrophic
    h. dendriform epithelial lesion
    h. interstitial neuropathy
    h. rhinitis
hypertrophy
    epithelial h.
    follicular h.
    gelatinous-appearing limbal h.
    giant papillary h. (GPH)
    papillary conjunctival h.
    pigment epithelial h.
    retinal pigment epithelial h.
    RP h.
hypertropia (HT)
    alternating h.
    constant h.
    dissociated double h. (DDHT)
    double dissociated h.
    flick h.
    left h. (LHT)
    right h.
hyperviscosity syndrome
hypervitaminosis D
hypesthesia
    infraorbital h.
hyphema
    8-ball h.
    black ball h.
    layered h.
    microscopic h.
    postoperative h.
    postsurgical h.
    spontaneous h.
    total h.
    traumatic h.
    uveitis, glaucoma, h. (UGH)
hypnagogic hallucination
hypnopompic hallucination
hypocalcemic cataract
hypochromic

Hypoclear
hypocomplementemic urticarial vasculitis (HUV)
hypocyclosis
hypoesophoria
hypoesthesia
    corneal h.
hypoexophoria
hypofluorescent
    h. dark spot
    h. streak
hypogammaglobulinemia
hypoglobus
hypoglycemic cataract
hypointense foci image
hypointensity
hypokalemic periodic paralysis
hypometric saccade
hypoorbitism
hypophoria
hypophosphatasia
    congenital h.
hypophysial artery
hypopigmentation
    oculocutaneous h.
hypoplasia
    bow-tie h.
    chiasmal h.
    hemiopic h.
    homonymous hemiopic h.
    macular h.
    optic disc h.
    optic nerve h.
    segmental h.
    thymic h.
hypoplastic
    h. disc
    h. ocular nerve
hypopyon
    blood-streaked h.
    h. keratitis
    keratoiritis h.
    recurrent h.
    sterile h.
    h. ulcer
    h. uveitis
hyposcleral
HypoTears
    H. PF Solution
    H. Select lubricant eye drops
hypotelorism
    ocular h.
    orbital h.

NOTES

H

237

hypotension
  intracranial h.
  spontaneous intracranial h.
hypotensive
  h. agent
  h. anesthesia
  h. retinopathy
hypothalami
  pars optica h.
hypothalamic glioma
hypothalamic-pituitary-thyroid axis
hypothalamus
hypothesis
  Knudsen h.
  Lyon h.
  h. testing
hypothyroidism
hypotonia
hypotonic solution
hypotonus
hypotony
  bilateral h.
  chronic prephthisical ocular h.
  essential h.
  h. maculopathy
  ocular h.

  persistent postdrainage h. (PPH)
  postoperative h.
  subsequent h.
  h. syndrome
  transient h.
hypotropia
  alternating h.
  constant h.
hypoxia
  orbital h.
  retinal h.
hypoxic
  h. corneal stress
  h. eyeball syndrome
  h. preconditioning
hypsiconchous
Hyrexin-50 Injection
hysteresis
  corneal h.
hysterical
  h. amblyopia
  h. blindness
  h. constricted field
  h. nystagmus
  h. visual field defect
Hyzine-50

I
luminous intensity
I/A
irrigation/aspiration
I/A cannula
I/A machine
steerable I/A
I&A
irrigating/aspirating
irrigation and aspiration
Simcoe I&A system
IAH
immune adherence hemagglutination
IALD
interocular axial length difference
iatrogenic
i. cataract
i. keratectasia
i. keratoconus
i. limbal stem cell deficiency
i. retinal break
i. retinal hole
i. retinal tear
ibuprofen
ICAM-1 antigen
ICaps
Alcon I.
I. Lutein & Zeaxanthin Formula
I. ocular vitamins
I. Plus
I. TR dietary supplement
ICCE
intracapsular cataract extraction
ICD
intercanthal distance
ICE
iridocorneal endothelial
ICE syndrome
ice
i. ball
i. pack test
ICG
indocyanine green
ICG angiography
ICGA
indocyanine green angiography
IC-Green kit
I-Chlor
ichthyosis
congenital i.
i. corneae
ICK
infectious crystalline keratopathy

ICL
implantable collamer lens
implantable contact lens
ICP
intracranial pressure
IC-PC
internal carotid-posterior communicating
IC-PC artery aneurysm
ICROP
International Classification of
Retinopathy of Prematurity
ICRS
intrastromal corneal ring segment
ICSC
idiopathic central serous
chorioretinopathy
icteric
icterus
scleral i.
IDDM
insulin-dependent diabetes mellitus
identical point
identification acuity
idiocy
amaurotic familial i. (AFI)
idiopathic
i. acquired retinal telangiectasia
i. amblyopia
i. arteritis of Takayasu
i. central serous chorioretinopathy
(ICSC)
i. choroidal fold
i. congenital esotropia
i. corneal endotheliopathy
i. demyelinating optic neuritis
i. epiretinal membrane (IERM)
i. facial palsy
i. inflammatory disease
i. inflammatory pseudotumor
i. intracranial hypertension (IIH)
i. juxtafoveal retinal telangiectasis
i. lacrimal gland inflammation
i. lipid keratopathy
i. macular cyst and hole
i. macular hole surgery
i. myositis
i. nongranulomatous optic neuritis
i. orbital inflammation
i. orbital inflammatory syndrome
(IOIS)
i. perifoveal telangiectasis (IPT)
i. perioptic neuritis
i. polypoidal choroidal vasculopathy
(IPCV)
i. preretinal membrane

idiopathic *(continued)*
    i. pseudotumor cerebri
    i. retinal vasculitis
    i. retinal vasculitis, aneurysms and
       neuroretinitis (IRVAN)
    i. scleritis
    i. sclerosing inflammation of orbit
    i. vitreitis
    i. vitreomacular traction syndrome
idioretinal light
idoxuridine (IDU)
I-Drops
IDU
    idoxuridine
IEBI
    intereye blink interval
IERM
    idiopathic epiretinal membrane
IFIS
    intraoperative floppy iris syndrome
ignipuncture
I-Homatrine
IIH
    idiopathic intracranial hypertension
IK
    interstitial keratitis
Ikeda microcapsulorrhexis forceps
IL-1
    interleukin-1
illacrimation
illaqueation
illiterate
    i. E
    i. E chart
    i. eye chart
illness
    high altitude i.
illuminance
illuminated
    i. hand magnifier
    i. near card (INC)
    i. stand magnifier
    i. suction needle
illumination
    axial i.
    background i.
    central i.
    coaxial i.
    contact i.
    critical i.
    dark-field i.
    dark-ground i.
    diffuse i.
    direct i.
    erect i.
    focal i.
    Ganzfeld i.
    incoherent i.
    indirect i.

    Köhler i.
    lateral i.
    Macbeth i.
    maximal i.
    narrow-slit i.
    oblique i.
    photopic i.
    sclerotic scatter i.
    slit i.
    tangential i.
    i. test
    vertical i.
    vision in reduced i.
illuminator
    high intensity i.
    Luxo surgical i.
    OPMI VISU 200 BrightFlex i.
    Synergetics endo i.
illusion
    frequency doubling i.
    Hermann grid i.
    i. of movement
    oculogravic i.
    oculogyral i.
    optic i.
    optical i.
    passive i.
illusory visual spread
ILM
    internal limiting membrane
    ILM maculorrhexis
Ilotycin Ophthalmic
image
    accidental i.
    aerial i.
    i. analysis
    i. artifact
    astigmatic i.
    bidimensional i.
    catatropic i.
    i. degradation
    digitized video fundus i.
    3-dimensional retinal i.
    direct i.
    i. displacement
    false i.
    formed i.
    foveal i.
    ghost i.
    gray-scale i.
    heteronymous i.
    homonymous i.
    hyperintense foci i.
    hypointense foci i.
    incidental i.
    inversion of i.
    inverted i.
    i. jump
    mirror i.

negative i.
ocular i.
optical i.
outside-world i.
i. plane
i. point
pseudostereo i.
Purkinje i.
Purkinje-Sanson mirror i.
real i.
retinal i.
Sanson i.
Scheimpflug slit i.
spectacular i.
specular i.
stigmatic i.
Tracey wavefront i.
true i.
unequal retinal i.
videooculographic i.
virtual i.
visual i.
IMAGEnet 2000 series digital imaging system
imager
Digital fundus i.
Digital slit-lamp i.
Humphrey retina i.
Photoshop 6.0 digitized i.
image-space focus
imaging
cine-magnetic resonance i.
color Doppler i.
diffusion-weighted imaging/magnetic resonance i. (DWI/MRI)
digital nonmydriatic fundus i.
i. element
high-resolution in vivo fundus autofluorescence i.
laser light i.
magnetic resonance i. (MRI)
ocular i.
off-axis i.
on-axis i.
ophthalmic retroillumination i.
optic i.
orbital i.
orbitocranial i.
polarization-sensitive i.
posterior visual pathway i.
Raman i.
stereoscopic i.
i. technology

ultra-high-resolution ophthalmic i.
ultra-high-speed ophthalmic i.
imbalance
binocular i.
central vestibular i.
Imbert-Fick
I.-F. law
I.-F. principle
imbricate
imbrication
eyelid i.
retinal i.
iMedConsent ophthalmology software program
imidazole derivative
immature cataract
immediate elevation
immersion
i. lens
i. method
imminens
glaucoma i.
immitis
Coccidioides i.
coccidioidomycosis i.
immune
i. adherence hemagglutination (IAH)
i. complex
i. compromise
i. mechanism
i. mediated
i. reaction
i. recovery uveitis
i. recovery vitreitis
i. recovery vitreitis syndrome
i. response
i. stromal keratitis (ISK)
i. system
i. Wessely ring
immunity
adaptive i.
cell-mediated i.
humoral i.
immunoadsorption therapy
immunochromatography analysis
immunodiagnostic method
immunodominant antibody
immunofluorescence
anticomplement i.
immunofluorescent
i. assay
i. staining
immunogenic inflammation

NOTES

immunohistochemical technique
immunohistochemistry
immunologic
    i. memory
    i. reaction
immunological conjunctivitis
immunology
    ocular i.
immunomodulator
immunomodulatory therapy
immunoperoxidase staining
immunoreactive adrenomedullin
  concentration
immunoreactivity
immunosuppressant-induced head tremor
immunosuppression
    triple-agent i.
immunosuppressive
    i. drug
    i. effect
impact
    i. resistance
    i. of vision impairment (IVI)
impaired
    i. perfusion
    i. vergence eye movement
impairment
    adduction i.
    cortical visual i.
    impact of vision i. (IVI)
    sensation i.
    visual i. (VI)
impatency
    congenital i.
impending macular hole
imperfection
    optical i.
impetigo contagiosa
impingement
implant
    absorbable i.
    accommodative i.
    ACIOL i.
    acorn-shaped eye i.
    acrylic hydroxyapatite i.
    acrylic lens i.
    Ahmed valve i.
    Allen orbital i.
    Alumina i.
    aluminum oxide i.
    anophthalmic i.
    anterior chamber intraocular lens i.
    Arroyo i.
    Arruga i.
    artificial iris diaphragm i.
    aspheric i.
    Baerveldt glaucoma i.
    Baerveldt seton i.
    Barkan infant i.

Barraquer i.
Berens conical i.
Berens pyramidal i.
Berens-Rosa scleral i.
Binkhorst collar stud lens i.
Binkhorst 2-loop intraocular lens i.
Binkhorst 4-loop iris-fixated i.
bioceramic i.
Bio-Eye ocular i.
biomatrix ocular i.
Bionic eye microdetector
  subretinal i.
Boberg-Ans lens i.
Boyd orbital i.
Brawner orbital i.
build-up i.
Bunker i.
Castroviejo acrylic i.
CE/IOL i.
Choyce Mark VIII i.
ciliary neurotrophic factor capsule
  protein eye i.
collagen i.
conical i.
conus shell-type eye i.
conventional shell i.
Cooper i.
Copeland i.
corneal i.
cosmetic contact shell i.
Crystalens model AT-45 i.
CTNF capsule protein eye i.
curlback shell i.
Cutler i.
45-degree bent reform i.
Dermostat i.
Doherty sphere i.
encircling i.
Endotine TransBleph i.
enophthalmos wedge i.
i. entry
Envision TD intravitreal i.
Epstein collar stud acrylic i.
expanded polytetrafluoroethylene
  SoftForm facial i.
Extend absorbable synthetic
  punctal i.
i. extrusion
facial i.
Federov 4-loop iris clip lens i.
Federov type I, II lens i.
Ferguson i.
filtering i.
Fine magnetic i.
FluidVision i.
fluocinolone acetonide intravitreal i.
foldable silicone i.
Fox sphere i.
front build-up i.

full-dimpled Lucite i.
ganciclovir intravitreal i.
Garcia-Novito eye i.
Gelfilm retinal i.
glass sphere i.
gold eyelid load i.
Goldmann 3-mirror i.
gold sphere i.
gonioscopic i.
grooved silicone i.
hemisphere eye i.
Herrick silicone lacrimal i.
hollow-sphere i.
hook-type i.
Hruby i.
Hughes i.
hydrophilic hydrogel i.
hydroxyapatite ocular i.
hydroxyapatite orbital i.
hydroxyapatite spherical
  enucleation i.
hydroxyethyl methacrylate i.
i. infection
intracanalicular collagen i.
intracorneal i.
intraocular lens i.
intraorbital i.
intravitreal bioerodible
  dexamethasone i.
intravitreal ganciclovir i.
Iowa orbital i.
Ivalon sponge i.
Jordan i.
24-karat gold biocompatible i.
keratolens i.
King orbital i.
Koeppe gonioscopic i.
Krupin i.
Krupin-Denver long-valve i.
lens i.
i. lens
Levitt i.
Lincoff scleral sponge i.
4-loop iris clip i.
4-loop iris fixated i.
Lucite sphere i.
i. magnet
magnetic i.
MedDev i.
Medical Optics PC11NB intraocular
  lens i.
Medpor MCOI i.
meridional i.

methylmethacrylate i.
i. migration
Molteno i.
motility i.
Mueller i.
Mules i.
multifocal i.
NewIris ocular i.
Oculo-Plastik ePTFE ocular i.
O'Malley self-adhering lens i.
Ophtec occlusion i.
optic i.
orbital floor i.
pars plana seton i.
peanut i.
piggyback i.
i. placement
plastic sphere i.
Plexiglas i.
pneumatically stented i. (PSI)
polyethylene i.
Porex i.
porous orbital i.
posterior chamber lens i. (PCLI)
posterior tube shunt i.
Precision Cosmet intraocular lens i.
primary lens i.
protein eye i.
pseudophake i.
i. radiotherapy
refractive floating i.
refractive phakic i.
ReSTOR vision i.
retinal Gelfilm i.
Retisert intravitreal i.
reverse-shape i.
Ridley anterior chamber lens i.
Ridley Mark II lens i.
Rodin orbital i.
Schocket tube i.
scleral i.
secondary lens i.
segmental i.
semishell i.
Severin i.
Shearing posterior chamber
  intraocular lens i.
shelf-type i.
shell i.
Silastic scleral buckler i.
silicone mesh i.
i. sleeve
sleeve i.

NOTES

implant *(continued)*
    sling for i.
    Smith orbital floor i.
    Snellen conventional reform i.
    SoftForm facial i.
    solid silicone with Supramid
      mesh i.
    sphere i.
    spherical i.
    sponge i.
    i. sponge
    2-staged Baerveldt glaucoma i.
    subperiosteal i.
    SupraFOIL i.
    Supramid-Allen i.
    Supramid lens i.
    surface i.
    sustained release intravitreal
      helical i.
    SutureGroove gold eye weight i.
    tantalum mesh i.
    Teflon i.
    temporary intracanalicular
      collagen i.
    Tennant i.
    Tensilon i.
    ThinProfile eyelid i.
    tire i.
    i. tire
    TransBleph i.
    Troutman i.
    tunneled i.
    ultrasmall incision i.
    Universal i.
    unpegged hydroxyapatite i.
    Uribe orbital i.
    VA magnetic orbital i.
    Varilux lens i.
    vitallium i.
    Vitrasert intravitreal i.
    Volk conoid lens i.
    Wheeler eye sphere i.
    wire mesh i.
implantable
    i. collamer lens (ICL)
    i. contact lens (ICL)
    i. miniaturized telescope (IMT)
implantation
    Ahmed glaucoma valve i.
    Artisan lens i.
    endocapsular balloon i.
    i. forceps
    gold microshunt i.
    gold weight i.
    in-the-bag i.
    intraocular lens i.
    keratoprosthesis i.
    i. of lens
    multifocal intraocular lens i.

    pediatric intraocular i.
    phakic IOL i.
    PHEMA KPro i.
    piggyback i.
    precise i.
    radon seed i.
implanter
impletion
implicit time
impression
    basilar i.
    i. cytology
    i. débridement
    i. tonometer
imprint
improved vision
improvement
    no i.
    pinhole no i. (PHNI)
    visual field i.
improvised explosive device
IMT
    implantable miniaturized telescope
Imuran
in
    base in (BI)
    in situ DNA nick end-labeling
    in situ DNA nick end-labeling
      staining
    in vitro toxicology assay
inactive
    i. ingredient
    i. trachoma
INAD
    infantile neuroaxonal dystrophy
inadequacy
    blink i.
Inamura
    I. race chopper
    I. small incision capsulorrhexis
      forceps
I-Naphline Ophthalmic
inattention
    visual i.
inborn error
INC
    illuminated near card
Inc.
    Ophthalmic Technologies I. (OTI)
incandescent lamp
incapacitating injury
incarceration
    iris i.
incidence
    angle of i.
    cataract i.
    plane of i.
incident
    i. angle

flux i.
i. point
ray i.
i. ray of light
incidental
   i. color
   i. image
incipient cataract
incision
   Agnew-Verhoeff i.
   arcuate i.
   buttonhole i.
   centrifugal i.
   centripetal i.
   chevron i.
   clear corneal step i.
   clear corneal tunnel i.
   conjunctival i.
   corneal relaxing i.
   cornea tunnel i.
   corneoscleral i.
   corridor i.
   cruciate i.
   cutdown i.
   eyelid crease i.
   gray-line i.
   grooved i.
   host i.
   i. into eyelid
   lateral canthal i.
   leaking i.
   limbal relaxing i. (LRI)
   Lynch medial canthal i.
   nasal buttonhole i.
   paracentesis i.
   phaco i.
   posterior i.
   relaxing i.
   scleral-limbal-corneal i.
   scleral tunnel i.
   side port i.
   i. spreader
   stab i.
   subciliary i.
   sutureless clear corneal i.
   Swan i.
   tangential i.
   temporal self-sealing clear
     corneal i.
   i. terminus
   trap i.
   trapezoid single-plane clear
     corneal i.

tunnel i.
i. viewing instrument
von Noorden i.
incision-related complication
incisura
   i. ethmoidalis ossis frontalis
   i. lacrimalis
   i. maxillae
   i. supraorbitalis
incisure
   ethmoidal i.
   frontal i.
   lacrimal i.
   supraorbital i.
inclinometer
inclusion
   i. blennorrhea
   i. body
   i. conjunctivitis
   i. cyst
   epithelial i.
   intranuclear i.
   mascara particle i.
incoherent illumination
incomitance
incomitant
   i. esodeviation
   i. vertical deviation
   i. vertical strabismus
incomplete
   i. achromatopsia
   i. hemianopia
   i. hemianopsia
   i. pupil-sparing oculomotor nerve
     paresis
incongruent nystagmus
incongruous
   i. field defect
   i. hemianopia
   i. hemianopsia
incontinentia pigmenti
incorrect
   i. lens power
   i. power IOL
increased
   i. myopic shift
   i. tension (T+)
   i. vertical fusional amplitude
increment
   half-diopter i.
   i. threshold spectral sensitivity
incrementally

NOTES

incubation
    lens i.
incycloduction
incyclophoria
incyclorotation
incyclotorsion
incyclotropia
incyclovergence
IND
    investigational new drug
indapamide
indentation
    globe i.
    i. gonioscopy
    i. operation
    prominent i.
    scleral i.
    i. tonometer
    i. tonometry
independence
    actual degree of i.
independent
    i. event
    i. risk factor
    spectacle i.
index, pl. **indices, indexes**
    i. amblyopia
    i. ametropia
    color confusion i.
    disability glare i. (DGI)
    Glaucoma Health Perceptions I.
      (GHPI)
    i. hypermetropia
    hyperopia i.
    i. hyperopia
    keratoconus prediction i. (KPI)
    modified Rabinowitz-McDonnell i.
    myopia i.
    i. myopia
    Ocular Surface Disease I. (OSDI)
    ophthalmic confidence i. (OCI)
    recession i. (RI)
    i. of refraction (IR, n)
    refractive i.
    resistive i.
    surface asymmetry i. (SAI)
    surface regularity i. (SRI)
    visual field i.
Indiana bleb appearance grading scale
indicator
    Berens-Tolman ocular
      hypertension i.
    quality i.
    i. yellow
indices (*pl. of* index)
indinavir sulfate
indirect
    i. argon laser drainage
    i. choroidal rupture

    i. fluorescent antibody
    i. illumination
    i. lens
    i. ophthalmoscope
    i. ophthalmoscopic laser
      photocoagulation
    i. ophthalmoscopy
    i. pupillary reaction
    i. vision
individualized mapping
Indocin ophthalmic solution
indocyanine
    i. green (ICG)
    i. green angiography (ICGA)
    i. green dye
indolent
    i. ulceration
    i. ulceration of cornea
indoltheticum
    Flavobacterium i.
indomethacin toxicity keratopathy
induced
    i. anisophoria
    i. astigmatism
    i. prism
inducing
    remission i.
induction
industrial
    i. eye protector
    i. spectacles
inelastic eyelid
I-Neocort
inert material for intraocular lens
infant
    I. Aphakia Treatment Study
    blind i.
    i. Karickhoff laser lens
    i. 3-mirror laser lens
    premature i.
    retinopapillitis of premature i.
infantile
    i. botulism
    i. cataract
    i. esotropia
    i. glaucoma
    i. neuroaxonal dystrophy (INAD)
    i. nystagmus
    i. nystagmus syndrome
    i. optic atrophy
    i. poikiloderma subgroup 1-2-3
    i. purulent conjunctivitis
    i. Refsum disease
    i. strabismus syndrome
infarct
    choroidal i.
    nerve fiber layer i.
infarction
    cerebral i.

eye i.
lateral medullary i.
orbital i.
paramedian thalamopeduncular i.
retinochoroidal i.
infarctive necrosis
infection
anaerobic ocular i.
bacterial i.
Borrelia burgdorferi i.
chlamydial i.
extended wear i.
eyelid molluscum contagiosum i.
fungal eyelid i.
gonococcal i.
graft i.
Gram-positive i.
herpetic ocular i.
implant i.
mycotic i.
ocular cryptococcal i.
ocular vaccinia i.
opportunistic i.
orbital i.
secondary ocular i.
Serratia marcescens i.
Toxoplasma gondii i.
trematode i.
vaccinia i.
viral i.
infectiosus
conjunctivitis necroticans i.
infectious
i. conjunctivitis
i. corneal ulcer
i. crystalline keratopathy (ICK)
i. dacryoadenitis
i. disease
i. endophthalmitis
i. epithelial keratitis
i. ophthalmoplegia
i. retinochoroiditis
infective myositis
inferior
i. altitudinal defect
i. arcuate bundle
arcus palpebralis i.
arteriola macularis i.
arteriola nasalis retinae i.
arteriola temporalis retinae i.
i. canaliculus
i. conjunctival fornix
i. conus

i. cornea
fissura orbitalis i.
i. fornix reformation
glandula lacrimalis i.
i. lacrimal gland
i. longitudinal fasciculus
i. macula
i. macular arteriole
musculus tarsalis i.
i. nasal artery
i. nasal quadrant
i. nasal vein
i. oblique
i. oblique extraocular muscle
i. oblique overaction (IOOA)
i. oblique palsy
i. olivary nucleus
i. ophthalmic vein
i. orbital fissure
i. orbital rim
i. orbital septum
i. palpebral vein
i. pole
i. punctum
i. rectus (IR)
i. rectus extraocular muscle
i. retinal arcade
i. salivary nucleus
i. steepening
i. symblepharon
i. tarsal muscle
i. tarsus
i. temporal arcade
i. temporal artery
i. temporal quadrant
i. temporal vein
vena ophthalmica i.
venula macularis i.
venula nasalis retinae i.
venula temporalis retinae i.
i. zone of retina
i. zygomatic foramen
inferiores
venae palpebrales i.
inferioris
pars orbitalis gyri frontalis i.
inferiorly
eye rotated i.
inferonasal artery
inferonasally
inferotemporal
i. arcade
i. artery

NOTES

inferotemporally
infiltrate
anular i.
bacterial infectious corneal i.
central stromal i.
i. in cornea
corneal punctate i.
crystalline i.
inflammatory cellular i.
leukemic i.
patchy anterior stromal i.
peripheral ring i.
plasmacytoid i.
ring i.
ring-shaped stromal i.
i. size
stromal anular i.
stromal ring i.
subepithelial punctate corneal i.
white stromal i.
wreath pattern stromal i.
infiltration
branching i.
choroidal i.
conjunctival i.
dermal amyloid i.
inflammatory cell i.
linear i.
lymphocytic i.
lymphoid i.
mononuclear cell i.
perivascular neutrophil i.
radial i.
sarcoidosis i.
infiltrative
i. keratitis
i. optic neuropathy
Infinitech
I. fiber optics
I. laser probe
infinite distance
infinity
infirmary
eye i.
Massachusetts Eye & Ear I.
Inflamase
I. Forte
I. Forte Ophthalmic
I. Mild
I. Mild Ophthalmic
inflamed pinguecula
inflammation
acute sterile i.
anterior chamber i.
anterior segment i.
apical orbital i.
ciliary body i.
i. control
corneal nerve i.

i. of eyelid
idiopathic lacrimal gland i.
idiopathic orbital i.
immunogenic i.
intraocular i.
noninfectious i.
ocular i.
orbital i.
persistent postoperative i.
postoperative i.
sight-threatening ocular i.
systemic marker of i.
vitreous i.
inflammatory
i. cascade
i. cell
i. cell infiltration
i. cellular infiltrate
i. change of retina
i. chemical mediator
i. dacryoadenitis
i. ectropion
i. glaucoma
i. marker
i. mediator
i. meibomian gland disease
i. membrane
i. myopathy
i. optic neuritis
i. optic neuropathy
i. orbital pseudotumor
i. retinal margin
i. retinopathy
i. syndrome
i. target site of eye
inflammatory-related parameter
inflection
infliximab
inflow
aqueous i.
influence
i. of an Artisan lens
genetic i.
influenzae
Haemophilus i.
influenza virus
influx
fibrin i.
infolding
macular translocation with
macular i.
macular translocation with scleral i.
(MTSI)
scleral i.
information
spatial i.
i. supply
informed consent
infraciliary

infraduct
infraduction
infraepitrochlear nerve
infranasal
infranuclear
    i. disorder
    i. ophthalmoplegia
    i. pathway
infraorbital
    i. anesthesia
    i. artery
    i. canal
    i. foramen
    i. groove
    i. hypesthesia
    i. margin
    i. margin of maxilla
    i. nerve
    i. region
    i. sulcus of maxilla
    i. suture
infraorbitalis
    nervus i.
    sutura i.
infrapalpebral sulcus
infrared
    i. cataract
    i. heater
    i. image analysis
    i. oculography
    i. optometer
    i. pupillometry
    i. radiation
    i. slit lamp
infratentorial arteriovenous malformation
infratrochlear nerve
infravergence
infraversion
infundibular cyst
infusion
    i. cannula
    i. capacity
    detachment i.
    i. flow rate
    i. light pipe
    microcatheter urokinase i.
    i. suction cutter vitreous cutter
    vented gas forced i. (VGFI)
ingredient
    inactive i.
ingrowth
    epithelial i.

    fibroblastic i.
    stromal i.
inhalation anesthetic
inheritance
    polygenic i.
    X-linked i.
inhibition
    intraoperative miosis i.
    lateral i.
    paradoxic levator i.
    vascular i.
inhibitional
    i. palsy
    i. palsy of contralateral antagonist
inhibitor
    carbonic anhydrase i. (CAI)
    mast cell i.
    matrix metalloproteinase i.
    plasminogen activator i. (PAI)
    T-cell i.
inion
initial trabeculectomy
injection
    antiangiogenesis i.
    anti-VEGF i.
    autologous blood i.
    botulinum toxin A i.
    ciliary i.
    circumcorneal i.
    conjunctival ciliary i.
    Cytoxan I.
    episcleral i.
    Hydrate I.
    Hyrexin-50 I.
    intracameral air i.
    intralesional triamcinolone i.
    intraocular gas i.
    intravenous i.
    intravitreal gas i.
    intravitreal SOD2 i.
    juxtascleral i.
    i. molding
    Neosar I.
    Osmitrol i.
    peribulbar i.
    periocular triamcinolone i.
    posterior sub-Tenon i.
    Predcor-TBA I.
    retrobulbar alcohol i.
    retrobulbar corticosteroid i.
    retroocular i.
    silicone oil i.
    subarachnoid i.

NOTES

injection *(continued)*
    subconjunctival i.
    sub-Tenon corticosteroid i.
    i. technique
    Toradol I.
    Van Lint i.
injector
    automatic twin syringe i.
    Dyonics syringe i.
    Monarch II i.
    plunger-type i.
    preloaded i.
    Royale intraocular lens i.
    SofPort easy-load i.
injector-aspirator
    double-barreled i.-a.
injury
    battle casualty i.
    chemical i.
    closed globe i.
    concomitant i.
    concussion i.
    contrecoup i.
    coup i.
    dehydration i.
    devastating ocular adnexal i.
    eye i.
    eyelid i.
    gestational i.
    head i.
    high-velocity projectile i.
    Hughes classification of chemical i.
    incapacitating i.
    iris i.
    lenticular i.
    levator i.
    microwave radiation i.
    ocular adnexal i.
    ocular bullet i.
    ocular chemical i.
    ocular paint-ball i.
    ocular war i.
    open globe i.
    optic nerve i.
    penetrating ocular i.
    perforating i.
    radiation i.
    rocket-propelled grenade i.
    scalpel i.
    shearing i.
    Taser penetrating ocular i.
    thermal i.
    ultraviolet-induced i.
    war-related i.
in-lab lens casting technology
inlay
    corneal i.
inner
    i. canthus

    i. limiting lamina
    i. limiting membrane
    i. molecular layer of retina
    i. nuclear layer
    i. nuclear layer of retina
    i. plexiform layer
    i. punctate choroidopathy
    i. segment
innervate
innervation
    eyelid i.
    Hering law of equal i.
    Hering law of equivalent i.
    Hering law of simultaneous i.
    levator i.
    reciprocal i.
    regeneration of i.
    Sherrington law of reciprocal i.
innocens
    diabetes i.
innominate steal syndrome
Innovar
Innovatome microkeratome
InnoVit
    I. 1800 probe
    I. vitrectomy probe
INO
    internuclear ophthalmoplegia
inoculum
input
    nerve i.
    i. nerve
    supranuclear i.
insert
    Intacs prescription i.
inserter
    AC tube i.
    AMO PhacoFlex lens and i.
    Fine III i.
    Lens-Eze i.
insertion
    contact lens i.
    Jones tube i.
    tendinous i.
    tensor i.
inside-out core vitrectomy
insipidus
    diabetes i.
insonification
    ultrasonic i.
inspired gas
instability
    tear film i.
instillation
    drop i.
    silicone oil i.
institute
    American National Standards I.
    (ANSI)

Dartmouth Eye I.
National Eye I. (NEI)
Wilmer Eye I.
Wilmer Ophthalmological I.
instrument
Accurate Surgical and
Scientific I.'s (ASSI)
Alcon Surgical i.
American Hydron i.
Argyll Robertson i.
Auto Ref-keratometer i.
Biophysic Ophthascan S i.
Carl Zeiss i.
Daisy irrigation/aspiration i.
DORC backflush i.
fixation i.
Grieshaber ultrasharp
microsurgery i.
guillotine vitrectomy i.
head-mounted i.
incision viewing i.
Iolab titanium i.
IOLMaster optical i.
IVI i.
Mastel Precision surgical i.
matte black i.
ophthalmic i.
optical centering i.
phacofracture ophthalmic i.
preschool vision screening i.
Rank-Taylor-Hobson-Talysurf i.
Retinomax refractometry i.
Rumex titanium i.
single-use i.
Sonomed 1500 A-scan i.
Sutherland rotatable microsurgery i.
topographic scanning/indocyanine
green angiography combination i.
UTAS 2000 electroretinography i.
vitrectomy i.
instrumentation
insufficiency
accommodation i.
accommodative i. (AI)
convergence i. (CI)
cortical visual i.
divergence i.
dynamic accommodation i.
i. of eyelid
i. of eyelid closure
muscular i.
static accommodation i.
vertebrobasilar artery i.

insular scotoma
insulin-deficient diabetes
**insulin-dependent diabetes mellitus
(IDDM)**
insulin resistance
Intacs
I. corneal ring segment
I. intrastromal corneal ring
I. prescription insert
intact
i. anterior hyaloid face
extraocular movement i. (EOMI)
integration
visual-motor i.
Integre 532 delivery system
integrity
break in retinal i.
corneal epithelial i.
epithelial i.
intelligence
artificial i.
intensity
luminous i. (I)
i. profile
radiant i.
unit of luminous i.
interaction
bipolar horizontal i.
contour i.
drug i.
electrostatic i.
Fas i.
FasL i.
rod-cone i.
spatial i.
intercalary staphyloma
intercanthal distance (ICD)
intercanthic
intercellular
i. adhesion molecule
i. space
intercept
corneal i.
interchangeable plate
interciliary fiber
intercilium
intereye blink interval (IEBI)
interface
graft-host i.
i. haze
laminar i.
macular vitreoretinal i.
membrane-corneal i.

NOTES

interface *(continued)*
    i. opacity
    parallel i.
    i. phenomena
    vitreomacular i.
    vitreoretinal i.
interfasciale
    spatium i.
interfascial space
interference
    electromagnetic i. (EMI)
    i. filter
    i. fringe
    i. visual acuity test
interferometer
    electron i.
    Zeiss IOL Master laser i.
interferometry
    electron i.
    laser i.
    low-coherence i.
    partial coherence i. (PCI)
interferon
    i. alfa-2a
    i. alfa-2b
    i. beta-1a
interior eye tumor
interlacing of collagen lamellae
interlamellar space
interleukin-1 (IL-1)
intermedia
    uveitis i.
intermediate
    i. posterior curve (IPC)
    i. uveitis
Intermedics
    I. intraocular tonometer
    I. lens
    I. Phaco I/A unit
intermedius
    nervus i.
    Staphylococcus i.
intermittent
    i. angle-closure glaucoma
    i. deviation
    i. esotropia (E(T))
    i. exotropia (X(T))
    i. strabismus
    i. tropia
intermuscular
    i. membrane
    i. septum
interna
    axis oculi i.
    membrana limitans i.
    ophthalmoplegia i.
internal
    i. axis of eye
    i. capsule syndrome

    i. carotid artery
    i. carotid-posterior communicating (IC-PC)
    i. carotid-posterior communicating artery aneurysm
    i. corneal ulcer of von Hippel
    i. hordeolum
    i. lacrimal fistula
    i. limiting membrane (ILM)
    i. limiting membrane peeling
    i. limiting membrane of retina
    i. nucleus hydrodelineation needle
    i. ophthalmopathy
    i. ophthalmoplegia
    i. ostium
    i. palsy
    i. rectus muscle
    i. reflectivity
    i. squint
    i. strabismus
International Classification of Retinopathy of Prematurity (ICROP)
internuclear
    i. ophthalmoparesis
    i. ophthalmoplegia (INO)
    i. paralysis
internuclearis
    ophthalmoplegia i.
internum
    hordeolum i.
internus
    axis bulbi i.
interobserver
interocular
    i. axial length difference (IALD)
    i. differential blur
interosseous wiring
interpalpebral
    i. fissure
    i. stromal disease
    i. zone
interpeduncular fossa
interphotoreceptor retinoid-binding protein (IRBP)
interplexiform cell
interpolation
interpupillary distance (IPD)
interrogans
    Leptospira i.
interrupted nylon suture
Intersol
Interspace YAG laser lens
interstitial
    i. keratitis (IK)
    i. neovascularization
    i. nucleus of Cajal
interthalamic commissure
intervaginale
    spatium i.

intervaginal space of optic nerve
interval
    confidence i.
    focal i.
    intereye blink i. (IEBI)
    Sturm i.
    i. of Sturm
intervention
    surgical i.
interventional
    i. case report
    i. procedure
interwave-guided multipass
interweaving
    collagen fibril i.
Interzeag bowl perimeter
in-the-bag
    i.-t.-b. implantation
    i.-t.-b. lens
intorsion
intort
intortor muscle
intoxication amaurosis
intraarterial cytoreductive chemotherapy
intraaxonal
intracameral
    i. administration
    i. air injection
    i. anesthesia
    i. lidocaine
    i. medication
    i. suture
intracanalicular
    i. anatomy
    i. collagen implant
    i. optic nerve
    i. punctum plug
intracapsular
    i. cataract extraction (ICCE)
    i. extraction of cataract
    i. ligament
intracavernous
    i. aneurysm
    i. carotid artery
intracellular
    i. cytoplasm
    i. target
intraconal space
intracorneal
    i. cyst
    i. implant
    i. ring

intracranial
    i. anatomy
    i. aneurysm
    i. glioma
    i. granuloma
    i. hypertension
    i. hypotension
    i. mass
    i. optic nerve
    i. optic nerve decompression
    i. pressure (ICP)
intracytoplasmic inclusion body
intradermal nevus
intraepithelial
    i. cyst
    i. dyskeratosis
    i. epithelioma
    i. microcyst
    i. neoplasia
    i. neoplasm
    i. plexus
intralacrimal papilloma
intralamellar
    i. autopatch
    i. pocket procedure
Intralase
    I. eye correction procedure
    I. FS30 laser
IntraLASIK procedure
intralenticular hemorrhage
intralesional triamcinolone injection
intraluminal suture
intramarginal sulcus
intramedullary segment
intranasal endoscopic
    dacryocystorhinostomy
intranuclear
    i. eosinophilic inclusion body
    i. inclusion
intraocular (IO)
    acetylcholine i.
    i. administration
    i. air
    i. anatomy
    i. anesthetic agent
    i. cataract extraction
    i. cilia
    i. coccidioidomycosis
    i. cowhitch knot
    i. cowhitch knot for dislocated lens
    i. cysticercus
    i. distance

NOTES

intraocular *(continued)*
 i. fistula
 i. fluid
 i. forceps
 i. foreign body (IOFB)
 i. foreign body trauma
 i. gas
 i. gas bubble
 i. gas injection
 i. hemorrhage
 i. inflammation
 i. involvement
 i. irrigating solution
 i. lens (IOL)
 i. lens decentration
 i. lens dialer
 i. lens dislocation
 i. lens exchange
 i. lens glide
 i. lens implant
 i. lens implantation
 i. lens manipulation
 i. lens power (IOLP)
 i. lidocaine
 i. lymphoma
 i. melanoma
 i. muscle (IOM)
 i. myelination of retinal nerve fiber
 i. optic nerve
 i. optic neuritis
 i. oxygen tension
 i. penetration
 i. pressure (IOP)
 i. pressure control
 i. pressure goal
 i. pressure level
 i. pressure-lowering docosanoid compound
 i. pressure-lowering medication
 i. pressure spike
 i. retinal prosthesis
 i. retinoblastoma
 i. silicone oil tamponade
 i. tamponade
 i. tuberculosis
 i. tumor
intraoperative
 i. adjustable suture surgery
 i. bleeding
 i. blood loss
 i. B-scan echogram
 i. complication
 i. floppy iris syndrome (IFIS)
 i. frozen section assessment
 i. miosis inhibition
 i. suture adjustment (ISA)
intraorbital
 i. air

 i. anatomy
 i. anesthesia
 i. foreign body
 i. hemorrhage
 i. implant
 i. margin of orbit
 i. nerve dysfunction
intraosseous optic nerve
intrapapillary drusen
intraretinal
 i. bleeding
 i. cystoid
 i. fleck
 i. hemorrhage
 i. lipid deposit
 i. microvascular abnormality (IRMA)
 i. separation
 i. space
intrascleral
 i. nerve loop
 i. plexus
intrasellar tumor
intrasheath tenotomy
intrastromal
 i. corneal ring
 i. corneal ring segment (ICRS)
 i. laser
intratemporal segment
intravenous (I.V., IV)
 i. fluorescein
 i. fluorescein angiography (IVFA)
 i. injection
 i. thyrotropin-releasing hormone test
intraventricular hemorrhage (IVH)
intravitreal
 i. administration
 i. antibiotic
 i. bioerodible dexamethasone implant
 i. fibrin
 i. ganciclovir implant
 i. gas injection
 i. hemorrhage
 i. pressure
 i. SOD2 injection
 i. steroid
 i. TPA
 i. triamcinolone
 i. triamcinolone acetonide
intrinsic
 i. light
 i. ocular muscle
 i. sympathomimetic activity
 i. vascularity
introducer
 Carter sphere i.
 silicone i.

sphere i.
Weaver trocar i.
Intron A
intrusion
saccadic i.
intubation
Crawford tubing i.
endotracheal i.
lacrimal i.
monocanalicular i.
O'Donoghue silicone i.
Silastic i.
silicone nasolacrimal i.
in-tumbling fashion
intumescent cataract
invasion
epithelial i.
invasive adenoma
inventory
Color Screening I.
Multiple Sclerosis Quality of
Life I. (MSQLI)
inversa
retinitis pigmentosa i.
inverse
i. astigmatism
i. axicon
i. ocular bobbing
inversion of image
inversus
canthus i.
epicanthal i.
epicanthus i.
situs i.
inverted image
inverter
stereoscopic diagonal i.
I. vitrectomy system
investigation
neuroophthalmological i.
scientific i.
investigational new drug (IND)
invisible bifocal
involutional
i. blepharoptosis
i. entropion
i. laxity
i. lower eyelid entropion
i. ptosis
i. senile ectropion
i. senile entropion
i. senile ptosis
i. stenosis

involvement
intraocular i.
vesicular i.
inward rectifier
IO
intraocular
IO muscle
iodide
echothiophate i.
metubine i.
Phospholine I.
potassium i.
iodine
radioactive i.
iodochlorhydroxyquin
iodopsin
iodoquinol
IOFB
intraocular foreign body
IOFB-caused defect
IOIS
idiopathic orbital inflammatory syndrome
IOL
intraocular lens
accommodating IOL
accommodative IOL
AcrySof IQ IOL
AcrySof Natural IOL
AcrySof single-piece IOL
AMO Array SA40N multifocal
IOL
AMO Clariflex IOL
anterior chamber IOL
apodized diffractive IOL
AquaSense IOL
Artisan iris-fixated phakic IOL
blue-filtering IOL
blue filtration hydrophobic IOL
IOL cartridge holder
CeeOn Edge foldable IOL
C-loop IOL
Collamer 3-piece IOL
Crystalens IOL
CV232 square-round-edge IOL
IOL decentration
disc IOL
IOL exchange
IOL explantation
foldable iris-claw phakic IOL
foldable 3-piece silicone IOL
IOL formula
Hydroview foldable IOL
incorrect power IOL

NOTES

IOL *(continued)*
    iris claw phakic IOL
    Kearney side-notch IOL
    KH-3500 IOL
    light-adjustable IOL
    MemoryLens prefolded IOL
    modified prolate anterior surface IOL
    monofocal IOL
    Morcher iris diaphragm IOL, type 67G
    multifocal phakic IOL
    multifocal silicone IOL
    NewLife IOL
    non-blue filtering IOL
    NuLens accommodating IOL
    optimal IOL
    parent spherical IOL
    Phakic 6 H2 IOL
    3-piece IOL
    1-piece hydrophilic acrylic IOL
    3-piece hydrophilic acrylic IOL
    piggybacked toric IOL
    plate-haptic IOL
    IOL position
    IOL power
    IOL power calculation
    presbyopia-correcting IOL
    ReZoom multifocal refractive IOL
    SC60B-OUV IOL
    Sensar OptiEdge AR40e IOL
    Sensar OptiEdge foldable acrylic IOL
    sharp-edged IOL
    silicone toric IOL
    single-piece acrylic IOL
    single-piece SN60AT IOL
    SoFlex IOL
    soft acrylic IOL
    spherical IOL
    Staar IOL
    Staar toric IOL
    Synchrony Dual Optic Accommodating IOL
    Tecnis acrylic IOL
    Tecnis foldable IOL
    IOL tilting
    traditional IOL
    UV-absorbing IOL
    Verisyse phakic IOL
    Visian IOL
    wavefront-corrected IOL
    well-centered IOL

Iolab
    I. 108 B lens
    I. I&A photocoagulator
    I. intraocular lens
    I. irrigating/aspirating photocoagulator
    I. irrigating/aspirating unit
    I. irrigating needle
    I. taper-cut needle
    I. titanium instrument
    I. titanium needle

IOLMaster optical instrument

IOLP
    intraocular lens power

IOM
    intraocular muscle

ION
    ischemic optic neuropathy

ion
    i. laser
    i. ratio

IONDT
    Ischemic Optic Neuropathy Decompression Trial

ionizing radiation

IOOA
    inferior oblique overaction

IOP
    intraocular pressure
        baseline IOP
        circadian pattern of IOP
        IOP control
        IOP curve
        foldable IOP
        mean IOP
        IOP monitor
        peak IOP
        IOP reduction
        sitting IOP
        IOP spike
        supine IOP

Iopidine

IOP-lowering drug

Ioptex
    I. laser intraocular lens
    I. TabOptic lens

Iowa
    I. orbital implant
    I. State fixation forceps

I/P
    iris and pupil

I-Paracaine

I-Parescein

IPC
    intermediate posterior curve

IPCV
    idiopathic polypoidal choroidal vasculopathy

IPD
    interpupillary distance

IPE
    iris pigment epithelium

I-Pentolate

I-Phrine Ophthalmic Solution

I-Picamide

I-Pilocarpine
I-Pilopine
I-Pred
I-Prednicet
ipsilateral
    i. antagonist
    i. centrocecal scotoma
    i. inferior oblique muscle
    i. iris
    i. medial rectus
    i. proptosis
IPT
    idiopathic perifoveal telangiectasis
IR
    index of refraction
    inferior rectus
IRBP
    interphotoreceptor retinoid-binding
      protein
Irene lens
I-Rescein
iridal
iridalgia
iridectasis
iridectome
iridectomesodialysis
iridectomize
iridectomy
    argon laser i.
    basal i.
    buttonhole i.
    Castroviejo i.
    central i.
    Chandler i.
    complete i. (CI)
    Elschnig central i.
    laser i.
    i. operation
    optic i.
    optical i.
    patent i.
    peripheral i. (PI)
    preliminary i.
    preparatory i.
    pupil-to-root i.
    i. scissors
    sector i.
    stenopeic i.
    superior sector i.
    therapeutic i.
    total i.
iridectopia
iridectropium

iridemia
iridencleisis
    Holth i.
    i. operation
iridentropium
irideremia
irides (*pl. of* iris)
iridescent
    i. lens particle
    i. spot
    i. vision
iridesis
iridiagnosis
iridial
    i. angle
    i. fold
    i. muscle
iridic, iridian
iridica
    stella lentis i.
iridis
    angulus i.
    anulus i.
    atresia i.
    coloboma i.
    ectropion i.
    epithelium pigmentosum i.
    facies anterior i.
    facies posterior i.
    heterochromia i.
    ligamentum pectinatum i.
    margo ciliaris i.
    margo pupillaris i.
    melanosis i.
    plicae i.
    rubeosis i.
    vitiligo i.
iridization
iridoavulsion
iridocapsular intraocular lens
iridocapsulitis
iridocapsulotomy scissors
iridocele
iridochoroiditis
iridociliary
    i. process contact
    i. sulcus
iridocoloboma
iridoconstrictor
iridocorneal
    i. angle
    i. endothelial (ICE)
    i. endothelial syndrome

NOTES

iridocorneal *(continued)*
    i. mesenchymal dysgenesis
    i. mesodermal dysgenesis
    i. synechia
    i. touch
iridocornealis
    angulus i.
iridocorneosclerectomy
iridocyclectomy
iridocyclitis
    Fuchs heterochromic i.
    granulomatous i.
    herpes simplex i.
    herpes zoster i.
    herpetic i.
    heterochromic i.
    hypertensive i.
    i. masquerade syndrome
    nongranulomatous i.
    posttraumatic i.
    i. septica
    varicella i.
iridocyclochoroidectomy
iridocyclochoroiditis
iridocycloretraction
iridocystectomy
iridodesis
iridodiagnosis
iridodialysis
    i. operation
    i. spatula
iridodiastasis
iridodilator
iridodonesis
iridoendothelial syndrome
iridogoniocyclectomy
iridogoniodysgenesis
iridokeratitis
iridokinesis, iridokinesia
iridokinetic
iridolenticular contact
iridoleptynsis
iridology
iridomalacia
iridomesodialysis
iridomotor
iridoncosis
iridoncus
iridoparalysis
iridopathy
iridoperiphakitis
iridoplasty
    argon laser peripheral i. (ALPI)
    laser i.
iridoplegia
    i. accommodation
    complete i.
    reflex i.

    i. reflex
    sympathetic i.
iridoptosis
iridopupillary
iridorrhexis
iridoschisis
iridoschisma
iridosclerotomy
iridosteresis
iridotasis operation
iridotomy
    Abraham i.
    Castroviejo radial i.
    laser i. (LPI)
    i. lens
    i. operation
    patent i.
    prophylactic laser i.
    radial i.
    i. scissors
iridozonular contact
I-Rinse
iris, pl. **irides**
    angle of i.
    anterior surface of i.
    i. architecture
    arterial circle of greater i.
    arterial circle of lesser i.
    i. atrophy
    i. bicolor
    i. bipolar forceps
    i. bombé
    i. capture
    i. chafing
    ciliary margin of i.
    circle of greater i.
    circle of lesser i.
    i. claw phakic IOL
    i. collarette
    i. coloboma
    coloboma of i.
    i. concavity
    congenital cleft of i.
    i. contour
    i. contraction reflex
    cosmetic i.
    crypt of i.
    i. crypt
    i. cyst
    i. dehiscence
    detached i.
    i. diameter
    i. diastasis
    i. dilator
    i. dysfunction
    i. ectasia
    embryonal epithelial cyst of i.
    i. epithelial hyperplasia
    essential progressive atrophy of i.

i. eye
i. fixation technique
i. freckle
i. frill
greater ring of i.
hernia of i.
i. heterochromia
heterochromia of i.
i. hook
i. hook cannula
hydrops of i.
i. incarceration
i. injury
ipsilateral i.
ischemic necrosis of i.
i. knife needle
leiomyoma of i.
lesser ring of i.
major arterial circle of i.
i. malformation
malignant melanoma of i.
i. manipulation
I. Medical OcuLight green laser
  system
I. Medical OcuLight infrared laser
  system
I. Medical OcuLight SLx
i. melanocytoma
melanoma of i.
i. melanoma
i. microscissors
i. neovascularization
neovascularization of i. (NVI)
i. nervus
i. neurofibroma
i. nevus
i. nodule
notch of i.
I. OcuLight SLx indirect
  ophthalmoscope delivery system
I. OcuLight SLx MicroPulse laser
i. pearl
pectinate ligament of i.
i. pigment dusting
pigmented epithelium of i.
pigmented layer of i.
i. pigment epithelium (IPE)
i. pit
plateau i.
i. process
prolapse of i.
i. prolapse
i. and pupil (I/P)

pupillae muscle of i.
pupillary margin of i.
i. registration system
i. repositor
i. retractor
retroflexion of i.
i. ring
ring of i.
i. roll
i. root
i. scissors
shredded i.
i. spatula
i. sphincter
i. sphincter muscle
i. sphincter tear
i. strand
i. stroma
stroma of i.
i. support
i. suture
i. sweep
i. synechia
i. tissue
torn i.
transfixion of i.
i. transillumination
i. transillumination defect (ITD)
tremulous i.
i. tuck
umbrella i.
iris-block glaucoma
iris-claw intraocular lens
iris-fixated lens
iris-lens diaphragm
**IrisMate flexible translimbal iris
  retractor**
iris-nevus syndrome
iris-supported lens
iris-suture technique
iritic
iritis

diabetic i.
Doyne guttate i.
fibrinous i.
follicular i.
i. glaucomatosa
gouty i.
hemorrhagic i.
leukemic i.
i. nodosa
nodular i.
nongranulomatous i.

NOTES

iritis *(continued)*
    i. obturans
    plastic i.
    postoperative i.
    purulent i.
    quiet i.
    serous i.
    spongy i.
    sympathetic i.
    syphilitic i.
    traumatic i.
    tuberculous i.
    uratic i.
iritoectomy
iritomy
Irlen syndrome
IRMA
    intraretinal microvascular abnormality
iron
    i. deposit
    i. deposition
    i. Fleischer ring
    i. line
    Pineda LASIK Flap I.
iron-ferry line
irotomy
irradiation
    i. cataract
    gamma i.
    heavy ion i.
    sham i.
    ^{90}Sr-plaque i.
irregular
    i. astigmatism
    i. cup floor
    i. nystagmus
    i. pupil
irregularity
    corneal i.
    flap i.
    surface i.
irreversible amblyopia
Irrigate eye wash
irrigating
    i. anterior chamber vectis
    i. C-hook extractor
    i. cortex extractor
    i. cystotome
    i. grasping forceps with curved
      shaft
    i. IOL positioner
    i. J-hook cannula
    i. pupil expander
    i. scissors with straight shaft
    i. solution
    i. vectis loop
irrigating/aspirating (I&A)
    i./a. cannula
    i./a. vectis

irrigation
    dilation and i. (D&I)
    fluorescein i.
    laminar interface i.
    ocular i.
    orbital i.
irrigation/aspiration (I/A)
    bimanual i./a.
    i./a. cannula
    i./a. system
    i./a. unit
irrigator
    anterior chamber i.
    Bishop-Harman anterior chamber i.
    cul-de-sac i.
    Dougherty i.
    Fox i.
    Gibson i.
    LASIK flap i.
    olive tip i.
    Randolph i.
    Seibel LASIK flap i.
    Vidaurri i.
irritation
    computer-related eye i.
    ocular i.
irritative
    i. hallucination
    i. miosis
IRVAN
    idiopathic retinal vasculitis, aneurysms
    and neuroretinitis
    IRVAN syndrome
Irvine
    I. irrigating/aspirating unit
    I. probe-pointed scissors
Irvine-Gass syndrome
ISA
    intraoperative suture adjustment
I-scan
ischemia
    anterior segment i.
    carotid i.
    choroidal i.
    foveal i.
    limbal i.
    i. of optic nerve
    i. retinae
    retinal i.
    transient vertebrobasilar i.
ischemic
    i. atherosclerosis
    i. bleb
    i. chiasmal syndrome
    i. choroidal atrophy
    i. disc
    i. edema
    i. episode
    i. maculopathy

i. necrosis
i. necrosis of chorioid
i. necrosis of ciliary body
i. necrosis of iris
i. ocular syndrome
i. oculomotor palsy
i. optic atrophy
i. optic neuropathy (ION)
I. Optic Neuropathy Decompression Trial (IONDT)
i. orbital compartment syndrome
i. papillitis
i. papillopathy
i. retina
i. retinal whitening
i. retinopathy
iScreen photoscreener
iseikonia
iseikonic lens
isethionate
dibromopropamidine i.
hydroxystilbamidine i.
pentamidine i.
propamidine i.
Ishihara
I. character
I. color plate
I. IV slit lamp
I. pseudoisochromatic plate
I. test
I. test for color blindness
ISK
immune stromal keratitis
island
central i.
isolated i.
Traquair i.
Ismotic
isobutyl 2-cyanoacrylate
Isocaine
isochromatic plate
isocoria
isoflurophate
isoiconia
isoiconic lens
isolated
i. colobomatous microphthalmia
i. cyclovertical muscle palsy
i. fixed dilated pupil
i. fourth nerve palsy
i. hereditary cataract
i. high hyperopia
i. inferior oblique paresis

i. island
i. oculomotor nerve dysfunction
i. sclerocornea
i. seventh nerve palsy
i. sixth nerve palsy
i. third nerve palsy
isomerase
retinal i.
retinene i.
isomerization
isometropia
isophoria
isopropyl
unoprostone i.
isopter
nasal i.
sloping i.
Isopto
I. Atropine
I. Carbachol
I. Carbachol Ophthalmic
I. Carpine
I. Carpine Ophthalmic
I. Cetamide
I. Cetamide Ophthalmic
I. Cetapred
I. Cetapred ophthalmic
I. Cetapred suspension
I. Eserine
I. Frin
I. Homatropine
I. Homatropine Ophthalmic
I. Hyoscine
I. Hyoscine Ophthalmic
I. Plain
I. Plain Solution
I. Prednisolone
I. Sterofrin
I. Tears
I. Tears Solution
isoscope
isosorbide
isothiocyanate
fluorescein i.
isotonic solution
isotope scan
isotretinoin
Ispan intraocular gas
israelii
Actinomyces i.
Istalol QD
I-Sulfacet

NOTES

itching
  ocular i.
itchy eye
ITD
  iris transillumination defect
25-Item Visual Function Questionnaire (VFQ-25)
itraconazole
I-Tropine
I.V., IV
  intravenous
    IV retinal fluorescein angiography
    IV slit lamp

Ivalon sponge implant
ivermectin
IVFA
  intravenous fluorescein angiography
IVH
  intraventricular hemorrhage
IVI
  impact of vision impairment
    IVI instrument
Ixodes dammini
iZon wavefront-guided lens

J

joule

J loop

jack-in-the-box phenomenon

Jacko Low Vision Interaction Assessment (JLVIA)

Jackson

J. cross cylinder

J. lacrimal intubation set

Jacob

J. capsule fragment forceps

J. membrane

J. ulcer

Jacobson

J. hemostatic forceps

J. retinitis

Jacoby

border tissue of J.

Jacod syndrome

Jacquart angle

Jadassohn-Lewandowski syndrome

Jadassohn-type anetoderma

Jaeger

J. acuity

J. acuity card

J. grading system

J. keratome

J. lid plate

J. notation

J. retractor

J. test type

J. visual test

Jaffe

J. capsulorrhexis forceps

J. Cilco lens

J. intraocular spatula

J. iris hook

J. laser blepharoplasty and facial resurfacing set

J. lens-manipulating hook

J. lens spatula

J. lid retractor

J. lid retractor set

J. lid speculum

J. microiris hook

J. needle holder

J. suturing forceps

Jaffe-Bechert nucleus rotator

Jahnke syndrome

Jamaican optic neuropathy

jamb

sphenoid door j.

Jameson

J. caliper

J. muscle forceps

J. muscle hook

Janelli clip

Jannetta procedure

Jansen-Middleton septotomy forceps

Jansky-Bielschowsky

J.-B. disease

J.-B. syndrome

Jardon eye shield

Jarisch-Herxheimer reaction

Jarrett side port manipulator

Javal

J. keratometer

J. ophthalmometer

J. rule

Javal-Schiotz ophthalmometer

jaw

end-gripping forceps with standard j.

j. muscle pain

j. winking

jaw-winking

j.-w. phenomenon

j.-w. syndrome

JCAHPO

Joint Commission on Allied Health Personnel in Ophthalmology

JC virus

Jedmed A-scan

Jedmed/DGH A-scan

jellied gasoline

Jellinek sign

jelly bump lipid deposit

jelly-like consistency

Jenning test

Jensen

J. capsule polisher cannula

J. capsule scratcher

J. disease

J. jerk nystagmus

J. juxtapapillary choroiditis

J. operation

J. polisher/scratcher

J. retinitis

J. transposition procedure

jerk

macro square-wave j.

j. nystagmus

quick adducting-retraction j.

square-wave j.

Jervey

J. capsule fragment forceps

J. iris forceps

Jeune syndrome

jeweled eye case

jeweler's
    j. bipolar forceps
    j. tweezers
jewelry
    optical j.
J-loop
    J-l. PC lens
    J-l. posterior chamber intraocular lens
JLVIA
    Jacko Low Vision Interaction Assessment
JNCL
    juvenile neuronal ceroid lipofuscinosis
JOAG
    juvenile open-angle glaucoma
Joffroy sign
Johnson
    J. double cannula
    J. evisceration knife
    J. hydrodelineation cannula
    J. hydrodissection cannula
    J. operation
    J. syndrome
Johnston
    J. fixation ring
    J. LASIK flap applanator
joint
    J. Commission on Allied Health Personnel in Ophthalmology (JCAHPO)
    J. Review Committee for Ophthalmic Medical Personnel (JRCOMP)
Jones
    J. forceps
    J. I, II dye test
    J. keratome
    J. operation
    J. Pyrex tube
    J. repair
    J. tear duct tube
    J. towel clamp
    J. tube insertion
    J. tube procedure
Jordan implant
Joseph
    J. device
    J. periosteal elevator
Joslin
    J. Vision Network (JVN)
    J. Vision Network Telehealth program
Joubert syndrome
joule (J)
JRCOMP
    Joint Review Committee for Ophthalmic Medical Personnel

J-shaped
    J-s. irrigating/aspirating cannula
    J-s. sella
JSM-54 IOLV microscope
JSM-6400 scanning electron microscope
Judd forceps
Judson-Smith manipulator
jump
    image j.
jumping eye
junction
    basal j.
    corneoscleral j.
    craniocervical j.
    host-graft j.
    mucocutaneous j.
    myoneural j.
    parietooccipital-temporal j.
    sclerocorneal j.
    scotoma j.
    j. scotoma
junctional
    j. bay
    j. nevus
    j. scotoma
    j. scotoma of Traquair
    j. zone
just
    J. Tears
    J. Tears Solution
juvenile
    j. corneal epithelial dystrophy
    j. developmental cataract
    j. diabetes
    j. diabetes mellitus
    j. glaucoma
    j. iris xanthogranuloma
    j. macular degeneration
    j. melanoma
    j. neuronal ceroid lipofuscinosis (JNCL)
    j. nevoxanthoendothelioma
    j. open-angle glaucoma (JOAG)
    j. optic atrophy
    j. pilocytic astrocytoma
    j. reflex
    j. retinoschisis
    j. systemic granulomatosis
    j. xanthogranuloma (JXG)
    j. X-linked retinoschisis (JXRS)
juvenile-onset
    j.-o. high pressure glaucoma
    j.-o. open-angle glaucoma
juvenilis
    angiopathia retinae j.
    arcus j.
juxtacanalicular
juxtafoveal
    j. choroidal neovascularization

j. lesion
j. microaneurysm
juxtalimbal suture
juxtapapillaris
retinochoroiditis j.
juxtapapillary
j. endophytic capillary hemangioma
j. leakage
j. nerve fiber layer
j. perfusion
j. retina

juxtaposition
juxtapupillary choroiditis
juxtascleral injection
JVN
Joslin Vision Network
JXG
juvenile xanthogranuloma
JXRS
juvenile X-linked retinoschisis

J

NOTES

K

corneal curvature
kelvin
phylloquinone
   K readings
   K Sol preservation solution
K-1
   Canon Auto Keratometer K-1
Kainair Ophthalmic
Kalt
   K. corneal needle
   K. forceps
   K. needle holder
   K. needle holder clamp
Kamdar microscissors
Kamppeter anomaloscope
kanamycin
Kandori
   flecked retina of K.
Kanizsa figure
Kansas fragment lens forceps
Kaplan-Meier
   K.-M. estimation technique
   K.-M. method
Kaposi
   K. sarcoma
   xeroderma of K.
kappa
   k. angle
   K. CTD finishing system
   k. light chain
   positive-angle k.
   K. SP lens finishing system
   k. statistic
karate chop technique
24-karat gold biocompatible implant
Karickhoff
   K. double cannula
   K. laser lens
KARNS
   Krypton-Argon Regression of
   Neovascularization Study
Kartagener syndrome
Kasabach-Merritt syndrome
Katena
   K. boat hook
   K. capsulorrhexis forceps
   K. depth gauge
   K. double-edged sapphire blade
   K. iris spatula
   K. MicroFinger tip irrigating
   chopper
   K. product
   K. quick switch I/A system
   K. scleral shield

K. soft IOL cutter
K. speculum
K. trephine
katophoria
katotropia
Katzen flap unzipper
Katzin-Barraquer forceps
Kaufman
   K. medium
   K. type II retractor
   K. type II vitrector
   K. vitreophage
**Kaufman-Capella cryopreservation
technique**
Kawai capsulorrhexis forceps
Kawasaki disease
Kayser-Fleischer cornea ring
KCS
   keratoconjunctivitis sicca
Kearney
   K. side-notch IOL
   K. side-notch lens
Kearns-Sayre syndrome (KSS)
Keeler
   K. binocular indirect
   ophthalmoscope
   K. cryosurgical unit
   K. extended round tip forceps
   K. intraocular foreign body
   grasping forceps
   K. intravitreal scissors
   K. lancet tip
   K. micro round tip
   K. microscissors
   K. micro spear tip
   K. panoramic lens
   K. panoramic loupe
   K. pantoscope
   K. prism
   K. Pulsair tonometer
   K. puncture tip
   K. razor tip
   K. retinoscope
   K. ruby knife
   K. specular microscope
   K. Tearscope
   K. and Teller card
   K. triple facet tip
Keeler-Konan Specular microscope
Keflex
Kehrer-Adie syndrome
Keith-Wagener (KW)
   K.-W. retinal change
Keith-Wagener-Barker (KWB)
   K.-W.-B. classification

K

Keith-Wagener-Barker *(continued)*
  K.-W.-B. hypertensive retinopathy
    staging (grade 1–4))
Keizer-Lancaster eye speculum
Kellan
  K. capsular sparing system
  K. hydrodissection
Kelly-Descemet membrane punch
Kelly hemostat
Kelman
  K. air cystotome
  K. aspirator
  K. cryoextractor
  K. cryosurgical unit
  K. cyclodialysis cannula
  K. Duet phakic lens
  K. flexible tripod lens
  K. iris retractor
  K. irrigating/aspirating unit
  K. irrigating handpiece
  K. knife
  K. Multiflex II lens
  K. Omnifit II intraocular lens
  K. operation
  K. PC 27LB CapSul lens
  K. phacoemulsification (KPE)
  K. phacoemulsification unit
  K. Quadriflex anterior chamber
    intraocular lens
  K. tip
Kelman-Mackool flare tip
Kelman-McPherson
  K.-M. corneal forceps
  K.-M. lens-holding forceps
  K.-M. suturing forceps
  K.-M. tying forceps
kelvin (K)
Kenacort
Kenaject-40
Kenalog
Kenalog-10, -40
Kennedy syndrome
Keracor laser
Kerasoft DuraWave lens
keratalgia
keratan sulfate
keratectasia
  iatrogenic k.
keratectomy
  automated lamellar k.
  Castroviejo k.
  deep lamellar k.
  excimer laser photorefractive k.
  excimer laser phototherapeutic k.
  laser-assisted subepithelial k.
    (LASEK)
  laser-scrape photorefractive k.
  no-touch transepithelial
    photorefractive k.

  k. operation
  photoastigmatic refractive k.
    (PARK)
  photorefractive k. (PRK)
  photorefractive astigmatic k.
  phototherapeutic k. (PTK)
  k. scissors
  superficial lamellar k.
  surface photorefractive k.
  tracker-assisted photorefractive k.
    (T-PRK)
keratic precipitate (KP)
keratinization
  canthal k.
keratin layer
keratinoid degeneration
keratitic precipitate
keratitis
  Acanthamoeba k.
  acne rosacea k.
  actinic k.
  aerosol k.
  AIDS-related k.
  alphabet k.
  amebic k.
  ameboid k.
  anular k.
  arborescent k.
  artificial silk k.
  avascular k.
  bacterial k.
  k. band
  band k.
  k. bandelette
  band-shaped k.
  k. bullosa
  Candida k.
  candidal k.
  chronic superficial k.
  classic dendritic k.
  Cogan interstitial k.
  confocal microscopy identification
    of *Acanthamoeba* k.
  contact lens-related microbial k.
  corneal k.
  Corynebacterium k.
  Cryptococcus laurentii k.
  deep punctate k.
  deep pustular k.
  dendriform k.
  dendrite k.
  dendritic herpes zoster k.
  desiccation k.
  diffuse deep k.
  diffuse lamellar k.
  Dimmer nummular k.
  disciform herpes simplex k.
  k. disciformis
  epithelial diffuse k.

epithelial punctate k.
exfoliative k.
exposure k.
farinaceous epithelial k.
fascicular k.
filament k.
filamentary k. (FK)
k. filamentosa
Fuchs k.
fungal k.
furrow k.
geographic k.
gonococcal k.
Gram-positive bacterial k.
herpes simplex k.
herpes zoster disciform k.
herpetic fungal k.
herpetic stromal k.
HSV epithelial k.
hypopyon k.
immune stromal k. (ISK)
infectious epithelial k.
infiltrative k.
interstitial k. (IK)
lagophthalmic k.
lamellar keratectomy for
  nontuberculous mycobacterial k.
lattice k.
k. lesion
letter-shaped k.
k. linearis migrans
luetic interstitial k.
Lyme disease k.
Lymphogranuloma venereum k.
marginal k.
metaherpetic k.
microbial k.
mixed bacterial-fungal k.
mixed fungal k.
Moraxella k.
mumps k.
Mycobacterium k.
mycotic k.
necrogranulomatous k.
necrotizing interstitial k.
necrotizing stromal k.
necrotizing ulcerative k.
neuroparalytic k.
neurotrophic k.
Nocardia k.
non-*Acanthamoeba* amebic k.
nontuberculous mycobacterial k.
nonulcerative interstitial k.

nummular k.
k. nummularis
onchocercal sclerosing k.
oyster shuckers' k.
paddy k.
parenchymatous k.
pediatric presumed microbial k.
k. periodica fugax
peripheral ulcerative k. (PUK)
k. petrificans
phlyctenular k.
pneumococcal/suppurative k.
polymorphic superficial k.
k. post vaccinulosa
presumed microbial k.
primary herpes simplex k.
protozoan k.
pseudodendritic k.
k. punctata (KP)
k. punctata profunda
k. punctata subepithelialis
punctate epithelial k.
purulent k.
k. pustuliformis profunda
pyknotic k.
radiation k.
reaper's k.
red coral k.
reticular k.
ribbon-like k.
ring k.
rosacea k.
k. rosacea
rubeola k.
sands of Sahara k.
Schmidt k.
sclerosing k.
scrofulous k.
secondary k.
serpiginous k.
k. sicca
stellate k.
striate k.
stromal k.
subepithelial k.
superficial linear k.
superficial punctate k. (SPK)
suppurative k.
syphilitic stromal k.
Thygeson superficial punctate k.
trachomatous k.
trophic k.
tuberculous k.

K

NOTES

keratitis *(continued)*
    ulcerative k.
    k. urica
    UV k.
    k. vaccinia
    vaccinial k.
    varicella k.
    vascular k.
    vasculonebulous k.
    vesicular k.
    viral interstitial k.
    vulnificus k.
    xerotic k.
    zonular k.
keratitis-ichthyosis-deafness (KID)
keratoacanthoma
    eruptive k.
keratocele
keratoconjunctivitis
    adenoviral k.
    allergic k.
    atopic eczema k.
    bilateral k.
    blinding k.
    epidemic k. (EKC)
    epizootic k.
    flash k.
    granulomatous k.
    herpes follicular k.
    herpes simplex k.
    herpes zoster k.
    herpetic k.
    limbic vernal k.
    microsporidial k.
    phlyctenular k.
    shipyard k.
    k. sicca (KCS)
    staphylococcal allergic k.
    superior limbic k. (SLK)
    Theodore k.
    ultraviolet k.
    UV k.
    vernal k. (VKC)
    viral k.
    virus k.
    welder's k.
keratoconus
    anterior k.
    circumscribed posterior k.
    Collaborative Longitudinal
      Evaluation of K. (CLEK)
    k. contact lens
    k. cornea
    k. dystrophy
    k. fruste
    iatrogenic k.
    posterior k.
    k. prediction index (KPI)

Sato k.
suspected k.
keratocyte transformation
keratoderma
    k. blennorrhagica
    palmoplantar k.
    punctate k.
keratodermatocele
keratoectasia
keratoepithelin
keratoepitheliomileusis
keratoepitheliopathy
    diabetic k.
keratoepithelioplasty
keratoglobus cornea
keratograph corneal topography system
keratography
    lamellar stromal k.
    video k.
keratohelcosis
keratohemia
keratohyaline granule
keratoid
keratoiridocyclitis
keratoiritis hypopyon
keratokyphosis
keratolens implant
keratolenticuloplasty
keratoleptynsis
keratoleukoma
keratolimbal allograft (KLA)
keratolysis
keratoma, pl. **keratomas, keratomata**
    solar k.
keratomalacia
keratome
    Accutome black diamond clear
      cornea k.
    Agnew k.
    Bard-Parker k.
    Beaver k.
    Berens partial k.
    Castroviejo angled k.
    Castroviejo electro k.
    Czermak k.
    Draeger modified k.
    k. excimer laser system
    filamentary k.
    Fuchs lancet-type k.
    Grieshaber k.
    k. guard
    HydroBrush k.
    Jaeger k.
    Jones k.
    Kirby k.
    Storz k.
    Tri-Beeled trapezoidal k.
    UltraShaper K.

UniShaper K.
Wiener k.

keratometer
Bausch & Lomb manual k.
k. calibrator
Canon auto refraction k.
Haag-Streit k.
Helmholtz k.
Javal k.
manual k.
Marco manual k.
k. mire
Osher surgical k.
10 SL/O Zeiss k.
Storz k.
Terry k.
Topcon k.

keratometric
k. astigmatism
k. flattening
k. power (KP)
k. readings

keratometry
extended range k.
handheld k.
surgical k.
k. value

keratomileusis (KM)
automated laser k. (ALK)
autoshaped lamellar k.
Barraquer k.
bilateral simultaneous laser in
  situ k.
epithelial laser-assisted
  intrastromal k. (E-LASIK)
homoplastic k.
hyperopic k.
laser-assisted epithelial k.
laser-assisted epithelium k.
  (LASEK)
laser-assisted intrastromal k.
  (LASIK)
laser-assisted in situ k. (LASIK)
laser epithelial k. (LASEK)
laser intrastromal k.
laser in situ k. (LASIK)
laser subepithelial k. (LASEK)
myopic k. (MKM)
k. operation
topographically guided therapeutic
  laser in situ k.

keratomycosis

keratoneuritis
pathognomonic radial k.

keratonosis

keratonyxis

keratopathia guttata

keratopathy
aphakic bullous k. (ABK)
band k.
band-shaped k.
Bietti k.
bullous k.
calcific band k.
central striate k.
chloroquine k.
chronic actinic k.
climatic droplet k.
climatic proteoglycan stromal k.
contact lens-induced k.
crystalline k.
dendritic k.
discrete colliquative k.
elastotic band k.
epithelial infectious crystalline k.
exposure k.
filamentary k.
fine punctate k.
Fuchs aphakic k.
HSV trophic k.
hurricane k.
idiopathic lipid k.
indomethacin toxicity k.
infectious crystalline k. (ICK)
Labrador k.
lamellar k.
linear k.
lipid k.
neuroparalytic k.
neurotrophic k.
pearl diver's k.
phenothiazine k.
plaque k.
postinfectious epithelial k.
pseudophakic bullous k. (PBK)
punctate epithelial k. (PEK)
spheroidal k.
striate k.
superficial punctate k.
Thygeson superficial punctate k.
transient k.
trigeminal neuropathic k.
trophic k.
ultraviolet k.
urate band k.

K

NOTES

keratopathy *(continued)*
    uveitic band k.
    vesicular k.
    vortex k.
keratophakia lens
keratophakic keratoplasty
keratopigmentation
Keratoplast tip
keratoplasty
    allopathic k.
    Arroyo k.
    Arruga k.
    autogenous k.
    autologous ipsilateral rotating
      penetrating k.
    automated lamellar therapeutic k.
      (ALTK)
    conductive k. (CK)
    deep lamellar k. (DLK, DLKP)
    deep lamellar endothelial k.
      (DLEK)
    Descemet-stripping automated
      endothelial k. (DSAEK)
    Elschnig k.
    endothelial lamellar k. (ELK)
    epikeratophakic k.
    Filatov k.
    fluid lamellar k.
    full penetrating k.
    full-thickness k.
    heterogenous k.
    homogenous k.
    homologous penetrating central
      limbo k.
    hyperopic automated lamellar k.
      (HALK)
    keratophakic k.
    lamellar k. (LKP)
    lamellar refractive k.
    laser-assisted epithelial k.
    laser thermal k. (LTK)
    layered k.
    manual lamellar k.
    Morax k.
    noncontact laser thermal k.
    nonpenetrating k.
    k. operation
    optic k.
    optical k.
    partial depth k.
    penetrating k. (PK, PKP)
    perforating k.
    photorefractive k. (PRK)
    posterior lamellar k.
    punctate epithelial k.
    refractive k.
    repeat penetrating k.
    k. scissors
    superficial lamellar limbo k.

    surface lamellar k.
    tectonic k.
    thermal k. (TKP)
    total k.
    total anterior lamellar k. (TALK)
keratoprosthesis
    Dohlman k.
    Eckardt temporary k.
    k. implantation
    Landers wide-field temporary k.
    PHEMA core-and-skirt k.
    temporary k. (TKP)
keratorefractive
    k. procedure
    k. surgery
keratorhexis, keratorrhexis
keratorus
keratoscleritis
keratoscope
    Klein k.
    Polack k.
    wire-loop k.
keratoscopy
keratosis
    actinic k.
    eyelid k.
    k. follicularis
    k. follicularis spinulosa decalvans
    seborrheic k.
    senescent k.
    senile k.
    solar k.
keratostomy
keratotome
keratotomy
    arcuate transverse k.
    astigmatic k. (AK)
    delimiting k.
    full-arc depth-dependent
      astigmatic k.
    hexagonal k.
    laser k.
    k. operation
    partial depth astigmatic k. (PDAK)
    Prospective Evaluation of
      Radial K. (PERK)
    radial k. (RK)
    refractive k.
    Ruiz trapezoidal k.
    trapezoidal k.
keratotorus
keratouveitis
    herpes simplex k.
    stromal k.
Keratron
    K. corneal topographer
    K. scout topographer
    K. Scout topography system
    K. videokeratoscope

KeraVision ring
kerectasis
kerectomy
Kerlone Oral
kerotome
Kerrison
- K. forceps
- K. mastoid rongeur

Kershner
- K. butterfly capsulorrhexis forceps
- K. LASIK flap forceps
- K. LRI marker
- K. One-Step Micro capsulorrhexis forceps
- K. reversible eyelid speculum

Kestenbaum
- K. number
- K. procedure
- K. rule
- K. sign

ketoconazole
ketorolac
- k. tromethamine
- k. tromethamine ophthalmic solution

ketosis-prone diabetes
ketosis-resistant diabetes
ketotifen
- k. fumarate
- k. fumarate ophthalmic solution

Keuch pupil dilator
Kevorkian-Younge forceps
keyhole
- k. bridge
- k. field
- lacrimal k.
- k. pupil
- k. vision

Keystone
- K. multi-stereo test
- K. view stereopsis test

KH-3500 IOL
Khodadoust line
kibisitome cystotome
KID
- keratitis-ichthyosis-deafness
- KID syndrome

Kikuchi-Fujimoto disease
killer cell
Kiloh-Nevin syndrome
Kilp lens
Kimmelstiel-Wilson
- K.-W. disease
- K.-W. syndrome

Kimura platinum spatula
kindergarten eye chart
kinematogram
- random-dot k.

kinematography
kinescope
kinetic
- k. echography
- k. perimeter
- k. perimetry
- k. strabismus
- k. ultrasound
- k. visual field testing

king
- K. clamp
- K. corneal trephine
- K. Khaled Eye Specialist Hospital (KKESH)
- K. operation
- K. orbital implant

kingae
- *Haemophilus, Actinobacillus actinomycetemicomitans, Cardiobacterium hominis, Eikenella corrodens, Kingella k.* (HACEK)

King-Devick saccade test
Kirby
- K. angulated iris spatula
- K. capsule forceps
- K. cataract knife
- K. corneoscleral forceps
- K. cylindrical zonal separator
- K. flat zonal separator
- K. hook expressor
- K. intracapsular lens expressor
- K. intracapsular lens loupe
- K. intracapsular lens spoon
- K. intraocular lens loupe
- K. intraocular lens scoop
- K. iris forceps
- K. keratome
- K. lens
- K. lens dislocator
- K. lid retractor
- K. muscle hook
- K. operation
- K. refractor
- K. scissors
- K. tissue forceps

Kirby-Bauer
- K.-B. disc-diffusion method
- K.-B. disc sensitivity test

K

NOTES

Kirisawa uveitis
Kirschner wire
Kishi lens
kissing
    k. puncta
    k. suprachoroidal hemorrhage
kit
    eyeglass repair k.
    E-Z mount disinfectant k.
    IC-Green k.
    Lacrimedics occlusion starter k.
    Lobob GP Starter K.
    Massachusetts Vision K. (MVK)
    Optimum rigid gas permeable
      starter k.
    Refrax corneal repair k.
    Shearing cortex suction k.
    sterile indocyanine green k.
    Tearscope Plus tear film k.
Kjellin syndrome
Kjer
    K. disease
    K. dominant optic atrophy
KKESH
    King Khaled Eye Specialist Hospital
KLA
    keratolimbal allograft
Klebsiella
    K. endophthalmitis
    K. oxytoca
    K. pneumoniae
Kleen
    Velva K.
Klein keratoscope
Klippel-Feil anomaly
Kloepfer syndrome
Kloti radiofrequency diathermy needle
Klumpke paralysis
Klyce-Wilson scale
KM
    keratomileusis
Knapp
    K. cataract knife
    K. classification
    K. eye speculum
    K. forceps
    K. iris hook
    K. iris probe
    K. iris repositor
    K. iris scissors
    K. iris spatula
    K. knife needle
    K. lacrimal sac retractor
    K. law
    K. lens loop
    K. lens spoon
    K. operation
    K. procedure
    K. refractor

    K. rule
    K. scoop
    K. strabismus scissors
    K. streak
    K. stria
Knies sign
knife, pl. **knives**
    Accutome LRI diamond k.
    Accutome side-port diamond k.
    Agnew canaliculus k.
    Alcon A-OK crescent k.
    Alcon A-OK ShortCut k.
    Alcon A-OK slit k.
    Alcon I k.
    angled sapphire k.
    ASICO multiangled diamond k.
    Bard-Parker k.
    Barkan goniotomy k.
    Barraquer keratoplasty k.
    BD safety k.
    Beaver goniotomy needle k.
    Beaver Xstar k.
    Beer canaliculus k.
    Beer cataract k.
    Berens cataract k.
    Berens glaucoma k.
    Berens keratoplasty k.
    Berens ptosis k.
    Bishop-Harman k.
    blade k.
    BRVO k.
    Castroviejo discission k.
    Castroviejo twin k.
    cataract k.
    Celita elite k.
    Celita sapphire k.
    central retinal vein occlusion k.
    clear cornea angled CVD
      diamond k.
    ClearCut dual-bevel line k.
    ClearCut ophthalmic dual bevel k.
    ClearCut SatinSlit k.
    Clearpath corneal diamond k.
    corneal k.
    crescent CVD diamond k.
    CRVO k.
    CVD diamond k.
    Dean iris k.
    Desmarres k.
    Diamatrix trapezoidal diamond k.
    diamond blade k.
    diamond-dusted k.
    diamond laser k.
    diamond phaco k.
    Diamontek k.
    discission k.
    dissector k.
    DORC illuminated diamond k.
    3D stainless steel k.

Duredge k.
EdgeAhead crescent k.
EdgeAhead microsurgical k.
EdgeAhead phaco slit k.
Elschnig cataract k.
Elschnig corneal k.
Elschnig pterygium k.
Feaster radial keratotomy k.
Feather clear cornea k.
Fugo plasma k.
Gill corneal k.
Gill-Fine corneal k.
Gills pop-up arcuate diamond k.
Gills-Welsh k.
Goldmann serrated k.
goniotomy k.
Graefe cataract k.
Graefe cystotome k.
Grieshaber ruby k.
Grieshaber ultrasharp k.
k. guard
Haab scleral resection k.
House myringotomy k.
Huco diamond k.
Johnson evisceration k.
Keeler ruby k.
Kelman k.
Kirby cataract k.
Knapp cataract k.
Koi diamond k.
Laseredge microsurgical k.
LRI diamond k.
Martinez k.
Maumenee goniotomy k.
McPherson-Ziegler k.
McReynolds pterygium k.
metal k.
Meyer Swiss diamond lancet k.
Meyer Swiss diamond mini-
  angled k.
Meyer Swiss diamond wedge k.
micrometer k.
microsurgical k.
Multi-System incision k.
k. needle
Optima diamond k.
Paton corneal k.
Paufique graft k.
Paufique keratoplasty k.
Phaco-4 diamond step k.
preset diamond k.
ptosis k.

pulsed electron avalanche k.
  (PEAK)
radial keratotomy k.
razor blade k.
Reese ptosis k.
Rhein Advantage II diamond
  limbal-relaxing incision k.
Rhein clear corneal diamond k.
Rhein 3D angled trapezoid
  diamond k.
Rizzuti-Spizziri cannula k.
ruby diamond k.
sapphire k.
Sato corneal k.
scarifier k.
Scheie goniopuncture k.
Scheie goniotomy k.
scleral resection k.
Seibel LRI diamond k.
self-fixating sideport diamond k.
Sharpoint microsurgical k.
Sharpoint slit k.
Shorti limbal relaxing incision
  diamond k.
Shorti LRI diamond k.
side port fixation k.
slit blade k.
Smith k.
Smith-Green cataract k.
Spizziri cannula k.
spoon k.
Stealth DBO freehand diamond k.
Step-Knife diamond blade k.
stiletto k.
stitch-removing k.
Storz cataract k.
straight sapphire k.
swift-cut phaco incision k.
Thornton triple micrometer k.
Tooke corneal k.
Tooke cornea-splitting k.
trapezoid angled CVD diamond k.
Troutman corneal k.
Troutman-Tooke corneal k.
Unicat diamond k.
Universal Pathfinder k.
V-lancet k.
von Graefe cataract k.
wave-edge k.
Weber k.
Weck k.
Wheeler discission k.
Wilder cystotome k.

NOTES

K

275

knife *(continued)*
    Zaldivar k.
    ZAP diamond k.
    Ziegler k.
knife/dissector
    Morlet lamellar k./d.
knife-edged lens
knife-needle
knives (*pl. of* knife)
Knobloch syndrome
Knolle
    K. anterior chamber irrigating
      cannula
    K. capsule polisher
    K. capsule scraper
    K. capsule scratcher
    K. lens cortex spatula
    K. lens nucleus spatula
    K. lens speculum
Knolle-Kelman cannulated cystotome
Knolle-Pearce irrigating lens loop
Knolle-Shepard lens-holding forceps
Knoll refraction technique
knot
    bow-tie k.
    cowhitch k.
    embedded suture k.
    intraocular cowhitch k.
    partial throw surgeon's k.
knuckle
    k. of choroid
    k. of loose vitreous
Knudsen hypothesis
Koch
    K. LRI marker
    K. nucleus hydrolysis
    K. nucleus manipulator
    K. phaco manipulator
Kocher sign
Koch-Minami chopper
Koch-Weeks
    K.-W. bacillus
    K.-W. conjunctivitis
Kodak Surecell Chlamydia test
Koebner phenomenon
Koeller illumination system
Koenen tumor
Koeppe
    K. diagnostic lens
    K. goniolens
    K. gonioscopic implant
    K. gonioscopy
    K. nodule
Koerber-Salus-Elschnig syndrome
KOH
    potassium chloride
    KOH smear
Köhler illumination

Koi diamond knife
Kölliker layer
Kollmorgen element
Kollner
    K. law
    K. rule
Kolmer crystalloid structure
Kolmogorov-Smirnov test
Konan
    K. fixed-frame method
    K. Noncon ROBO CA SP-8000
      noncontact specular microscope
    K. SP-5500 contact specular
      microscope
Konig bar chart
koniocellular retinal ganglion cell
Koo
    K. foldable intraocular lens cutter
    K. foldable IOL cutter
Kooijman eye model
Korb contact lens
koroscope
koroscopy
Kowa
    K. fluorescein system
    K. FM-500
    K. FM-500 laser flare meter
    K. hand-held slit lamp
    K. laser flare-cell photometer
    K. laser flare photometer
    K. Optimed slit lamp
    K. PRO II retinal camera
    K. RC-XV fundus camera
Koyter muscle
KP
    keratic precipitate
    keratitis punctata
    keratometric power
KPE
    Kelman phacoemulsification
KPI
    keratoconus prediction index
K-Plus
    Retinomax K-P. 2
Krabbe disease
Kraff
    K. capsule polisher
    K. capsule polisher curette
    K. fixation forceps
    K. hyperopic fixation ring
    K. intraocular utility forceps
    K. lens-holding forceps
    K. lens-inserting forceps
    K. LRI marker
    K. nucleus lens loupe
    K. nucleus splitter
    K. suturing forceps
    K. tying forceps

Kraff-Utrata
  K.-U. capsulorrhexis forceps
  K.-U. intraocular utility forceps
Kraft forceps
Krahn exophthalmometry
Kratz
  K. angled cystotome
  K. aspirating speculum
  K. capsule polisher
  K. capsule scraper
  K. capsule scratcher
  K. diamond-dusted needle
  K. elliptical-style lens
  K. K push-pull iris hook
  K. lens-inserting forceps
  K. lens needle
  K. polisher/scratcher
  K. posterior chamber intraocular
  lens
  K. "soft" J-loop intraocular lens
Kratz-Barraquer wire eye speculum
Krause
  K. lacrimal gland
  K. syndrome
  transverse suture of K.
  K. valve
K-reading
Kremer
  K. corneal fixation forceps
  K. excimer laser
  K. 2-point fixation forceps
Krill
  K. disc
  K. disease
Krimsky
  K. measurement
  K. method
  K. prism test
Kritzinger-Updegraff (K-U)
  K.-U. corneal marker
  K.-U. manipulator/elevator
Krönlein
  K. operation
  K. procedure
Krönlein-Berke operation
KR 7000-P cycloplegic refractor
Krukenberg
  K. corneal spindle
  K. pigment spindle
  K. sponge
Krumeich-Barraquer microkeratome
Krupin
  K. device

  K. eye disc
  K. implant
  K. valve
Krupin-Denver
  K.-D. long-valve implant
  K.-D. valve
krusei
  Candida k.
Kruskal-Wallis test
Kryptok
  K. bifocal
  K. lens
krypton
  k. photocoagulation
  k. red laser
**Krypton-Argon Regression of
  Neovascularization Study (KARNS)**
K-Sol medium
K-Sponge II
KSS
  Kearns-Sayre syndrome
K-tome microkeratome
KTP
  potassium-titanyl-phosphate
  KTP laser
K-U
  Kritzinger-Updegraff
  K-U corneal marker
  K-U manipulator/elevator
Kufs syndrome
Kuglen
  K. irrigating lens manipulator
  K. manipulating hook
  K. nucleus manipulator
  K. push/pull hook
  K. refractor
  K. retractor
Kuhnt
  K. corneal scarifier
  K. dacryostomy
  K. fixation forceps
  K. meniscus
  K. postcentral vein
  K. space
  K. tarsectomy
Kuhnt-Junius
  K.-J. disease
  K.-J. macular degeneration
  K.-J. maculopathy
  K.-J. repair
Kuhnt-Szymanowski
  K.-S. operation
  K.-S. procedure

K

NOTES

Kuler panoramic lens
Kveim
    K. antigen
    K. test
KW
    Keith-Wagener

KWB
    Keith-Wagener-Barker
    KWB classification
Kwitko conjunctival spreader
Kyrle disease

L
    lambert
LA
    Dexone LA
L&A
    light and accommodation
L.A.
    Dexasone L.A.
    Solurex L.A.
La
    lambert
lab
    optical l.
labeling
    terminal deoxynucleotidyl
        transferase-mediated dUTP-
        digoxigenin nick-end l. (TUNEL)
laboratory
    glaucoma sleep l.
Labrador keratopathy
Labtician oval sleeve
labyrinthine nystagmus
lacerate
    l. anterior foramen
    l. middle foramen
    l. posterior foramen
laceration
    canalicular l.
    central stellate l.
    complex l.
    conjunctival l.
    corneal l.
    corneoscleral l.
    eyebrow l.
    eyelid l.
    full-thickness corneal l.
    lid margin l.
    partial-thickness corneal l.
    stellate corneal l.
    tarsal l.
lachrymal (*var. of* lacrimal)
lacquer crack
Lacramore
LacriCATH
    L. balloon catheter
    L. lacrimal duct catheter
Lacrigel
Lacril Ophthalmic Solution
Lacri-Lube
    L.-L. NP
    L.-L. SOP
lacrimal, lachrymal
    l. abscess
    l. acinar lobule
    l. angle duct anomaly

l. anterior crest
l. apparatus
l. artery
l. awl
l. balloon catheter
l. bay
l. calculus
l. canal
l. canaliculus
l. caruncle
l. conjunctivitis
l. dilator
l. drainage
l. duct
l. ductal cyst
l. duct anlage
l. duct T-tube
l. fistula
l. fold
l. fornix
l. functional unit
l. gland
l. gland acinus
l. gland adenoid cystic carcinoma
l. gland cyst
l. gland epithelial tumor
l. gland fossa
l. gland gallium uptake
l. gland lesion
l. gland mass
l. gland repair
l. groove
l. incisure
l. intubation
l. intubation probe
l. irrigating cannula
l. irrigation test
l. keyhole
l. lake
l. lens
l. nerve
l. notch
l. nucleus aplasia
l. osteotome
l. outflow
l. papilla
l. point
l. posterior crest
l. power
l. probing
l. process
l. pump failure
l. punctal stenosis
l. punctum
l. reflex

L

lacrimal *(continued)*
    l. sac
    l. sac bur
    l. sac chisel
    l. sac diverticulum
    l. sac fossa
    l. sac gouge
    l. sac hemangiopericytoma
    l. sac massage
    l. sac retractor
    l. sac rongeur
    l. scintillography
    l. sound
    l. stent
    l. sulcus
    l. sulcus of lacrimal bone
    l. sulcus of maxilla
    l. surgery
    l. syringe
    l. system
    l. testing
    l. transit time
    l. trephine
    l. tubercle
    l. vein
lacrimale
    os l.
    punctum l.
lacrimales
    ductus l.
lacrimalis
    ampulla canaliculi l.
    ampulla ductus l.
    apparatus l.
    avulsion of caruncula l.
    canaliculus l.
    caruncula l.
    fistula l.
    fornix sacci l.
    Förster sacci l.
    fossa glandulae l.
    fossa sacci l.
    glandula l.
    hamulus l.
    incisura l.
    lacus l.
    nervus l.
    pars orbitalis glandulae l.
    pars palpebralis glandulae l.
    plica l.
    rivus l.
    sacculus l.
    saccus l.
    vena l.
lacrimation
    l. disorder
    excessive l.
    gustatory l.
    l. reflex

lacrimator
lacrimatory
Lacrimedics occlusion starter kit
lacrimo-auriculo-dento-digital syndrome
lacrimoconchalis
    sutura l.
lacrimoconchal suture
lacrimoethmoidal suture
lacrimomaxillaris
    sutura l.
lacrimomaxillary suture
lacrimonasal duct
lacrimotome
lacrimotomy
lacrimoturbinal suture
Lacrisert
Lacrivial
Lacrytest strip
lactate
    ammonium l.
    l. dehydrogenase
    squalamine l.
lacteal cataract
lactoferrin test
Lactoplate test
lacuna, pl. **lacunae**
    Blessig lacunae
    vitreous l.
lacunata
    Moraxella l.
lacus lacrimalis
LADAR 6000 excimer laser
LADARTracker closed-loop tracking system
LADARVision
    L. 4000 excimer laser system
    L. Platform
LADARWave CustomCornea wavefront system
Ladd-Franklin theory
LaFaci surgical system
LaForce knife spud
lag
    adduction l.
    dilation l.
    lid l.
Lagleyze operation
lagophthalmia, lagophthalmos, lagophthalmus
    blink out l.
    l. conjunctivitis
    nocturnal l.
    spastic l.
lagophthalmic keratitis
lagophthalmos
lagophthalmus *(var. of* lagophthalmia)
Lagrange
    L. operation

L. sclerectomy scissors
L. test
lake
lacrimal l.
tear l.
LAL
laser-adjustable lens
Lalonde hook forceps
LAM-B
lipoarabinomannan-B
lambda
l. angle
l. light-chain marker
L. phacoemulsification technique
L. Physik EMG 103 laser
lambert (L, La)
L. chalazion forceps
L. hook forceps
Lambert-Eaton myasthenic syndrome
lamella, pl. **lamellae**
collagen l.
corneal l.
corneoscleral l.
donor l.
l. of Fuchs
interlacing of collagen lamellae
Rabl l.
lamellar
l. calcification
l. channel
l. corneal graft
l. corneal transplant
l. developmental cataract
l. groove
l. haptic
l. hole
l. keratectomy for nontuberculous
mycobacterial keratitis
l. keratopathy
l. keratoplasty (LKP)
l. patch graft
l. refractive keratoplasty
l. separation of lens
l. stromal keratography
l. tattooing
l. zonular perinuclear cataract
lamellation
lamina, pl. **laminae**
anterior limiting l.
basal l.
basalis choroideae l.
basalis corporis ciliaris l.
Bowman l.

l. choriocapillaris
l. choroidocapillaris
l. cribrosa
l. cribrosa sclerae
l. densa
l. dot
l. elastica anterior
l. elastica posterior
episcleral l.
l. fusca sclerae
inner limiting l.
l. limitans anterior corneae
l. limitans posterior corneae
limiting l.
l. lucida
orbital l.
l. orbitalis ossis ethmoidalis
l. papyracea
posterior limiting l.
l. superficialis musculi
suprachoroid l.
l. suprachoroidea
l. vasculosa choroideae
l. vitrea
vitreal l.
vitreous l.
laminar
l. flow
l. interface
l. interface irrigation
laminated
l. acellular mass
l. spectacle lens
laminin
laminin-P1
serum l.-P1
lamp
Birch-Hirschfeld l.
Burton l.
Campbell slit l.
Canon RO-4000 slit l.
Canon RO-5000 slit l.
carbon arc l.
Coherent LaserLink slit l.
Duke-Elder l.
Eldridge-Green l.
fluorescent l.
gas discharge l.
Gullstrand slit l.
Haag-Streit Biomicroscope 900
slit l.
Hague cataract l.
Heine HSL 100 hand-held slit l.

L

NOTES

lamp *(continued)*
    incandescent l.
    infrared slit l.
    Ishihara IV slit l.
    IV slit l.
    Kowa hand-held slit l.
    Kowa Optimed slit l.
    Lumenis 950 slit l.
    Marco slit l.
    Nikon zoom photo slit l.
    Posner slit l.
    Reichert slit l.
    Rodenstock slit l.
    Specular reflex slit l.
    Thorpe slit l.
    Topcon SL-7E photo slip l.
    Topcon SL-E Series slit l.
    Topcon SL-1E slit l.
    tungsten-halogen l.
    Universal slit l.
    V-slit l.
    Wood l.
    Zeiss carbon arc slit l.
    Zeiss-Comberg slit l.
Lancaster
    L. eye magnet
    L. eye speculum
    L. lid speculum
    L. operation
    L. red-green projector
    L. red-green test
    L. screen test
Lancaster-O'Connor speculum
lance
    Rolf l.
Lancereaux diabetes
lancet
    Meyer Swiss diamond knife l.
    suture l.
    l. suture
    Swan l.
    ultrasonic cataract-removal l.
lancing pain
Landers
    L. biconcave lens
    L. contact lens
    L. irrigating vitrectomy ring
    L. sew-on lens
    L. subretinal aspiration cannula
    L. wide-field temporary
        keratoprosthesis
Landers-Foulks temporary
  keratoprosthesis lens
landmark
    eyelid l.
    retinal vessel l.
Landolt
    L. broken ring
    L. C acuity chart

    L. C optotype test
    L. C ring
    L. operation
Landry ascending paralysis
Landström muscle
Lane quick chopper
Lang
    L. speculum
    L. stereotest
Lange
    L. blade
    L. fold
Langer-Giedion trichorhinophalangeal
  syndrome
Langerhans granule
Langerman
    L. bi-directional phaco chopper
    L. diamond knife system
lanolin
    l. alcohol
    l. oil
Lanoxin
lantern test
Lanthony desaturated D15 test
LaPlace law
Largactil
large
    l. capsulotomy
    l. kappa angle
    l. nasal zonular dialysis
    l. physiologic cup
    l. print access
    l. print reading practice
    l. pupil diameter
    l. spot slit lamp adapter
large-angle
    l.-a. exotropia
    l.-a. infantile esotropia
large-bore aspiration tube
large-cell lymphoma
Larsen syndrome
larva, pl. **larvae**
    ocular l.
larval conjunctivitis
laryngeal and ocular granulation tissue
  in children from the Indian
  subcontinent (LOGIC)
Lasag
    L. Micropter II laser
    L. Microruptor
Laschal precision suture tome
lase
LASEK
    laser-assisted epithelium keratomileusis
    laser-assisted subepithelial keratectomy
    laser epithelial keratomileusis
    laser subepithelial keratomileusis
        LASEK alcohol well

LASEK alcohol well and epithelial trephine
LASEK bow dissector
LASEK epithelial detaching spatula
LASEK epithelial flap repositioning spatula
LASEK epithelial micro hoe

laser

l. ablation
l. activity
Aesculap argon ophthalmic l.
Aesculap excimer l.
Aesculap-Meditec excimer l.
Allegretto Wave excimer l.
Allergan Humphrey l.
AMO YAG 100 l.
Apex Plus excimer l.
ArF excimer l.
argon blue l.
argon fluoride excimer l.
argon green l.
argon-pumped tunable dye l.
Atlas-Elite l.
Atlas ophthalmic l.
Autonomous Technologies l.
l. biomicroscopy
Biophysic Medical YAG l.
l. blepharoplasty
blue-green argon l.
Britt argon/krypton l.
Britt argon pulsed l.
Britt BL-12 l.
Britt krypton l.
l. burn
l. burst
candela l.
l. capsulotomy
l. capsulotomy treatment
carbon dioxide l.
Carl Zeiss YAG l.
l. cavity
l. cell and flare meter (LCFM)
Ceralas I l.
Cilco argon l.
Cilco Frigitronics l.
Cilco krypton l.
Cilco YAG l.
Coherent 7910 l.
Coherent 900, 920 argon l.
Coherent 920 argon/dye l.
Coherent dye l.
Coherent krypton l.
Coherent Medical YAG l.

Coherent Novus Omni multiwavelength l.
Coherent radiation argon/krypton l.
Coherent radiation argon model 800 l.
Coherent Schwind Keraton 2 l.
Coherent Selecta 7000 l.
confocal scanning l. (CSL)
continuous l.
continuous-wave argon l.
continuous-wave diode l.
Cool Touch l.
Cooper 2000, 2500 l.
Cooper Laser Sonics l.
CooperVision argon l.
CooperVision YAG l.
l. corepraxy
CO_2 Sharplan l.
l. cyclotherapy
Derma-K l.
diode l.
diode-pumped solid-state photocoagulation l.
l. Doppler flowmeter
l. Doppler signal
l. Doppler velocimeter
l. Doppler velocimetry
dye yellow l.
EC-5000 excimer l.
l. epithelial keratomileusis (LASEK)
l. equipment
erbium l.
Er:YAG l.
ExciMed UV200 excimer l.
ExciMed UV200LA l.
excimer l.
excimer l., 193193-nm
Feather Touch CO_2 l.
femtosecond l.
l. flare-cell meter
l. flare-cell photometry
l. flare photometry
flashlamp-pumped microsecond pulse-dye l.
FS30 femtosecond l.
GentleLASE l.
green l. (GL)
helium-ion aiming l.
helium-neon aiming l.
HeNe l.
HGM argon green l.
HGM intravitreal l.
HGM ophthalmic l.

NOTES

laser *(continued)*
    holmium l.
    Ho:YAG l.
    l. indirect ophthalmoscope (LIO)
    L. Institute of America (LIA)
    l. interferometry
    Intralase FS30 l.
    intrastromal l.
    l. intrastromal keratomileusis
    ion l.
    l. iridectomy
    l. iridoplasty
    l. iridotomy (LPI)
    Iris OcuLight SLx MicroPulse l.
    Keracor l.
    l. keratotomy
    Kremer excimer l.
    krypton red l.
    KTP l.
    LADAR 6000 excimer l.
    Lambda Physik EMG 103 l.
    Lasag Micropter II l.
    Laserex Era 4106 YAG l.
    LaserHarmonic l.
    laser interferometer l.
    Lasertek l.
    l. lens
    l. light imaging
    Lightlas 532 green l.
    LightMed Lpulsa SYL9000 YAG l.
    liquid organic dye l.
    LPK-80 II argon l.
    Lumonics l.
    l. manipulation
    MC-7000 multi-wavelength l.
    MC-7000 ophthalmic l.
    Meditec Mel-60 excimer l.
    Mel 60. 80 excimer l.
    Mel 70 flying spot l.
    Mel 60 scanning l.
    Microlase transpupillary diode l.
    MicroProbe ophthalmic l.
    l. microtome
    miniature excimer l.
    mode-locked Nd:YAG l.
    molectron l.
    Nanolas Nd:YAG l.
    Nd:YAG l.
    Nd:YLF l.
    neodymium:YAG l.
    neodymium:yttrium aluminum
      garnet l.
    neodymium:yttrium-lithium-fluoride
      photodisruptive l.
    Nidek EC-1000 excimer l.
    Nidek EC-5000 excimer l.
    Nidek Laser System l.
    193-nm excimer l.
    Novus Spectra l.

    OcuLight SL diode l.
    OcuLight SLx ophthalmic l.
    oculocutaneous l.
    OmniMed argon-fluoride excimer l.
    Ophthalas argon l.
    Ophthalas argon/krypton l.
    Ophthalas krypton l.
    Opmilas 144 surgical l.
    l. optometer
    orange dye l.
    l. panretinal photocoagulation
    pattern scan l. (PASCAL)
    photocoagulation l.
    l. photocoagulator
    photodisrupting l.
    photon l.
    PhotoPoint l.
    photovaporation l.
    photovaporizing l.
    l. polarimetry
    l. presbyopia reversal
    Prima KTP/532 l.
    pulsed-dye l.
    Pulsion FS L.
    Q-switched Er:YAG l.
    Q-switched Nd:YAG l.
    Q-switched neodymium:YAG l.
    Q-switched ruby l.
    l. refractometry
    l. reversal of presbyopia
    l. ridge
    ruby l.
    scanning excimer l.
    S4 excimer l.
    Sharplan argon l.
    short-pulse l.
    l. in situ keratomileusis (LASIK)
    l. speckle flowgraphy
    l. speckle phenomenon
    Star excimer l.
    l. subepithelial keratomileusis
      (LASEK)
    Summit Apex Plus excimer l.
    Summit OmniMed excimer l.
    Summit SVS Apex l.
    Summit UV 200 ExciMed l.
    superpulsed l.
    l. surgery
    l. suture lysis
    Takata l.
    Technolas 217 excimer l.
    Technolas 217z excimer l.
    TEMoo mode beam l.
    THC:YAG l.
    l. therapy
    l. thermal keratoplasty (LTK)
    l. thermal keratoplasty procedure
    l. thermokeratoplasty (LTK)
    l. tomography scanner (LTS)

T-PRK l.
l. trabeculoplasty (LTP)
tracker-assisted PRK l.
transpupillary l.
l. transscleral cyclophotocoagulation
l. trap
l. tube
tunable dye l.
l. tweezers
UltraPulse l.
Uram E2 compact MicroProbe l.
Visulas 532 l.
Visulas argon C l.
Visulas argon/YAG l.
Visulas Combi 532/YAG l.
Visulas Nd:YAG l.
Visulas 690s PDT l.
Visulas YAG C, E, S l.
Visulas YAG II plus l.
VisuMed MEL60 l.
Visx 2020 excimer l.
Visx S2, S3 excimer l.
Visx Star S2 l.
Visx Star S3 ActiveTrak l.
Visx Twenty/Twenty excimer l.
VitaLase Er:YAG l.
white l.
YAG l.
yellow dye l.
yttrium-aluminum-garnet l.
Zeiss Visulas 532, 532s l.
Zeiss Visulas 690s l.
Zeiss Visulas YAG II l.
Zyoptix Infinity l.
laser-adjustable lens (LAL)
laser-argon device
laser-assisted
    l.-a. epithelial keratomileusis
    l.-a. epithelial keratoplasty
    l.-a. epithelium keratomileusis
      (LASEK)
    l.-a. epithelium keratomileusis pump
    l.-a. intrastromal keratomileusis
      (LASIK)
    l.-a. in situ keratomileusis (LASIK)
    l.-a. subepithelial keratectomy
      (LASEK)
lasered
Laseredge microsurgical knife
Laserex Era 4106 YAG laser
laser-filtering surgery

Laserflex
    L. coagulator
    L. lens
LaserHarmonic laser
laser-induced glaucoma
lasering
laser-ruby device
LaserScan LSX excimer laser system
laser-scrape
    l.-s. photorefractive keratectomy
    l.-s. technique
Lasertek laser
laser-treated eye
lash
    l. abrasion of cornea
    brow, lids, l.'s (BLL)
    l. margin
    misdirected l.
LASIK
    laser-assisted intrastromal keratomileusis
    laser-assisted in situ keratomileusis
    laser in situ keratomileusis
        LASIK aspiration spoon
        bilateral simultaneous LASIK
        bitoric LASIK
        CustomCornea wavefront-guided
          LASIK
        Dishler Excimer Laser System for
          LASIK
        LASIK enhancement
        epithelial LASIK
        LASIK eye guard
        LASIK eyelid drape
        LASIK flap irrigator
        LASIK flap manipulator
        hyperopic LASIK
        presbyopic LASIK
        LASIK spear
        topographically guided therapeutic
          LASIK
        topography-guided LASIK
        LASIK vision correction surgery
        wavefront-guided LASIK
lasing
Lasiodiplodia theobromae
lasso
    lens l.
LAT
    latency associated transcript
    limbal autograft transplantation
**latanoprost timolol maleate ophthalmic
solution**

NOTES

L

late
l. endothelial failure
l. phase detachment
l. postoperative suture adjustment (LPSA)

latency
l. analysis
l. associated transcript (LAT)
l. deficit

latent
l. angle-closure glaucoma
l. deviation
l. diabetes
l. endophthalmitis
l. hyperopia (Hl)
l. nystagmus
l. squint
l. strabismus

late-onset
l.-o. corneal haze
l.-o. epiphora
l.-o. esotropia
l.-o. exotropia
l.-o. glaucoma
l.-o. myopia

late-phase reaction
lateral
l. aberration
l. angle
l. angle of eye
l. canthal incision
l. canthal tendon
l. canthotomy
l. canthus
l. commissure of eyelid
l. gaze
l. geniculate body (LGB)
l. geniculate body lesion
l. geniculate nucleus (LGN)
l. hemianopsia
l. horn
l. illumination
l. inhibition
l. margin of orbit
l. medullary infarction
l. medullary syndrome
l. nystagmus
l. oblique conus
l. orbital decompression
l. orbital tubercle
l. orbitotomy
l. orbit tubercle
l. palpebral ligament
l. palpebral raphe
l. palpebral tubercle
l. phoria
l. rectus (LR)
l. rectus extraocular muscle
l. rectus muscle resection

l. rectus palsy
l. rectus recession
l. tarsal strip procedure

lateralis
angulus oculi l.
commissura palpebrarum l.
raphe palpebralis l.

laterodeviation
lateroduction
lateropulsion
laterotorsion
lathe-cut contact lens
lathe lens
lathing
corneal l.
l. procedure

lattice
l. corneal dystrophy
l. corneal dystrophy type I
l. corneal dystrophy type IIIA (LCDIIIA)
l. degeneration of retina
l. dystrophy of cornea
l. keratitis
l. retinal degeneration

Lauber disease
laughing gas
Laurence-Biedl syndrome
Laurence-Moon-Bardet-Biedl syndrome
Laurence-Moon-Biedl syndrome
Laurence-Moon syndrome
laurentii
Cryptococcus l.
Lauth canal
lavage
Lavoptik eye wash
law
Alexander l.
Ångström l.
Beer l.
Bernoulli l.
Bunsen-Roscoe l.
Descartes l.
Donders l.
Ewald l.
Ferry-Porter l.
Flouren l.
Friedenwald l.
Gullstrand l.
Herring l.
Horner l.
Imbert-Fick l.
Knapp l.
Kollner l.
LaPlace l.
Listing l.
Pascal l.
Plateau-Talbot l.
Poiseuille l.

Prentice l.
l. of refraction
Ricco l.
Roscoe-Bunsen l.
Sherrington l.
Snell l.
Stefan l.
Talbot l.
Weber l.
Wundt-Lamansky l.

Lawford syndrome
Lawton corneal scissors
laxa
cutis l.
laxity
horizontal l.
involutional l.
lid l.
lower lid l.
vertical l.
Layden infant lens
layer
aqueous tear l.
bacillary l.
basal l.
Bowman l.
Bruch l.
choriocapillary l.
columnar l.
cuticular l.
epithelial basement l.
fibrin l.
ganglion cell l.
grading of retinal nerve fiber l.
Haller l.
Henle fiber l.
inner nuclear l.
inner plexiform l.
juxtapapillary nerve fiber l.
keratin l.
Kölliker l.
limiting l.
lipid tear l.
molecular external l.
molecular inner l.
molecular internal l.
molecular outer l.
mucin l.
mucous tear l.
nerve fiber l. (NFL)
nerve fiber bundle l.
nuclear external l.

nuclear inner l.
nuclear internal l.
nuclear outer l.
oil l.
outer nuclear l.
outer plexiform l. (OPL)
peripapillary nerve fiber l.
peripapillary retinochoroidal l.
photoreceptor l.
pigment l.
plexiform external l.
plexiform inner l.
plexiform internal l.
plexiform outer l.
posterior collagenous l. (PCL)
retinal ganglion cell l.
retinal nerve fiber l. (RNFL)
retinochoroidal l.
l. of rods and cones
Sattler l.
suprachoroid l.
tear l.
layered
l. hyphema
l. keratoplasty
lazy eye
LC-65 Daily Contact Lens Cleaner
L-Caine
LCAT
limbal-conjunctival autograft
transplantation
LCDIIIA
lattice corneal dystrophy type IIIA
LCDVA
low-contrast distance visual acuity
LCFM
laser cell and flare meter
LCG
liquid crystal glasses
l-cone excitation
LCSLC
Low-Contrast Sloan Letter Chart
LD
local deviation
L/D
light-dark
L/D ratio
LDD
light-dark discrimination
LE
left eye
lens extraction

NOTES

L

Le
Le Grand-Geblewics phenomenon
Le Grand-Gullstrand eye model
lead
l. encephalopathy
l. incrustation of cornea
lead-filled mallet
Leahey chalazion forceps
leak
eyelash-induced l.
filtering bleb l.
glue patch l.
macular l.
pinpoint l.
point l.
leakage
capillary l.
corneal l.
juxtapapillary l.
microaneurysmal l.
parafoveal microvascular l.
peripheral l.
progressive fluorescein l.
leaking
l. bleb
l. glaucoma filtering bleb
l. incision
least
l. confusion circle
l. diffusion circle
Lea system
leaves of capsule
Lebensohn
L. reading chart
L. visual acuity chart
Leber
amaurosis congenita of L.
L. cell
L. congenital amaurosis
L. corpuscle
L. disease
L. hereditary optic atrophy
L. hereditary optic atrophy reverse
dot-blot assay
L. hereditary optic neuropathy
(LHON)
L. idiopathic stellate neuroretinitis
L. idiopathic stellate retinopathy
L. lymphangiectasia hemorrhagica
L. miliary aneurysm
L. optic atrophy
L. plus syndrome
LEC
lens epithelial cell
lecithin-cholesterol acyltransferase
deficiency
Lecythophora mutabilis
LED
light-emitting diode

LED-illuminated ring
left
l. bi-plate placement
l. deorsumvergence
l. esotropia
l. exotropia
l. eye (LE, OS)
l. gaze
l. hyperphoria
l. hypertropia (LHT)
l. inferior oblique recession
l. inferior rectus muscle
l. port
l. superior oblique tuck
l. superior rectus muscle
l. sursumvergence
left-beating nystagmus
left-handed cornea scissors
left-to-right shunting
legacy
AdvanTec L.
L. cataract surgical system
L. Series 2000 Cavitron/Kelman
phacoemulsifier aspirator
legal blindness
legally blind
Lehner-Utrata capsulorrhexis forceps
Leigh
L. capsule forceps
L. disease
L. encephalopathy
leiomyoma
l. of iris
l. of uveal tract
Leishman classification
Leishman-Donovan body
leishmaniasis
American l.
Leishmania tropica
Leiske lens
Leitz microscope
Leland refractor
lemniscus, pl. **lemnisci**
optic l.
lemon-drop nodule
Lempert rongeur
Lenercept
length
axial l. (AL)
chord l.
eye axial l.
focal l.
hinge cord l.
primary focal l.
secondary focal l.
temple l.
lens, pl. **lenses**
l. aberration
Abraham iridectomy laser l.

Abraham peripheral button iridotomy l.
Abraham YAG laser l.
absent l.
l. accessory
accommodation of crystalline l.
Accugel l.
achromatic spectacle l.
acrylic foldable intraocular l.
AcrySof foldable intraocular l.
AcrySof haptic l.
AcrySof MA60 l.
AcrySof Natural intraocular l.
AcrySof ReSTOR apodized diffractive optic posterior chamber intraocular l.
Acuvue Advance contact l.
Acuvue bifocal contact l.
Acuvue brand toric contact l.
Acuvue 1-day disposable l.
Acuvue disposable contact l.
Acuvue Etafilcon A l.
Acuvue toric contact l.
Acuvue 2-week UV-blocking disposable l.
adherent l.
AIRLens contact l.
Airy cylindric l.
Alan-Thorpe l.
Alcon AcrySof SA30AL single-piece l.
Alcon MA30BA optic AcrySof l.
Alges bifocal contact l.
Allen-Thorpe l.
Allergan AMO Array S155 l.
all-PMMA intraocular l.
l. alone
American Medical Optics Baron l.
AMO Array foldable intraocular l.
AMO Array multifocal ultraviolet-absorbing silicone posterior chamber intraocular l.
AMO Ioptex Model ACR 360 foldable acrylic l.
AMO PhacoFlex II foldable intraocular l.
amorphic l.
AMO Sensar intraocular l.
Amsoft l.
anastigmatic l.
angle-fixated l.
angle-supported l.
aniseikonic l.

Anis staple l.
anterior chamber intraocular l. (ACIOL)
anterior pole of l.
anular bifocal contact l.
AO l.
aphakic contact l.
aplanatic l.
apochromatic l.
apodized diffractive l.
Aquaflex contact l.
Aquasight l.
Arlt l.
Array multifocal intraocular l.
Arruga l.
artificial l.
Artisan myopia l.
aspherical ophthalmoscopic l.
aspheric cataract l.
aspheric spectacle l.
aspheric-viewing l.
aspiration of l.
l. assignment
astigmatic l.
auxiliary l.
l. axis
axis of cylindric l. (x)
Azar l.
back surface toric contact l.
Bagolini l.
Baikoff l.
balafilcon A contact l.
ballistic protective l.
bandage soft contact l.
Barkan gonioscopic l.
Barkan goniotomy l.
Baron l.
Barraquer l.
baseball l.
Bausch & Lomb Optima l.
Bausch & Lomb Surgical L161U l.
8.4 BC disposable l.
Bechert 7-mm l.
Beebe l.
beveled-edge l.
bicentric spectacle l.
biconcave contact l.
biconvex l.
bicurve contact l.
bicylindrical l.
Bietti l.
bifocal contact l.

NOTES

L

lens *(continued)*

bifocal intracorneal l.
bifocal spectacle l.
Binkhorst intraocular l.
Binkhorst iridocapsular l.
Binkhorst 2-loop l.
Binkhorst 4-loop iris-fixated l.
BIOM l.
Biomedics contact l.
biomicroscopic indirect l.
Bi-Soft l.
bispherical l.
bitoric contact l.
l. blank
blooming of l.
blooming spectacle l.
blue-blocking l.
blue filtering l.
blue light-absorbing intraocular l.
Boberg-Ans l.
Boston 7 contact l.
Boston Envision contact l.
Boston EO, ES contact l.
Boston II, IV contact l.
Boston RXD contact l.
Boston XO contact l.
Brücke l.
Burian-Allen contact l.
l. capsule
capsule of l.
l. capsule opacification
Carl Zeiss l.
cast resin l.
cataract l.
cataract extraction with
    intraocular l. (CE/IOL)
CeeOn heparin surface-modified l.
CeeOn Model 920 foldable
    intraocular l.
cellulose acetate butyrate contact l.
central posterior curve of
    contact l.
central retinal l.
central thickness of contact l.
Charles handheld infusion l.
Charles intraocular l.
Charles irrigating contact l.
chemically treated spectacle l.
child's l.
Chiroflex C11UB l.
Choyce intraocular l.
Choyce Mark VIII l.
CibaSoft Visitint contact l.
Clariflex foldable silicone
    intraocular l.
Clariflex OptiEdge foldable
    intraocular l.
l. clarity
clariVit central mag l.

clariVit central magnification
    vitrectomy l.
clariVit wide angle vitrectomy l.
Clayman intraocular l.
Clayman posterior chamber l.
l. cleaner
L. Clear
clear crystalline l.
ClearView contact l.
l. clip
l. clock
C-loop intraocular l.
C-loop posterior chamber l.
coating for spectacle l.
Coburn intraocular l.
collagen bandage l.
Collamer 1-piece intraocular l.
Collamer 3-piece intraocular l.
coloboma of l.
colored contact l.
Comberg contact l.
ComfortKone l.
composition of spectacle l.
compound l.
concave spectacle l.
concavoconcave l.
concavoconvex l.
condensing l.
congenital subluxated crystalline l.
conoid l.
constructional ability contact l.
contact l. (CL)
contact bandage l.
contact low-vacuum l.
contact side field l.
l. contamination
contour contact l.
convergent l.
converging meniscus l.
convexoconcave l.
convexoconvex l.
convex plano l.
convex spectacle l.
Cooper Clear DW contact l.
Cooper Toric contact l.
CooperVision PMMA-ACL Flex l.
Copeland radial panchamber
    intraocular l.
Copeland radial panchamber UV l.
coquille plano l.
corneal contact l.
corrected spectacle l.
cortex of l.
cortical substance of l.
cosmetic shell contact l.
coupling of progressive power l.
CR-39 l.
crocodile l.
Crookes l.

crossed l.
crown glass l.
l. crystallina
crystalline l.
CSI toric contact l.
curvature of l.
curve of spectacle l.
cylinder spectacle l.
cylindric l.
cylindrical l. (C, cyl.)
Dailies contact l.
daily wear contact l. (DWCL)
decentered l.
l. decentration
decentration of contact l.
Definity contact l.
diagnostic contact l.
diagnostic fiberoptic l.
diffractive multifocal l.
66-diopter iridectomy laser l.
direct gonioscopic l.
disc intraocular l.
l. discoloration
dislocated crystalline l.
dislocated intraocular l.
l. dislocation
dispersing l.
disposable contact l.
distance between lenses (DBL)
distortion of l.
divergent l.
diverging meniscus l.
dot-like l.
double concave l.
double convex l.
double slab-off contact l.
l. dressing
Drews l.
L. Drops lubricating and rewetting
  drops
dual l.
dual mechanism l.
Dulaney l.
Durasoft 2 ColorBlends l.
Durasoft 3 Optifit Toric
  ColorBlends contact l.
Durasoft 2 Optifit Toric for light
  eyes contact l.
Dura-T l.
Dyer nomogram system of ordering
  contact l.
E Clips prescription computer l.
Edge III hydrogel contact l.

edging of spectacle l.
El Bayadi-Kajiura l.
embryonic l.
Encore monthly disposable
  contact l.
EndoView sapphire l.
l. epithelial cell (LEC)
l. epithelium
Epstein collar stud acrylic l.
l. equator
equator of crystalline l.
ERG-Jet disposable contact l.
Eschenbach Optik l.
etafilcon A l.
l. exchange
executive spectacle l.
exfoliation of l.
l. exfoliation glaucoma
l. expressor
extended wear contact l. (EWCL)
l. extraction (LE)
eye l.
EZ.1 multifocal contact l.
EZVue violet haptic intraocular l.
Falcon l.
Feaster Dualens l.
Federov type I, II intraocular l.
l. fiber
fiberoptic diagnostic l.
field l.
finished contact l.
first definite apical clearance l.
  (FDACL)
Fisher-Price polycarbonate l.
l. fixation
flat contact l.
flat-edge l.
flexible contact l.
flexible-wear contact l.
Flexlens l.
l. flexure effect
flint glass l.
fluid contact l.
fluidless contact l.
fluid-ventilated l.
Fluorex 300, 500 contact l.
fluorocarbon in contact l.
Focus Dailies Toric contact l.
Focus Night & Day contact l.
foldable acrylic l.
foldable disc intraocular l.
foldable plate-haptic silicone
  intraocular l.

L

NOTES

lens *(continued)*
  FormFlex l.
  Franklin-style bifocal lenses
  Frenzel l.
  Frequency 38 monthly disposable
    contact l.
  FreshLook ColorBlends l.
  FreshLook contact l.
  Fresnel l.
  Friedman handheld Hruby l.
  front surface toric contact l.
  fundus contact l.
  fundus focalizing l.
  fundus laser l.
  fused bifocal l.
  fused multifocal l.
  Galin intraocular implant l.
  gas-permeable contact l. (GPCL)
  generating spectacle l.
  Gentex PDQ polycarbonate l.
  Gill intraocular implant l.
  glass l.
  l. glide
  glued-on hard contact l.
  Goldmann diagnostic contact l.
  Goldmann fundus contact l.
  Goldmann macular contact l.
  Goldmann 3-mirror contact
    diagnostic l.
  Goldmann multi-mirror l.
  goniolens l.
  gonioscopic l.
  Gould intraocular implant l.
  Gradal individual customized
    progressive l.
  Gray photochromic l.
  handheld Hruby l.
  handheld infusion l.
  hand-painted l.
  haptic plate l.
  hard contact l. (HCL)
  hardened spectacle l.
  hardening of l.
  Hart pediatric 3-mirror l.
  heparin surface-modified
    intraocular l. (HSM-IOL)
  Hessburg l.
  highly oxygen permeable contact l.
  high-power l.
  holk high-resolution aspherical l.
  honey bee l.
  Hoskins l.
  Hoskins-Barkan goniotomy infant l.
  Hruby contact l.
  Hunkeler l.
  Hydracon contact l.
  Hydrasoft contact l.
  Hydrocurve II l.
  hydrogel contact l.

  hydrogel disc intraocular l.
  hydrogel intraocular l.
  Hydron l.
  hydrophilic acrylic intraocular l.
  hydrophilic contact l.
  hydrophobic contact l.
  Hydroview intraocular l.
  hypermature l.
  immersion l.
  l. implant
  implant l.
  implantable collamer l. (ICL)
  implantable contact l. (ICL)
  implantation of l.
  l. incubation
  indirect l.
  inert material for intraocular l.
  infant Karickhoff laser l.
  infant 3-mirror laser l.
  influence of an Artisan l.
  l. insertion technique
  Intermedics l.
  Interspace YAG laser l.
  in-the-bag l.
  intraocular l. (IOL)
  intraocular cowhitch knot for
    dislocated l.
  Iolab 108 B l.
  Iolab intraocular l.
  Ioptex laser intraocular l.
  Ioptex TabOptic l.
  Irene l.
  iridocapsular intraocular l.
  iridotomy l.
  iris-claw intraocular l.
  iris-fixated l.
  iris-supported l.
  iseikonic l.
  isoiconic l.
  iZon wavefront-guided l.
  Jaffe Cilco l.
  J-loop PC l.
  J-loop posterior chamber
    intraocular l.
  Karickhoff laser l.
  Kearney side-notch l.
  Keeler panoramic l.
  Kelman Duet phakic l.
  Kelman flexible tripod l.
  Kelman Multiflex II l.
  Kelman Omnifit II intraocular l.
  Kelman PC 27LB CapSul l.
  Kelman Quadriflex anterior
    chamber intraocular l.
  Kerasoft DuraWave l.
  keratoconus contact l.
  keratophakia l.
  Kilp l.
  Kirby l.

Kishi l.
knife-edged l.
Koeppe diagnostic l.
Korb contact l.
Kratz elliptical-style l.
Kratz posterior chamber
  intraocular l.
Kratz "soft" J-loop intraocular l.
Kryptok l.
Kuler panoramic l.
lacrimal l.
lamellar separation of l.
laminated spectacle l.
Landers biconcave l.
Landers contact l.
Landers-Foulks temporary
  keratoprosthesis l.
Landers sew-on l.
laser l.
laser-adjustable l. (LAL)
Laserflex l.
l. lasso
lathe l.
lathe-cut contact l.
Layden infant l.
Leiske l.
L. Fresh
lenticular contact l.
lenticular-cut contact l.
lenticular spectacle l.
Lewis l.
light adjustable l.
lighthouse l.
l. localizer
long-wearing contact l.
l. loop
4-loop l.
loose contact l.
lotrafilcon A contact l.
l. loupe
Lovac gonioscopic l.
l. lubricant
luxated l.
luxation of l.
MA30BA intraocular l.
Machemer flat l.
Machemer infusion contact l.
Machemer magnifying vitrectomy l.
macular contact l.
magnifying l.
Mainster-HM retinal laser l.
Mainster retinal laser l.
Mainster-S retinal laser l.

Mainster Ultra Field PRP laser l.
Mainster-WF retinal laser l.
Mainster wide field l.
Mandelkorn suture laser lysis l.
l. manipulator
March laser l.
Mark II Magni-Focuser l.
Mark IX l.
L. Mate
mature l.
Maxsight sport-tinted contact l.
McGhan 3M intraocular l.
McLean prismatic fundus laser l.
Medallion l.
Medical Optics PC11NB
  intraocular l.
Meditec bandage contact l.
membranous l.
Menicon Z rigid gas permeable
  contact l.
meniscus concave l.
Meso contact l.
meter l.
microbevel edge l.
microincision intraocular l.
microthin contact l.
mid-coquille l.
MiniQuad XL l.
minus carrier contact l.
minus spectacle l.
3-mirror contact l.
105-mm Micro Nikkor l.
modified C-loop intraocular l.
modified C-loop UV l.
modified J-loop intraocular l.
modified J-loop UV l.
mold-injected l.
Momose l.
Morgan l.
multicurve contact l.
multidrop l.
Multiflex anterior chamber l.
multifocal spectacle l.
Multi-Optics l.
multipiece l.
nasal crystalline l.
negative meniscus l.
Neolens l.
New Orleans l.
NewVues sterile contact l.
Nike Max Rx prescription sun l.
Nikon aspheric l.
noncontact l.

L

NOTES

lens *(continued)*
Nova Aid l.
Nova Curve broad C-loop posterior chamber l.
Nova Curve Omnicurve l.
Nova Soft II l.
nuclear sclerosis of l.
l. nucleus
nucleus of l.
NuVita l.
objective l.
occupational l.
Oculaid l.
ocular l.
Omnifit intraocular l.
omnifocal l.
on-eye performance of l.
O2OPTIX breathable contact l.
L. Opacities Case-Control Study
l. opacities classification system (LOCS)
l. opacities classification system III grading
open l.
Ophtec Co. l.
ophthalmic progressive-power l.
optical center of spectacle l.
optical contact l.
Optical Radiation l.
optical zone of contact l.
optic 3-piece intraocular l.
optics of intraocular l.
Optiflex l.
Optima contact l.
Optycryl 60 contact l.
Opus III contact l.
orbital l.
ORC intraocular l.
Orthogon l.
orthokeratology contact l.
orthoscopic l.
O'Shea l.
Osher pan-fundus l.
Osher surgical gonio/posterior pole l.
Lenses and Overnight Orthokeratology (LOOK)
panchamber UV l.
Pannu intraocular l.
Pannu type II l.
Paraperm O2 contact l.
l. particle glaucoma
PBII blue loop l.
Pearce posterior chamber intraocular l.
pediatric Karickhoff laser l.
pediatric 3-mirror laser l.
Percepta progressive l.
peripheral curve on contact l.

periscopic concave l.
periscopic convex l.
Permaflex l.
Permalens l.
PermaVision intracorneal l.
Perspex CQ-Shearing-Simcoe-Sinskey l.
Petrus single-mirror laser l.
Peyman-Green vitrectomy l.
Peyman wide-field l.
PhacoFlex II SI30NB intraocular l.
Phakic 6 l.
Phakic intraocular l.
Pharmacia intraocular l.
Pharmacia Visco J-loop l.
photochromic l.
photogray l.
photosensitive l.
photosun l.
3-piece acrylic intraocular l.
3-piece hydrophobic acrylic Sensar l.
3-piece monofocal silicone l.
1-piece multifocal l.
3-piece plate haptic intraocular l.
1-piece plate haptic silicone intraocular l.
3-piece silicone intraocular l.
piggyback contact l.
piggyback intraocular l.
pigmentary deposits on l.
l. pit
l. placode
placode l.
l. plane
1-plane l.
2-plane l.
planoconcave l.
planoconvex nonridge l.
Plano T l.
plastic l.
plate-haptic intraocular l.
plate-haptic silicone l.
Platina clip l.
L. Plus
plus l.
L. Plus-Allergan
L. Plus daily cleaner
L. Plus Oxysept
L. Plus Oxysept System
L. Plus rewetting drops
L. Plus saline
plus spectacle l.
L. Plus Sterile Saline Solution
PMMA custom-made calibration contact l.
polarized l.
polarizing l.
polycarbonate l.

Polycon I, II contact l.
Polymacon l.
polymethyl methacrylate contact l.
positive meniscus l.
Posner diagnostic l.
posterior chamber intraocular l.
  (PCIOL, PC-IOL)
posterior pole of l.
posterior surface of l.
l. power
l. power calculation
Precision Cosmet l.
Prelex presbyopic l.
presbyopic intraocular l.
press-on Fresnel l.
primary l.
prismatic contact l.
prismatic effect by l.
prismatic gonioscopic l.
prismatic gonioscopy l.
prismatic goniotomy l.
prismatic spectacle l.
progressive addition l.
progressive additional lenses
progressive multifocal l.
progressive spectacles lenses
prolonged wear contact l.
prosthetic l.
protective l.
l. protein glaucoma
punctal l.
pupillary l.
PureVision extended-wear contact l.
PureVision toric l.
QuadPediatric fundus l.
radius of l.
Rayner l.
Red Reflex Lens Systems l.
l. refilling
refractive contact l.
removable keratophakia l.
l. removal
l. replacement
retroscopic l.
Revolution l.
RGP contact l.
ridge l.
Ridley l.
rigid gas-permeable contact l.
Ritch contact l.
Ritch nylon suture laser l.
Ritch trabeculoplasty laser l.
Rodenstock panfundus l.

rudiment l.
SA60AT intraocular l.
safety l.
Sarfarazi dual optic intraocular l.
SaturEyes contact l.
Saturn II contact lenses
Sauflon PW l.
Schlegel l.
scleral contact l.
scratched contact l.
scratch-resistant spectacle l.
secondary curve on contact l.
secondary intraocular l.
segmental l.
self-stabilizing vitrectomy l.
semifinished contact l.
semiscleral contact l.
Sensar acrylic intraocular l.
Sensar OptiEdge intraocular l.
Severin l.
sewn-in l.
sew-on l.
Shearing planar posterior chamber
  intraocular l.
Sheets l.
short C-loop l.
Signet Optical l.
silicone acrylate contact l.
silicone elastomer l.
silicone hydrogel contact l.
silicone intraocular l.
Silsoft contact l.
Simcoe II PC l.
simple plus l.
l. simulation sales tool
single-cut contact l.
single-vision l.
Sinskey intraocular l.
l. size
slab-off l.
Slant haptic single-piece
  intraocular l.
SlimFit ovoid intraocular l.
SlimFit small-incision ovoid l.
Snellen soft contact l.
SofLens 66 l.
SofLens contact l.
SoFlex series l.
SofPort AO aspheric l.
SofPort L161 AO l.
soft contact l. (SCL)
soft intraocular l.

NOTES

lens *(continued)*

SoftSITE high add aspheric multifocal contact l.
Sola Optical USA Spectralite high index l.
Soper cone contact l.
Sovereign bifocal l.
special spectacle l.
spectacle l.
Spectralite Transitions l.
spheric l.
spherical equivalent l.
spherocylindrical l.
spin-cast l.
l. sponge
spontaneous extrusion of l.
l. spoon
Staar AA 4207 l.
Staar implantable contact l.
Staar intraocular l.
Staar toric l.
Staar 4203VF l.
Staar 4207VF l.
Stableflex anterior chamber l.
l. star
star l.
steep contact l.
stigmatic l.
Stokes l.
Strampelli l.
Style S2 clear-loop l.
styrene contact l.
subluxated crystalline l.
subluxation of l.
subluxed l.
substance of l.
Super Field NC slit lamp l.
Surefit AC 85J l.
Surevue contact l.
Surgidev PC BUV 20-24 intraocular l.
Sussman l.
Sutherland l.
suture of l.
T l.
Tano double-mirror peripheral vitrectomy l.
Tecnis foldable intraocular l.
Tecnis Z9000 l.
Tek-Clear accommodating intraocular l.
telescopic l.
Tennant Anchorflex AC l.
therapeutic contact l.
thick l.
thickness of contact l.
thin l.
Thorpe 4-mirror vitreous fundus laser l.

tight contact l.
Tillyer bifocal l.
tilting l.
tinted contact l.
tinting of spectacle l.
Tolentino prism l.
Tolentino vitrectomy l.
Topcon aspheric l.
toric contact l.
toric intraocular l.
Toric-Optima series l.
toric spectacle l.
toroidal contact l.
Touchlite zoom l.
transition l.
transscleral fixation of dislocated intraocular l.
transsclerally sutured posterior chamber l. (TS-SPCL)
trial case and l.
trial contact l.
tricurve contact lenses
trifocal l.
Trokel l.
truncated contact l.
Trupower aspherical l.
TruVision l.
Ultex l.
Ultra mag l.
Ultra view SP slit lamp l.
UltraVue l.
uncut spectacle l.
Uniplanar style PC II l.
Univis l.
Univision low-vision microscopic l.
unstained l.
Urrets-Zavalia retinal surgical l.
Uvex l.
UV Nova Curve l.
Varilux Pangamic thin plastic l.
l. vault
vaulting of contact l.
vergence of l.
l. vesicle
Viscolens l.
Visian implantable collamer l.
vision-correcting contact l.
Vision Tech l.
Visitec Company l.
Vistakon contact l.
Volk aspheric l.
Volk coronoid l.
Volk G Series l.
Volk high-resolution aspherical l.
Volk 3 mirror ANF+ l.
Volk 3 mirror gonio fundus laser l.
Volk quadraspheric l.

Volk SuperMacula 2.2 focal
laser l.
Volk SuperQuad 160 contact l.
Volk SuperQuad 160 panretinal l.
Volk Transequator l.
Wang l.
Wesley-Jessen l.
L. Wet
wetting angle of contact l.
whorl l.
Wild l.
Wise iridotomy laser l.
Wise iridotomy-sphincterotomy
laser l.
with contact lenses (c̄cl)
Wood l.
Woods Concept l.
working l.
Worst Claw l.
Worst goniotomy l.
Worst medallion l.
Worst Platina iris-fixated l.
X-Chrom contact l.
Yannuzzi fundus laser l.
l. to yield
Youens l.
Y-suture of crystalline l.
Z-alpha l.
Zeiss l.
zero power l.
l. zone
zone of contact l.
l. zonule

LensCheck Advanced Logic lensometer
lensectomy
Charles l.
clear l.
coal-mining l.
pars plana l.
primary l.
Lensept
lenses (*pl. of* lens)
Lens-Eze inserter
lens-holding forceps
lens-induced
l.-i. secondary open-angle glaucoma
l.-i. UGH syndrome
l.-i. uveitis
lens-iris diaphragm
lens-maker formula
Lensmeter
L. 701

Nagel L.
Zeiss LA 110 projection L.
lensometer
Allergan Humphrey l.
AO Reichert Instruments l.
Carl Zeiss l.
Coburn l.
Hardy l.
LensCheck Advanced Logic l.
Marco l.
Topcon LM P5 digital l.
lensometry
lensopathy
lens-plus-eye system
Lensrins
lens-sparing vitrectomy
lens-threading forceps
Lens-Wet
lenticle
lenticonus
anterior l.
posterior l.
lenticula
lenticular
l. astigmatism
l. bowl
l. cataract
l. contact lens
l. degeneration
l. fibroxanthomatous nodule
l. fossa
l. fossa of vitreous body
l. ganglion
l. glaucoma
l. injury
l. myopia
l. nucleus
l. opacity
l. ring
l. spectacle lens
l. vesicle
lenticular-cut contact lens
lenticule
epikeratoplasty l.
lenticuli (*pl. of* lenticulus)
lenticulocapsular
lenticulo-optic
lenticulostriate
lenticulothalamic
lenticulus, pl. **lenticuli**
lentiform
l. nodule
nucleus l.

NOTES

L

lentigines, electrocardiogram abnormalities, ocular hypertelorism, pulmonary stenosis, abnormal genitalia, retardation of growth, and deafness (LEOPARD)
lentiglobus
lentis
    apparatus suspensorius l.
    axis l.
    capsula l.
    chalcosis l.
    coloboma l.
    cortex l.
    ectopia l.
    epithelium l.
    equator l.
    facies anterior l.
    facies posterior l.
    fibrae l.
    nucleus l.
    polus anterior l.
    polus posterior l.
    radius of l.
    siderosis l.
    spontaneous ectopia l.
    substantia corticalis l.
    tunica vasculosa l.
    vortex l.
Lenz syndrome
leonine appearance
LEOPARD
    lentigines, electrocardiogram abnormalities, ocular hypertelorism, pulmonary stenosis, abnormal genitalia, retardation of growth, and deafness
    LEOPARD syndrome
leopard
    l. fundus
    l. retina
    l. spot
leprae
    Mycobacterium l.
leprotica
    alopecia l.
leptomeningeal metastasis
Leptospira interrogans
leptospiral uveitis
leptospirosis
    ocular l.
leptotrichosis conjunctivae
lesion
    acquired abducens nerve l.
    acquired cranial nerve l.
    amelanotic l.
    Archer l.
    basal ganglia l.
    benign l.
    bilateral occipital lobe l.
    birdshot l.

    boomerang-shaped l.
    l. boundary
    brainstem l.
    branching l.
    bull's-eye macular l.
    central l.
    cerebellar l.
    cerebellopontine angle l.
    cerebral hemisphere l.
    cervical l.
    chiasmal l.
    chorioretinal l.
    choroidal l.
    concentric l.
    congenital abducens nerve l.
    congenital III nerve l.
    conjunctival melanotic l.
    corneal punctate l.
    corpus callosum l.
    CPA l.
    cracked windshield stromal l.
    dendritic epithelial l.
    diencephalic l.
    early l.
    epibulbar l.
    extrastriate cortex l.
    eyelid l.
    facial nerve l.
    frontal lobe unilateral cerebral hemisphere l.
    frontoparietal bilateral cerebral hemisphere l.
    geographic l.
    hamartomatous l.
    hemorrhagic disciform l.
    herpetoid l.
    hypertrophic dendriform epithelial l.
    juxtafoveal l.
    keratitis l.
    lacrimal gland l.
    lateral geniculate body l.
    LGB l.
    linear streak l.
    lipocytic l.
    lymphoepithelial l.
    lytic l.
    macular l.
    malignant pituitary l.
    medial longitudinal fasciculus l.
    medulla l.
    melanocytic conjunctival l.
    melanotic l.
    mesencephalic l.
    mesencephalon l.
    microcystic l.
    MLF l.
    neural l.
    nonenhancing mass l.

occipital lobe unilateral cerebral hemisphere l.
occult l.
oculomotor nerve l.
optic chiasmal l.
optic nerve l.
optic radiation l.
optic tract l.
orange-red l.
l. of orbit
orbital l.
osseous l.
parasellar l.
parietal lobe bilateral cerebral hemisphere l.
parietal lobe unilateral cerebral hemisphere l.
patchy inflammatory l.
peripheral l.
periventricular l.
phototoxic l.
pigmented l.
pigmented conjunctival l.
pons l.
pontine l.
poorly demarcated l.
precancerous l.
preganglionic l.
pseudocancerous l.
punched-out l.
recurrent corneal l. (RCL)
retinal l.
retrobulbar compressive l.
retrogeniculate l.
satellite l.
serpiginous l.
l. severity
sonolucent l.
space-occupying l.
subarachnoid oculomotor nerve l.
subfoveal l.
sunburst-type l.
supranuclear l.
suprasellar l.
temporal lobe unilateral cerebral hemisphere l.
trochlear nerve l.
ulcerated l.
unifocal optic nerve l.
unilateral l.
vision-compromising l.
VZV disciform l.
waxy l.

weeping eczematous l.
white laser l.
lesser
l. ring of iris
l. wing of sphenoid
Lester
L. fixation forceps
L. IOL manipulator
L. lens dialer
L. lens manipulator
Lester-Burch speculum
lethal midline granuloma
letter
l. blindness
l. chart accommodative facility
l. size
Sloan l.
Snellen l.
test l.
l. test
letterbox technique
letter-shaped keratitis
leucitis
leukemia
acute lymphoblastic l.
leukemic
l. cell
l. infiltrate
l. infiltration of optic disc
l. iritis
l. retinitis
l. retinopathy
Leukeran
leukocoria, leukokoria
leukocyte
l. adhesion
l. function associated antigen-1 (LFA-1)
leukocytoclastic vasculitis
leukoderma
periorbital l.
leukodystrophy
metachromatic l.
leukokoria (*var. of* leukocoria)
leukoma, pl. **leukomata**
l. adherens
adherent l.
l. corneae
corneal l.
leukomatous corneal opacity
leukopathia, leukopathy
congenital l.
leukopsin

NOTES

L

leukotomy
　　transorbital l.
Leustatin
Levaquin
levator
　　l. advancement
　　l. aponeurosis defect
　　l. aponeurosis disinsertion
　　l. aponeurosis repair
　　l. dehiscence repair
　　l. function testing
　　l. injury
　　l. innervation
　　l. muscle dehiscence
　　l. muscle of upper eyelid
　　l. palpebrae superioris
　　l. palpebrae superioris muscle
　　l. ptosis
　　l. resection
　　l. tendon
　　l. trochlear muscle
level
　　aqueous concentration l.
　　Brems astigmatism marker with l.
　　elevated glutamine l.
　　glutamine l.
　　haze l.
　　intraocular pressure l.
　　Mohs l.
level-dependent
　　blood oxygenation l.-d. (BOLD)
4-level severity rating scale
leventinese
　　malattia l.
Levine spud
Levitt implant
levobetaxolol hydrochloride
levobunolol
　　l. HCl
　　l. hydrochloride
levocabastine
　　l. HCl
　　l. hydrochloride
levoclination
levocycloduction
levodopa
levodopa-carbidopa
levoduction
levofloxacin ophthalmic solution
levotorsion
levoversion
Lewicky
　　L. formed cystotome
　　L. lens manipulating hook
　　L. needle
　　L. self-retaining chamber maintainer
　　L. threaded infusion cannula
Lewis
　　L. lens

　　L. lens loupe
　　L. scoop
Lewy body
Lexan polycarbonate resin
lexipafant
LFA-1
　　leukocyte function associated antigen-1
LGB
　　lateral geniculate body
　　LGB lesion
LGN
　　lateral geniculate nucleus
LHON
　　Leber hereditary optic neuropathy
LHT
　　left hypertropia
LIA
　　Laser Institute of America
library temple
Librium
lichenification
　　eyelid l.
lichenified lid
lid
　　l. agglutination
　　l. block
　　l. clamp
　　l. crease
　　l. crusting
　　l. crutch spectacles
　　l. droop
　　droopy l.
　　l. ectropion
　　l. edema
　　l. eversion
　　l. everter
　　l. fissure
　　l. forceps
　　granular l.
　　l. imbrication syndrome
　　l. lag
　　l.'s, lashes, lacrimals, lymphatics
　　　(LLLL)
　　l. lash loss
　　l. laxity
　　lichenified l.
　　l. loading
　　lower l. (LL)
　　l. margin
　　l. margin laceration
　　l. notching
　　l. nystagmus
　　l. plate
　　l. reflex
　　l. resection
　　l. retraction
　　l. scrub
　　l. scurf
　　l. speculum

l. splinting
l. thrush
tonic l.
l. trephine
upper l. (UL)
l. vesicle
l. wiper epitheliopathy
L. Wipes-SPF
lid-closure
l.-c. reaction
l.-c. reflex
lidocaine
l. hydrochloride
intracameral l.
intraocular l.
l. with epinephrine
Lidoject
Lidoject-1 with epinephrine
lid-triggered synkinesia
Lieberman
L. aspirating speculum
L. K-Wire speculum
L. lens-holding forceps
L. MicroFinger
L. MicroFinger manipulator
L. micro-ring lens forceps
L. wire aspirating speculum with
V-shape blade
Lieberman-type
L.-t. speculum, reversible thin solid
blade
L.-t. speculum with Kratz open
wire blade
Liebreich symptom
Lieppman cystotome
LIF
local intraarterial fibrinolysis
life
Health-Related Quality of L.
(HRQOL)
Low Vision Quality of L.
(LVQOL)
vision-related quality of l.
life-belt cataract
lifestyle factor
Li-Fraumeni syndrome
lift
SOOF l.
suborbicularis oculi fat l.
lifter
Weinstein fixation ring and flap l.
ligament
canthal l.

check l.
ciliary l.
cribriform l.
Hueck l.
hyaloideocapsular l.
intracapsular l.
lateral palpebral l.
Lockwood l.
medial canthal l.
medial palpebral l.
palpebral l.
pectinate l.
pectineal l.
suspensory l.
Weigert l.
Whitnall l.
Wieger l.
Zinn l.
ligamentum pectinatum iridis
light
l. and accommodation (L&A)
l. adaptation
l. adjustable lens
l. argon laser burn
autokinesis visible l.
axial ray of l.
back-scattered l.
Barkan l.
L. Blade laser workstation
blur anatomy point source of l.
central l.
l. coagulation
cobalt blue l.
coherent l.
convergent l.
dichromatic l.
l. difference
l. differential threshold
l. discrimination
divergent l.
emergent ray of l.
ether theory of l.
fixation l.
flashes of l.
halo around l.
idioretinal l.
incident ray of l.
intrinsic l.
l. loss
marginal ray of l.
l. microscope
l. microscopy
minimum l.

L

NOTES

light *(continued)*
    monochromatic red HeNe laser l.
    movable fixation l.
    near reaction to l.
    oblique ray of l.
    ophthalmoscopy with reflected l.
    l. optometer reflex
    paraxial ray of l.
    perception of l. (PL)
    l. perception (LP)
    l. perception cataract
    l. perception only (LPO)
    peripheral ray of l.
    pipe l.
    l. pipe
    l. pipe pick
    polarized l.
    polychromatic l.
    l. projection
    l. projection test
    pupils equal, react to l. (PERL)
    ray of l.
    l. ray
    l. reaction
    reflected l.
    l. reflex ring
    refracted l.
    l. response of pupil
    l. scatter
    l. scattering
    scleral fixation l.
    l. sensation
    l. sense
    l. sensitivity
    Serdarevic Circle of L.
    standard ambient l.
    l. stimulus
    subthreshold l.
    L. Touch technique
    l. toxicity
    l. transmission
    transmitted l.
    ultraviolet A l.
    unit of l.
    white l.
    Young theory of l.
light-activated drug
light-adapted eye
light-adjustable IOL
LightBlade
    Novatec L.
light-dark (L/D)
    l.-d. amplitude ratio
    l.-d. discrimination (LDD)
2-light discrimination
lighted flute needle
light-emitting diode (LED)
lighthouse
    L. distance visual acuity test

L. ET-DRS acuity chart
l. lens
L. Low Vision Service
lighting
    continuous ambient l.
    paraxial l.
Lightlas 532 green laser
LightMed Lpulsa SYL9000 YAG laser
light-near dissociation
lightning
    l. cataract
    l. eye movement
    l. streak
light-optometer
light-peak to dark-trough ratio
light-stress test
ligneous conjunctivitis
lignocaine hydrochloride
lilacinus
    Paecilomyces l.
limbal
    l. allograft
    l. approach
    l. arcade
    l. autografting
    l. autograft transplantation (LAT)
    l. bleeding
    l. cell allografting
    l. choristoma
    l. compression
    l. conjunctiva
    l. conjunctivitis
    l. dermoid
    l. follicle
    l. girdle
    l. girdle of Vogt
    l. groove
    l. guttering
    l. ischemia
    l. neurofibroma
    l. palisades of Vogt
    l. papillae
    l. parallel orientation
    l. rejection
    l. relaxing incision (LRI)
    l. stem cell
    l. stem cell deficiency
    l. stem-cell transplantation
    l. stroma
    l. tissue
    l. vasculitis
    l. zone
limbal-conjunctival
    l.-c. autograft
    l.-c. autograft transplantation (LCAT)
limbi (*pl. of* limbus)
limbic vernal keratoconjunctivitis
limbitis

Limbitrol
limbus, pl. **limbi**
    blue l.
    circumferential vascular plexus
      of l.
    congenital dermoid of l.
    conjunctival l.
    l. of cornea
    corneal inferior l.
    corneal scleral l.
    corneoscleral l.
    cystoid cicatrix of l.
    l. girdle
    l. guttering
    l. mass
    l. parallel orientation straddling
      tattoo mark
    l. of perception
    l. of sclera
    scleral l.
limbus-based conjunctival flap
limit
    Rayleigh l.
limitation
    eccentric l.
limited gallium scan
limiting
    l. angle
    l. lamina
    l. lamina anterior
    l. layer
    l. membrane
Lincoff
    L. balloon
    L. balloon catheter
    L. lens sponge
    L. scleral sponge implant
Lindau-von Hippel disease
Lindner spatula
Lindsay operation
Lindstrom
    L. arcuate incision marker
    L. astigmatic marker
    L. LASIK flap roller
    L. LASIK spatula
    L. lens-insertion forceps
    L. small incision marker
    L. Star
    L. Star nucleus manipulator
    L. Trident ophthalmic splitter
line
    absorption l.
    angular l.

Arlt l.
atopic l.
blue l.
Brücke l.
chatter l.
corneal iron l.
CVD black diamond keratome l.
datum l.
dendritic l.
l. of direction
Egger l.
Ehrlich-Türk l.
endothelial rejection l.
epithelial iron l.
face l.
Ferry l.
fingerprint l.
l. of fixation
flat demarcation l.
Fraunhofer l.
frown l.
glabellar frown l.
gray l.
Helmholtz l.
Hudson l.
Hudson-Stähli l.
iron l.
iron-ferry l.
Khodadoust l.
linear regression l.
mare's-hair l.
mare's-tail l.
nasolabial l.
nonius l.
Paton l.
pigment demarcation l.
principal l.
pupillary l.
rejection l.
retinal stress l.
Sampaolesi l.
Schwalbe l. (SL)
l. of sight
skin tension l.
Snellen l.
Stähli pigment l.
Stocker l.
stromal l.
superficial corneal l.
l. test
triradiate l.
Turk l.
l. of vision

NOTES

line *(continued)*
> visual l.
> l. of visual acuity
> Vogt l.
> Zöllner l.

linea, pl. **lineae**
> l. corneae senilis

linear
> l. basal cell carcinoma
> l. endotheliitis
> l. infiltration
> l. keratopathy
> l. regression line
> l. scar
> l. scarring
> l. sebaceous nevus sequence
> l. streak lesion
> l. subcutaneous atrophy
> l. vision
> l. visual acuity test

linezolid
linkage analysis
lint-free sponge
LIO
> laser indirect ophthalmoscope
> Coaxial Multicolor LIO

Lions Doheny Eye and Tissue Transplant Bank
lip
> anterior l.
> scleral l.

lipemia retinalis
lipemic
> l. retina
> l. retinopathy

lipid
> l. accumulation
> l. cell
> l. degeneration
> l. deposit
> l. exudate
> l. keratopathy
> l. layer thickness
> ocular hypotensive l.
> subretinal l.
> l. tear layer

lipoarabinomannan-B (LAM-B)
lipoatrophic diabetes
lipocytic lesion
lipodermoid
> conjunctival l.

lipofuscin
lipofuscinogenesis
lipofuscinosis
> ceroid l.
> juvenile neuronal ceroid l. (JNCL)
> neuronal ceroid l.

lipoides
> arcus l.

lipoidosis corneae
lipoma
> orbital l.

lipomatosis
> ptosis l.

lipophilicity
lipoplethoric diabetes
Lipo-Tears Forte
lippitude, lippitudo
Lipschütz inclusion body
lipuric diabetes
liquefaciens
> *Serratia* l.

liquefaction
> contraction and l.
> l. device
> vitreal l.

liquid
> l. crystal glasses (LCG)
> Lumigan ocular hypotensive l.
> l. organic dye laser
> perfluorocarbon l.
> l. perfluorocarbon
> L. Pred
> reservoir of l.
> l. vitreous-aspirating cannula

liquified vitreous
Liquifilm
> Albalon L.
> Betagan L.
> Bleph-10 L.
> L. Forte
> L. Forte Solution
> Herplex L.
> HMS L.
> Prefrin Z L.
> PV Carpine L.
> L. Rewetting Solution
> L. Tears
> L. Tears Solution
> L. Wetting

liquor
> l. corneae
> Morgagni l.

Lisch
> L. corneal dystrophy
> L. nodule
> L. spot

lisinopril
lissamine
> l. green
> l. green stain

Lister
> L. forceps
> L. scissors

Listing
> L. law
> L. plane
> L. primary position

L. reduced eye
L. torsion
Lite
Angiofluor L.
literal alexia
literature
ophthalmic l.
l. search
lithiasis
l. conjunctivae
conjunctival l.
l. conjunctivitis
lithotriptor
candela laser l.
Littauer
L. cilia forceps
L. dissecting scissors
Littler dissecting scissors
Littmann Galilean magnification changer
Live/Dead Kit stain
Livernois
L. lens-holding forceps
L. pickup and folding forceps
living-related conjunctival limbal allograft (lr-CLAL)
Livingston peribulbar wedge
Living Water Eye Lotion
Livostin
LKP
lamellar keratoplasty
maximum depth lamellar keratoplasty (MD-LKP)
LL
lower lid
LLLL
lids, lashes, lacrimals, lymphatics
Lloyd stereocampimeter
LMX1B gene
loading
lid l.
loafer temple
lobe
frontal l.
occipital l.
palpebral l.
parietal l.
temporal l.
temporoparietal l.
Lobob
L. GP Starter Kit
L. Hard Contact Lens Wetting Solution

Optimum by L.
L. Rigid Hard Contact Lens Soaking Solution
lobule
lacrimal acinar l.
lobulus, pl. lobuli
coloboma lobuli
local
l. anesthetic
l. deviation (LD)
l. intraarterial fibrinolysis (LIF)
l. outgrowth
l. tic
l. tonic pupil
localization
Comberg l.
spatial l.
localized
l. albinism
l. amyloidosis
l. carboplatin therapy
l. erythema
l. transient burning
localizer
lens l.
location
l. anomaly
tunnel l.
locator
Berman foreign body l.
foreign body l.
Sweet l.
loci (*pl. of* locus)
lock
Luer cannula l.
Lockwood
L. ligament
L. light reflex
superior tendon of L.
L. tendon
LOCS
lens opacities classification system
locus, pl. loci
l. of fixation
gene l.
GLC1A l.
preferred retinal l. (PRL)
retinoblastoma l.
trained retinal l.
lodoxamide
l. tromethamine
l. tromethamine ophthalmic solution
Löfgren syndrome

L

NOTES

log
    l. rank test
    l. unit
logadectomy
logarithmic Minimum Angle of Resolution (logMAR)
LOGIC
    laryngeal and ocular granulation tissue in children from the Indian subcontinent
    LOGIC syndrome
logistic discriminant analysis
logMAR
    logarithmic Minimum Angle of Resolution
    logMAR chart
Lombart
    L. radioscope
    L. tonometer
lomustine
long
    l. ciliary nerve
    l. posterior ciliary artery
    l. root of ciliary ganglion
    l. sight
long-acting
    l.-a. gas
    l.-a. gas tamponade
longi
    nervi ciliares l.
longitudinal
    l. aberration
    l. axis
    l. axis of Fick
    l. ciliary muscle
    l. fasciculus
    l. fiber
    L. Optic Neuritis Study (LONS)
    L. Study of Ocular Complications of AIDS (LSOCA)
long-scale contrast
long/short occluder
longsightedness
long-term
    l.-t. comparative study
    l.-t. graft
    l.-t. outcome
    l.-t. remyelination
    l.-t. suppressive therapy
long-wearing contact lens
LONS
    Longitudinal Optic Neuritis Study
LOOK
    Lenses and Overnight Orthokeratology
Look
    L. capsule polisher
    L. cortex extractor
    L. cystotome
    L. irrigating lens loop
    L. irrigating vectis

    L. micropuncture device
    L. retrobulbar needle
    L. suture
looking
    forced choice preferential l.
loop
    acquired prepapillary venous l.
    2-angled polypropylene l.
    Axenfeld nerve l.
    C l.
    Clayman-Knolle irrigating lens l.
    closed l.
    congenital prepapillary vascular l.
    expressor l.
    flexible l.
    Flynn lens l.
    haptic l.
    intrascleral nerve l.
    irrigating vectis l.
    J l.
    Knapp lens l.
    Knolle-Pearce irrigating lens l.
    lens l.
    Look irrigating lens l.
    Meyer-Archambault l.
    Meyer temporal l.
    modified J l.
    nerve l.
    nylon l.
    open l.
    prepapillary arterial l.
    prepapillary vascular l.
    temporal l.
    vascular l.
    venous l.
4-loop
    4-l. iris clip implant
    4-l. iris fixated implant
    4-l. lens
loose
    l. contact lens
    l. lens accommodative facility
    l. packing
    l. zonule
loperamide
loratadine
Lordan chalazion forceps
lorgnette occluder
Loring ophthalmoscope
loss
    altitudinal visual field l.
    amiodarone-related vision l.
    axonal l.
    blood l.
    central field l. (CFL)
    chiasmal visual field l.
    endothelial cell l.
    eyelash l.
    field l.

functional visual l.
glaucomatous visual field l.
hemisensory l.
hidden visual l.
intraoperative blood l.
lid lash l.
light l.
migrainous vision l.
nasal field l.
nonorganic visual l.
nonphysiologic visual field l.
painless visual l.
plug l.
progressive hearing l.
retinal ganglion cell l.
retrochiasmal visual field l.
scintillating vision l.
scotopic sensitivity l.
self-inflicted visual l.
sudden visual l.
transient monocular visual l.
unilateral hearing l.
vascular optical disc swelling
  without visual l.
l. of vision
vision l.
visual field l.
vitreous l.
l. of vitreous

lost rectus muscle
Lotemax ophthalmic suspension
loteprednol
l. etabonate
l. etabonate ophthalmic solution
l. etabonate ophthalmic suspension
l. and tobramycin ophthalmic

lotion
Living Water Eye L.

Lotmar Visometer
lotrafilcon A contact lens
Lo-Trau side-cutting needle
Lotze local sign
louchettes
loupe
angled lens l.
angled nucleus removal l.
Arlt lens l.
Atwood l.
Beebe l.
Berens lens l.
binocular l.
Castroviejo lens l.
Elschnig-Weber l.

Keeler panoramic l.
Kirby intracapsular lens l.
Kirby intraocular lens l.
Kraff nucleus lens l.
lens l.
Lewis lens l.
magnifying l.
Mark II Magni-Focuser l.
New Orleans lens l.
nucleus delivery l.
nucleus removal l.
Ocular Gamboscope l.
operating l.
panoramic l.
Simcoe l.
Simcoe double-end lens l.
Simcoe II PC nucleus delivery l.
Simcoe nucleus lens l.
Snellen lens l.
Troutman lens l.
Visitec nucleus removal l.
Weber-Elschnig lens l.
Wilder lens l.
Zeiss-Gullstrand l.
Zeiss operating field l.

Lovac gonioscopic lens
lover's eye concept
low
l. blink rate
l. contrast
l. convex
l. myopia
l. profile R-K marker
l. scleral rigidity
l. total spherical aberration
l. viscosity artificial tears
l. vision
l. vision care
L. Vision Functional Status
  Evaluation (LVFSE)
L. Vision Quality of Life
  (LVQOL)
L. Vision Quality of Life
  Questionnaire (LVQOLQ)
l. vision refraction

low-coherence interferometry
low-contrast
l.-c. distance visual acuity
  (LCDVA)
L.-c. Sloan Letter Chart (LCSLC)

Lowe
oculocerebrorenal syndrome of L.

L

NOTES

Lowe *(continued)*
    L. oculocerebrorenal syndrome
    L. ring
Löwenstein-Jensen medium
Löwenstein operation
lower
    l. canaliculus
    l. eyelid
    l. eyelid spacer
    l. hemianopsia
    l. lid (LL)
    l. lid laxity
    l. lid retractor
    l. lid sling procedure
    l. punctum
    l. retina
Lowe-Terrey-MacLachlan syndrome
low-humidity environment
low-pressure glaucoma
Lowry assay
low-tension glaucoma
low-vision
    l.-v. aid
    l.-v. enhancement system (LVES)
low-weight tonometer
loxophthalmus
LP
    light perception
LPI
    laser iridotomy
LPK-80 II argon laser
LPO
    light perception only
LPSA
    late postoperative suture adjustment
LR
    lateral rectus
lr-CLAL
    living-related conjunctival limbal
      allograft
LRI
    limbal relaxing incision
      LRI diamond knife
LSK
    LSK One disposable microkeratome
    LSK One standard microkeratome
LSM-2100C
    L. eye bank specular microscope
LSOCA
    Longitudinal Study of Ocular
      Complications of AIDS
LTK
    laser thermal keratoplasty
    laser thermokeratoplasty
      noncontact LTK
      LTK procedure
LTP
    laser trabeculoplasty

LTS
    laser tomography scanner
Lube-free petrolatum, mineral oil
   lubricant
lubricant
    lens l.
    Lube-free petrolatum, mineral oil l.
    ocular l.
    silicone l.
lubricating
    l. drops
    l. medication
lubrication
    ocular l.
    surface l.
    tear film l.
Lubricoat
Lubrifair
LubriTears
    L. Lubricant Eye Ointment
    L. Solution
Lucae dressing forceps
lucency, pl. **lucencies**
Lucentis
lucida
    camera l.
    lamina l.
lucidum
    tapetum l.
Lucite
    L. frame
    L. sphere implant
Luedde exophthalmometer
Luer
    L. cannula lock
    L. connection
    L. syringe tip
    L. tube
Luer-Lok
    L.-L. syringe
    Yale L.-L.
luetic
    l. chorioretinitis
    l. interstitial keratitis
    l. neuropathy
lugdunensis
    Staphylococcus l.
lumbricoides
    Ascaris l.
lumen, pl. **lumina, lumens**
    capillary l.
Lu-Mendez
    L.-M. LRI guide
    L.-M. LRI guide and fixation ring
Lumenis 950 slit lamp
lumens (*pl. of* lumen)
Lumigan
    L. ocular hypotensive liquid
    L. ophthalmic solution

lumina (*pl. of* lumen)
luminance
    l. acuity
    background l.
    l. rivalry
    l. setting
    l. size threshold perimetry
    Smith-Kettlewell Institute low l.
      (SKILL)
luminometer
    Packard l.
luminosity curve
luminous
    l. flux
    l. intensity (I)
    l. retinoscope
lumirhodopsin
Lumonics laser
lunata
    Curvularia l.
    plica l.
Lundsgaard sclerotome
Luneau retinoscopy rack
Luntz-Dodick punch
lupus
    l. erythematosus cell test
    l. oculopathy
Lurocoat
luster
    binocular l.
    corneal l.
    polychromatic l.
lusterless
lustrous central yellow point
lutea
    macula l.
lutein
    FloraGLO l.
    Ocuvite L.
lutetium
    motexafin l.
    l. texaphyrin (lu-tex)
luteum
    punctum l.
lu-tex
    lutetium texaphyrin
lux (lx)
    l. setting
luxated lens
luxation
    l. of eyeball
    l. of globe
    l. of lens

    superior oblique muscle and
      trochlear l.
Luxo surgical illuminator
luxurians
    ectropion l.
luxury perfusion
LVES
    low-vision enhancement system
    head-mounted video magnifier
      LVES
LVFSE
    Low Vision Functional Status Evaluation
LVQOL
    Low Vision Quality of Life
LVQOLQ
    Low Vision Quality of Life
      Questionnaire
lx
    lux
Lyle syndrome
Lyme
    L. disease
    L. disease keratitis
lymphangioma
    conjunctival l.
    eyelid l.
lymphatic
    l. drainage
    l. sinusoid chorioid
lymphatics
    lids, lashes, lacrimals, l. (LLLL)
lymphoblastic lymphoma
lymphocytic
    l. aggregation
    l. choriomeningitis virus
    l. infiltration
lymphoepithelial lesion
lymphoepithelioma
Lymphogranuloma
    L. venereum conjunctivitis
    L. venereum keratitis
lymphoid
    l. follicle
    l. hyperplasia
    l. infiltration
    l. pseudotumor
    l. tumor
lymphoma
    anterior chamber l.
    conjunctival MALT l.
    histiocytic l.
    intraocular l.
    large-cell l.

L

NOTES

lymphoma *(continued)*
    lymphoblastic l.
    MALT l.
    mucosa-associated lymphoid
      tissue l.
    non-Hodgkin l.
    ocular adnexal l.
    oculocerebral l.
    orbital l.
    porcupine l.
    primary central nervous system l.
      (PCNSL)
    primary intraocular l.
    primary ocular l.
    reticulum cell l.
    signet-ring l.
    T-cell l.
    well-differentiated small-cell l.
      (WDSCL)
    zone B-cell l.

lymphomatosis
    ocular l.
lymphophagocytosis
lymphoproliferative tumor
Lynch
    L. approach
    L. medial canthal incision
Lyon hypothesis
lysed
lysis
    cell l.
    laser suture l.
    l. of restricting strand
    symblepharon l.
lysosomal storage disease
lysozyme
    serum l.
    l. stabilization
lytic lesion

M

myopia
myopic
  M band
  M cell
  M cone excitation

3M

  3M small aperture Steri-Drape
  3M Steri-Drape drape

M4-400 freedom blade
MA30BA intraocular lens
MAC

monitored anesthesia care

Macbeth

  M. ColorChecker
  M. illumination

MacCallan

  M. classification
  M. classification of trachoma

Macewen sign
Machado-Joseph disease
Machat

  M. adjustable aspirating wire
    speculum
  M. double-ended marker
  M. superior flap LASIK marker

Machat-type adjustable aspirating LASIK speculum
Mach band
Machemer

  M. diamond-dust-coated foreign
    body forceps
  M. flat lens
  M. infusion contact lens
  M. magnifying vitrectomy lens
  M. vitreous cutter

machine

  CooperVision I/A m.
  I/A m.
  Stat Scrub handwasher m.
  Visual-Tech m.

Mackay-Marg

  M.-M. electronic tonometer
  M.-M. principle

Mackool

  M. capsule retractor
  M. system

macroaneurysm

  arterial m.
  retinal arterial m.

macroblepharia
macroblepharon
macrocornea
macrocupping

  pseudoglaucomatous m.

macrocyst
macrocytic anemia
macroerosion
macromovement
macroperforation
macrophage migration inhibitory factor (MMIF)
macrophthalmia
macrophthalmic
macrophthalmous
macropia
macropsia
macroptic
macroreticular dystrophy
macrosaccadic oscillation
macro square-wave jerk
macrostereognosis
macrovessel

  congenital retinal m.

MACRT

Monoclonal Antibody Cytomegalovirus
Retinitis Trial

Macugen
macula, pl. maculae

  m. adherens
  maculae ceruleae
  cherry-red spot in m.
  maculae corneae
  dragged m.
  drusen of m.
  ectopia maculae
  false m.
  graying of m.
  Henle layer of m.
  heterotopia maculae
  heterotropia maculae
  honeycomb m.
  inferior m.
  m. lutea
  m. lutea pigment
  parafoveal m.
  m. retinae
  superonasal m.
  temporal m.
  transcutaneous electrical nerve
    stimulation of m.
  vitelliform degeneration of m.

macula-off rhegmatogenous retinal detachment
macula-on rhegmatogenous retinal detachment
macular, maculate

  m. abnormality
  m. anatomy
  m. aplasia

M

macular *(continued)*
m. area
m. arteriole
m. arteriole occlusion
m. binocular vision
m. branch retinal vein occlusion (MBRVO)
m. buckling procedure
m. choroiditis
m. cluster
m. CMV
m. coloboma
m. computerized psychophysical test (MCPT)
m. contact lens
m. corneal dystrophy
m. cytomegalovirus
m. disciform degeneration
m. disease
m. displacement
m. dragging
m. drusen
m. dysplasia
m. ectopia
m. edema
m. epiretinal membrane
m. evasion
m. exudate
m. fold
m. graying
m. heredodegeneration
m. heterotopia
m. hole (MH)
m. hole formation
m. hole surgery
m. hypoplasia
m. laser grid photocoagulation
m. leak
m. lesion
m. neuroretinopathy
m. ocular histoplasmosis syndrome
m. OHS
m. pathology
M. Photocoagulation Study (MPS)
m. photostress
m. photostress testing
m. pigment density
m. pseudohole (MPH)
m. pucker
m. puckering
m. retinal detachment
m. retinal dystrophy
m. retinoblastoma
m. retinopathy
m. sparing
m. splitting
m. star
m. stereopsis
m. suppression

m. suppression amblyopia
m. surface wrinkling
m. telangiectasia
m. traction
m. traction detachment
m. translocation
m. translocation surgery
m. translocation with macular infolding
m. translocation with retinotomy and retinal rotation
m. translocation with scleral infolding (MTSI)
m. venule
m. vitreoretinal interface
MacularProtect multivitamin
MaculaRx Plus nutritional supplement
maculary fasciculus
maculate *(var. of* macular)
macule
maculocerebral
maculopathy
age-related m. (ARM)
atrophic degenerative m.
bull's-eye m.
cellophane m.
chloroquine/hydroxychloroquine m.
cystic m.
cystoid m.
diabetic m.
dry senile degenerative m.
exudative senile m.
familial pseudoinflammatory m.
Groenouw type II m.
heredity m.
histoplasmosis m.
hypotony m.
ischemic m.
Kuhnt-Junius m.
myopic m.
niacin m.
nicotinic acid m.
operating microscope-induced phototoxic m.
photic m.
phototoxic m.
pigment epithelial detachment m.
serous detachment m.
solar m.
Sorsby m.
m. staging system
Stargardt m.
toxic m.
unilateral acute idiopathic m.
vitelliform m.
maculorrhexis
ILM m.
maculosa
atrophia striata et m.

MaculoScope
maculovesicular
madarosis
Maddox
    M. LASIK spatula
    M. prism
    M. rod
    M. rod method
    M. rod occluder
    M. rod test
    M. wing test
madurae
    Actinomadura m.
Madurai Intraocular Lens Study IV
mafilcon A
Magendie-Hertwig
    M.-H. sign
    M.-H. syndrome
Magendie sign
magnae
    facies orbitalis alae m.
magnesium chloride hexahydrate
magnet
    eye m.
    Haab m.
    handheld eye m.
    Hirschberg m.
    implant m.
    Lancaster eye m.
    original Sweet eye m.
    Schumann giant type eye m.
    Storz-Atlas hand eye m.
    Storz Microvit m.
    Sweet original m.
magnetic
    m. extraction
    m. field-search coil test
    m. implant
    m. resonance angiography (MRA)
    m. resonance imaging (MRI)
    m. resonance imaging scan
    m. resonance spectroscopy (MRS)
    m. resonance venography (MRV)
magnification
    m. aid
    high m. (HM)
    meridional m.
    relative spectacle m.
    screen m.
magnifier
    bright-field m.
    circline m.
    hand m.

    handheld m.
    illuminated hand m.
    illuminated stand m.
    model 1559 m.
    optical m.
    projection m.
    right-angle prism m.
    spectacle m.
    stand m.
    Visolett m.
magnifying
    m. glasses
    m. lens
    m. loupe
    m. power
magnitude of ptosis
magnocellular
    m. cell
    m. visual pathway
Maguire-Harvey vitreous cutter
Maier
    sinus of M.
    M. sinus
main fiber
Mainster
    M. retinal laser lens
    M. Ultra Field PRP laser lens
    M. wide field lens
Mainster-HM retinal laser lens
Mainster-S retinal laser lens
Mainster-WF retinal laser lens
maintained
    central, steady and m. (CSM)
    good, central, m. (GCM)
    good, central, not m. (GCNM)
maintainer
    anterior chamber m. (ACM)
    Blumenthal anterior chamber m.
    Lewicky self-retaining chamber m.
maintenance
    binocularity m.
major
    m. amblyoscope
    m. amblyoscope test
    anulus iridis m.
    m. arterial circle of iris
    m. basic protein (MBP)
    camera oculi m.
    circulus arteriosus iridis m.
    erythema multiforme m.
    m. histocompatibility antigen
    m. histocompatibility complex
      (MHC)

M

NOTES

major *(continued)*
    m. meridian
    m. vascular arcade
majoris
    facies orbitalis alae m.
Maklakoff tonometer
malalignment
malattia leventinese
maleate
    chlorpheniramine m.
    naphazoline and pheniramine m.
    pilocarpine and timolol m.
    timolol m.
malformation
    Arnold-Chiari m.
    arteriovenous m.
    Chiari m.
    congenital brain m.
    dural arteriovenous m.
    infratentorial arteriovenous m.
    iris m.
    orbital arteriovenous m.
    retinal arteriovenous m.
    retinal vascular m.
    supratentorial arteriovenous m.
Malherbe calcifying epithelioma
malignancy
    eyelid m.
malignant
    m. choroidal melanoma
    m. ciliary epithelioma
    m. dyskeratosis
    m. epithelial tumor
    m. exophthalmos
    m. eyelid tumor
    m. glaucoma
    m. granular cell tumor metastatic
    m. hypertension
    m. hyperthermia
    m. melanoma of choroid
    m. melanoma of iris
    m. mesenchymoma
    m. myopia
    m. neurilemoma
    m. pituitary lesion
    m. schwannoma
    m. scleritis
malingering
Malis
    M. bipolar coagulating/cutting system
    M. forceps
Mallazine eye drops
mallet
    lead-filled m.
Mallett unit
Maloney nucleus rotator
malposition
    eyelid m.

malprojection
MALT
    mucosa-associated lymphoid tissue
    MALT lymphoma
maltophilia
    Stenotrophomonas m.
management
    anterior capsule m.
    cataract conservative m.
    filter m.
    medical m.
    m. strategy
    wound m.
Manche
    M. irrigation cannula
    M. LASIK forceps
    M. LASIK speculum
Manchester low-vision questionnaire
Manche-type LASIK irrigating cannula
mandatory eye exam
Mandelkorn suture laser lysis lens
maneuver
    driving m.
    Hallpike m.
    notch-and-roll m.
    Nylen-Barany m.
    oculocephalic m.
    Valsalva m.
    wall push m.
manganese superoxide dismutase
Manhattan
    M. Eye & Ear probe
    M. Eye & Ear spatula
    M. Eye & Ear suturing forceps
manifest
    m. deviation
    m. hyperopia (Hm)
    m. latent nystagmus
    m. refraction (MR)
    m. strabismus
manifestation
    neuroophthalmic m.
    neurovisual m.
    ocular m.
manipulation
    flap m.
    intraocular lens m.
    iris m.
    laser m.
    pharmacologic m.
    physical m.
manipulator
    Akahoshi nucleus m.
    angled m.
    button-tip m.
    Drysdale nucleus m.
    Friedman Phaco/IOL m.
    Grieshaber 2-function m.
    Grieshaber 3-function m.

Guimaraes ICL m.
Guimaraes implantable contact
  lens m.
Jarrett side port m.
Judson-Smith m.
Koch nucleus m.
Koch phaco m.
Kuglen irrigating lens m.
Kuglen nucleus m.
LASIK flap m.
lens m.
Lester IOL m.
Lester lens m.
Lieberman MicroFinger m.
Lindstrom Star nucleus m.
McIntyre irrigating iris m.
Sinskey IOL m.
Visitec m.
manipulator/elevator
Kritzinger-Updegraff m./e.
K-U m./e.
Mannis
M. probe
M. suture
mannitol
mannosidosis
Mann sign
Mann-Whitney U test
manometer
Honan m.
Tycos m.
manometry
manoptoscope
Manson-Aebli corneal section scissors
Manson double-ended strabismus hook
Mantel-Haenszel method
Mantoux test
manual
m. anterior capsulotomy
m. keratometer
m. kinetic perimetry
m. lamellar keratoplasty
m. vitrectomy
map
anisotropy m.
axial curvature m.
corneal keratometric m.
m. dystrophy
elevation topography m.
m. pattern
rasterstereography-based
  elevation m.
refractive eye m.

retinal thickness m.
wave aberration m.
wavefront m.
map-dot corneal dystrophy
map-dot-fingerprint (MDF)
m.-d.-f. corneal epithelial dystrophy
mapping
axial curvature m.
deletion m.
glaucomatous damage detection by
  retinal thickness m.
individualized m.
Orbscan pachymetry m.
Placido-based axial curvature m.
retinal m.
visually evoked potential m.
mapropsia
MAR
melanoma-associated retinopathy
MAR syndrome
marbleization
Marcaine
M. HCl
M. HCl with epinephrine
marcescens
Serratia m.
march
M. laser lens
M. laser sclerostomy needle
Marco
M. chart projector
M. lensometer
M. manual keratometer
M. perimeter
M. prism exophthalmometer
M. radius gauge
M. refractor
M. slit lamp
M. SurgiScope
Marcus
M. Gunn (MG)
M. Gunn dot
M. Gunn jaw-winking phenomenon
M. Gunn jaw-winking syndrome
M. Gunn pupil
M. Gunn pupillary sign
M. Gunn relative afferent defect
M. Gunn test
mare's-hair line
mare's-tail line
Marfan
M. disease

M

NOTES

Marfan *(continued)*
    M. sign
    M. syndrome
margin
    ciliary m.
    corneal m.
    eyelid m.
    fimbriated m.
    inflammatory retinal m.
    infraorbital m.
    lash m.
    lid m.
    orbital m.
    palpebral m.
    pupillary m.
    tumor-free m.
marginal
    m. blepharitis
    m. catarrhal ulcer
    m. chalazion forceps
    m. conjunctiva
    m. corneal degeneration
    m. corneal ulcer
    m. crystalline dystrophy
    m. degeneration of cornea
    m. entropion
    m. furrow
    m. furrow degeneration
    m. keratitis
    m. melt
    m. myotomy
    m. ray
    m. ray of light
    m. reflex distance (MRD)
    m. ring ulcer of cornea
    m. tear strip
marginalis
    blepharitis m.
marginoplasty
margo
    m. ciliaris iridis
    m. infraorbitalis orbitae
    m. lacrimalis maxillae
    m. lateralis orbitae
    m. medialis orbitae
    m. orbitalis
    m. palpebra
    m. pupillaris iridis
    m. supraorbitalis orbitae
    m. supraorbitalis ossis frontalis
Marie ataxia
Marinesco-Sjögren-Garland syndrome
Marinesco-Sjögren syndrome
Mariotte
    blind spot of M.
    M. blind spot
    M. experiment
    M. scotoma

mark
    M. II Magni-Focuser lens
    M. II Magni-Focuser loupe
    M. IX lens
    limbus parallel orientation
      straddling tattoo m.
    Nichamin fixation right with 10-
      degree m.'s
    periradial m.
    radial m.
marker
    Akura partial depth astigmatic
      keratotomy m.
    Amsler scleral m.
    Anis radial m.
    Anis suture placement m.
    Arrowsmith corneal m.
    ASSI triple m.
    astigmatic m.
    Bores axis m.
    Bores optic zone m.
    Bores radial m.
    Castroviejo corneal transplant m.
    Castroviejo scleral m.
    Chayet type corneal LASIK m.
    corneal transplant m.
    Dell astigmatism m.
    Dulaney LASIK m.
    Ellis astigmatism m.
    Feldman RK optical center m.
    Friedlander incision m.
    Gass scleral m.
    Geggel corneal transplant m.
    genetic m.
    Gonin m.
    Grandon T-incision m.
    Green-Kenyon corneal m.
    Hoffer optical center m.
    Hoffer optic zone m.
    Hofmann T-incision m.
    Hunkeler frown incision m.
    inflammatory m.
    Kershner LRI m.
    Koch LRI m.
    Kraff LRI m.
    Kritzinger-Updegraff corneal m.
    K-U corneal m.
    lambda light-chain m.
    Lindstrom arcuate incision m.
    Lindstrom astigmatic m.
    Lindstrom small incision m.
    low profile R-K m.
    Machat double-ended m.
    Machat superior flap LASIK m.
    Matos laser axis m.
    McDonald optic zone m.
    Mendez hexagon m.
    Mendez-type corneal LASIK m.
    microsatellite m.

Neumann-Shepard corneal m.
Neumann-Shepard oval optical
  center m.
Nordan-Ruiz trapezoidal m.
O'Brien m.
O'Connor m.
ocular m.
optical zone m.
Osher-Neumann corneal m.
Perone LASIK m.
Phillips gravity pivot axis m.
polymorphic microsatellite m.
Price radial m.
Probst Smiley LASIK m.
radial keratotomy m.
RK m.
Ruiz-Nordan trapezoidal m.
Ruminson astigmatic gauge and m.
scleral m.
Shepard optical center m.
Simcoe corneal m.
Soll suture and incision m.
Spivack axis m.
Storz radial incision m.
Thornton optical center m.
Thorton optic zone m.
Thurmond pachymetry m.
Visitec RK zone m.
Zaldivar LRI m.
m.'s for zone
marking pen
Markomanolakis aspirating speculum
Markwell
method of M.
Marlex mesh
Marlow test
Marmor
pattern dystrophy of pigment
  epithelium of Byers and M.
Marner cataract
Marshall syndrome
Marsh disease
Martegiani funnel
Martinez
M. corneal transplant centering ring
M. disposable corneal trephine
M. dissector
M. knife
mascara particle inclusion
mask
gel eye m.
masked diabetes

Masket
M. capsulorrhexis forceps
M. phaco spatula
mask-like facies
masque biliaire
masquerade
m. syndrome
m. technique
mass
cerebellopontine angle m.
choroidal m.
cicatricial m.
coalescent m.
contrast-enhancing m.
darkly pigmented nodular m.
gelatinous m.
hyaline m.
intracranial m.
lacrimal gland m.
laminated acellular m.
limbus m.
mulberry-shaped m.
mycelial m.
ochre m.
orbital apex m.
ovoid m.
subfoveal m.
subretinal m.
yellow-white choroidal m.
Massachusetts
M. Eye & Ear Infirmary
M. Vision Kit (MVK)
M. XII vitrectomy system (MVS)
massage
Crigler m.
eyelid m.
lacrimal sac m.
ocular m.
massaging
optic nerve m.
Masselon
M. glasses
M. spectacles
massive
m. granuloma of sclera
m. orbital trauma
m. osteolysis of Gorham
m. periretinal proliferation (MPP)
m. vitreous retraction (MVR)
Masson trichrome stain
mast
m. cell

M

NOTES

mast *(continued)*
    m. cell inhibitor
    m. cell stabilizer
Mastel
    M. compass-guided arcuate keratotomy system
    M. diamond compass
    M. Precision surgical instrument
    M. trifaceted diamond blade
master
    m. control gene
    m. eye
master-dominant eye
match
    color m.
    HLA m.
    human leucocyte antigen m.
mate
    Lens M.
    Soft M.
material
    alloplastic donor m.
    autogenous donor m.
    coating m.
    contrast m.
    cyanographic contrast m.
    donor m.
    exfoliative m.
    fibrillar m.
    gallium citrate contrast m.
    gelatinous m.
    heterogeneous donor m.
    homogeneous donor m.
    hyaline m.
    m.'s primary dye
    reading m.
    M.'s Testing System
    viscoelastic m.
Matos laser axis marker
matrix, pl. **matrices**
    acellular m.
    extracellular m. (ECM)
    glycocalyx m.
    Humphrey m.
    m. metalloproteinase (MMP)
    m. metalloproteinase inhibitor
    stromal m.
matte
    m. black forceps
    m. black instrument
matter
    particulate m.
    periaqueductal gray m.
Mattis corneal scissors
mattress suture
maturation
    delayed visual m.
    preinjury visual m.

mature
    m. cataphoria
    m. cataract
    m. lens
maturity-onset diabetes
Maumenee
    M. capsule forceps
    M. corneal forceps
    M. goniotomy knife
    M. goniotomy knife cannula
    M. iris hook
    M. knife goniotomy cannula
    M. vitreous-aspirating needle
    M. vitreous sweep spatula
Maumenee-Colibri corneal forceps
Maumenee-Park eye speculum
Maunoir iris scissors
Maurer spot
Maurice corneal depot technique
Mauthner test
Max
    M. Fine forceps
    M. Fine scissors
Maxidex
maxilla, pl. **maxillae**
    incisura maxillae
    infraorbital margin of m.
    infraorbital sulcus of m.
    lacrimal sulcus of m.
    margo lacrimalis maxillae
    processus zygomaticus maxillae
    sulcus infraorbitalis maxillae
    zygomaticoorbital process of m.
maxillaris
    nervus m.
maxillary
    m. bone
    m. nerve
    m. osteomyelitis
    m. sinusitis
maximal illumination
maximum
    m. depth lamellar keratoplasty (MD-LKP)
    m. tolerated medical therapy
Maxitrol suspension
MaxiVision
    M. dietary supplement
    M. ocular formula
    M. whole body formula
Maxsight sport-tinted contact lens
Maxwell
    M. ring
    M. spot
maxwellian view optical system
Mayo
    M. scissors
    M. stand
Mazzotti reaction

MBP
major basic protein
M-brace corneal trephine
MBRVO
macular branch retinal vein occlusion
MC
methylcellulose
Tears Again MC
MC-7000
MC-7000 multi-wavelength laser
MC-7000 ophthalmic laser
McCannel
M. ocular pressure reducer
M. suture
M. suture technique
McCarey-Kaufman
M.-K. preserved donor tissue
M.-K. transport medium
McCarthy reflex
McClure iris scissors
McCollough
M. effect
M. suturing forceps
McCune-Albright syndrome
McDonald
M. lens-folding forceps
M. optic zone marker
M. soft IOL folding forceps
McGannon retractor
McGhan 3M intraocular lens
McGill Pain Questionnaire
McGregor conjunctival forceps
McGuire corneal scissors
McIntyre
M. anterior chamber cannula
M. coaxial cannula
M. coaxial irrigating/aspirating
system
M. fish-hook needle holder
M. I/A needle
M. I/A system
M. III nucleus removal system
M. infusion set
M. irrigating/aspirating unit
M. irrigating hook
M. irrigating iris manipulator
M. irrigation/aspiration needle
M. irrigation/aspiration system
M. nylon cannula connector
M. reverse cystotome
M. spatula
M. truncated cone
McIntyre-Binkhorst irrigating cannula

McKinney
M. eye speculum
M. fixation ring
McLean
M. capsulotomy scissors
M. prismatic fundus laser lens
M. suture
McMonnies questionnaire
McNeill-Goldman
M.-G. blepharostat
M.-G. ring
McNemar chi-squared test
mCNV
myopic choroidal neovascularization
m-cone
MCP
multifocal choroiditis with panuveitis
MCP-1
monocyte chemotactic protein-1
McPherson
M. angled forceps
M. bent forceps
M. corneal forceps
M. corneal section scissors
M. irrigating forceps
M. microiris forceps
M. microsuture forceps
M. needle holder
M. spatula
M. speculum
M. suturing forceps
M. trabeculotome
M. tying iris forceps
McPherson-Castroviejo corneal section scissors
McPherson-Vannas microiris scissors
McPherson-Westcott
M.-W. conjunctival scissors
M.-W. stitch scissors
McPherson-Ziegler knife
MCPT
macular computerized psychophysical
test
McReynolds
M. lid-retracting hook
M. operation
M. pterygium knife
M. pterygium scissors
M. pterygium transplant
M. spatula
M. technique
MD
mean deviation

M

NOTES

MDF
    map-dot-fingerprint
    MDF corneal dystrophy
MD-LKP
    maximum depth lamellar keratoplasty
meal
    before m.'s (a.c.)
mean
    m. acuity
    m. corneal power
    m. deviation (MD)
    m. foveal thickness
    m. IOP
    m. spherical equivalent (MSE)
Means sign
measure
    Doppler flowmetry m.
    Geneva lens m.
    muscle imbalance m. (MIM)
    preventive m.
    visual performance m.
measurement
    A m.
    B m.
    baseline thickness m.
    box m.
    C m.
    circumpapillary m.
    color-contrast sensitivity m.
    criterion-free m.
    digital fitting m.
    direct m.
    diurnal intraocular pressure m.
    entopic foveal avascular zone m.
    1-eye m.
    glare disability m.
    Krimsky m.
    objective m.
    oxygen m.
    postocclusion m.
    prism cover m.
    psychophysical m.
    Rushton ocular m.
    sequential m.
    sitting m.
    Stenstrom ocular m.
    stress-strain m.
    thickness m.
    UBM m.
    vessel landmark m.
    white-to-white m.
measuring device
mechanical
    m. acquired ptosis
    m. corepraxy
    m. ectropion
    m. epithelial brush
    m. lid retraction
    m. scrape

    m. strabismus
    m. vitrector
mechanics
    fluid m.
mechanism
    m. of action
    blur-buffering m.
    cAMP mediated m.
    cholinergic m.
    fixation m.
    fogging m.
    graduated fine focus m.
    Hering after-image m.
    immune m.
    oculogyric m.
    primary m.
    pupillary block m.
    pursuit m.
    secondary m.
    self-adjusting m.
    trigger m.
mechanized scissors
Mecholyl test
Mectizan
MED
    minimal effective diameter
Medallion lens
Medcast epoxy resin
MedDev implant
media (*pl. of* medium)
    m. clearing
    ocular m.
    m. opacity
medial
    m. angle
    m. angle of eye
    m. arteriole of retina
    m. canthal ligament
    m. canthal repair
    m. canthal tendon
    m. canthus
    m. commissure of eyelid
    m. ectropion
    m. horn
    m. longitudinal fasciculus (MLF)
    m. longitudinal fasciculus lesion
    m. palpebral ligament
    m. rectus (MR)
    m. rectus extraocular muscle
    m. rectus function
    m. rectus palsy
    m. rectus transposition
    m. superior temporal (MST)
    m. superior temporal visual area
    m. venulae of retina
    m. vestibular nucleus (MVN)
medialis
    angulus oculi m.
    commissura palpebrarum m.

mediated
    immune m.
mediator
    inflammatory m.
    inflammatory chemical m.
medical
    m. adenomectomy
    m. management
    m. ophthalmoscopy
    M. Optics PC11NB intraocular lens
    M. Optics PC11NB intraocular lens implant
    m. tattooing
medicamentosa
    conjunctivitis m.
medication
    FDA-approved m.
    m. form
    intracameral m.
    intraocular pressure-lowering m.
    lubricating m.
    ophthalmic m.
    postoperative m.
    m. regimen
    systemic m.
medicine
    herbal m.
    National Center for Complementary and Alternative M.
    value-based m.
Medi-Duct ocular fluid management system
Meditec
    M. bandage contact lens
    M. Mel-60 excimer laser
Mediterranean anemia
medium, pl. **media**
    anaerobic m.
    chondroitin sulfate m.
    contrast m.
    corneal storage m.
    culture m.
    dextran m.
    dioptric m.
    Gram-negative m.
    Kaufman m.
    K-Sol m.
    Löwenstein-Jensen m.
    McCarey-Kaufman transport m.
    M-K m.
    ocular m.
    opaque m.
    Optisol m.

    Page m.
    refracting m.
    refractive m.
    Sabouraud m.
MedJet microkeratome
Med-Logics ML Microkeratome
Medmont
    M. E300 topographer
    M. M600 perimeter
medocromil sodium ophthalmic solution
Medpor MCOI implant
Medrol
medroxyprogesterone acetate
medrysone
medulla lesion
medullary
    m. cystic disease
    m. optic disease
    m. ray
medullated nerve fiber
medulloblastoma tumor
medulloepithelioma
    adult m.
    embryonal m.
    orbital m.
medusae
    caput m.
Medusa head
Meesmann
    M. epithelial corneal dystrophy
    M. juvenile epithelial dystrophy
megadose
megalocornea
    simple m.
megalopapilla
megalophthalmos
    anterior m.
megalopsia, megalopia
meglumine antimonate
megophthalmus
meibomian
    m. blepharitis
    m. conjunctivitis
    m. cyst
    m. duct
    m. gland carcinoma
    m. gland disease
    m. gland dysfunction (MGD)
    m. gland examination
    m. gland expressor
    m. gland obstruction
    m. gland orifice metaplasia
    m. sebaceous gland

M

NOTES

meibomian *(continued)*
> m. secretion
> m. sty

meibomianitis
> acne rosacea m.

meibomianum
> hordeolum m.

meibomitis

meibum oleic acid

Meige syndrome

Mel
> M. 60. 80 excimer laser
> M. 70 flying spot laser
> M. 60 scanning laser

melanin

melanin-containing cell

melaninogenicus
> *Bacteroides m.*

melanocyte
> uveal m.

melanocytic
> m. conjunctival lesion
> m. hamartoma
> m. iris tumor
> m. nevus

melanocytoma
> iris m.

melanocytosis
> congenital ocular m.
> congenital oculodermal m.
> ocular m.
> oculodermal m.

melanokeratosis
> striate m.

melanoma
> amelanotic m.
> amelanotic choroidal m.
> cavitary uveal m.
> choroidal amelanotic m.
> ciliary body m.
> ciliochoroidal m.
> conjunctival m.
> cutaneous m.
> m. of eyelid
> intraocular m.
> iris m.
> m. of iris
> juvenile m.
> malignant choroidal m.
> m. metastasis
> metastatic m.
> nodular m.
> ocular m.
> orbital m.
> pagetoid m.
> posterior uveal m.
> ring m.
> spindle A, B m.
> spindle cell m.

> tapioca iris m.
> uveal m.

melanoma-associated
> m.-a. retinopathy (MAR)
> m.-a. retinopathy syndrome

melanomalytic glaucoma

melanosis
> acquired m.
> m. bulbi
> diabetic m.
> epithelial congenital m.
> m. iridis
> ocular m.
> m. oculi
> oculodermal m.
> presenile m.
> primary acquired m. (PAM)
> m. sclerae

melanosome
> giant m.

melanotic
> m. lesion
> m. sarcoma
> m. schwannoma

Melkersson-Rosenthal syndrome

Melkersson syndrome

Mellaril

Meller operation

Mellinger speculum

mellitus
> adult-onset diabetes m. (AODM)
> diabetes m. (DM)
> gestational diabetes m.
> insulin-dependent diabetes m. (IDDM)
> juvenile diabetes m.
> non-insulin-dependent diabetes m.

melt
> corneal m.
> corneoscleral m.
> marginal m.
> sterile m.
> stromal m.

melting
> corneal m.
> scleral m.
> stromal m.

MEM
> monocular estimate method
> MEM retinoscopy

membrana, pl. **membranae**
> m. capsularis lentis posterior
> m. choriocapillaris
> m. hyaloidea
> m. limitans externa
> m. limitans interna
> m. nictitans
> m. pupillaris

m. ruyschiana
m. vitrea
membrane
  amniotic m.
  anterior basal m.
  anterior hyaloid m. (AHM)
  Barkan m.
  basement m. (BM)
  bilaminar m.
  Biopore m.
  Bowman m.
  Bruch m.
  choroidal neovascular m. (CNVM)
  conjunctival m.
  connective tissue m.
  contraction of cyclitic m.
  cryopreserved amniotic m.
  cyclitic m.
  Demours m.
  Descemet m.
  diabetic m.
  Duddell m.
  endothelial cell basement m.
  epimacular m.
  epipapillary m.
  epiretinal m. (ERM)
  epiretinal macular m.
  epithelial basement m.
  external limiting m.
  fibroglial m.
  fibroproliferative m.
  fibrovascular m.
  Fresnel m.
  glassy m.
  gliotic m.
  Haller m.
  Henle m.
  Hovius m.
  hyaline m.
  hyalitis of anterior m.
  hyaloid posterior m.
  idiopathic epiretinal m. (IERM)
  idiopathic preretinal m.
  inflammatory m.
  inner limiting m.
  intermuscular m.
  internal limiting m. (ILM)
  Jacob m.
  limiting m.
  m. lipid cell
  macular epiretinal m.
  mucous m.
  neovascular m.

nictitating m.
occult choroidal neovascular m.
ochre m.
onion skin-like m.
outer limiting m.
panretinal m.
m. peeler-cutter (MPC)
m. peeling
m. peeling forceps
periorbital m.
persistent pupillary m.
pigmented preretinal m.
posterior hyaloid m. (PHM)
preretinal m.
pupillary m.
purpurogenous m.
reduplication of Descemet m.
Reichert m.
retrocorneal m.
retroprosthetic m.
Ruysch m.
ruyschian m.
secondary m.
serous m.
stripping m.
subfoveal neovascular m.
subretinal m. (SRM)
subretinal neovascular m. (SRNVM)
tarsal m.
Tenon m.
trabecular m.
vitreal m.
vitreous m.
Wachendorf m.
wrinkling m.
Zinn m.
membrane-corneal interface
membranectomy
membranoproliferative glomerulonephritis
  type II
membranotomy
membranous
  m. cataract
  m. conjunctivitis
  m. lens
  m. rhinitis
memory
  immunologic m.
  visual m.
MemoryLens
  Mentor ORC M.
  M. prefolded IOL

M

NOTES

Mendez
- M. astigmatism dial
- M. cystotome
- M. degree gauge
- M. hexagon marker
- M. multipurpose LASIK forceps

Mendez-type corneal LASIK marker
Menicon Z rigid gas permeable contact lens
meningeal
- m. carcinomatosis
- m. cell
- m. hemangiopericytoma

meningioma
- angioblastic m.
- fibroblastic m.
- nerve sheath m.
- ocular m.
- optic nerve sheath m. (ONSM)
- orbital m.
- perioptic sheath m.
- psammomatous m.
- sphenoid wing m.
- suprasellar m.

meningitidis
- Neisseria m.

meningitis
- carcinomatous m.
- cryptococcal m.
- gummatous m.

meningocele
meningococcosis
meningococcus conjunctivitis
meningocutaneous angiomatosis
meningoencephalocele
meningosepticum
- Flavobacterium m.

meniscus, pl. **menisci**
- m. concave lens
- converging m.
- diverging m.
- m. floater
- Kuhnt m.
- negative m.
- negligible tear m.
- periscopic m.
- positive m.
- tear of m.

Mentor
- M. B-VAT II BVS contour circles distance stereoacuity test
- M. B-VAT II BVS random dot E distance stereoacuity test
- M. B-VAT II monitor
- M. B-VAT II video acuity tester
- M. curved eraser
- M. Exeter ophthalmoscope
- M. fine-focus microscope
- M. ORC MemoryLens
- M. precut drain
- M. wet-field cautery
- M. wet-field electrocautery
- M. wet-field eraser

meperidine hydrochloride
mepivacaine HCl
mercurialentis
mercurial preservative
mercuric oxide
mercury (Hg)
- m. bag
- millimeters of m. (mmHg)
- m. pressure

Meretoja syndrome
meridian
- m. of cornea
- corneal m.
- equatorial m.
- m. of eyeball
- horizontal m.
- major m.
- steepest m.
- vertical m.

meridional
- m. aberration
- m. amblyopia
- m. balance
- m. ciliary muscle fiber
- m. fold
- m. implant
- m. magnification
- m. refractometer

Merkel cell neoplasm
Mermoud nonpenetrating glaucoma forceps
Merocel
- M. lint-free sponge
- M. surgical spear

meropia
Mersilene suture
Mersilk black silk suture
mesangial cell
mesencephalic
- m. lesion
- m. lid retraction

mesencephalon lesion
mesenchymal
- m. dysgenesis
- m. ridge
- m. tumor

mesenchyme
- hemocytic m.
- neurogenic m.
- orbital m.

mesenchymoma
- malignant m.

mesh
- Marlex m.
- tantalum m.

meshwork
> m. dysfunction
> electron-dense m.
> trabecular m. (TM)

mesiris
mesoblastic tissue
mesochoroidea
Meso contact lens
mesocornea
mesoderm
> paraxial m.

mesodermal dysgenesis
mesodermalis
> primary dysgenesis m.

mesophryon
mesopia
mesopic
> m. condition
> m. perimetry
> m. pupil size

mesoretina
mesoridazine
mesoropter
Mestinon
mesylate
> nelfinavir m.
> ruboxistaurin m.

meta-analysis
metabisulfite
> sodium m.

metabolic
> m. coma
> m. syndrome cataract

metabolism
> amino acid m.

metachromatic leukodystrophy
metacognition
> visual m.

metacontrast
metaherpetic
> m. keratitis
> m. ulcer
> m. ulceration of cornea

metal knife
metalloproteinase
> matrix m. (MMP)

metallosis
> toxic retinal m.

metallothionein gene
metameric color
metamorphopsia
> cerebral m.
> m. varians

metaplasia
> conjunctival squamous m.
> meibomian gland orifice m.
> squamous m.

metaplastic epithelial cell
metarhodopsin
metastasis, pl. metastases
> chiasmal m.
> choroidal m.
> hematogenous m.
> hematopoietic m.
> leptomeningeal m.
> melanoma m.
> orbital m.
> pyogenic m.
> tumor m.
> m. of tumor
> uveal m.

metastatic
> m. carcinoma
> m. choroidal tumor
> m. choroiditis
> m. endophthalmitis
> malignant granular cell tumor m.
> m. melanoma
> m. neuroblastoma
> m. ophthalmia
> m. orbital tumor
> m. retinitis

Metcher speculum
Metenier sign
meter
> m. angle
> foot-candle m.
> functional visual acuity m.
> Guyton-Minkowski potential
>   acuity m.
> Kowa FM-500 laser flare m.
> laser cell and flare m. (LCFM)
> laser flare-cell m.
> m. lens
> potential acuity m. (PAM)
> retinal acuity m. (RAM)
> straylight m.
> van den Berg stray-light m.
> Vuero m.

meter-candle
methacholine chloride
methacrylate
> heparin surface-modified
>   polymethyl m.
> hydroxyethyl m. (HEMA)
> methyl m.

M

NOTES

methacrylate *(continued)*
    passivated polymethyl m.
    poly(2-hydroxyethyl m.) (PHEMA)
    polymethyl m. (PMMA)
methazolamide
methicillin
methicillin-resistant *Staphylococcus*
    aureus **(MRSA)**
method
    Barraquer m.
    Bio-Optics Bambi fixed-frame m.
    confrontation m.
    contact m.
    Coulter counter m.
    Crawford m.
    Credé m.
    Cuignet m.
    custom-contoured ablation
      pattern m.
    direct m.
    divide-and-conquer m.
    dot m.
    double K m.
    drifting-text m.
    fiber-tracking m.
    gradient m.
    grid m.
    Hanley and McNeil m.
    Hartmann-Shack wavefront m.
    heterophoria m.
    Hirschberg m.
    Holmgren m.
    immersion m.
    immunodiagnostic m.
    Kaplan-Meier m.
    Kirby-Bauer disc-diffusion m.
    Konan fixed-frame m.
    Krimsky m.
    Maddox rod m.
    Mantel-Haenszel m.
    m. of Markwell
    modified band lid m.
    monocular estimate m. (MEM)
    Mueller m.
    nonius m.
    optical density m.
    PCR-SSOP m.
    push-up m.
    rag-wheel m.
    Raman m.
    refractive screening m.
    Siepser m.
    m. of the sphere
    Sweet m.
    twirling m.
    Visx contoured ablation m.
    von Graefe prism dissociation m.
    von Kossa m.
    Westergren m.
    Wheeler m.
    Wolfe m.
methosulfate
    trimethidium m.
methotrexate
methoxsalen
methyl
    m. cyanoacrylate glue
    m. methacrylate
    m. propylparaben
methylcellulose (MC)
    hydroxypropyl m. (HPMC)
methylenetetrahydrofolate reductase
    (MTHFR)
methylergonovine
methylmethacrylate implant
methylparaben
methylpentynol
methylphenidate
    cocaine m.
methyl-phenyl-tetrahydropyridine (MPTP)
methylprednisolone
methylsulfate
    neostigmine m.
methysergide
Meticorten
metilprednisona
Metimyd
    M. Ophthalmic
    M. suspension
metipranolol
metoprolol
Metreton
metric
    m. ophthalmoscope
    m. ophthalmoscopy
metrics
    visual m.
metrizamide
MetroGel
metronidazole
metronoscope
metubine iodide
Metycaine
MEWDS
    multiple evanescent white-dot syndrome
Meyer
    M. Swiss diamond knife lancet
    M. Swiss diamond lancet knife
    M. Swiss diamond mini-angled
      knife
    M. Swiss diamond wedge knife
    M. temporal loop
Meyer-Archambault loop
Meyer-Schwickerath
    M.-S. coagulator
    M.-S. light coagulation
Meyhoefer chalazion curette
Meynert commissure

MFC
multifocal choroiditis
MFE
multifocal electroretinography
mfERG
multifocal electroretinogram
MG
Marcus Gunn
MG pupil
MGD
meibomian gland dysfunction
MGUS
monoclonal gammopathy of
undetermined significance
MH
macular hole
MHC
major histocompatibility complex
MHC gene
mica spectacles
micelles in vitreous
Michel
M. pick
M. spur
miconazole
Micra double-edged diamond blade
Micrins microsurgical suture
micro
m. bimanual irrigating handpiece
m. Colibri forceps
m. eye movement
105-mm M. Nikkor lens
M. One pneumatonometer
M. punctum plug
m. round-tip needle
m. vertical scissors
m. Westcott scissors
microadenoma
microaneurysm
capillary m.
hemorrhage and m. (h/ma)
juxtafoveal m.
microaneurysmal leakage
microangiography
microangiopathy
circumpapillary telangiectatic m.
occlusive m.
retinal m.
microanisocoria
microarray
tissue m.
microbacteria
atypical m.

microbevel edge lens
microbial
m. keratitis
m. virulence
microbiologic experience
microblepharia, microblepharism,
microblepharon
microcannula
Microcap scalpel
microcatheter urokinase infusion
microcautery unit
microchip
artificial silicone retina m.
microcirculation
retinal m.
microcoria
microcornea
microcyst
epithelial m.
intraepithelial m.
punctate epithelial m.
microcystic
m. corneal dystrophy
m. edema
m. epithelial dystrophy
m. lesion
microdot
microembolic episode
microembolism, pl. **microemboli**
retinal m.
microendoscope
ophthalmic laser m. (OLM)
microendoscopic test card
microenvironment
microfiber cleaning cloth
MicroFinger
Lieberman M.
microfold
retinal vascular m.
microforceps
Anis m. model 2-848
Colibri m.
Eckardt ILM m.
Sparta m.
microfuge tube
Micro-Glide corneal suture
microgonioscope
micrograsper
microhemagglutination test
microhook
Visitec m.
microhyphema
traumatic m.

M

NOTES

microhypopyon
microincision
    m. cataract surgery (MICS)
    corneal m.
    m. intraocular lens
microinfarct
    retinal m.
microinfarction
Microjet-based cutting and debriding device
microkeratome
    ALTK system m.
    Amadeus m.
    automated corneal shaper m.
    Barraquer m.
    BD K-3000 m.
    Carriazo-Barraquer m.
    Carriazo-Pendular m.
    Centurion SES m.
    Chiron ACS m.
    Chiron Hansatome m.
    Corneal Shaper m.
    Epi-K m.
    FlapMaker disposable m.
    Hansatome m.
    Innovatome m.
    Krumeich-Barraquer m.
    K-tome m.
    LSK One disposable m.
    LSK One standard m.
    MedJet m.
    Med-Logics ML M.
    MK-2000 m.
    Moria automated M2 m.
    Moria Model One m.
    SCMD m.
    SKBM m.
    Summit Krumeich-Barraquer m. (SKBM)
    Supratome m.
microKnife
    Ultrasharp round blade m. AU 681-21-3
microlaser
    diode m.
Microlase transpupillary diode laser
microloop curette polisher
microlymphocytotoxicity technique
micromanipulator
    self-centering m.
Micromatic ophthalmometer
micromegalopsia
micromesh sheeting
micrometer
    diamond m.
    m. disc
    m. knife
    Tolman m.
    ultrasonic m.

micromovement
    m. of eye
    retinal m.
micron
micronystagmus
micropannus
microperforation
microperimeter
microperimetry
    automated threshold m.
microphacoemulsification
    coaxial m.
    m. technique
microphakia
microphotography
microphthalmia, microphthalmos
    colobomatous m.
    complex m.
    cystic m.
    isolated colobomatous m.
    posterior m.
microphthalmoscope
micropia
micropick
    vitreoretinal m.
micropigmentation system
micropin
microplate fixation
micropoint
    m. needle
    m. suture
micropore
MicroProbe
    M. integrated laser endoscope
    M. integrated laser and endoscope system
    M. ophthalmic laser
microprocessor
microproliferation
micropsia
    cerebral m.
    convergence-accommodative m.
    psychogenic m.
    retinal m.
microptic
micropulse duty cycle
micropuncture
    anterior stromal m.
microruptor
    Lasag M.
microsaccade
microsatellite marker
microscalpel
    Oasis feather m.
microscissors
    DORC microforceps and m.
    iris m.
    Kamdar m.
    Keeler m.

microscope
> binocular m.
> Bio-Optics specular m.
> Bitumi monobjective m.
> confocal laser scanning m.
> ConfoScan 3 m.
> ConfoScan 2.0 slit corneal
>   confocal m.
> CooperVision m.
> corneal m.
> Czapski m.
> electron m.
> EM-1000 specular m.
> Fiberlite m.
> Galilean m.
> Heyer-Schulte specular m.
> JSM-54 IOLV m.
> JSM-6400 scanning electron m.
> Keeler-Konan Specular m.
> Keeler specular m.
> Konan Noncon ROBO CA SP-
>   8000 noncontact specular m.
> Konan SP-5500 contact specular m.
> Leitz m.
> light m.
> LSM-2100C eye bank specular m.
> Mentor fine-focus m.
> Moller m.
> Nikon NS-1 slit-lamp m.
> Olympus Vanox VH-2 m.
> operating m.
> OPMI pico i m.
> OPMI PRO magis m.
> OPMI VISU 200 m.
> OPMI VISU 210 m.
> Optiphot m.
> Project Research Ophthalmic
>   specular m.
> Pro-Koester wide-field SCM m.
> Reichert Zetopan m.
> scanning slit confocal m.
> slitlamp m.
> SMZ-10A zoom stereo m.
> specular m.
> Storz m.
> tandem scanning confocal m.
> Tomey ConfoScan confocal m.
> Topcon SP-1000 noncontact
>   specular m.
> transmission electron m.
> video specular m.
> Weck m.

> white light tandem-scanning
>   confocal m.
> Wild operating m.
> Zeiss-Barraquer cine m.
> Zeiss-Barraquer surgical m.
> Zeiss OM-3 operating m.
> Zeiss OpMi-6 FR m.

microscopic
> m. anomaly
> m. hyphema

microscopy
> confocal m.
> electron m.
> fluorescence m.
> fundus m.
> light m.
> specular m.
> transmission electron m.

MicroSeal ophthalmic handpiece
**microserrated Tano asymmetrical
  peeling forceps**
MicroShape keratome system
Micro-Sharp blade
microspectroscope
Microsphaeropsis olivacea
microspherophakia
microsponge
> Alcon m.

microsporidia
microsporidial keratoconjunctivitis
microstrabismic amblyopia
microstrabismus
microsurgery
> vitreous m.

microsurgical knife
microthin contact lens
Microtip phaco tip
microtome
> laser m.

microtrabeculectomy
MicroTrac direct specimen test
microtrauma
> blink-related m.

microtremor
> ocular m.
> superior oblique m.
> unilateral m.

microtrephine
microtropia
microtropic syndrome
microtubule
microvascular
> m. abnormality

M

NOTES

microvascular *(continued)*
    m. decompression
    m. ocular motor neuropathy
    m. sixth nerve palsy
microvasculopathy
    retinal m.
microvillus, pl. **microvilli**
Microvit
    M. probe
    M. probe system
    Storz Premiere M.
    M. vitrector
microvitrector
microvitreoretinal (MVR)
    m. blade
    m. spatula
microwave
    m. hyperthermia
    m. plaque thermotherapy
    m. radiation injury
MICS
    microincision cataract surgery
midazolam
midbrain
    m. corectopia
    m. disease
    m. ptosis
mid-coquille lens
middle
    m. cerebral artery
    m. temporal (MT)
    m. temporal visual area
midfacial fracture
midget system
midline
    m. granuloma
    m. position
    m. position of gaze
mid peripheral mottling pigmentation
midperiphery
midstromal
Mietens syndrome
migraine
    abdominal m.
    acephalgic m.
    acephalic m.
    basilar m.
    classic m.
    common m.
    complicated m.
    m. during pregnancy
    m. equivalent
    hemiplegic m.
    ocular m.
    ophthalmic m.
    m. ophthalmoplegia
    ophthalmoplegic m.
    retinal m.
    transformed m.

    m. with aura
    m. without aura
    m. without headache
migrainous
    m. hallucination
    m. ophthalmoplegia
    m. vision loss
    m. visual complaint
migrans
    erythema chronicum m.
    keratitis linearis m.
    ocular larva m.
    visceral larva m. (VLM)
migrating epithelium
migration
    bleb m.
    cell m.
    epithelial m.
    implant m.
    pigmentary m.
    m. theory
migratory ophthalmia
Mikamo double-eyelid operation
Mikulicz disease
Mikulicz-Radecki syndrome
Mikulicz-Sjögren syndrome
mild
    m. blurring
    m. chromic suture
    GenTeal M.
    Inflamase M.
    m. periocular hemorrhage
    Pred M.
milia
    eyelid m.
miliary
    m. aneurysm
    m. tuberculosis chorioretinitis
milieu
    proangiogenic m.
milk-alkali syndrome
milk-bag cataract
milky cataract
Millard-Gubler syndrome
Millennium
    M. CX, LX microsurgical system
    M. LX
    M. transconjunctival standard
      vitrectomy 25 system
    M. TSV25 light pipe
    M. TVS25 System
    M. vitreous cutter
Miller-Fisher
    M.-F. syndrome
    M.-F. variant
Miller-Nadler glare tester
Miller syndrome
Milles syndrome
millet seed nodule

Millex filter
millilambert
millimeters of mercury (mmHg)
Millipore filter
Milli-Q water purification system
Milroy Artificial Tears
MIM
    muscle imbalance measure
    MIM card
mimicking
    finger m.
Minardi phaco chopper
mind blindness
mineral oil
miner's
    m. blindness
    m. disease
    m. nystagmus
miniature
    m. blade
    m. excimer laser
    m. forceps
    m. glaucoma shunt
minicamera
    GD-LD-208C m.
minicircular capsulorrhexis
Mini-Drops eye therapy
miniflap
    scleral m.
mini-keratoplasty
    Castroviejo m.-k.
    m.-k. stitch scissors
minimal
    m. amplitude nystagmus
    m. brain dysfunction
    m. effective diameter (MED)
    m. pigment oculocutaneous albinism
minimum
    m. deviation
    m. light
    m. light threshold
    m. perceptible acuity
    m. separable acuity
    m. separable angle
    m. visible angle
    m. visual angle
miniophthalmic drape
miniplate
    titanium m.
    vitallium m.
MiniQuad XL lens
Mini-tip culturette

mini-trabulectomy
mini Westcott scissors
Minnesota low-vision reading test
Minocin
minocycline
Minolta LS 110 spot photometer
minor
    anulus iridis m.
    camera oculi m.
    circulus arteriosus iridis m.
Minsky
    M. circle
    M. intramarginal splitting
minus
    m. carrier
    m. carrier contact lens
    m. cyclophoria
    m. cylinder
    m. spectacle lens
Miocel
Miochol-E
Miochol solution
miosis
    congenital m.
    irritative m.
    paralytic m.
    pupil m.
    pupillary m.
    senescent m.
    senile m.
    spastic m.
    spinal m.
    traumatic pupillary m.
Miostat intraocular solution
miotic
    m. alkaloid
    m. pupil
    m. therapy
miotic-induced angle closure
Mira
    M. AGL-400
    M. cautery
    M. diathermy
    M. diathermy unit
    M. electrocautery
    M. encircling element
    M. endovitreal cryopencil
    M. photocoagulator
    M. silicone rod
MiraFlow
    M. Daily Cleaner
    M. Extra-Strength

M

NOTES

Miragel
    M. episcleral buckle
    M. exoplant
MiraSept system
mire
    keratometer m.'s
mirror
    m. area
    m. coating
    concave m.
    contact lens training m.
    convex m.
    m. haploscope
    head m.
    m. image
    power of m.
    m. rocking test
3-mirror
    3-m. contact lens
    3-m. prism
4-mirror goniolens
misalignment
    convergent m.
misdirected lash
misdirection
    aqueous m.
    facial nerve m.
    oculomotor nerve m.
    m. phenomenon
M.I.S. multi-port illumination system
missense variation
missing zonule
mist
    Nature's Tears all natural soothing
    eye m.
misty vision
Mitchell viscoelastic removal I/A tip
mitochondrial
    m. disease
    m. enzyme
    m. enzyme activity
    m. myopathy
mitomycin C (MMC)
mitosis
    epithelial m.
mitotic
Mitsubishi HL7955 CRT screen
Mitsuo phenomenon
Mittendorf dot
MityVac simple hand pump
mivacurium
mixed
    m. astigmatism
    m. bacterial-fungal keratitis
    m. cataract
    m. dyslexia
    m. esotropia
    m. fungal keratitis
    m. morphology bleb

    m. strabismus
    m. tumor
mixing
    color m.
    tear m.
mixture
    Neo-Synephrine cocaine m.
    Richardson methylene blue/aure
      II m.
Miyake
    M. photography
    M. technique
    M. view
Miyake-Apple posterior video technique
Miyoshi chopper
mizoribine (MZR)
Mizuo-Nakamura phenomenon
MK-2000
    MK-2000 keratome system
    MK-2000 microkeratome
MK IV ophthalmoscope
MKM
    myopic keratomileusis
M-K medium
MLF
    medial longitudinal fasciculus
    MLF lesion
MMC
    mitomycin C
    adjunctive MMC
mmHg
    millimeters of mercury
MMIF
    macrophage migration inhibitory factor
MMP
    matrix metalloproteinase
mobile eye unit
600XLE mobile surgery table
mobility
    outdoor m.
Möbius
    M. disease
    M. sign
    M. syndrome
MOBS
    modified binary search
mode
    m. of action
    free running m.
    function of Zernike m.
    hyperburst m.
    hyperpulse m.
    pulse m.
model
    Bohr m.
    m. eye
    floater eye m.
    Kooijman eye m.
    Le Grand-Gullstrand eye m.

m. 1559 magnifier
reduced eye m.
refractive growth m.
m. 177-33 viscocanalostomy
cannula
von Helmholtz eye m.
mode-locked Nd:YAG laser
moderate
m. amblyopia
GenTeal M.
m. myopia
modifiable risk factor
modification
Smith m.
surgical m.
Van Herick m.
modified
m. anterior capsulotomy
m. band lid method
m. binary search (MOBS)
M. Clinical Technique vision
screening
m. C-loop intraocular lens
m. C-loop UV lens
m. corncrib (inverted T) procedure
m. dandy criteria
m. Hughes flap
m. J loop
m. J-loop intraocular lens
m. J-loop UV lens
m. L loop haptic
m. monovision
m. prolate anterior surface
m. prolate anterior surface IOL
m. Rabinowitz-McDonnell index
m. Van Lint anesthesia
m. Van Lint block
m. Wies procedure
Modular One pneumatonometer
modulation transfer function
mofetil
Mohs
M. level
M. micrographic surgery
M. microsurgical resection
Moiré fringe
MoistAir humidifying chamber
moistened fine mesh gauze dressing
moisture
m. chamber
M. Eyes
M. Eyes liquid gel lubricant eye
drops

M. Eyes liquid gel preservative-
free eye drops
M. Eyes PM
M. Eyes PM eye ointment
m. goggles
M. ophthalmic drops
Mojave cataract extraction system
molded
m. frame
m. pressing
molding
cast m.
compression m.
injection m.
mold-injected lens
molectron laser
molecular
m. dissociation theory
m. external layer
m. inner layer
m. internal layer
m. outer layer
molecule
intercellular adhesion m.
proangiogenic m.
Moll
M. gland
M. gland cystadenoma
Moller microscope
Mollon-Reffin minimal test
molluscum
m. conjunctivitis
m. contagiosum
m. virus
Molteno
M. episcleral explant
M. implant
M. shunt tube
Momose lens
Monakow
M. fiber
M. syndrome
monarch
M. C cartridge
M. II injector
M. II intraocular lens delivery
system
M. II IOL delivery system
mongolian
m. fold
m. spot
mongoloid slant

M

NOTES

moniliforme
    Fusarium m.
monitor
    IOP m.
    Mentor B-VAT II m.
    Proview eye pressure m.
monitored anesthesia care (MAC)
monitoring
    electroretinographic m.
    refractive error m.
monoblepsia
monocanalicular
    m. intubation
    m. silicone stent
    m. stenting
monochromasia
monochromasy, monochromacy
    blue cone m.
    rod m.
monochromat
    atypical m.
    cone m.
    rod m.
monochromatic
    m. aberration
    m. cone
    m. eye
    m. radiation
    m. ray
    m. red HeNe laser light
monochromatism
    blue cone m.
    cone m.
    pi cone m.
    rod m.
    X-linked blue cone m.
monochromator
    grating m.
monochromic
monocle
monoclonal
    m. antibody
    M. Antibody Cytomegalovirus
      Retinitis Trial (MACRT)
    m. gammopathy of undetermined
      significance (MGUS)
monocular
    m. aphakia
    m. bandage
    m. blindness
    m. bobbing movement
    m. confrontation visual field test
    m. cue
    m. dazzle
    m. depth perception
    m. diplopia
    m. dressing
    m. electrooculogram

    m. estimate method (MEM)
    m. field defect
    m. fixation
    m. fixation target
    m. glaucoma
    m. heterochromia
    m. indirect ophthalmoscope
    m. nystagmus
    m. occlusion
    m. oscillopsia
    m. patch
    m. strabismus
    m. telescope
    m. temporal crescent
    m. vision
    m. visual acuity
monocular-estimate-method dynamic
  retinoscopy
monoculus
monocyte chemotactic protein-1 (MCP-1)
monodiplopia
monofilament nylon suture
monofixational phoria
monofixation syndrome
monofocal IOL
monograph
    Gullstrand m.
Monoka tube
monolateral strabismus
monolayered endothelium
mononuclear
    m. cell infiltration
    m. reaction
    m. response
monophosphate
    adenosine m. (AMP)
    cyclic adenosine m. (cAMP)
    cyclic guanidine m.
    cyclic guanosine m. (cGMP)
monophthalmica
    polyopia m.
monophthalmos
monopia
monostearate
    glyceryl m.
monotherapy
monovision
    modified m.
montage
    retinal m.
3-month postoperative refractive
  cylinder
Moody fixation forceps
moon blindness
Moore
    M. lens forceps
    M. lens-inserting forceps
    M. lightning streak

Mooren
    M. corneal ulcer
    M. ulceration
Moorfields bleb grading system
Moran
    M. enhancement spatula
    M. proptosis
Morax-Axenfeld conjunctivitis
Moraxella
    M. bovis
    M. catarrhalis
    M. conjunctivitis
    M. keratitis
    M. lacunata
    M. nonliquefaciens
Morax keratoplasty
morbidity
    ocular m.
morbillorum
    Gemella m.
Morcher
    M. Cionni endocapsular capsular
      tension ring
    M. iris diaphragm IOL, type 67G
    M. iris diaphragm ring, type 50C,
      type 96G
Morck
    M. cement
    M. cement bifocal
**Moretsky LASIK hinge protector
fixation ring**
Morgagni
    M. cataract
    M. globule
    M. liquor
    M. sphere
morgagnian
    m. cataract
    m. globule
Morgan lens
Moria
    M. automated M2 microkeratome
    M. Model One microkeratome
    M. obturator
    M. 1-piece speculum
    M. trephine
Morlet lamellar knife/dissector
morning
    m. discomfort
    m. glory disc
    m. glory optic atrophy
    m. glory optic disc anomaly
    m. glory retinal detachment

    m. glory syndrome
    m. ptosis
    m. stickiness
morpheaform pattern
morphine
morphologic variant
morphology
    cataract m.
morphometric analysis
morphometry
    endothelial cell m.
Morquio-Brailsford syndrome
Morquio syndrome
morrhuate
    sodium m.
Morris
    M. flexible cannula
    M. vertical scissors
Morse code pattern
mosaic
    m. fundus
    m. pattern
    m. pattern of dysfunction
    m. retinal dysfunction
    m. retinal dysfunction detection
    m. retinal dysfunction detection
      using multifocal electroretinogram
Mosher operation
Mosher-Toti operation
Mosler diabetes
mosquito
    m. clamp
    m. hemostatic forceps
moss
    M. operation
    M. traction
Motais operation
motexafin lutetium
motile scotoma
motility
    artificial eye m.
    extraocular m.
    m. implant
    ocular m.
    prosthesis m.
    restricted m.
    socket m.
motion
    m. automated perimetry
    m. detection perimetry
    m. and displacement perimetry
    hand m. (HM)
    m. parallax

M

NOTES

motion *(continued)*
    m. perception disorder
    m. photometry
    scissors m.
    scotoma for m.
    skew m.
    m. vision
    with m.
motoneuron
    ocular m.
motor
    m. function
    m. fusion
    m. nerve
    ocular m.
    m. oculi
    m. root
    m. root of ciliary ganglion
    m. tic
    Visuscope m.
motor-output disability
mottled appearance
mottling
    early receptor potential m.
    m. of fundus
    pigment m.
    retinal pigment epithelium m.
    subtle m.
mound
    pearl white m.'s
mount
    unstained wet m.
    wet m.
Mount-Reback syndrome
movable fixation light
movement
    cardinal ocular m.
    centripetal m.
    cogwheel ocular m.
    conjugate horizontal eye m.
    conjugate ocular m.
    corrective m.
    darting eye m.
    developmental eye m. (DEM)
    disconjugate roving eye m.
    disjugate m.
    disjunctive m.
    drift m.
    extraocular m. (EOM)
    eye m.
    eye-head m.
    facial m.
    fix-and-follow eye m.
    fixational ocular m.
    flick m.
    following m.
    fusional m.
    gaze m.
    hand m.

    illusion of m.
    impaired vergence eye m.
    lightning eye m.
    micro eye m.
    monocular bobbing m.
    nonoptic reflex eye m.
    nonrapid eye m.
    nystagmoid m.
    ocular m.
    perverted ocular m.
    prosthetic m.
    pursuit m.
    rapid eye m. (REM)
    reflex eye m.
    roving eye m.
    saccadic eye m.
    scissors m.
    slow conjugate roving eye m.
    smooth-pursuit m.
    synkinetic m.
    torsional m.
    vergence eye m. (VEM)
    vermiform m.
    version m.
    vertical m.
    voluntary eye m.
    yoke m.
moxifloxacin HCl ophthalmic solution
MPC
    membrane peeler-cutter
    MPC automated intravitreal scissors
MPF
    Polocaine MPF
    Sensorcaine MPF
MPH
    macular pseudohole
Mport lens insertion system
MPP
    massive periretinal proliferation
MPS
    Macular Photocoagulation Study
    multi-purpose solution
    Aquify MPS
MPTP
    methyl-phenyl-tetrahydropyridine
MR
    manifest refraction
    medial rectus
MRA
    magnetic resonance angiography
Mr. Color test
MRD
    marginal reflex distance
MRI
    magnetic resonance imaging
        FLAIR MRI
        MRI scan
MRS
    magnetic resonance spectroscopy

MRSA
> methicillin-resistant *Staphylococcus aureus*

MRV
> magnetic resonance venography

MSE
> mean spherical equivalent

MSFC
> Multiple Sclerosis Functional Composite

MSQLI
> Multiple Sclerosis Quality of Life Inventory

MST
> medial superior temporal
>> MST visual area

MT
> middle temporal
>> MT visual area

M-TEC 2000 surgical system

MTHFR
> methylenetetrahydrofolate reductase

MTI
>> MTI photoscreener
>> MTI photoscreener vision screening device

MTSI
> macular translocation with scleral infolding

mucin
> m. layer
> m. production
> m. strand
> m. of tear

mucin-like glycoprotein

mucinous
> m. adenocarcinoma tumor
> m. edema

mucocele
> sinus m.

mucocutaneous
> m. junction
> m. lymph node syndrome

mucoepidermoid carcinoma

mucoid discharge

mucolipidosis, pl. **mucolipidoses**
> m. type I–IV

Mucomyst

mucopurulent conjunctivitis

mucormycosis
> rhinoorbital m.
> rhinoorbital-cerebral m.

mucosa-associated
> m.-a. lymphoid tissue (MALT)
> m.-a. lymphoid tissue lymphoma

mucosae
> hyalinosis cutis et m.

mucosal
> m. neuroma
> m. pemphigoid

mucotome
> Castroviejo m.

mucous
> m. assay
> m. discharge
> m. membrane
> m. membrane graft
> m. membrane pemphigoid
> m. ophthalmia
> m. tear layer
> m. thread

mucous-like strand

mucus
> ropy m.
> m. strand
> stringy m.

Mueller
> M. cautery
> M. cell
> M. electric corneal trephine
> M. electrocautery
> M. electronic tonometer
> M. eye shield
> M. implant
> M. lacrimal sac retractor
> M. method
> M. operation
> radial cells of M.
> M. speculum
> M. trigone

mulberry-shaped mass

mulberry-type papilloma

Muldoon lacrimal dilator

Mules
> M. implant
> M. operation
> M. scoop
> M. vitreous sphere

mulibrey nanism

Müller
> M. cell
> M. cell footplate
> M. end feet
> M. fiber
> M. muscle

M

NOTES

multicore disease
multicorneal perfusion chamber
multicurve contact lens
multidrop lens
multifactorial disease
Multiflex anterior chamber lens
multifocal
    m. Best disease
    m. chorioretinal disease
    m. choroiditis (MFC)
    m. choroiditis with panuveitis
      (MCP)
    m. choroidopathy syndrome
    m. electroretinogram (mfERG)
    m. electroretinographic change
    m. electroretinography (MFE)
    m. fibrosclerosis
    m. hemorrhagic sarcoma
    m. implant
    m. intraocular lens implantation
    m. pattern dystrophy
    m. phakic IOL
    m. posterior pigment epitheliopathy
    m. silicone IOL
    m. spectacle lens
    m. visual evoked potential (mVEP)
multiforme
    erythema m.
    glioblastoma m.
multiincision 10-facet diamond blade
multilocular vesicle
multimodal approach
multinodularis
    episcleritis m.
multinucleated giant epithelial cell
Multi-Optics lens
multipass
    interwave-guided m.
multipiece lens
multiplanar reconstruction
multiple
    m. bottle regimen
    m. evanescent white-dot syndrome
      (MEWDS)
    m. lentigines syndrome
    m. myeloma
    m. ocular motor palsies
    m. sclerosis
    M. Sclerosis Functional Composite
      (MSFC)
    M. Sclerosis Quality of Life
      Inventory (MSQLI)
    m. vision
multiple-dose vial
multiple-quadrant hydrodissection
multipuncture capsulotomy
Multi-Purpose
    ReNu M.-P.
multi-purpose solution (MPS)

multiquadrant hydrodissection
multiscope
    roaming optical access m. (ROAM)
multistage correction
Multi-System incision knife
multivariate logistic regression analysis
multivesicular body
multivitamin
    MacularProtect m.
    OcularProtect m.
mumps keratitis
munitions fragment
Munsell color
Munson sign
mupirocin
mural cell
Murdock eye speculum
Murdock-Wiener eye speculum
Murdoon eye speculum
murine
    M. Plus Ophthalmic
    m. retina
    M. Solution
    M. sterile saline
    M. Tears
    M. Tears Plus
Muro
    M. 128
    M. Opcon
    M. Opcon A
    M. Tears
Murocel ophthalmic solution
Murocoll-2 Ophthalmic
musca, pl. muscae
muscarinic cholinergic side effect
muscle
    abductor m.
    adductor m.
    agonist m.
    m. belly
    bound-down m.
    Bowman m.
    Brücke m.
    ciliary body m.
    circular ciliary m.
    m. clamp
    common tendinous ring of
      extraocular m.
    m. cone
    congenital fibrosis of
      extraocular m.'s (CFEOM)
    m. contraction headache
    corrugator m.
    cyclorotary m.
    cyclovertical m.
    m. depressor
    dilator m.
    disinserted m.
    elevator m.

external rectus m.
extraocular m. (EOM)
extrinsic m.
m. of eye
eyelid m.
m. force
m. forceps
frontalis m.
m. hook
Horner m.
m. imbalance measure (MIM)
inferior oblique extraocular m.
inferior rectus extraocular m.
inferior tarsal m.
internal rectus m.
intortor m.
intraocular m. (IOM)
intrinsic ocular m.
IO m.
ipsilateral inferior oblique m.
iridial m.
iris sphincter m.
Koyter m.
Landström m.
lateral rectus extraocular m.
left inferior rectus m.
left superior rectus m.
levator palpebrae superioris m.
levator trochlear m.
longitudinal ciliary m.
lost rectus m.
medial rectus extraocular m.
Müller m.
oblique m.
ocular m.
oculorotatory m.
orbicularis oculi m.
orbicularis oris m.
orbital m.
palpebrae superioris m.
palsy of m.
m. paretic nystagmus
preseptal orbicularis m.
pupillary dilator m.
pupillary sphincter m.
radial dilator m.
recession of m.
rectus lateralis m.
rectus medialis m.
resection of m.
m. resection
Riolan m.
Rouget m.

m. sheath
sphincter m.
superciliary m.
superior oblique extraocular m.
superior rectus extraocular m.
superior tarsal m.
tarsal m.
temporalis m.
m. torque
m. transposition
trochlear m.
trochlea of superior oblique m.
vertical m.
vertical rectus m.
yoke m.

muscle-eye-brain disease
2-muscle surgery
muscular
    m. asthenopia
    m. balance
    m. dystrophy
    m. fascia
    m. funnel
    m. insufficiency
    m. strabismus
    m. vein
musculus, pl. **musculi**
    m. ciliaris
    m. corrugator supercilii
    m. depressor supercilii
    m. dilator pupilla
    lamina superficialis musculi
    m. levator palpebrae superioris
    m. obliquus inferior bulbi
    m. obliquus superior bulbi
    m. orbicularis
    m. orbicularis oculi
    m. orbitalis
    m. procerus
    m. rectus inferior bulbi
    m. rectus lateralis bulbi
    m. rectus medialis bulbi
    m. sphincter pupilla
    m. tarsalis inferior
    m. tarsalis superior
mushroom
    corneal m.
    m. corneal graft
mustache technique
Mustarde
    M. awl
    M. graft
    M. rotational cheek flap

M

NOTES

mustard gas
mutabilis
    Lecythophora m.
Mutamycin
mutation
    BIGH3 gene m.
    carbohydrate sulfotransferase
      gene m.
    crystalline protein m.
    frameshift m.
    Gln368Stop m.
    point m.
    retinoblastoma gene m.
    single-gene m.
mutton-fat
    m.-f. deposit
    m.-f. keratic precipitate
mutton fat
mVEP
    multifocal visual evoked potential
MVK
    Massachusetts Vision Kit
MVN
    medial vestibular nucleus
MVR
    massive vitreous retraction
    microvitreoretinal
      MVR blade
MVS
    Massachusetts XII vitrectomy system
My
    myopia
Myambutol
myasthenia
    focal m.
    m. gravis
    neonatal m.
    ocular m.
    pediatric m.
    m. syndrome
    transient neonatal m.
myasthenia-like syndrome
myasthenic
    m. crisis
    m. nystagmus
mycelial mass
Mycitracin
mycobacteria
    atypical m.
Mycobacteriaceae
mycobacterial disease
Mycobacterium
    M. africanum
    M. avium
    M. bovis
    M. chelonae
    M. fortuitum
    M. keratitis

    M. leprae
    M. smegmatis
    M. tuberculosis
Mycobutin
mycormycosis
Mycostatin
mycotic
    m. infection
    m. keratitis
    m. snowball opacity
mycotoxicity
Mydfrin ophthalmic solution
mydriasis
    accidental m.
    alternating m.
    amaurotic m.
    areflexical m.
    bounding m.
    congenital m.
    episodic unilateral m.
    factitious m.
    fixed m.
    paralytic m.
    permanent m.
    postoperative m.
    spasmodic m.
    spastic m.
    spinal m.
    springing m.
    transient unilateral m.
    traumatic m.
mydriatic
    m. ophthalmic solution
    m. provocative test
    m. rigidity
    m. test for angle-closure glaucoma
mydriatic-cycloplegic therapy
Mydrilate
myectomy
    m. operation
    orbicularis m.
    selective facial m.
myelinated retinal nerve fiber
myelination
    optic nerve m.
    m. of retinal nerve
    retinal nerve fiber m.
myelin disorder
myelitis
myeloidin
myeloma
    multiple m.
    osteosclerotic m.
myelomatosis
    disseminated nonosteolytic m.
myelooptic neuropathy
myeloperoxidase
    neutrophil m.

myiasis
    cutaneous m.
    ocular m.
MYOC
    myocilin
myocilin (MYOC)
    m. gene
    m. glaucoma
myoclonal
myoclonic epilepsy with ragged-red fiber
myoclonus
    m. nystagmus
    ocular m.
    oculopalatal m.
    startle m.
    vertical m.
myoculator
myocysticercosis
myodesopsia
myodiopter
myoepithelial cell
myoepithelioma
myofibril
myofibroblast
myogenic acquired ptosis
myoid visual cell
myo-inositol
myokymia
    eyelid m.
    facial m.
    superior oblique m.
myoneural junction
myopathic
    m. disorder
    m. eyelid retraction
    m. ptosis
myopathy
    centronuclear m.
    congenital m.
    dysthyroid m.
    endocrine m.
    fingerprint body m.
    inflammatory m.
    mitochondrial m.
    nemaline m.
    ocular m.
    proximal myotonic m.
    reducing body m.
    rod m.
    systemic m.
    thyrotoxic m.
    toxin-induced m.

    traumatic m.
    visceral m.
myope
    pathologic m.
myopia (M, My)
    abnormal nearwork-induced transient m.
    Artisan lens implantation for m.
    axial m.
    choroiditis m.
    chronic m.
    crescent m.
    curvature m.
    degenerative m.
    early-onset m.
    form-deprivation m.
    high m.
    m. index
    index m.
    late-onset m.
    lenticular m.
    low m.
    malignant m.
    moderate m.
    night m.
    nyctalopia with congenital m.
    pathologic m.
    peripheral m.
    pernicious m.
    physiologic m.
    prematurity m.
    primary m.
    prodromal m.
    progressive m.
    refractive m.
    school m.
    senile lenticular m.
    simple m.
    space m.
    transient m.
    vision deprivation m.
myopic (M)
    m. anisometropia
    m. astigmatism (AM, AsM)
    m. cave
    m. choroidal atrophy
    m. choroidal neovascularization (mCNV)
    m. choroidopathy
    m. conus
    m. crescent
    m. error
    m. foveoschisis

M

NOTES

myopic *(continued)*
  m. keratomileusis (MKM)
  m. macular hole detachment
  m. maculopathy
  m. reflex
  m. regression
  m. retinal degeneration
myorhythmia
  oculomasticatory m.
myoscope
myosin filament
myosis
myositis
  idiopathic m.
  infective m.
  orbital m.
  systemic m.
myotomy
  marginal m.

  m. operation
  Z m.
myotonia
  chondrodystrophic m.
  m. congenita
myotonic
  m. dystrophy
  m. dystrophy cataract
  m. dystrophy effect
  m. pupil
myReader low-vision auto-reading device
myringotomy blade
Mysoline
Mytrate
MZR
  mizoribine

N
  nasal
n
  index of refraction
NA
  numerical aperture
NA-AION
  nonarteritic anterior ischemic optic
  neuropathy
naboctate HCl
N1-acetylsulfanilamide
NaCl
  sodium chloride
Nadbath
  N. akinesia
  N. facial block
nadolol
Naegeli syndrome
Naegleria
  N. cyst
  N. fowleri
Nafazair Ophthalmic
nafcillin
Naffziger
  N. operation
  N. orbital decompression
NaFl
  sodium fluorescein
NAG
  narrow-angle glaucoma
Nagahara
  N. karate chopper
  N. phaco chopper
  N. quick chopper
Nagel
  N. anomaloscope
  N. Lensmeter
  N. test
Nager syndrome
NAION
  nonarteritic anterior ischemic optic
  neuropathy
naked
  n. eye
  n. vision (Nv)
nalorphine
naloxone hydrochloride
naming
  color n.
  picture n.
nana
  Hymenolepis n.
Nance-Horan syndrome
nanism
  mulibrey n.

Nanolas Nd:YAG laser
nanophthalmia, nanophthalmos
NANOS
  North American Neuro-Ophthalmology
  Society
Napha-A
Napha-Forte
naphazoline
  n. and antazoline
  n. and antazoline phosphate
  n. HCl
  n. and pheniramine maleate
Naphcon
  N. Forte
  N. Ophthalmic
Naphcon-A Ophthalmic
naphthyl ethylenediamine
napkin-ring peripapillary scarring
naproxen sodium
narcotic
  parenteral n.
narrow-angle glaucoma (NAG)
narrowed arteriole
narrowing
  angle n.
  arteriolar n.
  n. of retinal arteriole
narrow-slit illumination
Nasahist B
nasal (N)
  n. approach
  n. architecture
  n. arteriole of retina
  n. border of optic disc
  n. buttonhole incision
  n. canal
  n. canthus
  n. crystalline lens
  n. duct
  n. field loss
  n. hemianopsia
  n. isopter
  n. periphery
  n. speculum
  n. step
  n. step defect
  n. venule of retina
  n. vessel
  n. zone
nasal-hinged flap cornea
nasalization
nasi
  cancrum n.
nasion
nasoantritis

N

nasociliaris
    nervus n.
nasociliary
    n. nerve
    n. neuralgia
nasofrontalis
    vena n.
nasofrontal vein
nasojugal fold
nasolabial
    n. fold
    n. line
nasolacrimal
    n. blockade
    n. canal
    n. drainage system
    n. duct (NLD)
    n. duct obstruction (NLDO)
    n. duct probe
    n. gland
    n. groove
    n. occlusion
    n. reflex
    n. sac
nasolacrimalis
    ductus n.
nasoorbital fracture
Natacyn
natamycin
national
    N. Association for the Visually
       Handicapped (NAVH)
    N. Center for Complementary and
       Alternative Medicine
    N. Eye Institute (NEI)
    N. Eye Institute Visual Function
       Questionnaire (NEI-VFQ)
    N. Institute of Child Health and
       Human Development (NICHHD)
    N. Institute of Neurologic Diseases
       and Blindness (NINDB)
    n. stem cell bank
native vitreous collagen
natural
    n. cornea
    N. Tears
    n. UV radiation
Naturale
    Duratears N.
    Tears N.
Nature's
    N. Tears all natural soothing eye
       mist
    N. Tears Solution
NAVH
    National Association for the Visually
    Handicapped
navigation
    spatial n.

NBS
    nystagmus blockage syndrome
N-butyl-2-cyanoacrylate glue
NCCA
    noncontact corneal esthesiometer
NC-PAS
    noncontact photo-acoustic spectroscopy
NCT
    noncontact tonometer
Nd:YAG
    Nd:YAG laser
    Nd:YAG laser cyclophotocoagulation
    Nd:YAG Photon LaserPhaco system
Nd:YLF
    neodymium:yttrium lithium fluoride
    Nd:YLF laser
Neale
    N. analysis of reading ability
    N. reading analysis
near
    n. acuity testing
    n. add
    at distance and at n. (D/N)
    distance and n.
    esophoria at n. (E^1)
    n. esotropia (ET′)
    n. fixation
    n. fixation position of gaze
    n. light reflex
    n. Mallett unit
    n. phoria
    n. point
    n. point absolute
    n. point of accommodation (NPA,
       p.p.)
    n. point of convergence (NPC)
    n. reaction
    n. reaction to light
    n. response
    n. sight
    n. triad
    n. vision
    n. vision test
    n. vision testing
    n. visual acuity (NVA)
    n. visual point (NVP)
near-emmetropic eye
near-point
    n.-p. accommodation
    n.-p. esophoria
    n.-p. exophoria
    n.-p. phoria
    n.-p. relative
near-reflex spasm
nearsighted
nearsightedness
near-vision activity
nebula, pl. **nebulae**
    corneal n.

nebular stromal opacity
necrobiotic xanthogranuloma
necrogranulomatous keratitis
necrolysis
toxic epidermal n.
necrophorum
Fusobacterium n.
necrosis
acute retinal n. (ARN)
anterior segment n.
caseous n.
conjunctival n.
fibrinoid n.
infarctive n.
ischemic n.
perifascicular myofiber n.
progressive outer retinal n. (PORN)
retinal n.
scleral n.
stromal n.
white retinal n.
necrotic
n. adenocarcinoma
n. flap
n. follicle
n. infectious conjunctivitis
n. lymphomatous cell
n. occlusion
necrotizing
n. herpetic retinopathy
n. interstitial keratitis
n. nocardial scleritis
n. nodular scleritis
n. papillitis
n. retinitis
n. sclerocorneal ulceration (NSU)
n. stromal keratitis
n. ulcerative keratitis
n. vasculitis
nedocromil
n. sodium
n. sodium ophthalmic solution
needle
ACS n.
Agnew tattooing n.
Alcon CU-15 4-mil n.
Alcon irrigating n.
Alcon reverse cutting n.
Alcon spatula n.
Alcon taper cut n.
Alcon taper point n.
Amsler aqueous transplant n.
anesthesia n.

aqueous transplant n.
Atkinson peribulbar n.
Atkinson retrobulbar n.
Atkinson single-bevel blunt-tip n.
Atkinson tip peribulbar n.
Barraquer n.
BD n.
bent blunt n.
bent 22-gauge n.
blunt n.
Bowman cataract n.
Bowman stop n.
butterfly n.
BV100 n.
Calhoun n.
Castroviejo vitreous aspirating n.
cataract n.
cataract-aspirating n.
CD-5 n.
Charles flute n.
Charles vacuuming n.
Chiba eye n.
CIF4 n.
Cleasby spatulated n.
Colorado n.
CooperVision irrigating n.
CooperVision spatulated n.
corneal n.
couching n.
Crawford n.
Curran knife n.
Daily cataract n.
Davis knife n.
Dean knife n.
discission n.
Drews cataract n.
Ellis foreign body n.
Elschnig extrusion n.
Empire n.
enclavation n.
Ethicon BV-75-3 n.
extended round n.
extrusion n.
Fisher eye n.
flute n.
Flynn extrusion n.
foreign body n.
Fritz vitreous transplant n.
30-gauge n.
Girard anterior chamber n.
Girard cataract-aspirating n.
Girard phacofragmatome n.
Girard-Swan knife n.

N

NOTES

needle *(continued)*
> Graefe n.
> Grieshaber ophthalmic n.
> Haab knife n.
> Heyner double n.
> n. holder
> n. holder clamp
> illuminated suction n.
> internal nucleus hydrodelineation n.
> Iolab 108 B n.
> Iolab irrigating n.
> Iolab taper-cut n.
> Iolab titanium n.
> iris knife n.
> Kalt corneal n.
> Kloti radiofrequency diathermy n.
> Knapp knife n.
> knife n.
> Kratz diamond-dusted n.
> Kratz lens n.
> Lewicky n.
> lighted flute n.
> Look retrobulbar n.
> Lo-Trau side-cutting n.
> LX n.
> March laser sclerostomy n.
> Maumenee vitreous-aspirating n.
> McIntyre I/A n.
> McIntyre irrigation/aspiration n.
> micropoint n.
> micro round-tip n.
> nucleus hydrolysis n.
> peribulbar n.
> probe n.
> n. probe
> puncture n.
> puncture-tip n.
> razor n.
> razor-tip n.
> retrobulbar n.
> Reverdin suture n.
> reverse-cutting n.
> Riedel n.
> Rycroft n.
> Sabreloc n.
> Sato cataract n.
> Scheie cataract-aspirating n.
> sclerostomy n.
> Sharpoint Ultra-Guide ophthalmic n.
> side-cutting spatulated n.
> 4-sided cutting n.
> silicone brush back-flushed n.
> Simcoe II PC aspirating n.
> Simcoe suture n.
> ski n.
> spatula n.
> n. spatula
> spatulated n.
> n. spoon
> spoon n.
> n. spud
> n. stick
> Stocker n.
> Straus curved retrobulbar n.
> subconjunctival n.
> Surgicraft suture n.
> suturing n.
> Tano diamond dusted n.
> taper-cut n.
> taper-point n.
> tattooing n.
> TG-140 n.
> Thornton n.
> titanium n.
> translocation n.
> triple facet-tip n.
> ultrasonic cataract-removal lancet n.
> Universal soft tip cannulated
>   sliding extrusion n.
> vitreous aspirating n.
> vitreous transplant n.
> von Graefe knife n.
> Weeks n.
> Wright fascia n.
> Wright ophthalmic n.
> Yale Luer-Lok n.
> Ziegler iris knife n.

needle-and-syringe technique
needleless regional anesthesia
needling
> bleb n.

negative
> n. accommodation
> n. afterimage
> n. convergence
> n. dysphotopsia
> n. eyepiece
> false n.
> n. image
> n. meniscus
> n. meniscus lens
> n. predictive value
> n. scotoma
> n. vertical divergence
> n. vertical vergence
> n. visual phenomenon

neglect
> color n.
> n. dyslexia
> graphic n.
> visual n.

negligible tear meniscus
NEI
> National Eye Institute
> > NEI Visual Acuity Impairment
> > Survey study

Neisseria
- *N. gonorrhoeae*
- *N. meningitidis*

neisserial conjunctivitis

Neitz
- N. CT-R cataract camera
- N. Instruments Company

NEI-VFQ
- National Eye Institute Visual Function Questionnaire

nelfinavir mesylate

Nelson
- N. classification
- N. grading system

nemaline myopathy

nematode

Nembutal

Neocidin

Neo-Cobefrin

NeoDecadron
- N. Ophthalmic
- N. Solution
- N. Topical

Neo-Dexair

Neo-Dexameth Ophthalmic

Neodexasone

neodymium:YAG laser

neodymium:yttrium
- n.:y. aluminum garnet laser
- n.:y. lithium fluoride (Nd:YLF)

neodymium:yttrium-lithium-fluoride
- n.-l.-f. laser segmentation
- n.-l.-f. photodisruptive laser

Neo-Flow

neoformans
- *Cryptococcus n.*

Neofrin
- N. 2.5%
- N. 10%

Neo-Hydeltrasol

Neolens lens

Neolyte laser indirect ophthalmoscope

Neo-Medrol

Neomixin

neomycin
- n., polymyxin B, and dexamethasone
- n., polymyxin B, and gramicidin
- n., polymyxin B, and hydrocortisone
- n., polymyxin B, and prednisolone
- n. sulfate

Neomycin-Dex

neonatal
- n. corneal opacity
- n. erythroderma
- n. gliosis
- n. inclusion blennorrhea
- n. inclusion conjunctivitis
- n. intensive care unit
- n. myasthenia
- n. onset multisystem inflammatory disease (NOMID)
- n. ophthalmia
- n. period

neonatorum
- blennorrhea n.
- ophthalmia n.

neoplasia
- conjunctival intraepithelial n. (CIN)
- conjunctival squamous cell n.
- corneal conjunctival intraepithelial n.
- intraepithelial n.

neoplasm
- choroidal n.
- intraepithelial n.
- Merkel cell n.
- orbital n.
- parotid n.
- secondary malignant n.

neoplastic angioendotheliomatosis

Neo-Polycin

Neopolydex

Neoral

Neosar Injection

NeoSoniX
- N. handpiece
- N. system

Neosporin
- N. drops
- N. Ophthalmic Ointment
- N. Ophthalmic Solution

neostigmine
- n. methylsulfate
- n. test

Neo-Synephrine
- N.-S. cocaine mixture
- N.-S. Hydrochloride
- N.-S. Ophthalmic Solution
- N.-S. Viscous

Neotal

Neo-Tears

Neotricin HC Ophthalmic Ointment

neovascular
- n. angle-closure glaucoma

NOTES

neovascular *(continued)*
    n. iris vessel
    n. membrane
    n. net
    n. response
    retinal n.
    n. tuft
neovascularization
    choroidal n. (CNV)
    choroidovitreal n.
    classic choroidal n.
    corneal n.
    corneal stromal n.
    disc n.
    n. of disc (NVD)
    disseminated asymptomatic
      unilateral n.
    n. elsewhere (NVE)
    extraretinal n.
    flat n.
    hemorrhagic choroidal n.
    interstitial n.
    iris n.
    n. of iris (NVI)
    juxtafoveal choroidal n.
    myopic choroidal n. (mCNV)
    n. of new vessel ellipsometer
    occult choroidal n.
    pathologic n.
    peripapillary subretinal n.
    preretinal n.
    n. of retina
    retinal quadrant n.
    secondary n.
    stromal n.
    subfoveal choroidal n.
    subretinal n. (SRNV)
    type 1, 2 choroidal n.
    vitreous n.
Neovastat
nepafenac
    n. ophthalmic
    n. ophthalmic suspension
nephritica
    retinitis n.
nephropathic cystinosis
Neptazane
Nernst glower
nerve
    aberrant degeneration of third n.
    aberrant regeneration of n.
    aberrant reinnervation of
      oculomotor n.
    acoustic n.
    afferent n.
    aplasia of optic n.
    atrophy of optic n.
    basal epithelial n.
    block n.

n. block
cavernous portion of oculomotor n.
ciliary n.
coloboma of optic n.
n. core
corneal subbasal n.
cranial n. (CN)
n. cross section
cupping of optic n.
efferent n.
eighth cranial n.
facial n.
n. fiber
N. Fiber Analyzer laser
  ophthalmoscope
n. fiber axon
n. fiber bundle
n. fiber bundle defect
n. fiber bundle layer
n. fiber layer (NFL)
n. fiber layer analyzer
n. fiber layer dropout
n. fiber layer hemorrhage
n. fiber layer infarct
n. fiber technology
fifth cranial n.
fourth cranial n.
frontal n.
ganglionic layer of optic n.
ganglionic stratum of optic n.
ganglion layer of optic n.
ganglion stratum of optic n.
greater superficial petrosal n.
n. growth factor
n. head angioma
n. head drusen
hypoplastic ocular n.
infraepitrochlear n.
infraorbital n.
infratrochlear n.
n. input
input n.
intervaginal space of optic n.
intracanalicular optic n.
intracranial optic n.
intraocular optic n.
intraosseous optic n.
ischemia of optic n.
lacrimal n.
n. layer of retina
long ciliary n.
n. loop
maxillary n.
motor n.
myelination of retinal n.
nasociliary n.
normal optic n.
oculomotor n.
ophthalmic n.

optic n. (ON)
orbital optic n.
output n.
n. palsy
peripapillary retinal n.
peripheral oculomotor n.
petrosal n.
postganglionic short ciliary n.
prechiasmal optic n.
preganglionic oculomotor n.
prelaminar optic n.
n. regeneration
regeneration of n.
second cranial n.
secretomotor n.
sensory n.
seventh cranial n.
n. sheath
n. sheath meningioma
short ciliary n.
sixth cranial n.
supraorbital n.
supratrochlear n.
swollen n.
tentorial n.
third cranial n.
trigeminal n. (NV)
trochlear n.
tumor of optic n.
vascular circle of optic n.
vestibular n.
vidian n.
zygomatic n.
zygomaticofacial n.
zygomaticotemporal n.

nervea
tunica n.
nervous asthenopia
nervus, pl. **nervi**
n. infraorbitalis
n. intermedius
iris n.
n. lacrimalis
n. maxillaris
n. nasociliaris
n. oculomotorius
n. opticus
n. supraorbitalis
n. trigeminus
n. trochlearis
n. zygomaticus
Nesacaine
nests and strands of cells

net
neovascular n.
parafoveal capillary n.
Nettleship-Falls X-linked ocular albinism
Nettleship iris repositor
Nettleship-Wilder dilator
network
choriocapillaris vascular n.
Diabetic Retinopathy Clinical
Research N.
DRCR N.
Eye Cancer N.
Gerlach n.
Joslin Vision N. (JVN)
peritarsal n.
The Eye Cancer N.
trabecular n.
vascular n.
Neumann razor blade fragment holder
Neumann-Shepard
N.-S. corneal marker
N.-S. oval optical center marker
Neuprex
neural
n. crest
n. crest cell
n. ganglionic cell
n. lesion
n. retina
n. rim
n. transfer function
n. tube
neuralgia
nasociliary n.
postherpetic n.
Raeder paratrigeminal n.
supraorbital n.
trifacial n.
trigeminal n.
vidian n.
neurasthenic asthenopia
neurectomy
opticociliary n.
vidian n.
neurilemmosarcoma
neurilemoma
ameloblastic n.
eyelid n.
malignant n.
neuritic atrophy
neuritis, pl. **neuritides**
acute idiopathic demyelinating
optic n.

N

NOTES

neuritis *(continued)*
    anterior ischemic optic n.
    asymptomatic optic n.
    atherosclerotic ischemic n.
    chronic demyelinating optic n.
    demyelinating optic n.
    idiopathic demyelinating optic n.
    idiopathic nongranulomatous
      optic n.
    idiopathic perioptic n.
    inflammatory optic n.
    intraocular optic n.
    n. nodosa
    optic demyelinating n.
    orbital n.
    parainfectious optic n.
    paraneoplastic optic n.
    perioptic n.
    postocular n.
    postvaccination optic n.
    retrobulbar optic n.
    subclinical optic n.
neuro-Behçet disease
neuroblastic
neuroblastoma
    metastatic n.
    olfactory n.
neurochorioretinitis
neurochoroiditis
neurodealgia
neurodeatrophia
neurodegenerative syndrome
neuroectodermal
neuroepithelial layer of retina
neuroepithelioma
    orbital n.
neuroepithelium
neurofibroma
    eyelid n.
    iris n.
    limbal n.
    orbital n.
    plexiform n.
    n. type 1, 2
    uveal n.
neurofilament triplets antibody
neurogenic
    n. iris atrophy
    n. mesenchyme
    n. tumor
neurogenic-acquired ptosis
Neuroguard pulsed wave transducer
neuroimaging
neuroleptic malignant syndrome
neurologic
    n. deficit
    n. disorder
    n. dysfunction
    n. examination

neuroma
    acoustic n.
    facial n.
    mucosal n.
    orbital n.
    plexiform n.
neuromuscular
    n. blocking drug
    n. disorder
    n. disorder-causing drug
    n. effect
    n. eyelid retraction
    n. ptosis
neuromyelitis optica
neuromyotonia
    ocular n.
neuron
    abducens internuclear n.
    cholinergic n.
    Golgi I, II n.
    retinal n.
    sympathetic n.
    third order n.
neuronal
    n. ceroid lipofuscinosis
    n. plasticity
neuron-specific
    n.-s. enolase (NSE)
    n.-s. enolase antibody
neuroophthalmic manifestation
neuroophthalmologic
    n. abnormality
    n. case history
    n. diagnosis
    n. disease
    n. examination
neuroophthalmological investigation
neuroophthalmology
neuropapillitis
neuroparalytic
    n. keratitis
    n. keratopathy
    n. ophthalmia
neuropathic
    n. disease
    n. eyelid retraction
    n. tonic pupil
neuropathy
    anterior compressive optic n.
    anterior ischemic optic n. (AION)
    arteriosclerotic ischemic optic n.
    arteritic anterior ischemic optic n.
    autoimmune-related retinopathy and
      optic n. (ARRON)
    autosomal dominant hereditary
      optic n.
    autosomal recessive hereditary
      optic n.
    bilateral anterior ischemic optic n.

compressive optic n.
Cuban epidemic optic n.
demyelinating optic n.
distal optic n.
dominant optic n.
dysthyroid optic n.
giant axonal n.
glaucomatous optic n.
Graves optic n.
hereditary optic n.
hypertensive optic n.
hypertrophic interstitial n.
infiltrative optic n.
inflammatory optic n.
ischemic optic n. (ION)
Jamaican optic n.
Leber hereditary optic n. (LHON)
luetic n.
microvascular ocular motor n.
myelooptic n.
nonarteritic anterior ischemic
  optic n. (NA-AION, NAION)
nutritional optic n.
onion bulb n.
optic n.
parainfectious optic n.
paraneoplastic optic n.
peripheral n.
posterior ischemic optic n. (PION)
radiation-induced optic n.
radiation optic n. (RON)
retrobulbar compressive optic n.
retrobulbar ischemic optic n.
shock optic n.
subacute myelooptic n. (SMON)
toxic optic n.
traumatic optic n. (TON)
tropical optic n.
uremic optic n.
neurophakomatosis
neuroprotective antiglaucoma drug
neuroradiologic
neuroretinal rim
neuroretinitis
catscratch disease n.
diffuse unilateral subacute n.
  (DUSN)
idiopathic retinal vasculitis,
  aneurysms and n. (IRVAN)
Leber idiopathic stellate n.
stellate n.
subacute n.

neuroretinopathy
acute macular n. (AMN)
hypertensive n.
macular n.
neurosecretory granule
neurosensory
n. retina
n. retinal detachment
neurosyphilis
neurotomy
opticociliary n.
radial optic n.
neurotonic pupil
neurotransmitter
retinal n.
neurotrophic
n. keratitis
n. keratopathy
neurotropism
neurovisual manifestation
neutral
n. density filter
n. density filter test
n. point
n. zone
neutralization
neutralizer
AoDisc N.
neutrophil myeloperoxidase
Nevanac
nevi (*pl. of* nevus)
nevocyte
nevoid
nevoxanthoendothelioma
juvenile n.
nevus, pl. **nevi**
acquired n.
basal cell n.
blue n.
n. cell
choroidal n.
compound n.
conjunctival pigmented n.
cystic amelanotic n.
dermal n.
episcleral n.
epithelial n.
eyelid n.
n. flammeus
intradermal n.
iris n.
junctional n.
melanocytic n.

N

NOTES

nevus *(continued)*
    nonpigmented n.
    Ota n.
    n. of Ota
    n. pigmentation
    Spitz n.
    strawberry n.
    subepithelial n.
    uveal n.

Nevyas
    N. double sharp cystotome
    N. lens forceps
    N. retractor

new
    N. England Eye Bank
    N. Orleans Eye & Ear fixation forceps
    N. Orleans lens
    N. Orleans lens loupe
    n. physical finding
    N. York Eye & Ear Hospital fixation forceps
    N. York Lighthouse acuity test

newborn
    aniridia in n.
    Clinical Trial of Eye Prophylaxis in the N.
    conjunctivitis of n.
    n. conjunctivitis

Newcastle disease virus
NewIris ocular implant
NewLife IOL
Newman collagen plug inserter forceps
new-onset
    n.-o. internuclear ophthalmoplegia
    n.-o. nystagmus

Newton disc
newtonian aberration
NewVues sterile contact lens
Nexacryl
    N. cohesive product
    N. tissue adhesive

NFL
    nerve fiber layer

niacin maculopathy
Niamtu video imaging system
Nichamin
    N. fixation right with 10-degree marks
    N. fixation ring
    N. hydrodissection cannula
    N. I and II nucleus quick chopper
    N. LASIK irrigating cannula
    N. triple chopper
    N. vertical chopper

NICHHD
    National Institute of Child Health and Human Development

nicking
    arteriolar n.
    arteriovenous n.
    AV n.
    n. of retinal vein
    retinal venous n.

Nicol prism
nicotinic acid maculopathy
nictation *(var. of* nictitation*)*
nictitans
    membrana n.

nictitating
    n. membrane
    n. spasm

nictitation, nictation
Nidek
    N. AR-2000 Objective Automatic refractor
    N. combo laser system
    N. 3Dx stereodisk camera
    N. EC-1000 excimer laser
    N. EC-5000 excimer laser
    N. EC-5000 refractive laser system
    N. Laser System laser
    N. MK-2000 keratome system

Nieden syndrome
Niemann-Pick disease type A, B
niger
    Aspergillus n.

night
    n. blindness
    N. & Day Tears Again sterile lubricant gel
    n. myopia
    n. sight
    n. vision
    n. vision complaint

night-driving
    n.-d. performance
    n.-d. simulator

night-vision goggles
nigra
    cataracta n.

nigricans
    acanthosis n.
    pseudoacanthosis n.

nigroid body
nigrum
    pigmentum n.
    tapetum n.

Nike Max Rx prescription sun lens
Nikolsky sign
Nikon
    N. aspheric lens
    N. Auto Refractometer NR-1000F
    N. D100 digital camera
    N. FS-3 photo slitlamp biomicroscope
    N. NS-1 slit-lamp microscope

N. Retinomax K-Plus autorefractor
N. Retinopan fundus camera
N. zoom photo slit lamp

NINDB
National Institute of Neurologic Diseases and Blindness

NIPH
no improvement with pinhole

niphablepsia

niphotyphlosis

nitrate
cellulose n.
Grocott-Gomori methenamine silver n.
phenylmercuric n.
pilocarpine n.
silver n.

nitrocellulose filter paper

nivalis
ophthalmia n.

Nizoral

NLD
nasolacrimal duct

NLDO
nasolacrimal duct obstruction

NLP
no light perception

NM-1000 digital non-mydriatic fundus camera

NMG
no Marcus Gunn

no
no improvement
no improvement with pinhole (NIPH)
no light perception (NLP)
no light perception vision
no Marcus Gunn (NMG)
No Rub Opti-Free Express multi-purpose disinfecting solution

Noble forceps

Nocardia
N. asteroides
N. brasiliensis
N. caviae
N. dacryolith
N. keratitis

nocardial endophthalmitis

nocardiosis
ocular n.

nociceptive sensation

nociceptor
corneal n.

N₂O cryosurgical unit

noctograph

nocturnal
n. amblyopia
n. eye padding
n. intraocular pressure
n. lagophthalmia

nodal
n. plane
n. point

node
Rosenmüller n.

nodosa
conjunctivitis n.
endophthalmitis ophthalmia n.
iritis n.
neuritis n.
ophthalmia n.
periarteritis n. (PAN, PN)
polyarteritis n.

nodular
n. conjunctivitis
n. corneal degeneration
n. episcleritis
n. fasciitis
n. iritis
n. melanoma
n. scleritis
n. subtype

nodule
Busacca n.
conjunctival n.
Dalen-Fuchs n.
epibulbar Fordyce n.
episcleral rheumatic n.
Fordyce n.
iris n.
Koeppe n.
lemon-drop n.
lenticular fibroxanthomatous n.
lentiform n.
Lisch n.
millet seed n.
pseudorheumatoid n.
rheumatic n.
Sakurai-Lisch n.
Salzmann n.
subepidermal calcified n.

nodulus syndrome

Nolahist

Nolvadex

N

NOTES

NOMID
neonatal onset multisystem inflammatory disease
nomogram
Rochester n.
n. system
nonabsorbable suture
non-*Acanthamoeba* amebic keratitis
nonaccommodation
nonaccommodative
n. esodeviation
n. esophoria
n. esotropia
nonarteritic anterior ischemic optic neuropathy (NA-AION, NAION)
nonaspirating ultrasonic phaco chopper tip
nonatopic allergic conjunctivitis
non-blue filtering IOL
noncaseating conjunctival granuloma
noncentral ulcer
noncicatricial entropion
nonclearing hemorrhage
noncomitant
n. heterotropia
n. squint
n. strabismus
noncompliance
contact lens n.
nonconcomitant strabismus
nonconfluent plaque
noncongestive glaucoma
noncontact
n. corneal esthesiometer (NCCA)
n. corneal pachymetry
n. laser thermal keratoplasty
n. lens
n. LTK
n. photo-acoustic spectroscopy (NC-PAS)
n. pneumatic esthesiometer
n. tonometer (NCT)
noncycloplegic distance static retinoscopy
nondeposited tear coating
nondominant eye
nonenhancing mass lesion
nonepithelial tumor
nonfenestrated capillary
nonfilamentous fungus
nonfixed tissue
nongranulomatous
n. anterior uveitis
n. choroiditis
n. iridocyclitis
n. iritis
non-Hodgkin lymphoma

noninfectious
n. inflammation
n. retinopathy
non-insulin-dependent diabetes mellitus
noninvasive corneal redox fluorometry
noninvasively sectioning
nonischemic CRVO
nonius
n. bias
n. gap
n. line
n. method
n. offset
nonleaking bleb
nonliquefaciens
Moraxella n.
nonmechanical trephination
nonmembrane-bound vacuoles
nonmydriatic retinal photography
nonneovascular age-related macular degeneration
Nonne syndrome
nonneural ganglionic cell
nonnutrient agar
nonocular muscle group
nonoptic reflex eye movement
nonorbital childhood parameningeal embryonal rhabdomyosarcoma
nonorganic
n. blepharospasm
n. disorder diagnosis
n. paresis
n. visual loss
nonoxynol
nonparalytic strabismus
nonpenetrant gene
nonpenetrating
n. deep sclerectomy
n. filtering surgery
n. keratoplasty
nonperfusion
capillary n.
retinal capillary n.
nonphysiologic visual field loss
nonpigmented
n. ciliary epithelium
n. nevus
nonpreserved artificial tears
nonproliferative diabetic retinopathy (NPDR)
nonrapid eye movement
nonreactive pupil
nonreflex tearing
nonrefractive accommodative esotropia
nonrhegmatogenous retinal detachment
non-Sjögren keratoconjunctivitis sicca
nonsteroidal antiinflammatory drug (NSAID)
nonsurgical adjunct

nontuberculous mycobacterial keratitis
nonulcerative
  n. blepharitis
  n. interstitial keratitis
non-valve plate
Noonan syndrome
noradrenaline
Nordan-Ruiz trapezoidal marker
norepinephrine
norfloxacin
normal
  n. distribution
  n. eye
  n. fundus
  n. optic nerve
  n. retinal correspondence (NRC)
  n. tension (TN)
  n. upward corrective saccade
  n. viewing condition
normal-finger tension
normalized Zernike expansion
normal-looking retinal
normal-pressure glaucoma
normal-tension glaucoma (NTG)
normocytic hypochromic anemia
normokalemic periodic paralysis
Norrie disease
north
  N. American Neuro-Ophthalmology
  Society (NANOS)
  N. Carolina macular dystrophy
Norwood EyeCare epikeratome
Nosema corneum
no-stitch phacoemulsification surgery
no-suture vitrectomy
notation
  Jaeger n.
  Snellen n.
  standard n.
notch
  cerebellar n.
  n. of iris
  lacrimal n.
  supraorbital n.
notch-and-roll maneuver
notching
  lid n.
  rim n.
note blindness
Nothnagel syndrome
not invasive break-up time

no-touch
  n.-t. laser thermal keratoplasty
  procedure
  n.-t. transepithelial photorefractive
  keratectomy
Nott retinoscopy
nova
  N. Aid lens
  N. Curve broad C-loop posterior
  chamber lens
  N. Curve Omnicurve lens
  Dioptron N.
  N. Soft II lens
Novantrone
Novatec LightBlade
novel
  n. causative gene
  n. remedy
Novesine
Novocaine
Novus
  N. Omni 2000 photocoagulator
  N. 2000 ophthalmoscope
  N. 3000 photocoagulation device
  N. Spectra laser
Noyes
  N. forceps
  N. iridectomy scissors
  N. iris scissors
NP
  Lacri-Lube NP
NP-3S auto chart projector
NPA
  near point of accommodation
NPC
  near point of convergence
NPDR
  nonproliferative diabetic retinopathy
NRC
  normal retinal correspondence
NS
  nuclear sclerosis
  nuclear sclerotic
  NS cataract
NSAID
  nonsteroidal antiinflammatory drug
NSE
  neuron-specific enolase
NSU
  necrotizing sclerocorneal ulceration
NTG
  normal-tension glaucoma
nubecula

N

NOTES

nuclear
- n. antigen
- n. arc
- n. bronzing
- n. change
- n. cytoplasmic ratio
- n. developmental cataract
- n. expression
- n. external layer
- n. horizontal gaze paralysis
- n. inner layer
- n. internal layer
- n. layer of the retina
- n. ophthalmoplegia
- n. outer layer
- n. palsy
- n. ring
- n. sclerosis (NS)
- n. sclerosis of lens
- n. sclerotic (NS)
- n. sclerotic cataract
- n. tissue
- n. zone

nuclear-fascicular trochlear nerve palsy
nucleus, pl. **nuclei**
- abducens n.
- accessory n.
- adult n.
- brainstem motor n.
- n. cracker
- n. delivery loupe
- dense brunescent n.
- Edinger-Westphal n.
- n. expressor
- fetal n.
- geniculate n.
- 5195 n. hydrodissector/rotator
- n. hydrolysis needle
- inferior olivary n.
- inferior salivary n.
- lateral geniculate n. (LGN)
- n. of lens
- lens n.
- lenticular n.
- n. lentiform
- n. lentis
- medial vestibular n. (MVN)
- oculomotor n.
- opaque fetal n.
- Perlia n.
- n. of posterior commissure
- pretectal n.
- n. prolapse
- pyknotic nuclei
- n. removal loupe
- rostral interstitial n.
- n. rotator
- salivary n.
- n. segment

- n. spatula
- superior salivary n.
- suprachiasmatic n. (SCN)
- supraoptic n. (SON)
- trochlear nerve n.
- vestibular n.

nudge test
Nugent
- N. fixation forceps
- N. hook
- N. soft cataract aspirator
- N. superior rectus forceps

NuLens accommodating IOL
Nulicaine
null
- n. condition
- n. point
- n. zone

number
- Kestenbaum n.
- Snellen n.

numerical
- n. aperture (NA)
- n. visual acuity

numeric aperture
nummular
- n. atrophy
- n. keratitis

nummularis
- keratitis n.

Nurolon suture
nut
- retrocorneal n.

nutans
- spasmus n.

Nu-Tears II Solution
NutraTear
nutrient agar plate
nutritional
- n. amblyopia
- n. blindness
- n. deficiency
- n. deficiency cataract
- n. optic neuropathy
- n. supplement

NuVita lens
NV
- trigeminal nerve

Nv
- naked vision

NVA
- near visual acuity

NVD
- neovascularization of disc

NVE
- neovascularization elsewhere

NVI
- neovascularization of iris

NVP
near visual point
nyctalopia with congenital myopia
nyctanopia
Nylen-Barany maneuver
nylon
n. frame
n. loop
n. 66 suture
nystagmic
nystagmiform
nystagmogram
nystagmograph
nystagmography
nystagmoid-like oscillation
nystagmoid movement
nystagmus
acquired fixation n.
acquired jerk n.
acquired pendular n.
ageotropic n.
amaurosis n.
amaurotic n.
arthrokinetic n.
ataxic n.
aural n.
autokinetic n.
Baer n.
Bechterew n.
blockage n.
n. blockage syndrome (NBS)
Bruns n.
caloric n.
caloric-induced n.
central vestibular n.
centripetal n.
cervical n.
Cheyne n.
circular n.
compressive n.
congenital n.
conjugate n.
constant n.
convergence-evoked n.
convergence-retraction n.
deviational n.
disconjugate n.
disjunctive n.
dissociated vertical n.
divergence n.
downbeat n.
drug-induced n.
dysjunctive n.

elliptical n.
end-gaze n.
end-point n.
end-position n.
epileptic n.
eyelid n.
fatigue n.
fixation n.
galvanic n.
gaze-evoked n.
gaze paretic n.
geotropic n.
head n.
hemi-seesaw n.
horizontal jerk n.
hysterical n.
incongruent n.
infantile n.
irregular n.
Jensen jerk n.
jerk n.
labyrinthine n.
latent n.
lateral n.
left-beating n.
lid n.
manifest latent n.
miner's n.
minimal amplitude n.
monocular n.
muscle paretic n.
myasthenic n.
myoclonus n.
new-onset n.
oblique n.
occlusion n.
ocular n.
opticokinetic n.
optokinetic n. (OKN)
oscillating n.
paretic n.
pendular n.
periodic alternating windmill n.
peripheral vestibular n.
perverted n.
physiologic n.
positional n.
pseudocaloric n.
railroad n.
rebound n.
retraction n.
rhythmic n.
right-beating n.

N

NOTES

nystagmus *(continued)*
    rotational n.
    rotatory n.
    seesaw n.
    sensory deprivation n.
    strabismal n.
    n. test
    torsional n.
    undulatory n.

    upbeat n.
    upbeating n.
    vasculopathic downbeat n.
    vertical n.
    vestibular n.
    vibratory n.
    voluntary n.
    n. with demyelination
nystatin

OAD
overall diameter
OAG
open-angle glaucoma
OAO
ophthalmic artery occlusion
Oasis
O. Collagen Plug
O. feather microscalpel
OAV
oculoauriculovertebral
OAV dysplasia
obcecation
OBF
ocular blood flow
OBF tonometer
object
Berens test o.
o. blindness
o. displacement
o. distance
fixation on moving o.
o. of regard
o. size
o. space
test o.
object/image relationship
objective
achromatic o.
apochromatic o.
o. lens
o. measurement
o. noninvasive technology
o. optometer
o. perimetry
o. prism-neutralized cover test
o. refractor
o. vertigo
object-space focus
obligate carrier
obligatory suppression
oblique
o. aberration
o. astigmatism
o. fiber
o. illumination
inferior o.
o. muscle
o. muscle dysfunction
o. muscle hook
o. muscle palsy
o. nystagmus
o. palsy
o. position
o. prism

o. prism device
o. ray of light
obliterans
endarteritis o.
thromboangiitis o.
obliteration
ductal orifice o.
O'Brien
O. akinesia
O. akinesia technique
O. anesthesia
O. fixation forceps
O. lid block
O. marker
O. spud
O. stitch scissors
obscuration
transient visual o.
obscured fovea
obscure vision
Obstbaum
O. lens spatula
O. synechia spatula
obstruction
canalicular o.
carotid o.
congenital nasolacrimal o.
congenital nasolacrimal duct o.
meibomian gland o.
nasolacrimal duct o. (NLDO)
outflow o.
primary acquired nasolacrimal
duct o. (PANDO)
retinal venous o.
silent central retinal vein o.
obstructive
o. glaucoma
o. retinal vasculitis
obturans
iritis o.
obturator
Moria o.
occipital
o. apoplexy
o. cortex
o. lobe
o. lobe unilateral cerebral
hemisphere lesion
occipitofrontalis
venter frontalis musculi o.
occipitothalamica
radiatio o.
occipitothalamic radiation
occludable
occluded pupil

O

occludens
 zonula o.
occluder
 black/white o.
 clip-on/tie-on o.
 eye o.
 Halberg trial clip o.
 long/short o.
 lorgnette o.
 Maddox rod o.
 Odyssey Parasol punctal o.
 Parasol punctal o.
 pinhole o.
 Plus punctal o.
 Pram o.
 red lens o.
 single/double o.
 thumb o.
occlusion
 o. amblyopia
 branch retinal artery o. (BRAO)
 branch retinal vein o. (BRVO)
 o. of branch vein
 carotid artery o.
 central retinal artery o. (CRAO)
 central retinal vein o. (CRVO)
 choroidal vascular o.
 cilioretinal artery o.
 combined cilioretinal artery and
  central retinal vein o.'s
 macular arteriole o.
 macular branch retinal vein o.
  (MBRVO)
 monocular o.
 nasolacrimal o.
 necrotic o.
 o. nystagmus
 ophthalmic artery o. (OAO)
 peripheral branch retinal vein o.
  (PBRVO)
 punctal o.
 o. of pupil
 retinal arterial o.
 retinal artery o.
 retinal branch vein o.
 retinal central artery o.
 retinal central vein o.
 retinal vascular o.
 o. of retinal vein
 retinal vein o.
 retinal venous o.
 o. therapy
 thermal punctal o.
 tributary vein o.
 vascular o.
occlusive
 o. microangiopathy
 o. retinal arteritis

 o. retinal vasculopathy
 o. vascular disease
occlusor
 Elastoplast eye o.
OCCT
 Olson calibrated cornea trephine
occult
 o. anular ciliary body
 o. chorioretinal anastomosis
 o. choroidal neovascularization
 o. choroidal neovascular membrane
 o. lesion
 o. penetrating orbitocranial trauma
 o. scleral rupture
 o. temporal arteritis
 o. tumor cell
 Verteporfin with Altered Light
  in O. (VALIO)
occupational
 o. bifocal
 o. lens
 o. ophthalmology
ochre
 o. hemorrhage
 o. mass
 o. membrane
ochronosis
 exogenous o.
 ocular o.
Ochsner
 O. cartilage forceps
 O. hook
 O. tissue/cartilage forceps
 O. tissue forceps
OCI
 ophthalmic confidence index
OCLM
 oculomedin
 OCLM gene
o'clock
 o. position
 1–12 o. position
 3 o. staining
O'Connor
 O. depressor
 O. flat hook
 O. iris forceps
 O. lid forceps
 O. marker
 O. muscle hook
 O. operation
 O. sharp hook
 O. sponge forceps
 O. tenotomy hook
OCP
 ocular cicatricial pemphigoid
OCT
 optical coherence tomography

spectral-domain OCT
Visante OCT
OCT3
   optical coherence tomography-3
octafluoropropane gas
Octopus
   O. automated perimetry
   O. 101 bowl perimeter
   O. 500 EZ
   O. 1-2-3 perimeter
   O. 201 perimeter
   O. 201 perimeter test
   O. threshold perimetry
Ocu-Bath
Ocu-Caine
OcuCaps
   Akorn O.
Ocu-Carpine
Ocu-Chlor
OcuClear Ophthalmic
OcuCoat PF Ophthalmic Solution
Ocu-Cort
Ocu-Dex
Ocudose
   Timoptic O.
Ocu-Drop
Ocufen Ophthalmic
ocufilcon
Ocufit SR
Ocuflox ophthalmic
Ocugene glaucoma genetic test
Ocugestrin Ophthalmic
Ocu-Guard
OcuHist
Oculab Tono-Pen
Oculaid
   O. capsular tension ring
   O. lens
ocular
   o. adnexal burn
   o. adnexal injury
   o. adnexal lymphoma
   o. adnexal tumor
   o. albinism
   o. alignment
   o. allergy
   o. angle
   o. anomaly
   o. argyrosis
   o. ataxia
   o. axis
   o. ballottement
   o. barrier

o. bartonellosis
o. blepharospasm
o. blood flow (OBF)
O. blood flow analyzer
o. bobbing
o. bullet injury
o. burning
o. capsule
o. casualty
o. chemical injury
o. cicatricial pemphigoid (OCP)
o. circulation dislocated
o. coherence tomography
o. coloboma
o. cone
o. conjunctiva
o. contusion
o. crisis
o. cryptococcal infection
o. cul-de-sac
o. cup
o. decongestant
o. development
o. dipping
o. dominance
o. dominance column
o. duction
o. dysmetria
o. dysmotility
o. echography
o. erythema
o. flora
o. flutter
o. fundus pigmentation
O. Gamboscope loupe
o. gel
o. gunshot wound
o. gymnastics
o. hemodynamic assessment
o. hemodynamic value
o. herpes
o. histoplasmosis
o. histoplasmosis syndrome (OHS)
o. humor
o. hypertelorism
o. hypertension (OHT)
O. Hypertension Treatment Study (OHTS)
o. hypotelorism
o. hypotensive agent
o. hypotensive lipid
o. hypotony
o. image

NOTES

ocular *(continued)*

o. imaging
o. immunology
o. inflammation
o. irrigation
o. irritation
o. ischemic syndrome (OIS)
o. itching
o. larva
o. larva migrans
o. lens
o. leptospirosis
o. lubricant
o. lubrication
o. Lyme borreliosis
o. Lyme disease
o. lymphomatosis
o. manifestation
o. marker
o. massage
o. media
o. medium
o. melanocytosis
o. melanoma
o. melanosis
o. meningioma
O. Microcirculation View Analysis Treatment (OMVAT)
o. microtremor
o. migraine
o. morbidity
o. motility
o. motility disorder
o. motility effect
o. motility test
o. motoneuron
o. motor
o. motor apraxia
o. motor syndrome
o. motor system
o. movement
o. muscle
o. muscle palsy
o. muscle paralysis
o. muscle transplant
o. myasthenia
o. myasthenia ptosis
o. myiasis
o. myoclonus
o. myopathy
o. neuromyotonia
o. nocardiosis
o. nystagmus
o. ochronosis
o. ointment
o. onchocerciasis
o. oscillation
o. paint-ball injury
o. pathology

o. pemphigoid
o. pemphigus
o. perforation
o. perfusion pressure (OPP)
o. pharyngeal dystrophy
o. phthisis
o. plagiocephaly
o. pressure reducer
o. prosthesis
o. protection
o. pseudoexfoliation syndrome
o. refraction
o. region
o. response analyzer
o. rigidity
o. risk
o. rosacea
o. rosacea symptom
o. rotation
o. saccade
o. scoliosis
o. siderosis
o. sign
o. sparganosis
o. spectrum
o. surface
o. surface abnormality
o. surface disease (OSD)
O. Surface Disease Index (OSDI)
o. surface disorder
o. surface failure
o. surface reconstruction
o. surface restoration
o. surface vital staining
o. survival
o. syphilis
o. syphilitic disease
o. tension (Tn)
o. tilt reaction (OTR)
o. tolerability
o. torsion
o. torticollis
o. total higher order aberration (OTHA)
o. toxicity
o. toxocariasis
o. toxoplasmosis
o. trauma
o. tumor of childhood
o. ultrasound
o. vaccinia
o. vaccinia infection
o. vaccinial conjunctivitis
o. vergence and accommodation sensor (OVAS)
o. vertigo
o. vesicle
o. war injury

ocularist
American Society of O.'s
ocular-mucous membrane syndrome
OcularProtect multivitamin
oculentum
Oculex drug delivery system
oculi (*pl. of* oculus)
abducens o.
o. unitas
OcuLight
O. GL/GLx green laser photocoagulator
O. GL photocoagulator
O. GLx green laser photocoagulator
Iris Medical O. SLx
O. SL diode laser
O. SLx ophthalmic laser
oculist
oculistics
oculoauditory syndrome
oculoauricular dysplasia
oculoauriculovertebral (OAV)
o. dysplasia
oculobuccogenital syndrome
oculocardiac reflex
oculocephalic
o. maneuver
o. reflex
o. synkinesis
o. test
o. vascular anomaly
oculocephalogyric reflex
oculocerebral
o. lymphoma
o. syndrome
oculocerebrorenal
o. dystrophy
o. syndrome
o. syndrome of Lowe
oculocutaneous
o. albinism
o. albinoidism
o. hypopigmentation
o. laser
o. syndrome
oculodentodigital (ODD)
o. dysplasia
oculodermal
o. disorder
o. melanocytosis
o. melanosis
o. melanosis in children

oculodigital reflex
oculodynia
oculofacial paralysis
oculoglandular
o. conjunctivitis
o. disease
o. syndrome
o. tularemia
oculography
infrared o.
photoelectric o.
photosensor o.
oculogravic illusion
oculogyral illusion
oculogyration
oculogyria
oculogyric
o. auricular reflex
o. crisis
o. mechanism
oculomandibulodyscephaly
oculomasticatory myorhythmia
oculomedin (OCLM)
oculometer
oculometroscope
oculomotor
o. apraxia
o. apraxia of childhood
o. cranial nerve palsy
o. decussation
o. disorder
o. nerve
o. nerve fascicle
o. nerve lesion
o. nerve misdirection
o. nerve schwannoma
o. nerve synkinesis
o. nucleus
o. paresis with cyclic spasm
o. root
o. root of ciliary ganglion
o. system
oculomotorius
nervus o.
oculomycosis
oculonasal
Ocu-Lone
oculopalatal
o. myoclonus
o. myoclonus syndrome
o. tremor
oculopathy
hypertensive o.

O

NOTES

oculopathy *(continued)*
    lupus o.
    pituitarigenic o.
oculopharyngeal
    o. dystrophy
    o. reflex
    o. syndrome
oculoplastic
    o. surgeon
    o. surgery
oculoplastics
Oculo-Plastik ePTFE ocular implant
oculoplasty corneal protector
oculoplethysmography
oculopneumoplethysmography (OPG)
oculopupillary reflex
oculoreaction
oculorenal syndrome
oculorespiratory
    o. reflex
    o. syndrome
oculorotatory muscle
oculosensory cell reflex
oculospinal
oculosporidiosis
oculosympathetic
    o. dysfunction
    o. paresis
    o. pathway
oculotoxic
oculovertebral dysplasia
oculovestibular reflex
oculozygomatic
Ocu-Lube
oculus, pl. **oculi**
    adnexa oculi
    O. BIOM noncontact lens system
    bulbus oculi
    congenital melanosis oculi
    deprimens oculi
    o. dexter (right eye)
    O. Easyloupes
    equator bulbi oculi
    fundus oculi
    melanosis oculi
    motor oculi
    musculus orbicularis oculi
    pars lacrimalis musculi orbicularis oculi
    pars orbitalis musculi orbicularis oculi
    pars palpebralis musculi orbicularis oculi
    polus anterior bulbi oculi
    polus posterior bulbi oculi
    o. sinister (left eye)
    sphincter oculi
    tapetum oculi
    tendo oculi

    O. trial frame
    tunica albuginea oculi
    tunica vasculosa oculi
    tutamina oculi
    venae choroideae oculi
Ocumeter
Ocu-Mycin
Ocu-Pentolate
Ocu-Phrin
Ocu-Pred
    O.-P. A
    O.-P. Forte
Ocupress
    O. Ophthalmic
    O. Ophthalmic Solution
Ocuscan
    O. A-scan biometric ultrasound
    Sonometric O.
    O. 400 transducer
Ocusert
    O. device
    O. Pilo-20, -40
Ocusil
OCuSoft
    O. eyelid cleanser
    O. scrub
Ocu-Sol
Ocusporin
Ocusulf-10
Ocu-Tears PF
ocutome
    CooperVision o.
    disposable o.
    o. probe
    o. vitrectomy unit
Ocutricin HC
Ocu-Trol
Ocu-Tropic
Ocu-Tropine
Ocuvite
    O. Extra
    O. Lutein
    O. Lutein Antioxidant Supplement
    O. Lutein tablet
    O. PreserVision vitamins
Ocu-Zoline
OD
    right eye
ODD
    oculodentodigital
    ODD dysplasia
ODM
    ophthalmodynamometry
O'Donoghue
    O. angled DCR probe
    O. silicone intubation
odyssey
    O. Parasol Punctal Occluder
    O. phacoemulsification system

Oestrus ovis
off-axis imaging
off-center
    o.-c. ablation
    o.-c. bipolar cell
office-based surgery
off-label treatment
offset
    nonius o.
ofloxacin ophthalmic solution
O'Gawa
    O. cataract-aspirating cannula
    O. suture-fixation forceps
    O. 2-way aspirating cannula
OGPR
    OptiMed glaucoma pressure regulator
Ogston-Luc operation
Oguchi disease
Ogura
    O. cartilage forceps
    O. tissue/cartilage forceps
    O. tissue forceps
OHS
    ocular histoplasmosis syndrome
      macular OHS
OHT
    ocular hypertension
OHTS
    Ocular Hypertension Treatment Study
oil
    AdatoSil silicone o.
    o. droplet cataract
    lanolin o.
    o. layer
    mineral o.
    silicone o.
oily secretion
ointment (ung)
    AK-Poly-Bac O.
    AK-Spore H.C. Ophthalmic O.
    Akwa Tears lubricant
      ophthalmic o.
    anesthetic o.
    bland ophthalmic o.
    Cortisporin Ophthalmic O.
    Dexacine o.
    Dry Eyes lubricant o.
    LubriTears Lubricant Eye O.
    Moisture Eyes PM eye o.
    Neosporin Ophthalmic O.
    Neotricin HC Ophthalmic O.
    ocular o.

    ophthalmic o.
    petrolatum ophthalmic o.
    Polycin-B O.
    sty ophthalmic o.
    Tears Naturale PM lubricant
      eye o.
    Tears Renewed lubricant o.
    Terak Ophthalmic O.
    Terak with polymyxin B sulfate o.
    Terramycin w/polymyxin B
      Ophthalmic O.
    ticrynafen o.
    TobraDex ophthalmic o.
OIP
    ophthalmomyiasis interna posterior
OIS
    ocular ischemic syndrome
    OIS image digitizing system
    OIS WinStation 5000 Ophthalmic
      Imaging System
Oklahoma iris wire retractor
OKN
    optokinetic nystagmus
OKT3
    orthoclone
Okuma plate
old
    o. eye
    o. sight
oleosa
    blepharitis o.
olfactory neuroblastoma
oligonucleotide primer
olivacea
    Microsphaeropsis o.
olive
    o. tip
    o. tip cannula
    o. tip capsule polisher
    o. tip irrigator
olivopontocerebellar atrophy (OPCA)
Olk
    O. vitreoretinal pick
    O. vitreoretinal spatula
OLM
    ophthalmic laser microendoscope
olopatadine
    o. HCl ophthalmic solution
    o. hydrochloride ophthalmic
      solution
OLSAT
    Otis-Lennon School Ability Test

NOTES

Olson
- O. calibrated cornea trephine (OCCT)
- O. calibrated cornea trephine system
- O. phaco chopper
- O. quick chopper

Olympus
- O. fundus camera
- O. Vanox VH-2 microscope

O'Malley self-adhering lens implant

OMM
- ophthalmomandibulomelic
- OMM syndrome

Omnifit intraocular lens

omnifocal lens

OmniMed argon-fluoride excimer laser

OMP
- ophthalmic medical personnel

OMT
- optimal medical therapy

OMVAT
- Ocular Microcirculation View Analysis Treatment

ON
- optic nerve

on-axis imaging

on-center bipolar cell

onchocercal sclerosing keratitis

Onchocerca volvulus

onchocerciasis
- ocular o.

onchocercosis

one-and-a-half syndrome

on-eye
- o.-e. performance of lens
- o.-e. predicted power

ONH
- optic nerve head

ONHD
- optic nerve head drusen

onion
- o. bulb neuropathy
- o. ring-like posterior polar cataract
- o. skin-like membrane

only
- light perception o. (LPO)

Onodi cell

ONSD
- optic nerve sheath decompression

ONSF
- optic nerve sheath fenestration

ONSM
- optic nerve sheath meningioma

O2OPTIX breathable contact lens

oozing
- transconjunctival aqueous o.

OP
- oscillatory potential

opaca
- cornea o.

opacification
- anterior capsular o.
- capsular bag o.
- o. cherry-red spot
- corneal o.
- cortical o.
- delayed postoperative o.
- lens capsule o.
- polygonal stromal o.
- posterior capsular o.
- posterior capsule o. (PCO)
- recurrent visual axis o.
- subepithelial o.
- visual axis o.
- vitreous o.

opacified cuff

opacity
- calcium-containing o.
- capsular o.
- central unilateral lens o.
- congenital lens o.
- corneal o. (CO)
- corneal deep o.
- cortical o.
- crystalline o.
- deep corneal stromal o.
- dense o.
- disciform o.
- dust-like o.
- early lens o.
- fetal nuclear o.
- glistening o.
- interface o.
- lenticular o.
- leukomatous corneal o.
- media o.
- mycotic snowball o.
- nebular stromal o.
- neonatal corneal o.
- peripheral corneal o.
- posterior subcapsular o.
- posterior supine position capsular o.
- pulverulent o.
- punctate corneal o.
- snowball o.
- spotty corneal o.
- striate o.
- stromal o.
- subepithelial corneal o.
- vitreous o.
- whorled corneal o.'s

opalescent cornea

opaque
- o. canalicular plug
- o. fetal nucleus

o. Herrick lacrimal plug
o. medium

OPCA
olivopontocerebellar atrophy

Opcon
O. Maximum Strength Allergy Drops
Muro O.
O. Ophthalmic

Opcon-A

OPD-Scan
OPD-S. diagnostic system
OPD-S. refractometer

OPD-Station software

open
o. globe
o. globe injury
o. globe surgery
o. lens
o. loop

open-angle glaucoma (OAG)

open-funnel detachment

opening
apraxia of eyelid o. (AEO)
apraxia of lid o.
compulsive eye o.
dumbbell o.
orbital o.
o. of orbital cavity
palpebral o.
posterior capsule o.
punctal o.

open-loop accommodation

open-sky
o.-s. cataract wound
o.-s. cryoextraction
o.-s. cryoextraction operation
o.-s. dissection
o.-s. technique
o.-s. trephination
o.-s. vitrectomy

operating
o. loupe
o. microscope
o. microscope-induced phototoxic maculopathy

operation
ab externo filtering o.
Adams o.
Adler o.
Agnew o.
Allen o.
Allport o.

Alvis o.
Ammon o.
Amsler o.
Anagnostakis o.
Anel o.
Angelucci o.
anular corneal graft o.
Argyll Robertson o.
Arlt o.
Arroyo o.
Arruga o.
Bangerter pterygium o.
Barkan double cyclodialysis o.
Barkan goniotomy o.
Barraquer enzymatic zonulolysis o.
Barraquer keratomileusis o.
Beard-Cutler o.
Beer o.
Berens sclerectomy o.
Berens-Smith o.
Berke o.
Bielschowsky o.
Birch-Hirschfeld entropion o.
Blaskovics canthoplasty o.
Blaskovics dacryostomy o.
Blaskovics inversion of tarsus o.
Blaskovics lid o.
Böhm o.
Bonnet enucleation o.
Borthen iridotasis o.
Bowman o.
Boyd o.
Bridge o.
bridge pedicle flap o.
Bronson foreign body removal o.
Burch eye evisceration o.
Burow flap o.
Buzzi o.
Byron Smith ectropion o.
Callahan o.
Carter o.
Casanellas lacrimal o.
cataract extraction o.
cautery o.
cerclage o.
Chandler vitreous o.
cinching o.
Cleasby iridectomy o.
Collin-Beard o.
Comberg foreign body o.
Conrad orbital blowout fracture o.
Cooper o.
corneal graft o.

NOTES

operation *(continued)*

Crawford sling o.
crescent o.
cryoextraction o.
cryotherapy o.
Custodis o.
Cutler o.
Cutler-Beard o.
cyclodiathermy o.
Czermak pterygium o.
dacryoadenectomy o.
dacryocystectomy o.
Daviel o.
decompression of orbit o.
de Grandmont o.
Deiter o.
diathermy o.
Dieffenbach o.
dilation of punctum o.
discission of lens o.
D'Ombrain o.
drainage of lacrimal gland o.
drainage of lacrimal sac o.
Duke-Elder o.
Dupuy-Dutemps o.
Elliot o.
encircling of globe o.
encircling of scleral buckle o.
enucleation of eyeball o.
equilibrating o.
Esser inlay o.
Eversbusch o.
evisceration o.
excision of lacrimal gland o.
excision of lacrimal sac o.
exenteration of orbital contents o.
extracapsular cataract extraction o.
Faden o.
Fasanella-Servat ptosis o.
fascia lata sling for ptosis o.
filtering o.
Förster o.
Fox o.
Friedenwald-Guyton o.
Frost-Lang o.
Fuchs canthorrhaphy o.
Fuchs iris bombe transfixation o.
Fukala o.
Gifford delimiting keratotomy o.
Gillies scar correction o.
Girard keratoprosthesis o.
Gonin cautery o.
goniotomy o.
Graefe o.
Grossmann o.
Heine o.
Herbert o.
Hess eyelid o.
Hess ptosis o.

Hippel o.
Holth o.
Hughes o.
Hummelsheim o.
Hunt-Transley o.
indentation o.
iridectomy o.
iridencleisis o.
iridodialysis o.
iridotasis o.
iridotomy o.
Jensen o.
Johnson o.
Jones o.
Kelman o.
keratectomy o.
keratomileusis o.
keratoplasty o.
keratotomy o.
King o.
Kirby o.
Knapp o.
Krönlein o.
Krönlein-Berke o.
Kuhnt-Szymanowski o.
Lagleyze o.
Lagrange o.
Lancaster o.
Landolt o.
Lindsay o.
Löwenstein o.
McReynolds o.
Meller o.
Mikamo double-eyelid o.
Mosher o.
Mosher-Toti o.
Moss o.
Motais o.
Mueller o.
Mules o.
myectomy o.
myotomy o.
Naffziger o.
O'Connor o.
Ogston-Luc o.
open-sky cryoextraction o.
orbital implant o.
pars plana o.
pattern cut corneal graft o.
peripheral iridectomy o.
Peters o.
pocket o.
Power o.
probing lacrimonasal duct o.
reattachment of choroid o.
reattachment of retina o.
recession of ocular muscle o.
removal of foreign body o.
Saemisch o.

Sato o.
Scheie o.
scleral buckling o.
scleral fistulectomy o.
scleral shortening o.
scleroplasty o.
sclerotomy o.
sector iridectomy o.
seton o.
slant muscle o.
Smith eyelid o.
Smith-Indian o.
Snellen ptosis o.
1-snip punctum o.
3-snip punctum o.
splitting lacrimal papilla o.
step graft o.
Summerskill o.
suture of cornea o.
suture of eyeball o.
suture of iris o.
suture of muscle o.
suture of sclera o.
tattoo of cornea o.
tenotomy o.
Thomas o.
Toti o.
trabeculectomy o.
transfixion of iris o.
transplantation of muscle o.
trap-door scleral buckle o.
Troutman o.
tumbling technique o.
Vogt o.
von Graefe o.
von Hippel o.
Wheeler o.
Whitnall sling o.
Wies o.

operculated
o. retinal hole
o. retinal tear

operculum, pl. **opercula**
free o.
peripheral retinal o.

OPG
oculopneumoplethysmography

ophryosis

Ophtec
O. Co. lens
O. 9.0 mm trephine
O. occlusion implant

Ophthacet

Ophthaine

Ophthalas
O. argon/krypton laser
O. argon laser
O. krypton laser
O. photocoagulator

Ophthalgan Ophthalmic

ophthalmalgia

ophthalmectomy

ophthalmencephalon

ophthalmia
Brazilian o.
catarrhal o.
caterpillar-hair o.
o. eczematosa
Egyptian o.
o. electrica
flash o.
gonococcal o.
gonorrheal o.
granular o.
o. hepatica
metastatic o.
migratory o.
mucous o.
neonatal o.
o. neonatorum
neuroparalytic o.
o. nivalis
o. nodosa
periodic o.
purulent o.
scrofulous o.
spring o.
strumous o.
sympathetic o.
transferred o.
ultraviolet ray o.
varicose o.

ophthalmiatrics

ophthalmic
Acular O.
Akarpine O.
AK-Chlor O.
AK-Cide O.
AK-Con o.
AK-Dex O.
AK-Homatropine O.
AK-Neo-Dex O.
AK-Poly-Bac O.
AK-Pred O.
AKPro O.
AK-Sulf O.

NOTES

ophthalmic *(continued)*
    AKTob O.
    AK-Tracin O.
    Albalon-A O.
    Albalon Liquifilm O.
    alpha-2-adrenergic agonist agent, o.
    Antazoline-V O.
    o. artery
    o. artery aneurysm
    o. artery occlusion (OAO)
    Betimol O.
    Betoptic S O.
    o. blade
    Bleph-10 O.
    Blephamide O.
    bromfenac o.
    Carbastat O.
    Carboptic O.
    o. cautery
    Cetamide O.
    Cetapred o.
    Chloroptic O.
    Chloroptic-P O.
    Ciloxan O.
    Collyrium Fresh O.
    Comfort O.
    o. confidence index (OCI)
    o. corticosteroid
    o. cul-de-sac
    o. cup
    Cyclomydril O.
    o. disorder
    o. drill
    o. drug
    o. dye
    Econopred O.
    o. electrocautery
    o. endoscope
    Estivin II O.
    o. examination
    Floropryl O.
    o. ganglion
    Geneye O.
    Genoptic S.O.P. o.
    Gentacidin o.
    Gentak o.
    o. glucocorticoid
    o. Graves disease
    Herplex O.
    o. hook
    Humorsol O.
    o. hyperthyroidism
    Ilotycin O.
    I-Naphline O.
    Inflamase Forte O.
    Inflamase Mild O.
    o. instrument
    Isopto Carbachol O.
    Isopto Carpine O.

Isopto Cetamide O.
Isopto Cetapred o.
Isopto Homatropine O.
Isopto Hyoscine O.
Kainair O.
o. laser microendoscope (OLM)
o. literature
loteprednol and tobramycin o.
o. medical personnel (OMP)
o. medication
Metimyd O.
o. migraine
Murine Plus O.
Murocoll-2 O.
Nafazair O.
Naphcon O.
Naphcon-A O.
NeoDecadron O.
Neo-Dexameth O.
nepafenac o.
o. nerve
OcuClear O.
Ocufen O.
Ocuflox o.
Ocugestrin O.
Ocupress O.
o. ointment
Opcon O.
Ophthalgan O.
Opticaine o.
Optigene O.
OptiPranolol O.
Osmoglyn O.
Paremyd O.
Phospholine Iodide O.
O. Photographers Society (OPS)
Pilagan O.
Pilocar O.
Pilokair O.
Pilopine HS O.
Piloptic O.
Pilostat O.
o. plexus
Polysporin O.
Polytrim O.
Pred Forte O.
Pred-G O.
Pred Mild O.
o. problem
Profenal O.
o. progressive-power lens
Propine O.
o. reaction
o. retroillumination imaging
Sodium Sulamyd O.
o. solution
o. specialty
o. sponge
Sulf-10 O.

o. surgery
O. Technologies Inc. (OTI)
o. test
Tetrasine Extra O.
Timoptic O.
Timoptic-XE O.
TobraDex o.
Tobrex O.
Vasocidin O.
VasoClear O.
Vasocon-A O.
Vasocon Regular O.
Vasosulf O.
o. vein
o. vesicle
Vira-A O.
Viroptic O.
Visine Extra O.
Visine LR O.
o. vitreous surgical technique
Voltaren O.
ophthalmica
vesicula o.
zona o.
ophthalmicus
herpes zoster o.
varicella zoster o.
ophthalmitis
ophthalmoblennorrhea
ophthalmocarcinoma
ophthalmocele
ophthalmocopia
ophthalmodesmitis
ophthalmodiagnosis
ophthalmodiaphanoscope
ophthalmodonesis
ophthalmodynamometer
Bailliart o.
Reichert o.
suction o.
ophthalmodynamometry (ODM)
ophthalmodynia
ophthalmoeikonometer
ophthalmofunduscope
ophthalmogram
echo o.
ophthalmograph
ophthalmography
echo o.
ophthalmogyric
ophthalmoleukoscope
ophthalmolith
ophthalmologic surgery

ophthalmologist
Contact Lens Association of O.'s
(CLAO)
European Contact Lens Society
of O.'s
pediatric o.
Royal Australian College of O.'s
ophthalmology
American Academy of O. (AAO)
American Board of O. (ABO)
American Society of
Contemporary O. (ASCO)
Association for Research in Vision
and O. (ARVO)
Association of Technical Personnel
in O. (ATPO)
certified registered nurse in o.
(CRNO)
Fellow of the American Academy
of O. (FAAO)
Joint Commission on Allied Health
Personnel in O. (JCAHPO)
occupational o.
pediatric o.
prenatal o.
ophthalmomalacia
ophthalmomandibulomelic (OMM)
o. dysplasia
ophthalmomelanosis
ophthalmomeningea
vena o.
ophthalmomeningeal vein
ophthalmometer
Haag-Streit o.
Hertel o.
Javal o.
Javal-Schiotz o.
Micromatic o.
ophthalmometroscope
ophthalmometry
ophthalmomicroscope
binocular indirect o. (BIOM)
ophthalmomycosis
ophthalmomyiasis
Cuterebra o.
o. interna posterior (OIP)
ophthalmomyitis
ophthalmomyositis
ophthalmomyotomy
ophthalmoneuritis
ophthalmoneuromyelitis
ophthalmoparesis
internuclear o.

O

NOTES

ophthalmopathy
dysthyroid o.
endocrine o.
external o.
Graves o.
internal o.
thyroid o.
thyroid-associated o. (TAO)
ophthalmophacometer
ophthalmophantom
ophthalmophlebotomy
ophthalmophthisis
ophthalmoplasty
ophthalmoplegia
autosomal dominant o.
autosomal recessive o.
basal o.
binocular internuclear o.
chronic progressive external o.
(CPEO)
exophthalmic o.
o. externa
external o.
fascicular o.
infectious o.
infranuclear o.
o. interna
internal o.
internuclear o. (INO)
o. internuclearis
migraine o.
migrainous o.
new-onset internuclear o.
nuclear o.
orbital o.
painful o.
Parinaud o.
partial o.
o. partialis
posterior internuclear o.
o. progressiva
progressive external o. (PEO)
pseudointernuclear o.
Sauvineau o.
sensory ataxic neuropathy with
dysarthria and o. (SANDO)
supranuclear o.
thyrotoxicosis o.
total o.
o. totalis
wall-eyed bilateral internuclear o.
(WEBINO)
ophthalmoplegic
o. exophthalmos
o. migraine
o. muscular dystrophy
ophthalmoptosis
ophthalmoreaction
Calmette o.

ophthalmorrhagia
ophthalmorrhea
ophthalmorrhexis
ophthalmoscope
Alcon indirect o.
All Pupil II indirect o.
AO Reichert Instruments binocular
indirect o.
binocular indirect o.
Canon SLO scanning laser o.
confocal laser scanning o.
cordless monocular indirect o.
demonstration o.
direct o.
Exeter o.
Fison indirect binocular o.
Friedenwald o.
Ful-Vue o.
ghost o.
Gullstrand o.
halogen o.
Helmholtz o.
indirect o.
Keeler binocular indirect o.
laser indirect o. (LIO)
Loring o.
Mentor Exeter o.
metric o.
MK IV o.
monocular indirect o.
Neolyte laser indirect o.
Nerve Fiber Analyzer laser o.
Novus 2000 o.
Panoramic200 Non-Mydriatic O.
Panoramic200 scanning laser o.
polarizing o.
Polle pod attachment for o.
Propper-Heine o.
Propper indirect o.
Reichert binocular indirect o.
Reichert Ful-Vue binocular o.
Rodenstock scanning laser o.
scanning laser o. (SLO)
Schepens binocular indirect o.
Schepens-Pomerantzeff o.
stereo o.
TopSS scanning laser o.
Vantage o.
video binocular indirect o. (VBIO)
Visuscope o.
Welch-Allyn o.
Zeiss o.
ophthalmoscopic
o. detectability
o. examination
ophthalmoscopy
binocular indirect o.
confocal laser scanning o. (cLSO)
confocal scanning laser o.

direct o.
distant direct o.
dynamic scanning laser o.
indirect o.
medical o.
metric o.
slitlamp o.
o. with reflected light
ophthalmospectroscope
ophthalmospectroscopy
ophthalmostasis
ophthalmostat
ophthalmostatometer
ophthalmosteresis
ophthalmosynchysis
ophthalmothermometer
ophthalmotomy
ophthalmotonometer
ophthalmotonometry
ophthalmotoxin
ophthalmotrope
ophthalmotropometer
ophthalmotropometry
ophthalmovascular
ophthalmoxerosis
ophthalmoxyster
Ophthascan Mini-A scan
Ophthasonic pachometer
Ophthas subjective optometer
Ophthetic
Ophthimus
O. High-Pass Resolution perimeter
O. ring perimeter
Ophthochlor
Ophthocort
OPL
outer plexiform layer
OPMI
O. pico i microscope
O. PRO magis microscope
O. VISU 200 BrightFlex
illuminator
O. VISU 200 microscope
O. VISU 210 microscope
Opmi
Opmilas 144 surgical laser
OPP
ocular perfusion pressure
opponent
o. color
o. colors theory
opportunistic infection
Opraflex drape

OPS
Ophthalmic Photographers Society
opsin
cone o.
opsiometer
opsoclonia
opsoclonus
paraneoplastic o.
Optacon
Optacryl
Opt-Ease
Optec 3000 contrast sensitivity test
Optef
Op-Temp
O.-T. disposable cautery
O.-T. disposable electrocautery
optesthesia
optic
o. aberration
o. agnosia
o. angle
o. aphasia
o. artery
o. ataxia
o. axis
biconvex o.
o. canal
o. canal decompression
o. capture
o. center
o. chiasm
o. chiasmal lesion
o. chiasmal syndrome
o. coherence tomography
o. commissure
o. cul-de-sac
o. cup
o. cup-to-disc ratio
o. decussation
o. demyelinating neuritis
o. deposit
o. disc
o. disc anomaly
o. disc atrophy
o. disc change
o. disc colomba
o. disc cupping
o. disc dragging
o. disc drusen
o. disc drusen calcification
o. disc drusen retinopathy
o. disc dysplasia
o. disc edema

NOTES

O

optic *(continued)*
    o. disc hemifield test
    o. disc hypoplasia
    o. disc pallor
    o. disc pit
    o. disc size
    o. disc swelling
    o. disc topography
    o. disc tubercle
    o. edge
    o. evagination
    o. foramen
    o. fundus
    o. ganglion
    o. groove
    o. hyperesthesia
    o. illusion
    o. imaging
    o. implant
    o. iridectomy
    o. keratoplasty
    o. lemniscus
    o. muscle recession
    o. nerve (ON)
    o. nerve aplasia
    o. nerve atrophy
    o. nerve axon count
    o. nerve coloboma
    o. nerve congenital abnormality
    o. nerve cupping
    o. nerve damage
    o. nerve disease
    o. nerve disorder
    o. nerve dysfunction
    o. nerve dysplasia
    o. nerve fiber
    o. nerve glioma
    o. nerve head (ONH)
    o. nerve head appearance
    o. nerve head avulsion
    o. nerve head drusen (ONHD)
    o. nerve hemangioblastoma
    o. nerve hypoplasia
    o. nerve injury
    o. nerve lesion
    o. nerve massaging
    o. nerve myelination
    o. nerve pallor
    o. nerve pit
    o. nerve sheath
    o. nerve sheath decompression
        (ONSD)
    o. nerve sheath fenestration
        (ONSF)
    o. nerve sheath meningioma
        (ONSM)
    o. nerve tumor
    o. neuropathy
    o. pachymeter

    o. papilla (P)
    o. papilla cavity
    o. pathway glioma
    o. perineuritis
    o. 3-piece intraocular lens
    o. primordium
    o. radiation
    o. radiation lesion
    o. recess
    o. stalk
    o. strut
    o. sulcus
    o. sunscreen
    o. thalamus
    o. tract
    o. tract compression
    o. tract damage
    o. tract lesion
    o. tract syndrome
    o. tweezers
    o. vesicle
optica, pl. **opticae**
    hyperesthesia o.
    neuromyelitis o.
    radiatio o.
Opticaid spring clip
Opticaine ophthalmic
optical
    o. aberration
    o. accessory
    o. alexia
    o. allachesthesia
    American O. (AO)
    o. atrophy
    o. axis
    o. bench
    o. blur
    o. breakdown
    o. center
    o. centering instrument
    o. center of spectacle lens
    o. clarity
    o. coherence tomography (OCT)
    o. coherence tomography-3 (OCT3)
    o. contact lens
    o. correction
    o. cross
    o. density method
    o. disc swelling
    o. dispensary
    o. dispenser
    o. fossa
    o. frame
    o. glass
    o. heterogeneity
    o. illusion
    o. image
    o. imperfection
    o. iridectomy

o. jewelry
o. keratoplasty
o. lab
o. low vision aid
o. magnifier
o. nodal point
o. pachymeter
o. penalization
o. performance
o. power
o. quality
O. Radiation lens
o. ray tracing
o. rehabilitation
o. retinal cross-section
o. side effect
o. system
o. tilt
o. transfer function
o. zone (OZ)
o. zone centration
o. zone chamber
o. zone of contact lens
o. zone diameter
o. zone enlargement
o. zone marker
optically empty
Opticath
optici
circulus vasculosus nervi o.
discus nervi o.
radix lateralis tractus o.
radix medialis tractus o.
optician
opticianry
opticist
Opti-Clean II
Opti-Clear
opticoacoustic nerve atrophy
opticocerebral syndrome
opticochiasmatic, optochiasmic
o. arachnoiditis
opticociliary
o. neurectomy
o. neurotomy
o. shunt
o. shunt vein
o. shunt vessel
opticocochleodentate degeneration
opticofacial winking reflex
opticokinetic nystagmus
opticonasion
opticopupillary

opticopyramidal syndrome
Opticrom
Opticrom 4%
optics
Advanced Medical O. (AMO)
American Medical O. (AMO)
confocal o.
Fresnel o.
gaussian o.
geometric o.
Infinitech fiber o.
o. of intraocular lens
physical o.
physiologic o.
reverse o.
opticum
chiasma o.
foramen o.
opticus
axis o.
discus o.
nervus o.
porus o.
recessus o.
Opticyl
Optiflex lens
Opti-Free
O.-F. Daily Cleaner
O.-F. Enzymatic Cleaner
O.-F. Express Multi-Purpose
Solution
O.-F. Rewetting Drops
O.-F. Rinsing Disinfecting and
Storage
O.-F. Supraclens
Optigene
O. 3
O. Ophthalmic
**Optikon 2000 placido-based corneal
topography system Keratron Scout**
Optima
O. contact lens
O. diamond knife
optimal
o. IOL
o. medical therapy (OMT)
OptiMed
O. device
O. glaucoma pressure regulator
(OGPR)
Optimine
Optimize viscoelastic
Optimmune

O

NOTES

optimum
- O. blade
- O. cleaning, disinfecting, and storage solution
- O. extra-strength cleaner
- O. by Lobob
- O. by Lobob Daily Cleaner
- O. by Lobob wetting and rewetting drops
- O. rigid gas permeable starter kit

Optimyd
optineurin gene
option
- treatment o.

Opti-One
- O.-O. Conditioning Solution
- O.-O. Multi-Purpose Solution
- O.-O. Rewetting Drops

Optiphot microscope
OptiPranolol Ophthalmic
Optipress
Opti-Pure System
Optique 1 Eye Drops
Optised
Opti-Soak
- O.-S. Conditioning Solution
- O.-S. Daily Cleaner

Optisoap
Opti-Soft
Optisol-GS
Optisol medium
Opti-Tears
Optivar ophthalmic solution
OptiZen lubricating eye drops
Opti-Zyme enzymatic cleaner
OPTN gene
optochiasmatic
- o. arachnoiditis
- o. tuberculoma

optochiasmic (*var. of* opticochiasmatic)
optogram
optokinesis
optokinetic
- o. drum
- o. nystagmus (OKN)
- o. reflex
- o. stimulator
- o. stimulus
- o. system
- o. tape
- o. test

optomeninx
optometer
- automatic infrared o.
- infrared o.
- laser o.
- objective o.
- Ophthas subjective o.
- Vernier o.

optometric
- para o.
- o. practice
- o. vision training
- o. visual exercise

optometrist
optometry
- American Academy of O. (AAO)
- developmental o.
- Fellow of the American Academy of O. (FAAO)

optomotor reflex
optomyometer
optophone
optostriate
optotype
- picture o.
- Sloan o.
- Snellen letter o.

Optrin
Optycryl 60 contact lens
optyl frame
Opus III contact lens
OR
- overrefraction

ora (*pl. of* os)
- o. globule
- o. serrata
- o. serrata retinae

oral
- O. administration
- AllerMax O.
- Banophen O.
- Belix O.
- Benadryl O.
- Cartrol O.
- Cytoxan O.
- Dimetabs O.
- Kerlone O.
- Phendry O.
- Siladryl O.
- Toradol O.

orange
- o. dye laser
- o. punctate pigmentation

orange-red lesion
Oratrol
orb
orbiculare
- os o.

orbiculare
- *Pityrosporum o.*

orbicularis
- alopecia o.
- o. contraction
- musculus o.
- o. myectomy
- o. oculi muscle
- o. oris muscle

o. phenomenon
o. pupillary reflex
o. reaction
o. sign
o. strength
orbicular muscle of eye
orbiculoanterocapsular fiber
orbiculociliary fiber
orbiculoposterocapsular fiber
orbit
aneurysm of o.
o. blade
blowout fracture of o.
bony o.
contaminated o.
contusion of o.
CT scan of o.
dermoid of o.
emphysema of o.
fracture of o.
o. hamartoma
idiopathic sclerosing inflammation
 of o.
intraorbital margin of o.
lateral margin of o.
lesion of o.
roof of o.
supraorbital margin of o.
tight o.
orbitae
aditus o.
corpus adiposum o.
margo infraorbitalis o.
margo lateralis o.
margo medialis o.
margo supraorbitalis o.
paries inferior o.
paries lateralis o.
paries medialis o.
paries superior o.
orbital
o. adipose tissue
o. akinesia
o. amyloidosis
o. anesthesia
o. aneurysm
o. angiography
o. angioma
o. angiosarcoma
o. aperture
o. apex
o. apex mass
o. apex syndrome

o. arch
o. arch of frontal bone
o. arteriovenous malformation
o. axis
o. blowout fracture
o. border of sphenoid bone
o. canal
o. cavernoma
o. cavernous hemangioma
o. cavity
o. cellulite
o. cellulitis
o. conjunctiva
o. content
o. crest
o. CT scan
o. cyst
o. decompression
o. decompression surgery
o. depressor
o. dermoid
o. dimension
o. dystopia
o. echography
o. emphysema
o. encephalocele
o. enlargement
o. enucleation compressor
o. eosinophilic angiocentric fibrosis
o. exenteration
o. exit
o. extension
o. fascia
o. fasciitis
o. fat
o. fat pad
o. fat prolapse
o. fat suppression
o. fibroma
o. fibromatosis
o. fibrosarcoma
o. floor
o. floor fracture
o. floor implant
o. floor prosthesis
o. ganglion
o. glioma
o. granuloma
o. hamartoma
o. height
o. hemangioendothelioma
o. hemangiopericytoma
o. hematoma

NOTES

O

orbital *(continued)*
- o. hemorrhage
- o. hernia
- o. hypertelorism
- o. hypotelorism
- o. hypoxia
- o. imaging
- o. implant operation
- o. infarction
- o. infarction syndrome
- o. infection
- o. inferior rim
- o. inflammation
- o. inflammatory disease
- o. inflammatory pseudotumor
- o. irrigation
- o. lamina
- o. lens
- o. lesion
- o. lipoma
- o. lymphoma
- o. margin
- o. medulloepithelioma
- o. melanoma
- o. meningioma
- o. mesenchyme
- o. metastasis
- o. muscle
- o. myositis
- o. neoplasm
- o. neuritis
- o. neuroepithelioma
- o. neurofibroma
- o. neuroma
- o. opening
- o. ophthalmoplegia
- o. optic nerve
- o. palsy
- o. pathology
- o. periosteum
- o. periostitis
- o. pit
- o. plane
- o. plaque brachytherapy
- o. plate of ethmoid bone
- o. plate of frontal bone
- o. polymyositis
- o. portion of eyelid
- o. pseudotumor
- o. radiology
- o. radiotherapy
- o. region
- o. resilience
- o. rhabdomyosarcoma
- o. rim fracture
- o. roentgenogram
- o. roof
- o. schwannoma
- o. section
- o. septum
- o. structure
- o. subperiosteal abscess
- o. sulcus
- o. sulcus of frontal bone
- o. superior fissure
- o. syndrome
- o. teratoma
- o. tomography
- o. trauma
- o. tumor
- o. varix
- o. vasculitis
- o. vein thrombosis
- o. venography
- o. venous anomaly
- o. venous congestion
- o. venous pressure
- o. vessel
- o. volume
- o. wall fracture
- o. width
- o. wing of sphenoid bone
- o. x-ray

orbitale
- planum o.
- septum o.

orbitales
- fasciae o.

orbitalia
- cribra o.

orbitalis
- margo o.
- musculus o.

orbitectomy
- radical o.

orbitocranial
- o. imaging
- o. trauma

orbitography
- Graves o.
- positive contrast o.

orbitomalar foramen
orbitonasal
orbitonometer
orbitonometry
orbitopalpebral
orbitopathy
- acute o.
- congestive o.
- dysthyroid o.
- Graves o.
- thyroid o.
- thyroid-related o.

orbitostat
orbitotemporal
orbitotomy
- Berke-Krönlein o.
- lateral o.

Orbscan
    O. corneal topography
    O. II corneal diagnostic system
    O. II corneal topography system
    O. II multidimensional diagnostic
      system
    O. pachymetry mapping
    O. topography analysis system
    O. value
ORC intraocular lens
order
    random o.
ordered array
ordering
    Dyer nomogram system of lens o.
organ
    o. culture
    o. transplantation
    vestibular o.
    o. of vision
    visual o.
organic amblyopia
organism
    causative o.
    coliform o.
    endogenous surface o.
    excysting o.
    Gram-positive o.
    HACEK group o.
organized vitreous
organizer
    Richard Products fundus camera
      drug o.
organoid nevus syndrome
orientation
    epithelial o.
    false o.
    limbal parallel o.
oriented
    radially o.
original
    o. Sweet eye magnet
    Visine O.
oris
    pars marginalis musculi
      orbicularis o.
    sphincter o.
ornithine tolerance test
orodigitofacial dysplasia
orphan drug
orthoclone (OKT3)
orthogonal
Orthogon lens

ortho-K
orthokeratology
    o. contact lens
    Lenses and Overnight O. (LOOK)
    o. lens wear
Ortho-Lite
orthometer
orthophoria
orthophoric
orthopia
orthoposition
orthoptic
orthoptics
orthoptist
    certified o. (CO)
orthoptoscope
orthoscope
orthoscopic
    o. lens
    o. spectacles
orthoscopy
Ortopad orthoptic patch
OS
    left eye
os, pl. ora
    o. lacrimale
    o. orbiculare
    o. palatinum
    o. planum
    o. unguis
oscillating
    o. blade
    o. nystagmus
    o. vision
oscillation
    convergent-divergent pendular o.
    macrosaccadic o.
    nystagmoid-like o.
    ocular o.
    voluntary saccadic o.
oscillatory
    o. potential (OP)
    o. potential recording
oscillopsia
    monocular o.
    torsional o.
OSD
    ocular surface disease
OSDI
    Ocular Surface Disease Index
O'Shea lens
Osher
    O. foreign body forceps

O

NOTES

Osher *(continued)*
  O. hook
  O. pan-fundus lens
  O. surgical gonio/posterior pole
  lens
  O. surgical keratometer
Osher-Neumann corneal marker
Osmitrol injection
osmium
  o. tetroxide
  o. tetroxide solution
Osmoglyn Ophthalmic
osmolarity
  tear o.
  tear film o.
osmotherapy
  hypertonic o.
osmotic
  o. agent
  o. cataract
  o. pressure
  o. shock
osseous
  o. anomaly
  o. choristoma
  o. lesion
  o. metaplasia over choroidal
  hemangioma
  o. system
osseus
  tarsus o.
ossis
  bulla ethmoidalis o.
ossium
  fragilitas o.
osteitis deformans
osteoma
  choroidal o.
  uveal o.
osteomyelitis
  maxillary o.
osteoporosis-pseudoglioma syndrome
osteosclerotic myeloma
osteotome
  lacrimal o.
osteotomy
ostium
  internal o.
Ota
  nevus of O.
  O. nevus
  O. nevus syndrome
OTHA
  ocular total higher order aberration
OTI
  Ophthalmic Technologies Inc.
  OTI ultrasound B & A scan
oticus
  herpes zoster o.

Otis-Lennon
  O.-L. School Ability Test
  (OLSAT)
otolithic-ocular reflex
OTR
  ocular tilt reaction
OU
  both eyes
out
  base o. (BO)
  pericyte drop o.
outcome
  bleb o.
  cosmetic o.
  long-term o.
  predictive visual o.
  refractive o.
  visual o.
outdoor mobility
outer
  o. canthus
  o. limiting membrane
  o. nuclear layer
  o. nuclear layer of retina
  o. plexiform layer (OPL)
  o. retinal necrosis syndrome
  o. segment
outflow
  aqueous o.
  coefficient of facility of o.
  conventional o.
  o. disorder
  facility of o.
  lacrimal o.
  o. obstruction
  parasympathetic o.
  o. resistance
  trabecular o.
  unconventional o.
  uveoscleral o.
outfolding
  scleral o.
outgrowth
  extrascleral o.
  local o.
outpouching
output nerve
outside-world image
oval
  o. cornea
  o. eye
  o. eye patch
ovale
  Pityrosporum o.
oval-shaped vernal ulcer
OVAS
  ocular vergence and accommodation
  sensor

overaction
inferior oblique o. (IOOA)
overall diameter (OAD)
overcorrection
surgical o.
over-dipping
overflow diabetes
overhanging eyelid skin
overnight corneal reshaping
overrefraction (OR)
overriding
scleral o.
overripe cataract
overt diabetes
ovis
Oestrus o.
ovoid mass
oxidation of solution
oxidative
o. damage
o. stress
oxide
cocamidopropylamine o.
mercuric o.
oxidized cellulose
oxidopamine
oximetry sensor
oxprenolol
Oxsoralen
oxyblepsia

oxybuprocaine hydrochloride
oxycephaly
oxycodone
oxygen
o. flux
hyperbaric o. (HBO)
o. measurement
o. permeability (Dk)
o. saturation
o. transmissibility (Dk/L)
oxygenation
corneal o.
oxymetazoline HCl
oxymorphone hydrochloride
oxyopia
oxyopter
oxyphenbutazone
oxyphenonium
Oxysept
Lens Plus O.
oxysporum
Fusarium o.
oxytetracycline
o. and hydrocortisone
o. and polymyxin B
oxytoca
Klebsiella o.
oyster shuckers' keratitis
OZ
optical zone

NOTES

O

P

optic papilla
pupil
P2Y2 agonist
P55 Pachymetric Analyzer
PA
phakic-aphakic
Pachmate DGH55 pachymeter
pachometer
Alcon ultrasound p.
corneal p.
Humphrey ultrasonic p.
Ophthasonic p.
Sonogage ultrasound p.
ultrasound p.
Pach-Pen
P.-P. XL pachymeter
P.-P. XL tonometer
pachyblepharon
pachymeter
Advent p.
corneal p.
DGH 2000 AP ultrasonic p.
optic p.
optical p.
Pachmate DGH55 p.
Pach-Pen XL p.
PalmScan AP2000 portable p.
Villasenor ultrasonic p.
pachymetry
corneal p.
noncontact corneal p.
ultrasonic p.
p. value
Packard luminometer
Packer
P. tunnel silicone sponge
P. Wick extrusion handpiece
packing
loose p.
Packo pars plana cannula
PACT
prism and alternate cover test
pad
eye p.
fat p.
orbital fat p.
spectacle frame p.
Telfa p.
padding
eye p.
nocturnal eye p.
paddle
Rosen nucleus p.
p. temple

paddy keratitis
Paecilomyces lilacinus
Page medium
pagetoid
p. melanoma
p. spread
PAI
plasminogen activator inhibitor
pain
atypical facial p.
boring p.
p. control
facial p.
jaw muscle p.
lancing p.
postoperative p.
p. prevention strategy
p. reaction
trigeminal p.
painful
p. eye
p. ophthalmoplegia
painless
p. blurred vision
p. progressive loss of vision
p. visual loss
paint-ball
p.-b. game
p.-b. pellet
p.-b. projectile
palatine bone
palatinum
os p.
palatoethmoidalis
sutura p.
palatomaxillaris
sutura p.
palatomaxillary suture
pale
p. conjunctiva
p. optic disc
palinopsia
palisades of Vogt
palisading orbital granuloma
palladium
p. 103 ophthalmic plaque
brachytherapy
p. 103 ophthalmic plaque
radiotherapy
palliative therapy
pallidotomy
pallidum
Treponema p.
pallidus
globus p. (GP)

P

Pallin lens spatula
Pallister-Hall syndrome
pallor
    p. of conjunctiva
    disc p.
    discussion p.
    horizontal band p.
    optic disc p.
    optic nerve p.
    sector p.
    subtle disc p.
    temporal artery p.
    temporal optic disc p.
palmate
    vitamin A p.
Palmitate-A
palmoplantar keratoderma
PalmScan AP2000 portable pachymeter
palpable purpura
palpebra, pl. **palpebrae**
    margo p.
    paraphimosis palpebrae
    palpebrae superioris muscle
    tertius p.
palpebral
    p. adipose bag
    p. aperture
    p. cartilage
    p. commissure
    p. conjunctiva
    p. conjunctival hue (PCH)
    p. fascia
    p. fissure
    p. fissure widening
    p. fold
    p. furrow
    p. gland
    p. ligament
    p. lobe
    p. margin
    p. oculogyric reflex
    p. opening
    p. raphe
    p. slant
    p. vein
palpebrale
    coloboma p.
palpebrales
    venae p.
palpebralis
    epicanthus p.
palpebrarum
    dermatolysis p.
    facies anterior p.
    facies posterior p.
    pediculosis p.
    phthiriasis p.
    rima p.
    tunica conjunctiva p.

    xanthelasma p.
    xanthoma p.
palpebrate
palpebration
palpebritis
palpebromandibular reflex
palpebronasal fold
palsy, pl. **palsies**
    abducens nerve p.
    accommodative p.
    acquired superior oblique p.
    Bell p.
    brachial plexus p.
    cerebral p.
    complete p.
    congenital abducens nerve p.
    congenital oculomotor nerve p.
    congenital third nerve p.
    conjugate gaze p.
    cranial nerve p.
    cyclic oculomotor p.
    cyclovertical muscle p.
    double elevator p.
    elevator p.
    external p.
    extraocular muscle p.
    facial nerve p.
    fourth nerve p.
    gaze p.
    idiopathic facial p.
    inferior oblique p.
    inhibitional p.
    internal p.
    ischemic oculomotor p.
    isolated cyclovertical muscle p.
    isolated fourth nerve p.
    isolated seventh nerve p.
    isolated sixth nerve p.
    isolated third nerve p.
    lateral rectus p.
    medial rectus p.
    microvascular sixth nerve p.
    multiple ocular motor palsies
    p. of muscle
    nerve p.
    nuclear p.
    nuclear-fascicular trochlear nerve p.
    oblique p.
    oblique muscle p.
    ocular muscle p.
    oculomotor cranial nerve p.
    orbital p.
    progressive supranuclear p.
    pseudoabducens p.
    pseudobulbar p.
    saccade p.
    sector p.
    seventh cranial nerve p.
    sixth cranial nerve p.

stem p.
subarachnoid oculomotor nerve p.
superior division p.
superior oblique p.
superior rectus p.
supranuclear ocular p.
third cranial nerve p.
trochlear nerve p.
twelfth nerve p.
PAM
potential acuity meter
primary acquired melanosis
PAM procedure
pamoate
hydroxyzine p.
PAN
periarteritis nodosa
Panamax
pANCA
perinuclear antineutrophil cytoplasmic
antibody
panchamber UV lens
Pancoast
P. superior sulcus syndrome
P. tumor
pancreatic
p. diabetes
p. disease
pancuronium bromide
pancytokeratin antibody
PANDO
primary acquired nasolacrimal duct
obstruction
panel
Farnsworth D15 p.
panencephalitis
subacute sclerosing p.
panfundus
panfunduscope
Rodenstock p.
Panmycin
panni (*pl. of* pannus)
Pannu
P. intraocular lens
P. type II lens
Pannu-Kratz-Barraquer speculum
pannus, pl. **panni**
allergic p.
corneal p.
p. crassus
degenerative p.
p. degenerativus
p. eczematosus

eczematous p.
fibrovascular p.
glaucomatous p.
phlyctenular p.
trachomatous p.
panophthalmia
panophthalmitis
clostridial p.
Panoptic bifocal
Panoramic200
P. Non-Mydriatic Ophthalmoscope
P. scanning laser ophthalmoscope
P. Ultra-Widefield Ophthalmic
Imaging Device
panoramic loupe
panphotocoagulation
panretinal
p. ablation
p. argon laser photocoagulation
p. membrane
p. scatter photocoagulation
pansinusitis
panstromal
pantachromatic
pantankyloblepharon
pantoscope
Keeler p.
pantoscopic
p. angle
p. angling
p. effect
p. spectacles
p. tilt
Panum
P. fusional space
P. fusion area
panuveitis
granulomatous p.
herpes p.
multifocal choroiditis with p.
(MCP)
Papanicolaou stain
papaverine hydrochloride
paper
nitrocellulose filter p.
Schirmer filter p.
Whatman No. 1 qualitative-type
filter p.
papilla, pl. **papillae**
Bergmeister p.
cobblestone p.
conjunctival p.
drusen of optic p.

NOTES

P

papilla *(continued)*
> giant p.
> lacrimal p.
> limbal papillae
> optic p. (P)
> persistent Bergmeister p.
> splitting of lacrimal p.

papillary
> p. area
> p. capillary hemangioma
> p. conjunctival hypertrophy
> p. conjunctivitis
> p. stasis

papilledema
> acute p.
> asymmetric p.
> chronic p.
> diabetic p.
> unilateral p.

papilliform tumor
papillitis
> diabetic p.
> florid p.
> ischemic p.
> necrotizing p.

papilloma
> caruncular p.
> conjunctival p.
> eyelid p.
> intralacrimal p.
> mulberry-type p.
> pedunculated p.
> sessile p.
> squamous p.
> verruca vulgaris p.

papillomacular
> p. nerve fiber bundle
> p. retinal fold

papillomatosis
papillopathy
> diabetic p.
> ischemic p.

papillophlebitis
papillopruritic dermatosis
papilloretinitis
papyracea
> lamina p.

PAR
> posterior apical radius
> PAR CTS corneal topography
> system

parablepsia
paracentesis
> anterior chamber p.
> aqueous p.
> p. incision
> tunnel p.

paracentral
> p. cell

> p. defect
> p. nerve fiber bundle
> p. ring scotoma
> p. visual field

paracentric
paracetamol
parachroma
parachromatism
parachromatopsia
Paradigm ocular blood flow analyzer
paradoxic
> p. gustolacrimal reflex
> p. levator excitation
> p. levator inhibition
> p. pupil
> p. pupillary phenomenon
> p. pupillary reflex

paradoxical
> p. darkness reaction
> p. diplopia
> p. movement of eyelid
> p. pupil
> p. pupillary phenomenon
> p. pupillary reflex

paraequilibrium
paraffin block
paraflocculus syndrome
parafovea
parafoveal
> p. capillary net
> p. cystic space
> p. fluorescein
> p. halo
> p. macula
> p. microvascular leakage
> p. serous retinal elevation

paraganglioma
paragraph
> Gray Standardized Oral
> Reading P.'s

parainfectious
> p. optic neuritis
> p. optic neuropathy

parainfluenzae
> *Haemophilus p.*

parallactic
parallax
> binocular p.
> crossed p.
> direct p.
> heteronymous p.
> homonymous p.
> motion p.
> stereoscopic p.
> p. test
> vertical p.

parallel
> p. interface
> p. ray

parallelism
    eyelash p.
    p. of gaze
parallel-plate flow chamber
paralysis, pl. **paralyses**
    abducens nerve p.
    p. of accommodation
    amaurotic pupillary p.
    bulbar p.
    congenital abducens facial p.
    congenital abduction p.
    congenital bulbar p.
    congenital oculofacial p.
    conjugate p.
    convergence p.
    divergence p.
    Duchenne p.
    Duchenne-Erb p.
    Erb p.
    Erb-Duchenne p.
    facial p.
    familial periodic p.
    p. of gaze
    hyperkalemic periodic p.
    hypokalemic periodic p.
    internuclear p.
    Klumpke p.
    Landry ascending p.
    normokalemic periodic p.
    nuclear horizontal gaze p.
    ocular muscle p.
    oculofacial p.
    periodic p.
    psychogenic p.
    pupillary p.
    sectoral iris p.
    Todd p.
    upgaze p.
    vagus nerve p.
    Weber p.
paralytic
    p. ectropion
    p. heterotropia
    p. miosis
    p. mydriasis
    p. pontine exotropia
    p. strabismus
paramedian thalamopeduncular infarction
parameter
    inflammatory-related p.
    stereometric p.

    treatment p.
    visual p.
paramethasone acetate
paramyotonia congenita
paranasal
    p. sinus
    p. sinusitis
paraneoplastic
    p. cerebellar degeneration
    p. lichen planus
    p. opsoclonus
    p. optic neuritis
    p. optic neuropathy
    p. retinopathy
    p. syndrome
para optometric
Paraperm O2 contact lens
paraphimosis palpebrae
paraphrophilus
    Haemophilus p.
parapsilosis
    Candida p.
parasellar
    p. lesion
    p. syndrome
parasitic
    p. agent
    p. blepharitis
    p. uveitis
parasitica
    blepharitis p.
Parasol punctal occluder
parastriate area
parasympathetic
    p. fiber
    p. nerve system
    p. nervous system
    p. outflow
    p. pathway
parasympatholytic drug
parasympathomimetic drug
parathyroid
    p. adenoma
    p. disorder
paratrachoma
paraxial
    p. lighting
    p. mesoderm
    p. ray
    p. ray of light
Parcaine
Paredrine
Paremyd Ophthalmic

NOTES

P

parenchymatosus
    xerosis p.
parenchymatous
    p. corneal dystrophy
    p. keratitis
parenteral
    p. administration
    p. narcotic
parent spherical IOL
paresis
    abducens p.
    accommodation p.
    complete but pupil-sparing
      oculomotor nerve p.
    convergence p.
    cyclic oculomotor p.
    divergence p.
    incomplete pupil-sparing oculomotor
      nerve p.
    isolated inferior oblique p.
    nonorganic p.
    oculosympathetic p.
    vertical gaze p.
paretic nystagmus
paries
    p. inferior orbitae
    p. lateralis orbitae
    p. medialis orbitae
    p. superior orbitae
parietal
    p. eye
    p. lobe
    p. lobe bilateral cerebral
      hemisphere lesion
    p. lobe field defect
    p. lobe unilateral cerebral
      hemisphere lesion
parietooccipital artery
parietooccipital-temporal junction
Parinaud
    P. oculoglandular conjunctivitis
    P. oculoglandular syndrome
    P. ophthalmoplegia
Parinaud-plus syndrome
PARK
    photoastigmatic refractive keratectomy
Park
    P. speculum
    P. 3-step test
Park-Maumenee speculum
Parks-Bielschowsky 3-step head-tilt test
paromomycin
parophthalmia
parophthalmoncus
paropsia, paropsis
parotid neoplasm
Parrot sign
Parry disease

pars
    p. ciliaris retinae
    p. corneoscleralis
    p. iridica retinae
    p. lacrimalis musculi orbicularis
      oculi
    p. marginalis musculi orbicularis
      oris
    p. nervosa retinae
    p. optica hypothalami
    p. optica retinae
    p. orbitalis glandulae lacrimalis
    p. orbitalis gyri frontalis inferioris
    p. orbitalis musculi orbicularis
      oculi
    p. orbitalis ossis frontalis
    p. palpebralis glandulae lacrimalis
    p. palpebralis musculi orbicularis
      oculi
    p. pigmentosa retinae
    p. plana
    p. plana approach
    p. plana Baerveldt tube insertion
      with vitrectomy
    p. plana corporis ciliaris
    p. plana lensectomy
    p. plana operation
    p. plana posterior capsulectomy
    p. plana posterior vitrectomy
    p. plana seton implant
    p. planitis
    p. plicata
    p. plicata corporis ciliaris
    p. uvealis
partial
    p. accommodative esotropia
    p. albinism
    p. cataract
    p. coherence interferometry (PCI)
    p. conjunctival flap (PCF)
    p. depth astigmatic keratotomy
      (PDAK)
    p. depth keratoplasty
    p. limbal stem cell deficiency
    p. ophthalmoplegia
    p. response
    p. sclerectasia
    p. thickness macular hole
    p. throw surgeon's knot
    p. vitrectomy
partialis
    ophthalmoplegia p.
partially
    p. sighted
    p. sighted child
partial-thickness
    p.-t. corneal laceration
    p.-t. trephination

particle
    iridescent lens p.
particulate
    p. matter
    p. retinopathy
parvocellular
    p. binocular vision system
    p. cell
    p. pathway
parvum
    Chrysosporium p.
PAS
    periodic acid-Schiff
    peripheral anterior synechia
    Prism Adaptation Study
    PAS stain
PASCAL
    pattern scan laser
    PASCAL photocoagulator
Pascal law
Pascheff conjunctivitis
pass
    pupil p.
passant
    bouton en p.
Passarelli 1-pass capsulorrhexis forceps
passivated polymethyl methacrylate
passive
    p. duction
    p. forced duction test
    p. illusion
Passport disposable injection system
paster
past ocular history (POH)
past-pointing
PAT
    prism adaptation test
Patanol ophthalmic solution
patch
    binocular eye p.
    Bitot p.
    Cogan p.
    cotton-wool p.
    Donaldson eye p.
    p. eye
    glue p.
    p. graft
    histoacryl glue p.
    Hutchinson p.
    monocular p.
    Ortopad orthoptic p.
    oval eye p.
    salmon p.

    Snugfit eye p.
    venous sheath p.
    wicking glue p.
patching
    pressure p.
patchy
    p. anterior stromal infiltrate
    p. atrophy
    p. hyperfluorescence
    p. inflammatory lesion
    p. window defect
patency
    tear duct p.
patent
    p. iridectomy
    p. iridotomy
Paterson-Brown-Kelly syndrome
pathergy testing
PathFinder corneal analysis software
pathobiology
pathogen
    bacterial p.
pathognomonic radial keratoneuritis
pathologic
    p. cupping
    p. myope
    p. myopia
    p. neovascularization
pathological astigmatism
pathology
    epiretinal p.
    macular p.
    ocular p.
    orbital p.
    systemic p.
    vitreoretinal p.
pathometer attachment
pathway
    afferent visual p.
    anterior visual p.
    cAMP final common p.
    canalicular p.
    COX p.
    infranuclear p.
    magnocellular visual p.
    oculosympathetic p.
    parasympathetic p.
    parvocellular p.
    pregeniculate visual p.
    retinogeniculate p.
    retrochiasmal visual p.
    sensory visual p.
    supranuclear p.

NOTES

P

pathway *(continued)*
  sympathetic p.
  visual p.
patient
  p. compliance
  diabetic p.
  high-risk p.
  primary glaucoma p.
  straight-eyed p.
patient-based preference
Paton
  P. anterior chamber lens implant forceps
  P. capsule forceps
  P. corneal knife
  P. corneal transplant forceps
  P. corneal trephine
  P. double spatula
  P. eye shield
  P. line
  P. needle holder
  P. single spatula
  P. single speculum
  P. suturing forceps
  P. transplant spatula
  P. transplant speculum
  P. tying/stitch removal forceps
pattern
  A p.
  abnormal staining p.
  Antoni p.
  p. arborization
  arborization p.
  arteriovenous p.
  AV p.
  blur p.
  childhood blindness p.
  classic flower petal p.
  coarse vascular p.
  comedo p.
  contiguous p.
  contoured ablation p. (CAP)
  custom-contoured ablation p. (C-CAP)
  p. cut corneal graft operation
  p. discrimination perimetry
  p. distortion amblyopia
  p. dystrophy of pigment epithelium of Byers and Marmor
  p. electroretinogram
  flower petal p.
  fluorescein staining p.
  Harrington-Flocks multiple p.
  map p.
  morpheaform p.
  Morse code p.
  mosaic p.
  petaloid p.
  racquet-like p.

  p. recognition
  p. retinal dystrophy
  p. scan laser (PASCAL)
  scatter p.
  shagreen p.
  staining p.
  p. standard deviation (PSD)
  stippled p.
  surgical ablation p.
  umbrella-like p.
  V p.
  videokeratography p.
  p. visual-evoked response (PVER)
  Visx Contoured Ablation P.
  vortex p.
  wavefront ablation p.
  Zellballen p.
pattern-cut corneal graft
pattern-evoked electroretinogram (PERG)
Paufique
  P. graft knife
  P. keratoplasty knife
  P. suturing forceps
Paul lacrimal sac retractor
Pautler infusion cannula
paving-stone degeneration
Payne retractor
PBA
  Prevent Blindness America
PBC
  point of basal convergence
PBII blue loop lens
PBK
  pseudophakic bullous keratopathy
PBRVO
  peripheral branch retinal vein occlusion
PBZ-SR tablet
PBZ tablet
PC
  posterior chamber
P&C
  prism and cover
  P&C test
PcB
  point of basal convergence
PCD
  posterior corneal deposit
P-cell
PCF
  partial conjunctival flap
PCH
  palpebral conjunctival hue
PCI
  partial coherence interferometry
PCIOL, PC-IOL
  posterior chamber intraocular lens
PCL
  posterior collagenous layer

PCLI
posterior chamber lens implant
PCMD
pellucid corneal marginal degeneration
PCNSL
primary central nervous system
lymphoma
PCO
posterior capsule opacification
fibrotic PCO
sand dune PCO
wrinkling PCO
PCR
polymerase chain reaction
PCR-SSOP
polymerase chain reaction-sequence
specific oligonucleotide probe
PCR-SSOP method
PCV
polypoidal choroidal vasculopathy
PD
prism diopter
pupillary distance
frame PD
p.d.
prism diopter
PDAK
partial depth astigmatic keratotomy
PDR
proliferative diabetic retinopathy
PDS
pigment dispersion syndrome
PDT
photodynamic therapy
PDVR
proliferative diabetic vitreoretinopathy
PE
pigment epithelium
PE-400 ERG/VEP system
PEA
posterior ethmoidal artery
PeaceKeeper
P. cannula
P. extrusion aspiration cannula
eraser
PEAK
pulsed electron avalanche knife
peak
p. circadian intraocular pressure
p. IOP
p. latencies of pattern
electroretinogram
p. visual performance

peaking
temporal p.
peak-to-peak amplitude
peanut implant
pear cataract
Pearce
P. coaxial irrigating/aspirating
cannula
P. nucleus hydrodissector
P. posterior chamber intraocular
lens
P. trabeculectomy
pearl
p. cyst
p. diver's keratopathy
Elschnig p.
iris p.
p. white mounds
pear-shaped pupil
Pearson chi-square test
Pease-Allen Color test
pectinate
p. ligament
p. ligament of iris
pectineal ligament
PED
pigment epithelial detachment
PEDF
pigment epithelium-derived factor
PEDF gene
pediatric
p. aphakia
p. cataract
P. Eye Disease Investigator Group
(PEDIG)
p. eye examination
p. eye specialist
p. glaucoma
p. intraocular implantation
p. IOL calculator
p. Karickhoff laser lens
p. lid speculum
p. 3-mirror laser lens
p. myasthenia
p. ocular sarcoidosis
p. ophthalmologist
p. ophthalmology
p. orbital cellulitis
p. orbital floor fracture
p. presumed microbial keratitis
p. uveitis
p. vision screening
p. vitrectomy lens set

NOTES

P

pedicle
    p. cone
    p. flap
    tarsoconjunctival p.
pediculated flap
pediculosis palpebrarum
pediculous blepharitis
PEDIG
    Pediatric Eye Disease Investigator Group
pedigree
    p. analysis
    p. chart
peduncular hallucination
pedunculated
    p. congenital corneal dermoid
    p. papilloma
peek sign
peeler
peeler-cutter
    membrane p.-c. (MPC)
peeling
    internal limiting membrane p.
    membrane p.
    spontaneous p.
PEELS
    pigment epithelial endoscopic laser
    surgery
    endoscopic PEELS
pefloxacin
pegaptanib sodium
peg-coupled prosthesis
PEHO
    progressive encephalopathy with edema,
    hypsarrhythmia and optic atrophy
    PEHO syndrome
PEK
    punctate epithelial keratopathy
Pel crisis
Pel-Ebstein crisis
pellet
    p. extrusion
    paint-ball p.
Pelli-Robson
    P.-R. contrast sensitivity chart
    P.-R. letter chart
pellucid
    corneal p.
    p. corneal marginal degeneration
    (PCMD)
    p. marginal corneal degeneration
    p. marginal retinal degeneration
pellucidum
    septum cavum p.
pemirolast
    p. potassium
    p. potassium ophthalmic solution
pemphigoid
    benign mucosal p.
    Brunsting-Perry cicatricial p.

    bullous p.
    cicatricial p.
    mucosal p.
    mucous membrane p.
    ocular p.
    ocular cicatricial p. (OCP)
pemphigus
    ocular p.
pen
    Accu-Line surgical marking p.
    ASSI Accu-line surgical marking p.
    gentian violet marking p.
    marking p.
    piokutanin p.
    Rhein reusable cautery p.
    skin marking p.
    surgical marking p.
penalization
    atropine p.
    optical p.
Penbritin
pencil
    astigmatism of oblique p.'s
    cataract p.
    p. cautery
    20-gauge straight bipolar p.
    glaucoma p.
    p. push-ups
    p. push-up therapy
    retinal detachment p.
    vitreous p.
    Wallach cryosurgical p.
pendular-jerk waveform
pendular nystagmus
penetrant gene
penetrating
    p. corneal transplant
    p. full-thickness corneal graft
    p. keratoplasty (PK, PKP)
    p. keratoplasty astigmatism
    p. keratoplasty button
    p. keratoplasty and glaucoma
    (PKPG)
    p. ocular injury
    p. scleral wound
    p. trauma
penetration
    corneal p.
    intraocular p.
    vitreous p.
    zone of p.
penicillin
    acid-resistant p.
    antistaphylococcal p.
    aqueous crystalline p. G
    p. G
    p. G benzathine
    synthetic p.
penicillinase

peninsula pupil
penlight
    p. examination
    Heine p.
    Welch-Allyn halogen p.
pentafilcon A
pentagonal block excision
pentamidine isethionate
Penthrane
pentigetide
pentobarbital sodium
Pentolair
pentolinium
Pentostam
Pentothal
pentoxifylline
penumbra
PEO
    progressive external ophthalmoplegia
Pepper
pepper-and-salt
    p.-a.-s. fundus
    p.-a.-s. retinopathy
Pepper Visual Skills for Reading test
peptide-binding groove
Peptococcus
Peptostreptococcus
perborate
    sodium p.
Percepta progressive lens
perceptible acuity
perception
    binocular depth p.
    blur p.
    color p.
    contrast threshold for motion p.
    (CTMP)
    depth p.
    p. dissociation
    dissociation of visual p.
    facial p.
    flicker p.
    form p.
    Frostig Development Test of
    Visual P.
    light p. (LP)
    p. of light (PL)
    limbus of p.
    monocular depth p.
    no light p. (NLP)
    shape p.
    simultaneous p.
    simultaneous foveal p. (SFP)
    simultaneous macular p. (SMP)
    stereoscopic depth p.
    visual p.
perceptual
    p. challenge
    p. phenomenon
perennial rhinoconjunctivitis
perfect
    P. Pupil dilator
    P. Pupil expansion device
PerfectCapsule
    P. irrigation device
    P. system
perfilcon A
perfluorocarbon
    p. coaxial I/A cannula
    p. gas
    liquid p.
    p. liquid
perfluorodecalin
perfluorohexyloctane
Perfluoron
perfluoro-N-octane (PFO)
perfluoropropane (C3F8)
    p. gas
perforans
    scleromalacia p.
perforating
    p. injury
    p. keratoplasty
perforation
    conjunctival p.
    corneal p.
    flap p.
    globe p.
    ocular p.
performance
    clinically viable methods maximum
      optimization of visual p.
    closed road driving p.
    distance visual p.
    night-driving p.
    optical p.
    peak visual p.
    predictive of visual p.
Performa surface process
perfringens
    Clostridium p.
perfusion
    capillary p.
    impaired p.
    juxtapapillary p.

NOTES

P

perfusion *(continued)*
>   luxury p.
>   retinal artery p.

PERG
>   pattern-evoked electroretinogram

Periactin

periaqueductal
>   p. gray matter
>   p. syndrome

periarteritis
>   p. nodosa (PAN, PN)
>   regional p.

peribulbar
>   p. administration
>   p. anesthesia
>   p. anesthesia-related diplopia
>   p. injection
>   p. needle

pericanalicular connective tissue

pericecal scotoma

pericentral
>   p. rod-cone dystrophy
>   p. scotoma

perichiasmal

perichoroidal, perichorioidal
>   p. space

perichoroideale
>   spatium p.

periconchitis

pericorneal plexus

pericyte
>   p. drop out
>   tissue-specific p.

peridectomy

perifascicular myofiber necrosis

perifoveal
>   p. arteriole
>   p. edema
>   p. posterior vitreous detachment
>   (PPVD)

perifoveolar

perihemangioma subretinal hemorrhage

perikeratic

perilenticular

perilimbal
>   p. conjunctival vessel
>   p. stroma
>   p. suction
>   p. suction cup
>   p. ulceration
>   p. vitiligo

perilimbic circulation

perimacular vasculature

perimeter
>   AccuMap multifocal objective p.
>   Allergan Humphrey p.
>   arc and bowl p.
>   automated hemisphere p.
>   Brombach p.

Canon p.
CooperVision imaging p.
p. corneal reflex test
Ferree-Rand p.
Goldmann manual projection p.
Henson CFS 2000 p.
Humphrey p.
Interzeag bowl p.
kinetic p.
Marco p.
Medmont M600 p.
Octopus 1-2-3 p.
Octopus 201 p.
Octopus 101 bowl p.
Ophthimus High-Pass Resolution p.
Ophthimus ring p.
Peritest p.
p. projection
projection p.
Schweigger hand p.
static p.
Topcon p.
Tübinger p.

perimetric

perimetry
>   achromatic automated p. (AAP)
>   Aimark p.
>   arc p.
>   automated static threshold p.
>   binocular p.
>   blue-yellow p.
>   chromatic p.
>   color p.
>   computed p.
>   computerized static p.
>   conjunctival p.
>   conventional p.
>   FDT p.
>   flicker p.
>   frequency doubling p.
>   Goldmann kinetic p.
>   hemisphere projection p.
>   high-pass resolution p. (HRP)
>   kinetic p.
>   luminance size threshold p.
>   manual kinetic p.
>   mesopic p.
>   motion automated p.
>   motion detection p.
>   motion and displacement p.
>   objective p.
>   Octopus automated p.
>   Octopus threshold p.
>   pattern discrimination p.
>   profile p.
>   quantitative threshold p.
>   resolution acuity p.
>   ring p.
>   scanning laser ophthalmoscope p.

scotopic p.
short wavelength automated p.
  (SWAP)
standard automated p. (SAP)
static automated achromatic p.
suprathreshold static p.
tangent p.
temporal modulation p.
tendency-oriented p. (TOP)
Tübinger p.
white-on-white p.

perineural cell
perineuritis
optic p.
syphilitic optic p.
perinuclear
p. antineutrophil cytoplasmic
  antibody (pANCA)
p. cataract
periocular
p. administration
p. basal cell cancer
p. depigmentation
p. drug sensitivity
p. ecchymosis
p. hemangioma
p. surgery
p. syndrome
p. trauma
p. triamcinolone injection
period
amblyogenic p.
blink-free p.
critical p.
effective refractory p. (ERP)
hypertension p.
neonatal p.
preoperative p.
periodic
p. acid-Schiff (PAS)
p. alternating gaze deviation
p. alternating windmill nystagmus
p. esotropia
p. exotropia
p. ophthalmia
p. paralysis
p. strabismus
perioperative complication
periophthalmic
periophthalmitis
perioptic
p. cerebrospinal fluid
p. hygroma

p. neuritis
p. sheath meningioma
p. subarachnoid space
perioptometry
periorbit
periorbital
p. cellulitis
p. edema
p. fat atrophy
p. hemangioma
p. leukoderma
p. membrane
p. volume augmentation
periosteum
orbital p.
periostitis
orbital p.
peripapillary
p. central serous choroidopathy
p. choroid
p. choroidal arterial system
p. choroidal atrophy
p. coloboma
p. nerve fiber layer
p. retinal height
p. retinal nerve
p. retinal nerve fiber
p. retinochoroidal layer
p. scar
p. sclerosis
p. scotoma
p. staphyloma
p. subretinal neovascularization
periphacitis, periphakitis
peripheral
p. anterior chamber
p. anterior synechia (PAS)
p. branch retinal vein occlusion
  (PBRVO)
p. cataract
p. chorioretinal atrophic spot
p. chorioretinal atrophy
p. corneal opacity
p. corneal thinning
p. corneal ulcer
p. corneal ulceration
p. curve on contact lens
p. cystoid degeneration
p. detection test
p. disciform degeneration
p. endotheliitis
p. fusion
p. glare

NOTES

P

peripheral *(continued)*
- p. glioma
- p. granuloma
- p. intraretinal hemorrhage
- p. iridectomy (PI)
- p. iridectomy operation
- p. iris roll
- p. leakage
- p. lesion
- p. light focusing
- p. light scatter
- p. multifocal chorioretinitis (PMC)
- p. myopia
- p. necrotizing retinitis
- p. neuropathy
- p. oculomotor nerve
- p. placement
- p. proliferation
- p. ray of light
- p. retina
- p. retinal ablation
- p. retinal atrophy
- p. retinal operculum
- p. retinal pigment dispersion
- p. retinal vascular sheathing
- p. ring infiltrate
- p. rod function
- p. schisis
- p. scotoma
- p. silvery gloss
- p. tapetochoroidal degeneration
- p. ulcerative keratitis (PUK)
- p. uveitis
- p. vestibular nystagmus
- p. vision
- p. visual field
- p. vitreoretinal traction

peripherin/RDS gene

periphery
- nasal p.
- posterior pole and p. (PP&P)

periphlebitis
- p. retinae
- retinal p.

periphoria
periradial mark
periretinal edema
periscleral space
periscleritis
perisclerotic
periscopic
- p. concave lens
- p. convex lens
- p. meniscus
- p. spectacles

perisellar
perisilicone proliferation
peristaltic pump
peristriate visual cortex

peritarsal network
peritectomy
Peritest perimeter
peritomize
peritomy
perivascular
- p. neutrophil infiltration
- p. sheathing
- p. stromal cell

perivasculitis
- retinal p.

periventricular lesion
PERK
- Prospective Evaluation of Radial Keratotomy
- PERK Study

Perkins
- P. applanation tonometer
- P. brailler

PERL
- pupils equal, react to light

PERLA
- pupils equal, reactive to light and accommodation

Perlia nucleus
Permaflex lens
Permalens lens
permanent
- p. deficit
- p. mydriasis

PermaVision intracorneal lens
permeability
- corneal epithelial p.
- endothelial p.
- oxygen p. (Dk)

permeable
permethrin
pernicious
- p. anemia
- p. myopia

Perone
- P. LASIK Flap Forceps
- P. LASIK marker

peroxide
- hydrogen p.

peroxisomal disorder
PERRLA
- pupils equal, round, reactive to light and accommodation

perseveration
- visual p.

persistence of vision
persistent
- p. anterior hyperplastic primary vitreous
- p. Bergmeister papilla
- p. epithelial defect
- p. fetal vasculature
- p. hyaloid artery

p. hyperplastic primary vitreous (PHPV)
p. hypertrophic primary vitreous (PHPV)
p. postdrainage hypotony (PPH)
p. posterior hyperplastic primary vitreous
p. postoperative inflammation
p. primary hyperplastic vitreous
p. pupillary membrane
p. pupillary membrane remnant
Personna steel blade
personnel
Joint Review Committee for Ophthalmic Medical P. (JRCOMP)
ophthalmic medical p. (OMP)
Perspex
P. CQ
P. CQ-Shearing-Simcoe-Sinskey lens
P. CQ UV PMMA
P. frame
P. rod
pertussis
Bordetella p.
perverted
p. nystagmus
p. ocular movement
petaloid
p. accumulation of fluid
p. pattern
Peters
P. anomaly
P. operation
Petit canal
Petriellidium boydii
petrificans
conjunctivitis p.
keratitis p.
petrolatum ophthalmic ointment
petroleum
white p.
petrosal nerve
petrous
p. apex
p. bone
p. ridge
Petrus single-mirror laser lens
Pettigrove
P. irrigation cannula
P. LASIK irrigating cannula
P. LASIK set
Petzetakis-Takos syndrome
Petzval surface

PEXG
pseudoexfoliative glaucoma
Peyman
P. full-thickness eye-wall resection
P. wide-field lens
Peyman-Green
P.-G. vitrectomy lens
P.-G. vitreous forceps
PFO
perfluoro-N-octane
PGC
pontine gaze center
PGTP
primary glaucoma triple procedure
PH
pinhole
phacitis
phaco
phacoemulsification
p. burst
P. Cavitron irrigating/aspirating unit
p. cleanup
p. efficiency
P. Emulsifier Cavitron unit
p. incision
p. sleeve
p. time
p. tip
p. trabeculectomy
Phaco-4 diamond step knife
phacoanaphylactic
p. endophthalmitis
p. uveitis
phacoanaphylaxis
phacoantigenic
p. endophthalmitis
p. uveitis
phacoaspiration
phacocele
phacochop technique
phacocyst
phacocystectomy
phacocystitis
phacodonesis
phacoemulsification, phakoemulsification (phaco)
anterior chamber p.
bare-needle p.
bimanual microincision p.
p. cautery
choo-choo chop and flip p.
clear corneal p.
endocapsular p.

NOTES

P

phacoemulsification *(continued)*
    endolenticular p.
    Er:YAG laser p.
    extracapsular p.
    1-handed p.
    2-handed p.
    p. handpiece
    high-vacuum p.
    Kelman p. (KPE)
    sclerocorneal p.
    small-incision p.
    p. system
phacoemulsifier
phacoemulsify
phacoerysis
phacoexcavator
PhacoFlex
    P. II SI30NB intraocular lens
    Single-Stitch P.
phacofracture ophthalmic instrument
phacofragmatome
phacofragmentation
phacogenic, phakogenic
    p. glaucoma
    p. uveitis
phacoglaucoma
phacohymenitis
phacoid
phacoiditis
phacoidoscope
Phacojack Phaco System
phacolase
    Er:YAG p.
phacolysin
phacolysis
    calcific p.
phacolytic, phakolytic
    p. glaucoma
    p. uveitis
phacoma
phacomalacia
phacomatosis
phacometachoresis
phacometer
phacomorphic, phakomorphic
    p. glaucoma
phacopalingenesis
phacosclerosis
phacoscope
phacoscopy
phacoscotasmus
phacotoxic uveitis
phagocytosed cellular debris
Phakan
phakia
Phakic
    P. 6 H2 IOL
    P. intraocular lens
    P. 6 lens

phakic
    p. cystoid macular edema
    p. dysphotopsia
    p. eye
    p. glaucoma
    p. IOL implantation
    p. posterior chamber
    p. pupillary block
phakic-aphakic (PA)
phakitis
phakoemulsification *(var. of* phacoemulsification)
phakofragmatome
    Girard p.
phakogenic *(var. of* phacogenic)
phakolytic *(var. of* phacolytic)
phakoma
phakomatosis
    Bourneville p.
phakomatous
    p. choristoma
    p. choristoma tumor
phakomorphic *(var. of* phacomorphic)
Phakonit nucleus division technique
phalangosis
phantom vision
pharmaceutical agent
Pharmacia
    P. corneal trephine
    P. intraocular lens
    P. Visco J-loop lens
pharmacological
    p. blockade
    p. dilation
pharmacologic manipulation
pharyngoconjunctival fever
phase
    ascent p.
    p. difference haloscope
    ultra-late p.
    uveitic p.
PHEMA
    poly(2-hydroxyethyl methacrylate)
    PHEMA core-and-skirt
      keratoprosthesis
    PHEMA KPro implantation
phemfilcon A
phenacaine hydrochloride
phenacetin
Phenazine
phenazopyridine
phencyclidine hydrochloride
Phendry Oral
phenelzine sulfate
Phenergan
phenethyl alcohol
phengophobia
phenindamine

pheniramine maleate and naphazoline HCl
phenmetrazine hydrochloride
phenobarbital sodium
phenolphthalein
phenomenon, pl. **phenomena**
    Alder-Reilly p.
    aqueous influx p.
    Ascher aqueous influx p.
    Ascher glass-rod p.
    Aschner p.
    Aubert p.
    autokinetic visible light p.
    Becker p.
    Bell p.
    Bezold-Brücke p.
    Bielschowsky head-tilt p.
    blood-influx p.
    blue field entoptic p.
    break p.
    breakup p.
    Brücke-Bartley p.
    click p.
    crowding p.
    doll's head p.
    entoptic p.
    escape p.
    extinction p.
    fatigue p.
    Fick p.
    flicker p.
    Flynn p.
    Galassi pupillary p.
    Gartner p.
    glass-rod negative p.
    glass-rod positive p.
    Gunn jaw-winking p.
    halo p.
    hemifield slide p.
    Hertwig-Magendie p.
    interface phenomena
    jack-in-the-box p.
    jaw-winking p.
    Koebner p.
    laser speckle p.
    Le Grand-Geblewics p.
    Marcus Gunn jaw-winking p.
    misdirection p.
    Mitsuo p.
    Mizuo-Nakamura p.
    negative visual p.
    orbicularis p.
    paradoxical pupillary p.
    paradoxic pupillary p.
    perceptual p.
    phi p.
    Piltz-Westphal p.
    positive visual p.
    prostaglandin-mediated p.
    pseudo-Graefe p.
    Pulfrich stereo p.
    Purkinje p.
    Riddoch p.
    Schlieren p.
    setting-sun p.
    shot-silk p.
    Splendore-Hoeppli p.
    Tournay p.
    Tullio p.
    Tyndall p.
    Uhthoff p.
    Westphal p.
    Westphal-Piltz p.
    wipe-out p.
    wound healing p.
Phenoptic
phenothiazine
    p. keratopathy
    p. toxicity
phenoxybenzamine hydrochloride
phenylephrine
    p. hydrochloride
    sulfacetamide p.
phenylmercuric
    p. acetate
    p. nitrate
phenylpropanolamine hydrochloride
Phialophora
Philadelphia
    Wills Eye Hospital/Children's Hospital of P. (WEH/CHOP)
Phillips
    P. fixation forceps
    P. gravity pivot axis marker
phimosis
    capsular p.
phi phenomenon
phlebitis
    retinal p.
phlebophthalmotomy
phlebosclerosis
phlegmatous conjunctivitis
phlegmonous dacryocystitis
phlorhizin diabetes
phlyctenar
phlyctenula

NOTES

P

phlyctenular
    p. conjunctivitis
    p. keratitis
    p. keratoconjunctivitis
    p. pannus
phlyctenule
    conjunctival p.
    corneal p.
phlyctenulosis
    allergic p.
    conjunctival p.
    corneal p.
    tuberculous p.
PHM
    posterior hyaloid membrane
PHNI
    pinhole no improvement
phocomelia
    Roberts-SC p.
phoria
    basal p.
    decompensated p.
    far p.
    lateral p.
    monofixational p.
    near p.
    near-point p.
    vertical p.
phoriascope
phorometer
phorometry
phoro-optometer
Phoroptor
    P. retractor
    Ultramatic Rx Master P.
    P. vision tester
phoroscope
phorotone
phosphate
    Aralen P.
    dexamethasone sodium p.
    p. diabetes
    disodium hydrogen p.
    ganciclovir cyclic p.
    Hexadrol P.
    Hydrocortone P.
    naphazoline and antazoline p.
    potassium p.
    prednisolone sodium p.
    sodium p.
phosphate-buffered saline
phosphene
phospholine
    echothiophate p.
    P. Iodide
    P. Iodide Ophthalmic
phosphonoformic acid
phosphoric acid
photalgia

photerythrous
photesthesia
photic
    p. maculopathy
    p. retinal toxicity
photo
    fundus p. (FP)
    p. screening
photoablation
    excimer laser transepithelial p.
    stromal p.
    transepithelial p.
photoablative laser goniotomy (PLG)
photoastigmatic refractive keratectomy (PARK)
photoceptor
photochemical
    p. process
    p. visual pigment
photochemistry
photochromic
    p. lens
    p. spectacles
photocoagulation
    argon laser p.
    dye-enhanced p.
    ETDRS laser p.
    focal laser p.
    grid laser p. (GLP)
    indirect ophthalmoscopic laser p.
    krypton p.
    p. laser
    laser panretinal p.
    macular laser grid p.
    panretinal argon laser p.
    panretinal scatter p.
    retinal laser p.
    retinal scatter p.
    scatter laser p.
    subthreshold subfoveal diode laser p. (SSDLP)
    p. therapy
    transscleral retinal p.
    xenon arc p.
photocoagulator
    Coherent p.
    continuous-wave p.
    EyeLite p.
    green laser light p.
    Iolab I&A p.
    Iolab irrigating/aspirating p.
    laser p.
    Mira p.
    532nm Green laser p.
    Novus Omni 2000 p.
    OcuLight GL p.
    OcuLight GL/GLx green laser p.
    OcuLight GLx green laser p.
    Ophthalas p.

PASCAL p.
semiconductor GaAIAs infrared
    diode laser p.
Ultima 2000 p.
Viridis Lite p.
xenon arc p.
Zeiss p.
photodisrupting laser
photodisruptor
Aura Nd:YAG p.
photodynamic therapy (PDT)
photodynia
photodysphoria
photoelasticity
photoelectric oculography
photofrin
photogene
photograph
color fundus p.
endothelial p.
fundus p.
p. reading analysis
red free p.
stereoscopic fundus p.
photographer
Tearscope Plus p.
photography
central endothelial p.
cross-polarization p.
fluorescence retinal p.
Miyake p.
nonmydriatic retinal p.
red-free p.
retinal p.
Scheimpflug p.
slitlamp p.
ultraviolet fluorescence p.
photogray lens
photokeratitis
photokeratopathy
photokeratoscope
Allergan Humphrey p.
Allergan Medical Optics p.
computerized p.
CooperVision refractive surgery p.
Corneascope 9-ring p.
Tomey TMS-1 p.
photokeratoscopy
digital subtraction p.
photolysis
Dodick p.
photometer
Bunsen grease spot p.

flame p.
flicker p.
Förster p.
Kowa laser flare p.
Kowa laser flare-cell p.
Minolta LS 110 spot p.
Spectra-Pritchard 1980-PR p.
photometry
heterochromatic flicker p.
laser flare p.
laser flare-cell p.
motion p.
photon
P. cataract removal system
p. cloud
p. laser
P. Laser Phacolysis Probe
P. Ocular Surgery System
photonic
photophobia
psychogenic p.
photophobic
photophthalmia
photopia
photopic
p. adaptation
p. ERG
p. eye
p. illumination
p. vision
photopigment
cone p.
PhotoPoint
P. laser
P. laser therapy
P. treatment
photoprotection
retinal p.
photopsia, photopsy
transient p.
photopsin
photoptarmosis
photoptometer
Förster p.
photoptometry
photoreception
photoreceptive
photoreceptor
p. cell
p. degeneration
p. dysfunction
p. layer
p. preservation

NOTES

P

photoreceptor *(continued)*
    rod p.
    p. transplantation
    p. transplantation ineffective
      alternative
photoreceptor-bipolar synapse
photorefraction
    eccentric p.
photorefractive
    p. astigmatic keratectomy
    p. keratectomy (PRK)
    p. keratoplasty (PRK)
    p. surgery
photoretinitis
photoretinopathy
photoscopy
photoscreener
    iScreen p.
    MTI p.
    p. pediatric camera
photoscreening
photosensitive lens
photosensitivity
photosensitization
photosensitizer
photosensitizing drug
photosensor oculography
Photoshop 6.0 digitized imager
photostress
    macular p.
    p. recovery time (PRT)
    p. test
photosun lens
phototherapeutic keratectomy (PTK)
phototherapy
photothermolysis
    selective p.
Phototome System 2700
phototonus
phototoxic
    p. lesion
    p. maculopathy
phototoxicity
    blue-green photic p.
phototransduction cascade
photovaporation laser
photovaporization
photovaporizing laser
Photrex
PHPV
    persistent hyperplastic primary vitreous
    persistent hypertrophic primary vitreous
phthalocyanine
phthiriasis palpebrarum
phthiriatica
    blepharitis p.
Phthirus pubis
phthisical eye

phthisis
    p. bulbi
    essential p.
    ocular p.
phycomycosis
    cerebral p.
phylloquinone (K)
physical
    p. finding
    p. manipulation
    p. optics
physician
    Fellow of the Royal College
    of P.'s (FRCP)
physiologic
    p. anisocoria
    p. astigmatism
    p. blind spot
    p. cup
    p. excavation
    p. myopia
    p. nystagmus
    p. optic nerve cupping
    p. optics
    p. retina
    p. scotoma
physostigmine
    pilocarpine and p.
    p. and pilocarpine
    p. salicylate
    p. sulfate
phytohemagglutinin cell
PI
    peripheral iridectomy
pial
    p. arterial plexus
    p. sheath
    p. system
PIC
    punctate inner choroidopathy
pick
    Burch p.
    45-degree scissor with
      membrane p.
    Desmarres fixation p.
    fiberoptic p.
    fixation p.
    light pipe p.
    Michel p.
    Olk vitreoretinal p.
    P. retinitis
    Rice p.
    scleral p.
    P. sign
    Sinskey p.
    Synergetics Awh serrated p.
    P. vision
Pickford-Nicholson anomaloscope

pickup
> Shoch foreign body p.
> p. spatula suture

pi cone monochromatism

pictograph

picture
> p. chart
> p. naming
> p. optotype

piebald eyelash

piece
> preformed p.

1-piece
> 1-p. bifocal
> 1-p. hydrophilic acrylic IOL
> 1-p. multifocal lens
> 1-p. plate haptic silicone
>   intraocular lens

3-piece
> 3-p. acrylic intraocular lens
> 3-p. hydrophilic acrylic IOL
> 3-p. hydrophobic acrylic Sensar
>   lens
> 3-p. monofocal silicone lens
> 3-p. plate haptic intraocular lens
> 3-p. silicone intraocular lens

pie-in-the-sky
> p.-i.-t.-s. defect
> p.-i.-t.-s. quadrantanopia

pie-on-the-floor
> p.-o.-t.-f. defect
> p.-o.-t.-f. quadrantanopia

Pierre-Marie ataxia

Pierre Robin syndrome

Pierse
> P. corneal Colibri-type forceps
> P. eye speculum
> P. fixation forceps

Pierse-type Colibri forceps

piezoelectric transducer technique

piezometer

piggyback
> p. contact lens
> p. graft
> p. implant
> p. implantation
> p. intraocular lens
> p. probe

piggybacked toric IOL

pigment
> p. atrophy
> p. cell
> p. change

> clumped retinal p.
> p. clumping
> p. demarcation line
> p. deposit
> p. deposition
> p. derangement
> discoloration of p.
> p. dispersion
> p. dispersion syndrome (PDS)
> p. epithelial detachment (PED)
> p. epithelial detachment
>   maculopathy
> p. epithelial dystrophy
> p. epithelial endoscopic laser
>   surgery (PEELS)
> p. epithelial hypertrophy
> p. epitheliitis
> epitheliitis focal retinal p.
> p. epitheliopathy
> p. epithelium (PE)
> p. epithelium-derived factor (PEDF)
> p. floater
> gold tattoo p.
> p. granule
> p. layer
> p. layer ectropion
> macula lutea p.
> p. mottling
> photochemical visual p.
> placoid p.
> platinum tattoo p.
> p. precipitate
> p. seam
> silver tattoo p.
> tattoo p.
> trabecular membrane p.
> unwanted migration of p.
> visual p.
> white p.
> xanthophyll p.

pigmentary
> p. deposits on lens
> p. dilution
> p. dispersion glaucoma
> p. dispersion syndrome
> p. dropout
> p. halo
> p. migration
> p. perivenous chorioretinal
>   degeneration
> p. rarefaction and clumping
> p. retinopathy

NOTES

P

pigmentation
>clumped p.
>congenital optic disc p.
>hematogenous p.
>Hudson-Stähli line of corneal p.
>mid peripheral mottling p.
>nevus p.
>ocular fundus p.
>orange punctate p.
>p. rarefaction

pigmented
>p. chorioretinal scar
>p. conjunctival lesion
>p. epithelium of iris
>p. keratic precipitate
>p. layer of ciliary body
>p. layer of eyeball
>p. layer of iris
>p. layer of retina
>p. lesion
>p. line of cornea
>p. macular pucker
>p. paravenous chorioretinal atrophy
>p. paravenous retinochoroidal atrophy
>p. preretinal membrane
>p. stroma
>p. trabecular meshwork cell
>p. veil

pigmenti
>incontinentia p.

pigmento
>retinitis pigmentosa sine p.

pigmentosa
>autosomal dominant retinitis p.
>pseudoretinitis p.
>retinitis p. (RP)
>RP10 gene variant of retinitis p.
>sector retinitis p.
>X-linked retinitis p. (XLRP)

pigmentosum
>conjunctivitis xeroderma p.
>xeroderma p.

pigmentum nigrum
pigtail
>p. fixation
>p. probe

Pilagan Ophthalmic
PilaSite
Pillat dystrophy
pillow
>Richard p.

Pilo-20, -40
>Ocusert P.-20, -40

Pilocar Ophthalmic
pilocarpine
>epinephrine and p.
>p. and epinephrine
>p. HCl

>p. nitrate
>p. and physostigmine
>physostigmine and p.
>p. test
>timolol and p.
>p. and timolol maleate

Pilocel
pilocytic astrocytoma
Pilofrin
Pilokair Ophthalmic
pilomatrixoma tumor
Pilomiotin
Pilopine
>P. HS
>P. HS gel
>P. HS Ophthalmic

Piloptic Ophthalmic
Pilopto-Carpine
Pilostat Ophthalmic
pilot application
Piltz sign
Piltz-Westphal phenomenon
pimaricin
pimelopterygium
pin
>Walker micro p.

pince-nez
pincushion distortion
pineal
>p. blastoma
>p. eye
>p. gland

pinealoblastoma
pinealoma
Pineda LASIK Flap Iron
ping-pong gaze
pinguecula, pinguicula, pl. **pingueculae**
>inflamed p.

pinhole (PH)
>p. accommodation
>p. disc
>p. and dominance test
>p. goggles
>p. no improvement (PHNI)
>no improvement with p. (NIPH)
>p. occluder
>potential acuity p.
>p. pupil
>p. vision

pink
>sharp and p. (S&P)

pinkeye
>p. conjunctivitis
>p. disc

pinky ball
pinocytotic vesicle
pinpoint
>p. leak
>p. pupil

piokutanin pen
PION
posterior ischemic optic neuropathy
pipe
effusion light p.
flute p.
infusion light p.
light p.
p. light
Millennium TSV25 light p.
piperacillin
piperazine
piperocaine hydrochloride
pirenzepine ophthalmic gel
piroxicam
pisciform cataract
pit
congenital optic nerve p.
foveal p.
Herbert peripheral p.
iris p.
lens p.
optic disc p.
optic nerve p.
orbital p.
temporal p.
pituitarigenic
p. oculopathy
pituitary
p. ablation
p. adenoma
apoplexy of p.
p. apoplexy
p. body
p. gland
p. tumor
Pityrosporum
P. orbiculare
P. ovale
pivot point
pixel
PK
penetrating keratoplasty
PKC
protein kinase C
PKP
penetrating keratoplasty
PKPG
penetrating keratoplasty and glaucoma
PL
perception of light
placebo eye drops

placement
implant p.
left bi-plate p.
peripheral p.
right bi-plate p.
Placido
P. da Costa disc
P. ring
Placido-based axial curvature mapping
Placido-disc videokeratoscopy system
placode
lens p.
p. lens
placoid
p. pigment
p. pigmentation of epithelium
p. pigment epitheliopathy
pladaroma, pladarosis
plagiocephaly
ocular p.
plain
p. catgut suture
p. collagen suture
p. film
p. film radiography
p. gut suture
Isopto P.
plaited frill
plan
dominant action p.
treatment p.
plana
cornea p.
pars p.
trans pars p.
plane
Broca visual p.
Daubenton p.
Descemet p.
equivalent refracting p.
eye/ear p.
Frankfort horizontal p.
horizontal p.
image p.
p. of incidence
lens p.
Listing p.
nodal p.
orbital p.
p. parallel plate
principal p.
pupillary p.
p. of regard

NOTES

P

plane *(continued)*
 spectacle p.
 unity conjugacy p.'s
 vertical p.
 visual p.
1-plane lens
2-plane lens
plane-surface refraction
Plange spud
planitis
 cyclitis in pars p.
 pars p.
planned
 p. comparison test
 p. extracapsular cataract extraction
planner
 Visx refractive p.
planoconcave lens
planoconvex nonridge lens
planoconvex-shaped disc
Planoscan treatment system
Plano T lens
plant
 stereoscopic depth p.
planum
 p. orbitale
 os p.
 xanthoma p.
planus
 paraneoplastic lichen p.
plaque
 adherent p.
 avascular p.
 p. brachytherapy
 brachytherapy episcleral p.
 cholesterol p.
 cobalt-60 eye p.
 delayed mucous p.
 demyelinating p.
 endothelial p.
 episcleral eye p.
 eye p.
 eyelid p.
 gold eye p.
 gray p.
 Hollenhorst p.
 hyaline p.
 hyperkeratotic p.
 p. keratopathy
 nonconfluent p.
 preretinal p.
 radioactive eye p.
 p. radiotherapy
 red scaly p.
 ruthenium p.
 ruthenium-106 ophthalmic p.
 scaly p.
 subcapsular p.
 subepithelial p.

 subretinal pigment epithelial p.
 vascularized p.
plaque-type psoriasis
plasma
 p. blade
 p. cell
 p. cell tumor
 p. cloud
plasmacytoid infiltrate
plasmin
plasminogen
 p. activator
 p. activator inhibitor (PAI)
 tissue p.
plasmoid
 p. agglutination
 p. aqueous
 p. aqueous humor
plastic
 p. bifocal
 p. cyclitis
 p. disposable irrigating vectis
 p. eye shield
 p. frame
 p. iritis
 p. lens
 p. prism
 p. repair of eyelid
 p. sphere implant
plasticity
 neuronal p.
plate
 American Optical Hardy-Rand-
  Rittler color p.
 depth p.
 embryonic p.
 Gelfilm p.
 Hardy-Rand-Ritter color vision p.
 Hardy-Rand-Ritter
  pseudoisochromatic p.
 Hardy-Rand-Ritter screening p.
 HRR p.
 interchangeable p.
 Ishihara color p.
 Ishihara pseudoisochromatic p.
 isochromatic p.
 Jaeger lid p.
 lid p.
 non-valve p.
 nutrient agar p.
 Okuma p.
 plane parallel p.
 pseudoisochromatic color p.
 reticular p.
 scar p.
 Silastic p.
 Stahl caliper p.
 standard pseudoisochromatic p.
  (SPP)

standard pseudoisochromatic p. part
2 (SPP2)
Stilling p.
Storz lid p.
tarsal p.
Teflon p.
Thayer-Martin p.
plateau
cataract extraction p.
p. iris
p. iris configuration
p. iris syndrome
Plateau-Talbot law
plate-haptic
p.-h. intraocular lens
p.-h. IOL
p.-h. silicone lens
platelet-derived
p.-d. growth factor
p.-d. growth factor-B
platform
Alfonso cutting p.
LADARVision P.
Selecta 1064 laser p.
Platina
P. clip
P. clip lens
platinum
p. probe spatula
p. tattoo pigment
platymorphia
platysmal reflex
pledget
cotton p.
pleomorphic
p. adenoma
p. spindle cell tumor
pleoptic exercise
pleoptics
Bangerter method of p.
Cüppers method of p.
pleoptophor
plethysmographic goggles
plethysmography
plexiform
p. external layer
p. inner layer
p. internal layer
p. neurofibroma
p. neuroma
p. outer layer
Plexiglas
P. frame

P. implant
P. tube
plexus, pl. **plexus, plexuses**
angular aqueous sinus p.
anular p.
capillary p.
ciliary ganglionic p.
epithelial nerve p.
Hovius p.
intraepithelial p.
intrascleral p.
ophthalmic p.
pericorneal p.
pial arterial p.
scleral p.
stroma p.
subepithelial p.
sympathetic carotid p.
vascular p.
Pley extracapsular forceps
PLG
photoablative laser goniotomy
Pliagel
plica, pl. **plicae**
p. ciliaris
p. lacrimalis
p. lunata
p. semilunaris
p. semilunaris conjunctivae
plicata
pars p.
plication
retractor p.
Plitz reflex
plot
Bland-Altman p.
box-and-whisker p.
plug
p. anchorage
arrow-shaft silicone punctal p.
blue opaque Herrick lacrimal p.
brass scleral p.
capsular p.
collagen p.
EaglePlug tapered-shaft punctum p.
EagleVision Freeman punctum p.
epithelial p.
Extend punctal p.
FCI Ready-Set punctal p.
Form Fit intracanalicular p.
Freeman punctum p.
Herrick lacrimal p.
intracanalicular punctum p.

NOTES

P

plug *(continued)*
> p. loss
> Micro punctum p.
> Oasis Collagen P.
> opaque canalicular p.
> opaque Herrick lacrimal p.
> punctal p.
> punctum p.
> Ready-Set punctum p.
> Sharpoint UltraPlug punctum p.
> silicone punctal p.
> Smart Plug lacrimal p.
> Soft Plug punctal p.
> Super punctum p.
> tapered-shaft punctum p.
> TearSaver punctum p.
> Tears Naturale silicone punctum p.
> Teflon p.
> umbrella punctum p.
> Xsorb punctal p.

plugging
> follicular p.

plumes
> corneal ablation p.

plunger-type injector

plus
> Amvisc P.
> BSS P.
> p. cyclophoria
> p. disease
> Duramist P.
> Econopred P.
> ICaps P.
> Lens P.
> p. lens
> Murine Tears P.
> P. punctal occluder
> Refresh P.
> p. spectacle lens
> Tears P.
> Unisol P.
> Wet-N-Soak P.

Plus-Allergan
> Lens P.-A.

plus-minus syndrome

PMC
> peripheral multifocal chorioretinitis

PMMA
> polymethyl methacrylate
> Blue core PMMA
> PMMA custom-made calibration
> contact lens
> PMMA haptics
> Perspex CQ UV PMMA

PN
> periarteritis nodosa

PNET
> primitive neuroectodermal tumor

pneumatic
> p. displacement procedure
> p. retinopathy
> p. retinopexy
> p. tonometer
> p. trabeculoplasty
> p. vitrectomy

pneumatically stented implant (PSI)

pneumatonograph
> Alcon applanation p.

pneumatonometer
> Micro One p.
> Modular One p.

pneumococcal
> p. bacillus
> p. conjunctivitis
> p. endophthalmitis
> p. ulcer

pneumococcal/suppurative keratitis

pneumococcus ulcer

Pneumocystis
> *P. carinii*
> *P. carinii* choroidopathy
> *P. carinii* pneumonia

pneumoencephalography

pneumonia
> *Pneumocystis carinii* p.

pneumoniae
> *Klebsiella p.*
> *Streptococcus p.*

pneumotomography

pneumotonometer

pneumotonometry

POAG
> primary open-angle glaucoma

pocket
> corneal p.
> detachment p.
> p. operation
> p. red filter
> P. Starter device
> stromal p.

pocketing hook

POH
> past ocular history

POHS
> presumed ocular histoplasmosis
> syndrome

poikiloderma
> p. atrophicans and cataract
> p. congenitale
> infantile p. subgroup 1-2-3

point
> anterior focal p.
> axial p.
> p. of basal convergence (PBC,
> PcB)
> blur p.
> break p.

cardinal p.
central yellow p.
congruent p.
conjugate p.
p. of convergence
convergence p.
correspondence p.
corresponding retinal p.
diathermy p.
disparate retinal p.
p. of dispersion
p. of divergence
eye p.
far p.
fixation p.
p. of fixation
fixed p.
focal image p.
identical p.
image p.
incident p.
lacrimal p.
p. leak
lustrous central yellow p.
p. mutation
near p.
near visual p. (NVP)
neutral p.
nodal p.
null p.
optical nodal p.
pivot p.
posterior focal p.
principal p.
p. of regard
restoration p.
retinal p.
secondary focal p.
p. source
sphere end p.
p. spread function (PSF)
stereo-identical p.
supraorbital p.
p. system test type
virtual p.
visual p.
yellow p.
pointed cystotome tip
4-point fixation
The Pointing Game
point-of-purchase display
3-point touch
Poiseuille law

poisoning degenerative cataract
Polack keratoscope
Poladex
polar
p. bear tracks
p. cataract
Polaramine
polarimeter
confocal scanning laser p.
GDx Access scanning laser p.
GDx VCC scanning laser p.
scanning laser p.
polarimetry
confocal scanning laser p.
laser p.
scanning laser p. (SLP)
polariscope
polariscopic
polariscopy
polarization
angle of p.
polarization-sensitive imaging
polarize
polarized
p. lens
p. light
polarizer
polarizing
p. lens
p. ophthalmoscope
Polaroid
P. 3D Vectograph test
P. filter
P. vectograph slide
Polaron sputter coater
pole
anterior p.
inferior p.
posterior p.
superior p.
pol gene
polioencephalitis
superior p.
poliosis
canities p.
ciliary p.
polisher
capsule p.
Drews capsule p.
felt disc p.
Gills-Welsh capsule p.
Holladay posterior capsule p.
Knolle capsule p.

NOTES

P

polisher *(continued)*
        Kraff capsule p.
        Kratz capsule p.
        Look capsule p.
        microloop curette p.
        olive tip capsule p.
        squeegee capsule p.
        Terry silicone capsule p.
        Yaghouti LASIK p.
polisher/scratcher
        Jensen p./s.
        Kratz p./s.
polishing
        capsule p.
        diamond-bur p.
        posterior capsular p.
Polle pod attachment for ophthalmoscope
Pollock
        P. forceps
        P. punch
Polocaine
        P. MPF
poloxamer 282, 407
polus
        p. anterior bulbi oculi
        p. anterior lentis
        p. posterior bulbi oculi
        p. posterior lentis
polyacrylamide
polyaminopropyl biguanide
polyarteritis nodosa
polycarbonate
        p. ballistic protective eyewear
        p. lens
polychondritis
        atrophic p.
        relapsing p.
polychromatic
        p. light
        p. luster
Polycin-B Ointment
Polycon I, II contact lens
polycoria vera
Polydek suture
Poly-Dex Suspension
polydimethylsiloxane
polydystrophy
        pseudo-Hurler p.
polyester suture
polyethylene
        p. glycol
        p. implant
        p. T-tube
        p. tube
polygenic inheritance
polyglactin 910 suture
polyglycolate suture
polyglycolic acid suture

polygonal
        p. pigmented cell
        p. stromal opacification
polyhedral cell
polyhexamethylene biguanide
poly(2-hydroxyethyl methacrylate) (PHEMA)
Polymacon lens
polymegethism
polymerase
        p. chain reaction (PCR)
        p. chain reaction-sequence specific oligonucleotide probe (PCR-SSOP)
polymer ring
polymethyl
        p. methacrylate (PMMA)
        p. methacrylate contact lens
polymorphic
        p. cataract
        p. microsatellite marker
        p. superficial keratitis
polymorphism
        apolipoprotein E gene p.
        corneal endothelial p.
        single-stranded conformation p.
polymorphonuclear
        p. reaction
        p. response
polymorphous dystrophy
Polymox
polymyositis
        orbital p.
polymyxin
        p. B
        p. B sulfate
        p. B and Terramycin
        p. E
        oxytetracycline and p. B
        trimethoprim and p. B
polynomial
        Zernike p.
polyopia, polyopsia
        binocular p.
        cerebral p.
        p. monophthalmica
polyopy
polyoxyl 40 stearate
polyphaga
        Acanthamoeba p.
polypoidal choroidal vasculopathy (PCV)
Poly-Pred Ophthalmic Suspension
polypropylene suture
polypseudophakia
Polyquad
polyquaternium
polysorbate 20, 80
Polysporin Ophthalmic
polystichia
polytetrafluoroethylene (PTFE)

expanded p. (ePTFE)
p. suture
polytome x-ray
Polytracin
polytrichosis
Polytrim Ophthalmic
polyunsaturated fatty acid (PUFA)
polyurethane dilator
polyvinyl alcohol (PVA)
polyvinylpyrrolidone
pons lesion
pontine
p. gaze center (PGC)
p. lesion
Pontocaine Eye
pontomesencephalic dysfunction
pool
tear p.
pooling
p. of dye
fluorescein p.
poorly
p. controlled diabetes
p. demarcated lesion
poor vision from birth
population
geriatric p.
porcine eye
porcupine lymphoma
Porex implant
PORN
progressive outer retinal necrosis
porofocon
porous
p. hydroxyapatite sphere
p. orbital implant
port
butterfly needle infusion p.
Gills-Welsh guillotine p.
graduated side p.
left p.
right p.
sclerotomy p.
self-sealing side p.
side p.
p. vitrectomy
portable
p. device
p. PT100 noncontact tonometer
3-port pars plana vitrectomy
porus opticus
position
p. accommodation

p. ametropia
bipolar electrode p.
cardinal p.
convergence p.
p. cyclophoria
dissociated p.
p. error
eyelid p.
p. eyepiece
face-down p.
flap p.
fusion-free p.
heterophoric p.
IOL p.
Listing primary p.
midline p.
oblique p.
o'clock p.
1–12 o'clock p.
primary p.
Rhese p.
p. scotoma
secondary p.
sulcus fixated p.
tertiary p.
vertical divergence p.
positional
p. abnormality of retina
p. nystagmus
positioner
irrigating IOL p.
positive
p. accommodation
p. afterimage
p. contrast orbitography
p. convergence
cyclophoria p.
p. dysphotopsia
p. eyepiece
false p.
p. meniscus
p. meniscus lens
p. predictive value
p. scotoma
p. spherical aberration
p. vertical divergence
p. visual phenomenon
positive-angle kappa
Posner
P. diagnostic gonioprism
P. diagnostic lens
P. slit lamp
P. surgical gonioprism

NOTES

P

Posner-Schlossman syndrome
post
    p. chamber
    p. enucleation socket syndrome
    p. scrape
postbasic stare
postcanalicular system
postcataract
    p. bleb
    p. endophthalmitis
    p. pediatric glaucoma
postconceptual age
postequatorial retina
posterior
    p. amorphous corneal dysgenesis
    p. amorphous corneal dystrophy
    p. angle
    p. apical radius (PAR)
    p. blepharitis
    camera oculi p.
    p. capsular opacification
    p. capsular polishing
    p. capsular zonular barrier
    p. capsular zonular disruption
    p. capsule opacification (PCO)
    p. capsule opacification software
    p. capsule opening
    p. capsulotomy
    p. central curve
    p. cerebral artery
    p. chamber (PC)
    p. chamber intraocular lens
      (PCIOL, PC-IOL)
    p. chamber lens implant (PCLI)
    p. chiasmatic commissure
    p. choroiditis
    p. ciliary artery
    p. ciliary vein
    p. collagenous layer (PCL)
    p. conical cornea
    p. conjunctival artery
    p. conjunctival vein
    p. corneal curvature
    p. corneal defect
    p. corneal deposit (PCD)
    p. corneal depression
    p. corneal tissue
    p. discission
    p. dislocation
    p. embryotoxon
    p. epithelium of cornea
    p. ethmoidal artery (PEA)
    p. explant
    p. fixation suture
    p. focal point
    p. fossa nerve decompression
    p. hyaloid
    p. hyaloid membrane (PHM)
    p. hyaloid traction

    p. hydrophthalmia
    p. incision
    p. inferior cerebellar artery
      syndrome
    p. intermediate curve
    p. internuclear ophthalmoplegia
    p. ischemic optic neuropathy
      (PION)
    p. keratoconus
    p. lamellar disc
    p. lamellar keratoplasty
    lamina elastica p.
    p. lamina raphe
    p. lens cell
    p. lenticonus
    p. limiting lamina
    p. limiting ring
    membrana capsularis lentis p.
    p. microphthalmia
    ophthalmomyiasis interna p. (OIP)
    p. optical zone (POZ)
    p. peribulbar block
    p. peripheral curve (PPC)
    p. pigment epitheliopathy
    p. pituitary ectopia
    p. polar cataract
    p. pole
    p. pole of eye
    p. pole of eyeball
    p. pole granuloma
    p. pole of lens
    p. pole and periphery (PP&P)
    p. polymorphic dystrophy (of
      cornea) (PPMD)
    p. polymorphous corneal dystrophy
    p. scleral cartilage
    p. scleritis
    sclerochoroiditis p.
    p. sclerochoroiditis
    p. sclerotomy
    p. segment
    p. segment of eye
    p. staphyloma
    p. subcapsular cataract (PSC)
    p. subcapsular opacity
    p. sub-Tenon injection
    p. supine position capsular opacity
    p. surface of lens
    p. symblepharon
    p. synechia
    p. thermal sclerostomy
    p. toric
    p. tube shunt implant
    p. uveal melanoma
    p. uveitis
    p. visual pathway imaging
    p. vitrectomy
    p. vitreous
    p. vitreous detachment (PVD)

p. vitreous finding
p. vitreous findings in spontaneous
retinal reattachment
postganglionic
p. fiber
p. fiber regeneration
p. Horner syndrome
p. short ciliary nerve
**postgeniculate congenital homonymous
hemianopsia**
postherpetic
p. headache
p. neuralgia
posticum
staphyloma p.
postinfectious epithelial keratopathy
postinflammatory
p. atrophy
p. cataract
postinjection
p. infectious endophthalmitis
p. sterile endophthalmitis
postkeratoplasty
post-LASIK ectasia
postlensectomy
postlens tear film
postmarital amblyopia
postocclusion
p. measurement
p. surge
postocular neuritis
postoperative
p. aberrometry
p. adjustment
p. amblyopia
p. anterior uveitis
p. antibiotic
p. aphakic glaucoma
p. betamethasone
p. blindness
p. ciprofloxacin
p. complication
p. corticosteroid
p. diclofenac
p. endophthalmitis
p. flat anterior chamber
p. ghost cell glaucoma
p. hyphema
p. hypotony
p. inflammation
p. iritis
p. irregular astigmatism
p. medication

p. mydriasis
p. pain
p. sequela
p. steroid
p. topical anesthetic
p. treatment
p. vision quality
p. visual acuity
postorbital
postpapilledema atrophy
postplaced suture
postsaccadic drift
postsurgical hyphema
**postsynaptic congenital myasthenic
disorder**
posttraumatic
p. accommodative spasm
p. endophthalmitis
p. headache
p. iridocyclitis
postural exophthalmos
posture
abnormal head p.
head p.
postvaccination optic neuritis
postvitrectomy
p. cataract
p. fibrin
Posurdex
potassium
p. acetate
p. bicarbonate
p. borate
p. chloride (KOH)
p. citrate
p. hydroxide
p. iodide
pemirolast p.
p. phosphate
p. tetraborate
potassium-titanyl-phosphate (KTP)
potential
p. acuity meter (PAM)
p. acuity pinhole
compound muscle action p.
(CMAP)
early receptor p.
evoked p.
flash visual-evoked p. (fVEP)
multifocal visual evoked p.
(mVEP)
oscillatory p. (OP)
receptor p.

NOTES

P

potential *(continued)*
    S p.
    p. visual acuity
    visual-evoked p. (VEP)
    visual-evoked cortical p. (VECP)
POTF
    preocular tear film
Potter-Bucky diaphragm
Potter syndrome
pouch
    Rathke p.
Pourcelot ratio
pouting
    erythematous p.
povidone-iodine preparation
Powell wand
power
    add p.
    back vertex p. (BVP)
    bending p.
    p. calculation
    contact lens vertex p.
    dioptric p.
    equivalent p.
    front vertex p.
    incorrect lens p.
    intraocular lens p. (IOLP)
    IOL p.
    keratometric p. (KP)
    lacrimal p.
    lens p.
    magnifying p.
    mean corneal p.
    p. of mirror
    p. modulation technology
    on-eye predicted p.
    P. operation
    optical p.
    Prentice position p.
    radiant p.
    refractive p.
    resolving p.
    topographic simulated
      keratometric p. (TOPO)
    p. vergence
    vertex of p.
    zero optical p.
POZ
    posterior optical zone
PP
    punctum proximum of convergence
p.p.
    near point of accommodation
    punctum proximum
PPC
    posterior peripheral curve
PPDR
    preproliferative diabetic retinopathy

PPH
    persistent postdrainage hypotony
PPMD
    posterior polymorphic dystrophy (of
      cornea)
PP&P
    posterior pole and periphery
PPVD
    perifoveal posterior vitreous detachment
PR
    presbyopia
Pr
    prism
p.r.
    far point of accommodation
    punctum remotum
practice
    large print reading p.
    optometric p.
    reading p.
practitioner
    eyecare p.
prairie conjunctivitis
Pram occluder
Prausnitz-Kustner reaction
prebleached dark-adapted threshold
precancerous lesion
precapillary arteriole
prechiasmal
    p. compression
    p. disorder
    p. optic nerve
    p. optic nerve compression
      syndrome
prechopper
    Akahoshi hybrid combo p.
    Akahoshi phaco p.
    Akahoshi universal p.
pre-chopping forceps
precipitate
    granulomatous keratic p.
    keratic p. (KP)
    keratitic p.
    mutton-fat keratic p.
    pigment p.
    pigmented keratic p.
    punctate keratic p.
precise implantation
precision
    p. astigmatism reduction
    p. astigmatism reduction procedure
    P. Cosmet intraocular lens implant
    P. Cosmet lens
    P. refractor
    p. suture tome
PreClean soak system
preconditioning
    hypoxic p.
precorneal tear film

Pred
- P. Forte
- P. Forte Ophthalmic
- Liquid P.
- P. Mild
- P. Mild Ophthalmic

Predair
- P. A
- P. Forte

Predcor-TBA Injection
pre-Descemet corneal dystrophy
pre-descemetic dissection
Pred-G
- P.-G Ophthalmic
- P.-G SOP
- P.-G suspension

predictive
- p. factor
- p. value
- p. visual outcome
- p. of visual performance

predisposing condition
predisposition
- genetic p.

Prednefrin Forte
prednisolone
- p. acetate
- p. and atropine
- chloramphenicol and p.
- p. and gentamicin
- Isopto P.
- neomycin, polymyxin B, and p.
- p. sodium phosphate
- sulfacetamide and p.

prednisone
Predsulfair
preeclamptic hypertensive retinopathy
preexisting
- p. posterior capsule defect
- p. well-balanced cornea-lens

preference
- fixation p.
- patient-based p.

preferential-looking technique
preferred retinal locus (PRL)
Preflex for Sensitive Eyes
preformed piece
Prefrin
- P. Liquifilm Vasoconstrictor and Lubricant Eye Drops
- P. Ophthalmic Solution
- P. Z Liquifilm

preganglionic
- p. Horner syndrome
- p. lesion
- p. oculomotor nerve
- p. parasympathetic axon

pregeniculate visual pathway
pregnancy
- migraine during p.
- toxemic retinopathy of p.

preimplantation genetic diagnosis
preinjury visual maturation
prelaminar optic nerve
prelens tear film
Prelex presbyopic lens
preliminary iridectomy
preloaded injector
premacular
- p. fibrosis
- p. gliosis
- p. subhyaloid hemorrhage

premature
- p. birth
- p. infant
- p. presbyopia
- p. tear breakup

prematurity
- cataract of p.
- cicatricial retinopathy of p.
- Cryotherapy for Retinopathy of P. (CRYO-ROP)
- Early Treatment of Retinopathy of P. (ETROP)
- Effects of Light Reduction on Retinopathy of P.
- International Classification of Retinopathy of P. (ICROP)
- p. myopia
- retinopathy of p. (ROP)
- p. retinopathy
- Supplemental Therapeutic Oxygen for Prethreshold Retinopathy of P.
- threshold stage III of retinopathy of p. (TS III ROP)

premelanosome
prenatal
- p. diagnosis
- p. ocular trauma
- p. ophthalmology

Prentice
- P. law

NOTES

P

Prentice *(continued)*
P. position power
P. rule
preocular tear film (POTF)
preoperative
p. aberrometry
p. period
p. risk assessment
p. risk factor
p. visual acuity
p. workup
prepapillary
p. arterial loop
p. hemorrhage
p. vascular loop
preparation
povidone-iodine p.
preparatory iridectomy
preplaced suture
preponderance
directional p.
prepresbyopia
preproliferative diabetic retinopathy (PPDR)
preretinal
p. gliosis
p. hemorrhage
p. macular fibrosis
p. membrane
p. neovascularization
p. plaque
presbyope
presbyopia (PR)
p. glasses
laser reversal of p.
premature p.
pseudophakic p.
surgical reversal of p. (SRP)
presbyopia-correcting IOL
presbyopic
p. intraocular lens
p. LASIK
p. lens exchange
presbytia
presbytism
preschool
p. Randot stereoacuity test
p. screening
p. vision screening instrument
p. visiting screening test
preschooler
Vision in P.'s (VIP)
Prescott wireless foot switch
prescriber
contact lens p.
presenile
p. cataract
p. melanosis

presentation
rapid serial visual p. (RSVP)
vitreous p.
preseptal
p. cellulitis
p. orbicularis muscle
p. space
preservation
photoreceptor p.
visual p.
preservative
mercurial p.
p.'s in solution
preservative-free
p.-f. artificial tears
P.-f. Moisture Eyes
p.-f. saline solution
preserved saline solution
preset diamond knife
pressing
eye p.
molded p.
press-on
p.-o. Fresnel lens
p.-o. prism
pressure
p. amaurosis
applanation p.
p. bandage
circadian variation of intraocular p.
digital p.
episcleral venous p. (EVP)
exophthalmos due to p.
eye restored to normotensive p.
intracranial p. (ICP)
intraocular p. (IOP)
intravitreal p.
mercury p.
nocturnal intraocular p.
ocular perfusion p. (OPP)
orbital venous p.
osmotic p.
p. patch dressing
p. patching
peak circadian intraocular p.
p. phosphene tonometer
p. sensor
p. shield
p. transducer
white without p.
pressure-related damage
presumed
p. microbial keratitis
p. ocular histoplasmosis
p. ocular histoplasmosis syndrome (POHS)
presumptive diagnosis
presynaptic congenital myasthenic disorder

pretectal
    p. area
    p. nucleus
    p. region
    p. syndrome
prethreshold disease
prevalence
    cataract p.
    dry eye p.
    high p.
    p. of ocular trauma
Prevent Blindness America (PBA)
preventive measure
previous
    p. cataract surgery
    p. trauma
Prevost sign
prezonular space
Price
    P. corneal punch
    P. corneal transplant system
    P. donor cornea punch set
    P. radial marker
Priestley-Smith retinoscope
Prima KTP/532 laser
Primaria tissue culture flask
primary
    p. acetylcholine receptor deficiency
    p. acquired melanosis (PAM)
    p. acquired nasolacrimal duct
      obstruction (PANDO)
    p. action
    p. angle-closure glaucoma
    p. anophthalmia
    p. cataract
    p. central nervous system
      lymphoma (PCNSL)
    p. childhood glaucoma
    p. color
    p. cone dysfunction
    p. congenital open-angle glaucoma
    p. conjunctival chancre
    p. demyelinating disease
    p. deviation
    p. dye test
    p. dysgenesis mesodermalis
    p. excision
    p. eye
    p. eyelid chancre
    p. familial amyloidosis
    p. focal length
    p. gaze alignment
    p. glaucoma patient

    p. glaucoma triple procedure
      (PGTP)
    p. graft failure
    p. herpes simplex keratitis
    p. hydroxyapatite-coated sleeve
    p. infantile glaucoma
    p. infantile glaucoma blepharospasm
    p. intraocular lymphoma
    p. lens
    p. lensectomy
    p. lens implant
    p. line of sight
    p. mechanism
    p. myopia
    p. ocular disease
    p. ocular lymphoma
    p. open-angle glaucoma (POAG)
    p. optic atrophy
    p. perivasculitis of retina
    p. persistent hyperplastic vitreous
    p. pigmentary degeneration
    p. pigmentary degeneration of
      retina
    p. position
    p. position of gaze
    p. pupillary block
    p. retinal degeneration
    p. retinal fold
    p. visual cortex
Primbs suturing forceps
primer
    oligonucleotide p.
primitive neuroectodermal tumor
(PNET)
primordium, pl. **primordia**
    optic p.
Prince
    P. cautery
    P. muscle clamp
    P. muscle forceps
    P. rule
principal
    p. fiber
    p. focus
    p. line
    p. line of direction
    p. optic axis
    p. plane
    p. point
    p. visual direction
principle
    Carriazo-Barraquer p.
    Fresnel p.

NOTES

P

principle *(continued)*
    Imbert-Fick p.
    Mackay-Marg p.
    Scheimpflug p.
    Scheiner p.
prinomastat
printers' point system
print size
prion-mediated disease
Prio video display terminal vision tester
prism (Pr)
    p. adaptation
    P. Adaptation Study (PAS)
    p. adaptation test (PAT)
    Allen-Thorpe gonioscopic p.
    p. and alternate cover test (PACT)
    p. angle
    AO rotary p.
    apex of p.
    p. apex
    p. ballast
    p. ballast design
    p. bar
    bar p.
    p. base
    base-down p.
    4 p. base-out test
    BD p.
    Becker gonioscopic p.
    Berens p.
    BI p.
    p. correction
    p. and cover (P&C)
    p. cover measurement
    p. and cover test
    p. degree
    diopter p.
    p. diopter (PD, p.d.)
    dispersion p.
    p. dissociation test
    Drews inclined p.
    Fresnel press-on p.
    Goldmann contact lens p.
    Goldmann 3-mirror p.
    gonioscopic p.
    handheld rotary p.
    induced p.
    Keeler p.
    Maddox p.
    3-mirror p.
    Nicol p.
    oblique p.
    plastic p.
    press-on p.
    reflecting p.
    refracting angle of p.
    right-angle p.
    Risley rotary p.

    rotary p.
    scanning p.
    p. segment
    p. shift test
    p. spectacles
    square p.
    temporary p.
    p. test
    p. vergence test
prismatic
    p. contact lens
    p. dioptric value
    p. effect
    p. effect by lens
    p. fundus
    p. gonioscopic lens
    p. gonioscopy lens
    p. goniotomy lens
    p. spectacle lens
    p. spectacles
prism-neutralized cover test
prismoptometer
prismosphere
Prizm keratome blade
PRK
    photorefractive keratectomy
    photorefractive keratoplasty
PRL
    preferred retinal locus
proangiogenic
    p. milieu
    p. molecule
probe
    Accurus 2500 p.
    Alcon vitrectomy p.
    Anel p.
    angled p.
    p. beam
    Bodian lacrimal pigtail p.
    Bodian mini lacrimal p.
    Bowman lacrimal p.
    Castroviejo lacrimal sac p.
    p. cataract
    Clark p.
    cryopexy p.
    cryotherapy p.
    curved laser p.
    curved retinal p.
    Dodick photolysis p.
    Ellis foreign body spud needle p.
    French lacrimal p.
    Frigitronics freeze-thaw cryopexy p.
    Harms trabeculotomy p.
    Infinitech laser p.
    InnoVit 1800 p.
    InnoVit vitrectomy p.
    Knapp iris p.
    lacrimal intubation p.
    Manhattan Eye & Ear p.

Mannis p.
Microvit p.
nasolacrimal duct p.
p. needle
needle p.
ocutome p.
O'Donoghue angled DCR p.
Photon Laser Phacolysis P.
piggyback p.
pigtail p.
polymerase chain reaction-sequence specific oligonucleotide p. (PCR-SSOP)
Quickert-Dryden p.
Quickert lacrimal intubation p.
Ritleng p.
Rolf lacrimal p.
Rollet lacrimal p.
Simpson lacrimal p.
p. spatula
spatula p.
straight retinal p.
Synergetics directional laser p.
p. syringe
Theobald p.
trabeculotomy p.
Vygantas-Wilder retinal drainage p.
Werb right-angle p.
Williams p.
Worst pigtail p.
Ziegler p.

probing
diagnostic p.
lacrimal p.
p. lacrimonasal duct
p. lacrimonasal duct operation

problem
ophthalmic p.

Probst Smiley LASIK marker
procaine hydrochloride
procedure
acuity card p.
advancement p.
Anderson-Kestenbaum p.
artificial divergence p.
Baerveldt filtering p.
Beverly Douglas p.
Bick p.
buckling p.
burst hemiflip p.
chemical p.
ciliary p.
collagen wick p.

corrective p.
Custodis nondraining p.
CustomVue LASIK p.
cyclodestructive p.
encircling p.
epi-LASIK p.
eyelid-sparing p.
Faden p.
Fasanella-Servat p.
filtering p.
Girard p.
guarded filtration p.
hamular p.
Harada-Ito p.
hex p.
Hummelsheim p.
interventional p.
intralamellar pocket p.
Intralase eye correction p.
IntraLASIK p.
Jannetta p.
Jensen transposition p.
Jones tube p.
keratorefractive p.
Kestenbaum p.
Knapp p.
Krönlein p.
Kuhnt-Szymanowski p.
laser thermal keratoplasty p.
lateral tarsal strip p.
lathing p.
lower lid sling p.
LTK p.
macular buckling p.
modified corncrib (inverted T) p.
modified Wies p.
no-touch laser thermal keratoplasty p.
PAM p.
pneumatic displacement p.
precision astigmatism reduction p.
primary glaucoma triple p. (PGTP)
Quickert p.
Ruiz p.
Salleras p.
Sato p.
scleral buckling p.
scleral expansion band p.
sling p.
small-incision p.
2-stage p.
strip p.
Sunrise LTK p.

NOTES

P

procedure *(continued)*
  surgical decompression p.
  tarsal strip p.
  Thal p.
  Toti p.
  transciliary filtration p.
  triple p.
  tube-shunt p.
  tuck p.
  tumbling p.
  uncinate p.
  up-and-down staircases p.
  Visx p.
  Wheeler p.
  Wies p.
  Zaldivar anterior p. (ZAP)
procerus
  musculus p.
process
  ciliary p.
  complex visual p.
  disciform p.
  emmetropization p.
  fine iris p.
  iris p.
  lacrimal p.
  Performa surface p.
  photochemical p.
  Sand p.
  spin-cast p.
  visual p.
  zygomaticoorbital p.
processor
  talking word p.
processus
  p. ciliares
  p. zygomaticus maxillae
ProConcept
  P. Contact Lens Cleaner
  P. Wetting and Soaking Solution
Procyon digital infrared pupillometer
procyonis
  Baylisascaris p.
prodromal
  p. glaucoma
  p. myopia
product
  convolution p.
  Katena p.
  Nexacryl cohesive p.
  SPP color deficiency testing p.
  standard pseudoisochromatic plates
    color deficiency testing p.
  viscoelastic p.
  Xomed Surgical P.'s
production
  aqueous humor p.
  mucin p.

  reflex tear p.
  tear p.
Profenal Ophthalmic
professional
  eye care p.
profile
  p. analyzer
  intensity p.
  p. perimetry
  sickness impact p. (SIP)
profiling
  stereophotogrammetric p.
ProFinesse II ultrasonic handpiece
ProFree/GP weekly enzymatic cleaner
profunda
  keratitis punctata p.
  keratitis pustuliformis p.
prognosis
  visual p.
program
  birth defect monitoring p. (BDMP)
  Canny edge detection p.
  CRS-Master software p.
  diagnostic p.
  Hoffberger p.
  iMedConsent ophthalmology
    software p.
  Joslin Vision Network
    Telehealth p.
progression
  Contact Lens and Myopia P.
    (CLAMP)
  p. detection
  glaucoma p.
  rate of p.
  visual field p.
progressiva
  ophthalmoplegia p.
progressive
  p. additional lenses
  p. addition lens
  p. bifocal chorioretinal atrophy
  p. cataract
  p. choroidal atrophy
  p. cone degeneration
  p. cone dystrophy
  p. cone-rod dystrophy
  p. encephalopathy with edema,
    hypsarrhythmia and optic atrophy
    (PEHO)
  p. external ophthalmoplegia (PEO)
  p. fluorescein leakage
  p. foveal dystrophy
  p. hearing loss
  p. hemifacial atrophy
  p. herpetic corneal endotheliopathy
  p. macular dystrophy
  p. multifocal lens

p. myopathic upper eyelid blepharoptosis
p. myopia
p. myopic degeneration
p. optic atrophy
p. orbital edema
p. outer retinal necrosis (PORN)
p. outer retinal necrosis syndrome
p. spectacles lenses
p. supranuclear palsy
p. systemic sclerosis
p. tapetochoroidal dystrophy
p. vaccinia
p. visual failure
progressive-add bifocal
project
Cataract PPO p.
P. Research Ophthalmic specular microscope
projectile
paint-ball p.
projecting staphyloma
projection
erroneous p.
false p.
light p.
p. magnifier
perimeter p.
p. perimeter
retinocortical p.
retinogeniculostriate p.
visual p.
Project-O-Chart
AO Reichert Instruments P.-O.-C.
Ultramatic P.-O.-C. (UPOC)
projector
acuity visual p.
fiberoptic light p.
Lancaster red-green p.
Marco chart p.
NP-3S auto chart p.
Topcon chart p.
Ultramatic Project-O-Chart p.
UPOC p.
ProKera amniotic membrane graft
Pro-Koester wide-field SCM microscope
prolactin-secreting adenoma
prolapse
iris p.
p. of iris
nucleus p.
orbital fat p.
vitreous p.

Prolene suture
proliferans
fibrous p.
retinitis p.
proliferated cortex
proliferating retinitis
proliferation
anterior hyaloidal fibrovascular p.
conjunctival lymphoid p.
cortex p.
epimacular p.
epiretinal membrane p. (EMP)
extraretinal fibrovascular p.
fibrovascular p.
glial p.
hyaloidal fibrovascular p.
massive periretinal p. (MPP)
peripheral p.
perisilicone p.
regressed p.
retinal angiomatous p.
retinal glial p.
uveal melanocytic p.
proliferative
p. background diabetic retinopathy
p. choroiditis
p. diabetic retinopathy (PDR)
p. diabetic vitreoretinopathy (PDVR)
p. lupus retinopathy
p. retinitis
p. sickle-cell retinopathy
p. vitreoretinopathy (PVR)
prolificans
Scedosporium p.
prolonged
p. eyelid edema
p. wear contact lens
promethazine
prominence
Ammon scleral p.
prominent
p. buckle
p. indentation
p. Schwalbe ring
Pro-Ophtha
propamidine isethionate
proparacaine
p. HCl
p. hydrochloride
p. ophthalmic drops
prophylactic
p. antibiotic

NOTES

P

prophylactic *(continued)*
    p. laser iridotomy
    p. retinopexy
    p. treatment of age-related macular degeneration (PTAMD)
prophylaxis
    antibiotic p.
    Credé p.
    retinal p.
    steroid p.
    tetanus p.
Propine Ophthalmic
propionate
    clobetasol p.
    sodium p.
Propionibacterium
    P. acnes
    P. acnes endophthalmitis
    P. propionicus
propionic acid derivative
propionicus
    Propionibacterium p.
proportional fragmentation
Propper-Heine ophthalmoscope
Propper indirect ophthalmoscope
propria
    substantia p.
proprioception
proprioceptive
    p. head-turning reflex
    p. oculocephalic reflex
    p. stimulus
proptometer
proptosis
    axial p.
    ipsilateral p.
    Moran p.
    unilateral p.
proptotic
propylene glycol
propylparaben
    methyl p.
Prorex
Proshield collagen corneal shield
prosopagnosia
    apperceptive p.
    associative p.
    developmental p.
prospective
    P. Evaluation of Radial Keratotomy (PERK)
    P. Evaluation of Radial Keratotomy Study
prostaglandin analog
prostaglandin-mediated phenomenon
prosthesis, pl. **prostheses**
    intraocular retinal p.
    p. motility
    ocular p.

    orbital floor p.
    peg-coupled p.
    retinal p.
    shell p.
    socket p.
prosthesis-induced trachoma
prosthetic
    p. fit
    p. lens
    p. movement
prosthokeratoplasty
Prostigmin test
protan color blindness
protanomaly
protanope
protanopia, protanopsia
protanopic
protease
    coagulation cascade p.
    serine p.
protection
    ocular p.
    UV radiation p.
protective
    p. glasses
    p. lens
    p. spectacles
    p. sports eye wear
protector
    Arroyo p.
    Arruga p.
    Buratto flap p.
    eye p.
    industrial eye p.
    oculoplasty corneal p.
protein
    antiglial fibrillary acidic p.
    bactericidal permeability-increasing p. (BPI)
    C-reactive p.
    crystalline p.
    p. deposit
    eosinophil cationic p. (ECP)
    p. eye implant
    Fas liquid p.
    GCAP1 p.
    glial fibrillary acidic p. (GFAP)
    high-sensitivity C-reactive p. (hs-CRP)
    interphotoreceptor retinoid-binding p. (IRBP)
    p. kinase C (PKC)
    major basic p. (MBP)
    p. remover
    retained lens p.
    RNA III activating p. (RAP)
    silver p.
    tear p.

protein-1
    monocyte chemotactic p.-1 (MCP-1)
proteinaceous
    p. aqueous exudation
    p. coating
    p. cyst
proteinolipidic film
proteolytic enzyme
Proteus syndrome
protocol
    ETDRS p.
    FD2 testing p.
    surgical management p.
    treatment p.
    Yasuma p.
protometer
proton beam
ProTon portable tonometer
protozoan
    p. keratitis
    p. uveitis
protriptyline hydrochloride
protruding eyes
protrusion
    conical p.
    corneal p.
Proview eye pressure monitor
Provisc
provocative
    p. test
    p. testing
Prowazek-Greeff body
Prowazek-Halberstaedter body
Prowazek inclusion body
proximal
    p. convergence
    p. myotonic myopathy
proximum
    punctum p. (p.p.)
proxymetacaine HCl 0.5%
PRRE
    pupils round, regular, and equal
PRT
    photostress recovery time
prurigo
    actinic p.
    Hutchinson Summer p.
psammoma body
psammomatous meningioma
PSC
    posterior subcapsular cataract
PSD
    pattern standard deviation

Pseudallescheria boydii
pseudoabducens palsy
pseudoacanthosis nigricans
pseudoaccommodation
pseudo-Argyll Robertson pupil
pseudobaggy eyelid
pseudoblepsia, pseudoblepsis
pseudobulbar palsy
pseudocaloric nystagmus
pseudocancerous lesion
pseudochiasmal
pseudocoloboma
pseudo-CSF signal
pseudocyst
    foveal p.
pseudocystoid macular edema
pseudodendrites
    Acanthamoeba keratitis p.
pseudodendritic keratitis
pseudodiphtheriticum
    Corynebacterium p.
pseudodoubling
pseudodrusen
pseudoendothelial dystrophy
pseudoenophthalmos
pseudoephedrine
    carbinoxamine and p.
pseudoepitheliomatous hyperplasia
pseudoesotropia
pseudoexfoliation (PXF)
    p. of lens capsule
    p. syndrome
pseudoexfoliative
    p. capsular glaucoma
    p. glaucoma (PEXG)
pseudoexophoria
pseudoexophthalmos
pseudoexotropia
pseudo-Foster Kennedy syndrome
pseudoglaucoma
pseudoglaucomatous macrocupping
pseudoglioma
pseudo-Graefe
    p.-G. phenomenon
    p.-G. sign
pseudohemianopia, pseudohemianopsia
pseudohistoplasmosis
pseudohole
    macular p. (MPH)
pseudo-Hurler polydystrophy
pseudohypertelorism
pseudohypoparathyroidism
pseudohypopyon

NOTES

P

423

pseudoinflammatory
    p. macular dystrophy
    p. macular dystrophy of Sorsby
pseudointernuclear ophthalmoplegia
pseudoiritis
pseudoisochromatic
    p. chart
    p. color plate
    p. color test
pseudomelanoma
pseudomembrane
    conjunctival p.
pseudomembranous
    p. conjunctivitis
    p. rhinitis
Pseudomonas
    P. aeruginosa
    P. cepacia
    P. pyocyanea
    P. stutzeri
pseudomycosis
pseudomyopia
pseudonystagmus
pseudooperculum
pseudopannus
pseudopapilledema
pseudopapillitis
pseudopemphigoid
pseudophacos, pseudophakos
pseudophake implant
pseudophakia
pseudophakic
    p. bullous keratopathy (PBK)
    p. cystoid macular edema
    p. detachment
    p. dysphotopsia
    p. eye
    p. presbyopia
    p. spherical aberration
pseudophakodonesis
pseudophakos (*var. of* pseudophacos)
pseudopit
pseudopolycoria
pseudopresumed ocular histoplasmosis syndrome
pseudoprolactinoma
pseudoproptosis
pseudopseudohypoparathyroidism
pseudopsia
pseudopterygia
pseudopterygium
pseudoptosis
pseudoretinitis pigmentosa
pseudoretinoblastoma
pseudorheumatoid nodule
pseudorosette
pseudosarcomatous endothelial hyperplasia

pseudosclerosis
    spastic p.
pseudoscopic vision
pseudostereo image
pseudostrabismus
pseudotabes
    pupillotonic p.
pseudotemporal arteritis
pseudotrachoma
pseudotumor
    p. cerebri (PTC)
    idiopathic inflammatory p.
    inflammatory orbital p.
    lymphoid p.
    orbital p.
    orbital inflammatory p.
pseudovernal conjunctivitis
pseudoxanthoma
    elastic p.
    p. elasticum (PXE)
PSF
    point spread function
PSI
    pneumatically stented implant
psittaci
    Chlamydia p.
Psoralens
psoriasis
    plaque-type p.
psoriatic
    p. corneal abscess
    p. uveitis
psorophthalmia
psychic
    p. blindness
    p. paralysis of fixation of gaze
psychogenic
    p. micropsia
    p. paralysis
    p. photophobia
psychological disturbance
psychophysical measurement
psychophysics
    visual p.
psychosis
    black patch p.
    Wernicke-Korsakoff p.
PTAMD
    prophylactic treatment of age-related macular degeneration
PTC
    pseudotumor cerebri
pterion
pterygial tissue
pterygium, pl. **pterygia**
    active p.
    Arlt p.
    belly of p.
    cicatricial p.

congenital p.
conjunctival p.
double-headed p.
epitarsus p.
p. scissors
p. surgery
p. unguis
pterygium-induced astigmatism
pterygoid levator synkinesis
pterygomaxillary fissure
pterygopalatine
    p. fat
    p. ganglion
PTFE
    polytetrafluoroethylene
ptilosis
PTK
    phototherapeutic keratectomy
ptosis, pl. **ptoses**
    acquired myopathic p.
    p. adiposa
    age-related p.
    aponeurogenic p.
    aponeurotic p.
    Berke p.
    bilateral p.
    botulism-induced p.
    cerebral p.
    congenital dystrophic p.
    congenital myopathic p.
    cortical p.
    p. crutch spectacles
    developmental p.
    drug-induced p.
    eyelash p.
    eyelid p.
    false p.
    fatigable p.
    p. forceps
    guarding p.
    Horner p.
    involutional p.
    involutional senile p.
    p. knife
    levator p.
    p. lipomatosis
    magnitude of p.
    mechanical acquired p.
    midbrain p.
    morning p.
    myogenic acquired p.
    myopathic p.

neurogenic-acquired p.
neuromuscular p.
ocular myasthenia p.
p. scissors
senescent p.
snake bite-induced p.
p. sympathetica
traumatic p.
upside-down p.
waking p.
ptotic eyebrow
pubis
    Phthirus p.
pucker
    macular p.
    pigmented macular p.
puckering
    macular p.
puddler's cataract
PUFA
    polyunsaturated fatty acid
puff of loose vitreous
PUK
    peripheral ulcerative keratitis
Pulfrich
    P. effect
    P. stereo phenomenon
pulley
    heterotopic p.
    rectus muscle p.
pulpit spectacles
Pulsair tonometer
pulsating exophthalmos
pulsation
    spontaneous retinal venous p.
    venous p.
Pulsatome cataract emulsifier
pulse
    choroidal p.
    energetic p.
    fluid p.
    p. mode
    radiofrequency p.
    retinal venous p.
    saccadic p.
    sonic p.
    square-wave p.
pulsed-dye laser
pulsed electron avalanche knife (PEAK)
pulseless disease
pulsing
Pulsion FS Laser

NOTES

P

pulverulent
    p. cataract
    p. opacity
pulverulenta
    cataracta centralis p.
pump
    air p.
    AMO HPF 500 p.
    Carones LASEK p.
    p. chamber
    p. cycle
    flow-based p.
    frame-mounted p.
    laser-assisted epithelium
        keratomileusis p.
    MityVac simple hand p.
    peristaltic p.
    scroll p.
    tear p.
    vacuum-based p.
    Venturi p.
pump-leak system
punch
    Barron donor corneal p.
    Barron marking corneal p.
    Berens corneoscleral p.
    p. block
    bone p.
    bone-biting p.
    Carpel trabeculectomy p.
    Castroviejo corneoscleral p.
    corneal p.
    corneoscleral p.
    Descemet membrane p.
    donor p.
    Gass corneoscleral p.
    Gass scleral p.
    Gass sclerotomy p.
    Hardy p.
    Holth scleral p.
    Kelly-Descemet membrane p.
    Luntz-Dodick p.
    Pollock p.
    Price corneal p.
    Reiss punctal p.
    Rothman-Gilbard corneal p.
    scleral p.
    sclerectomy p.
    sclerotomy p.
    Storz corneoscleral p.
    Tanne corneal p.
    Tanne guillotine-style p.
    p. trephine
    Troutman p.
    Walser corneoscleral p.
    Walton p.
punched-out
    p.-o. chorioretinal scar
    p.-o. lesion

puncta (*pl. of* punctum)
    kissing p.
punctal
    p. abnormality
    p. cautery
    p. dilator
    p. ectropion
    p. lens
    p. occlusion
    p. opening
    p. plug
    p. stenosis
punctata
    p. albescens retinopathy
    keratitis p. (KP)
punctate
    p. cataract
    p. corneal epithelial defect
    p. corneal opacity
    p. epithelial erosion
    p. epithelial keratitis
    p. epithelial keratopathy (PEK)
    p. epithelial keratoplasty
    p. epithelial microcyst
    p. hemorrhage
    p. hyalitis
    p. hyalosis
    p. inner choroiditis
    p. inner choroidopathy (PIC)
    p. keratic precipitate
    p. keratitis of Thygeson
    p. keratoderma
    p. oculocutaneous albinism
    p. oculocutaneous albinoidism
    p. outer retinal toxoplasmosis
    p. retinitis
    p. staining
punctiform
punctograph
punctoplasty
punctum, pl. **puncta**
    p. aplasia
    p. cecum
    dilation of p.
    p. dilator
    erythematous pouting of p.
    eversion of p.
    everted p.
    inferior p.
    lacrimal p.
    p. lacrimale
    lower p.
    p. luteum
    p. plug
    p. proximum (p.p.)
    p. proximum of accommodation
    p. proximum of convergence (PP)
    p. remotum (p.r.)
    1-snip p.

3-snip p.
p. stenosis
superior p.
upper p.
punctumeter
puncture
anterior p.
anterior stromal p.
p. diabetes
diathermy p.
eyelid p.
globe p.
p. needle
self-sealing scleral p.
p. wound
Ziegler p.
puncture-tip needle
Puntenney forceps
pupil (P)
Adie tonic p.
amaurotic p.
Argyll Robertson p. (ARP)
artificial p.
attention reflex of p.
Behr p.
p. block
p. block glaucoma
blown p.
bounding p.
Bumke p.
catatonic p.
cat's-eye p.
cholinergic p.
cogwheel p.
constricted p.
contraction of p.
cornpicker's p.
p. cycle induction test
diabetic Argyll Robertson p.
diffraction-limited p.
dilated p.
p. dilation
p. dilator
dilator muscle of p.
p. dilator ring
p. disorder
elliptic p.
entrance p.
p.'s equal, reactive to light and
  accommodation (PERLA)
p.'s equal, react to light (PERL)
p.'s equal, round, reactive to light
  and accommodation (PERRLA)

exclusion of pupil
exit p.
fixed dilated p.
Gunn p.
hammock p.
Holmes-Adie p.
Horner p.
Hutchinson p.
iris and p. (I/P)
irregular p.
isolated fixed dilated p.
keyhole p.
light response of p.
local tonic p.
Marcus Gunn p.
MG p.
p. miosis
miotic p.
myotonic p.
neuropathic tonic p.
neurotonic p.
nonreactive p.
occluded p.
occlusion of p.
paradoxic p.
paradoxical p.
p. pass
pear-shaped p.
peninsula p.
pinhole p.
pinpoint p.
pseudo-Argyll Robertson p.
reverse Marcus Gunn p.
rigid p.
Robertson p.
p.'s round, regular, and equal
  (PRRE)
Saenger p.
scalloped p.
seclusion of p.
p. size
skew p.
small p.
sphincter muscle of p.
p. spreader/retractor forceps
spring p.
square p.
stiff p.
p. stretching
tadpole p.
tadpole-shaped p.
teardrop p.
tonic p.

NOTES

P

pupil *(continued)*
    updrawn p.
    Wernicke p.
    white p.
pupilla, pl. **pupillae**
    musculus dilator p.
    musculus sphincter p.
    sphincter pupillae
pupillaris
    membrana p.
pupillary
    p. aperture
    p. areflexia
    p. athetosis
    p. axis
    p. block
    p. block glaucoma
    p. block mechanism
    p. capture
    p. center
    p. diameter
    p. dilator muscle
    p. disorder
    p. distance (PD)
    p. effect
    p. entrapment
    p. escape
    p. floater
    p. hemiakinesia
    p. iris cyst
    p. lens
    p. light-near dissociation
    p. light reflex
    p. line
    p. margin
    p. margin of iris
    p. membrane
    p. membrane remnant
    p. miosis
    p. near response
    p. paradoxic reflex
    p. paralysis
    p. plane
    p. reaction
    p. ruff
    p. sparing
    p. sphincter akinesis
    p. sphincter contraction
    p. sphincter muscle
    p. zone
pupilloconstrictor fiber
pupillograph
pupillography
pupillometer
    Colvard handheld infrared p.
    corneal reflection p. (CRP)
    Procyon digital infrared p.
    Pupilscan II p.
    reflex p.

pupillometry
    infrared p.
pupillomotor fiber
pupilloplasty
    cerclage p.
pupilloplegia
pupilloscope
pupilloscopy
pupillostatometer
pupillotonia
pupillotonic pseudotabes
Pupilscan II pupillometer
pupil-to-root iridectomy
Puralube
    P. Tears
    P. Tears Solution
pure
    p. alexia
    p. color
    p. cyclitis
    P. Eyes Cleaner/Rinse
    P. Eyes Disinfection/Soaking
        Solution
    P. Eyes Soaking Solution
PureVision
    P. extended-wear contact lens
    P. toric lens
purified ovine hyaluronidase
Purilens UV Disinfection Solution
purinergic
    selective p.
Purisol
Purkinje
    P. effect
    P. figure
    P. image
    P. image tracker
    P. phenomenon
    P. shadow
    P. shift
Purkinje-Sanson mirror image
Purlytin
purple
    visual p.
purpura
    palpable p.
purpurea
    Digitalis p.
purpuriparous
purpurogenous membrane
pursuit
    p. disorder
    p. mechanism
    p. movement
    saccadic p.
    smooth p.
    p. testing
    p. tracking

Purtscher
>P. angiopathic retinopathy
>P. disease

Purtscher-like retinopathy
purulent
>p. conjunctivitis
>p. cyclitis
>p. discharge
>p. iritis
>p. keratitis
>p. ophthalmia
>p. retinitis
>p. rhinitis

push-and-pull hook
pusher
>Aker lens p.
>Visitec lens p.

push-plus refraction technique
push-up
>p.-u. method
>pencil p.-u.'s

pustular blepharitis
Putterman
>P. levator resection clamp
>P. ptosis clamp

PV
>PV Carpine
>PV Carpine Liquifilm

PVA
>polyvinyl alcohol
>PVA spear

p value
PVD
>posterior vitreous detachment

PVER
>pattern visual-evoked response

PVR
>proliferative vitreoretinopathy

PXE
>pseudoxanthoma elasticum

PXF
>pseudoexfoliation

pyknotic
>p. keratitis
>p. nuclei

pyocyanea
>*Pseudomonas p.*

pyocyaneus
>*Bacillus p.*

pyogenes
>*Streptococcus p.*

pyogenic
>p. granuloma
>p. metastasis

Pyopen
pyophthalmia
pyophthalmitis
pyramidal
>p. cataract
>p. system

pyrazolone derivative
Pyrex
>P. eye sphere
>P. T-tube
>P. tube

pyridostigmine
pyridoxine
pyrimethamine

NOTES

QALY
>quality-adjusted life year

q arm

Q-banding

Q-switched
>Q-s. Er:YAG laser
>Q-s. Nd:YAG laser
>Q-s. neodymium:YAG laser
>Q-s. ruby laser

QuadPediatric fundus lens

quad-ported LASIK irrigating cannula

quadrant
>q. hemianopsia
>inferior nasal q.
>inferior temporal q.

quadrantanopia
>crossed binasal q.
>crossed bitemporal q.
>heteronymous q.
>homonymous q.
>pie-in-the-sky q.
>pie-on-the-floor q.
>superior q.

quadrantic
>q. defect
>q. hemianopia
>q. hemianopsia
>q. sclerectomy with internal drainage
>q. scotoma

quality
>average retinal image q.
>q. indicator
>optical q.
>postoperative vision q.
>tear q.

quality-adjusted life year (QALY)

quantitative
>q. echography
>q. fluorescein angiography
>q. haze assessment
>q. static threshold
>q. threshold perimetry

quantity
>tear q.

quartic axicon

quaternary
>q. ammonium chloride
>q. ammonium compound

QUEST
>quick estimation by sequential testing

Questek laser tube

questionnaire
>allergic conjunctivitis quality of life q.
>current symptoms q.
>driving habits q. (DHQ)
>dry eye q.
>25-Item Visual Function Q. (VFQ-25)
>Low Vision Quality of Life Q. (LVQOLQ)
>Manchester low-vision q.
>McGill Pain Q.
>McMonnies q.
>National Eye Institute Visual Function Q. (NEI-VFQ)
>rhinoconjunctivitis quality of life q.
>VF-14 q.
>Virtual Reality Symptom Q. (VRSQ)
>Visual Activities Q. (VAQ)
>Visual Function Q. (VFQ)

quick
>q. adducting-retraction jerk
>q. estimation by sequential testing (QUEST)
>q. left/right component

Quickert
>Q. lacrimal intubation probe
>Q. procedure
>Q. suture
>Q. 3-suture technique

Quickert-Dryden
>Q.-D. probe
>Q.-D. tube

QuickRinse automated instrument rinse system

Quickswitch irrigation/aspiration ophthalmic system

quiescent
>q. eye
>q. stromal scarring

quiet
>q. chamber
>deep and q. (D&Q)
>eye was q.
>q. iritis

quinacrine hydrochloride

quinine
>q. amblyopia
>q. sulfate

Quire mechanical finger forceps

Quixin ophthalmic solution

Rabinowitz-McDonnell test
Rabl lamella
raccoon
    r. eyes
    r. sign
racemose
    r. aneurysm
    r. angioma
    r. hemangioma
    r. hemangiomatosis
racemosum
    staphyloma corneae r.
rack
    Luneau retinoscopy r.
racquet body
racquet-like pattern
radial
    r. astigmatism
    r. cells of Mueller
    r. dilator muscle
    r. drusen
    r. fiber
    r. infiltration
    r. iridotomy
    r. iridotomy scissors
    r. keratotomy (RK)
    r. keratotomy knife
    r. keratotomy marker
    r. mark
    r. optic neurotomy
    r. sponge
    r. transillumination defect
    r. vessel array
radially oriented
radiance
radiant
    r. absorptance
    r. emittance
    r. energy
    r. intensity
    r. and luminous flux
    r. power
    r. reflectance
radiata
    corona r.
radiatio
    r. occipitothalamica
    r. optica
radiation
    artificial UV r.
    beta r.
    r. burn
    r. cataract
    r. effect
    electromagnetic r.

    external beam r.
    geniculocalcarine r.
    Goldmann Coherent r.
    heavy ion r.
    infrared r.
    r. injury
    ionizing r.
    r. keratitis
    monochromatic r.
    natural UV r.
    occipitothalamic r.
    optic r.
    r. optic neuropathy (RON)
    r. retinopathy
    solar r.
    r. therapy
    ultraviolet r.
    visual r.
    Wernicke r.
radiation-induced
    r.-i. carcinoma
    r.-i. optic neuropathy
    r.-i. vasculopathy
radical orbitectomy
radicans
    Rhus r.
radices (*pl. of* radix)
radii (*pl. of* radius)
radioactive
    r. eye plaque
    r. iodine
    r. plaque brachytherapy
radiofrequency
    r. energy
    r. pulse
    r. wave
radiogenic vasculopathy
radiography
    plain film r.
radioimmunoassay technique
radioisotope scan
radiologic study
radiology
    orbital r.
radiopaque intraocular foreign body
radioscope
    Lombart r.
radiosurgery
    stereotactic r.
radiotherapy
    implant r.
    orbital r.
    palladium 103 ophthalmic plaque r.
    plaque r.
radius, pl. **radii**

radius *(continued)*
    apical r.
    axial length-corneal r. (AL/CR)
    back optic zone r. (BOZR)
    r. of curvature
    front optic zone r. (FOZR)
    r. gauge
    r. of lens
    r. of lentis
    posterior apical r. (PAR)
radix, pl. **radices**
    r. lateralis tractus optici
    r. medialis tractus optici
    r. oculomotoria ganglii ciliaris
    r. sympathica ganglii ciliaris
radon
    r. ring brachytherapy
    r. seed implantation
Raeder
    R. paratrigeminal neuralgia
    R. paratrigeminal syndrome
ragged-red fiber
ragged wound edge
rag-wheel method
railroad nystagmus
rainbow
    r. symptom
    r. syndrome
    r. vision
raindrop-shaped keratometric reflection
Rainin
    R. air injection cannula
    R. clip-bending spatula
    R. lens spatula
Raji cell assay
raking
    endoscopic r.
RAM
    retinal acuity meter
Raman
    R. effect
    R. imaging
    R. method
    R. signal
    R. spectroscopy
    R. spectrum
    R. stimulus
Ramsden eyepiece
ramus, pl. **rami**
Randolph
    R. cyclodialysis cannula
    R. irrigator
random
    r. dot E stereoacuity test
    r. dot stereopsis
    r. order
random-dot
    r.-d. kinematogram
    r.-d. stereogram (RDS)

Randot
    R. chart
    R. circle
    R. Dot E stereotest
    R. Stereo Smile test
range
    r. of accommodation
    r. of convergence
    vertical fusion r.
ranibizumab
Rank-Taylor-Hobson-Talysurf instrument
RAP
    RNA III activating protein
RAPD
    relative afferent pupillary defect
raphe
    canthal r.
    horizontal r.
    lateral palpebral r.
    palpebral r.
    r. palpebralis lateralis
    posterior lamina r.
    retinal r.
    temporal r.
rapid
    r. antibiotic susceptibility testing
      (RAST)
    r. eye movement (REM)
    r. plasma reagin test
    r. serial visual presentation (RSVP)
rarefaction
    pigmentation r.
Rasch analysis
rasp
RAST
    rapid antibiotic susceptibility testing
rasterstereography
rasterstereography-based elevation map
rate
    aspiration flow r.
    infusion flow r.
    low blink r.
    r. of progression
    reading r.
    r. of refractive growth
    seropositivity r.
    spontaneous eye blink r. (SEBR)
    susceptibility kill r.
    tear clearance r.
    variable repetition r. (VRR)
Rathke
    R. cleft cyst
    R. pouch
    R. pouch tumor
ratio
    accommodation-convergence r.
    accommodative convergence-
      accommodation r.
    AL/CR r.

aperture r.
Armaly cup/disc r.
arteriovenous r.
artery-to-vein r. (A/V)
axial length-corneal radius r.
CA/C r.
convergence-accommodation r.
cup-to-disc r. (C/D, CDR)
ion r.
L/D r.
light-dark amplitude r.
light-peak to dark-trough r.
nuclear cytoplasmic r.
optic cup-to-disc r.
Pourcelot r.
rim-to-disc r.
Strehl r.

Raven progressive matrices test

ray

convergent r.
converging r.
divergent r.
emergent r.
r. incident
light r.
r. of light
marginal r.
medullary r.
monochromatic r.
parallel r.
paraxial r.
r. tracing

Rayleigh

R. color matching test
R. equation
R. limit
R. scattering

Raymond-Cestan syndrome
Raymond syndrome
Rayner lens
razor

Bard-Parker r.
r. blade
r. blade knife
r. needle

razor-blade trephine
razor-tip needle
RBRVS

Resource-Based Relative Value Scale

RC-2 fundus camera
RCL

recurrent corneal lesion

RD

retinal detachment

RDS

random-dot stereogram

reaction

Alamar blue redox r.
anaphylactic r.
anterior chamber r.
Arthus r.
basophilic r.
Calmette conjunctival r.
Calmette ophthalmic r.
conjunctival r.
consensual r.
direct pupillary light r.
early-phase r.
eosinophilic r.
eye-closure pupil r.
Griess r.
hemiopic pupillary r.
hypersensitivity r.
immune r.
immunologic r.
indirect pupillary r.
Jarisch-Herxheimer r.
late-phase r.
lid-closure r.
light r.
Mazzotti r.
mononuclear r.
near r.
ocular tilt r. (OTR)
ophthalmic r.
orbicularis r.
pain r.
paradoxical darkness r.
polymerase chain r. (PCR)
polymorphonuclear r.
Prausnitz-Kustner r.
pupillary r.
toxic r.
vestibular pupillary r.
vitreous cellular r.
Weil-Felix r.
Wernicke r.

reactive lymphoid hyperplasia (RLH)
reader

bar r.
ready-made r.
screen r.

reading

r. ability
r. card

NOTES

reading *(continued)*
    r. chart
    r. glasses
    K r.'s
    keratometric r.'s
    r. material
    r. practice
    r. rate
    r. rectangle
    r. speed
    r. speed test
    r. task
    r. vision
ready-made reader
Ready-Set punctum plug
reagent
    Brücke r.
    r. strip
real
    r. focus
    r. image
reaper's keratitis
reattachment
    r. of choroid
    r. of choroid operation
    hydraulic retinal r.
    posterior vitreous findings in
      spontaneous retinal r.
    r. of retina
    r. of retina operation
    spontaneous retinal r.
Rebif
rebleeding
rebound
    r. conjunctival hyperemia
    r. nystagmus
recalcitrant
    r. anaerobic endophthalmitis
    r. diabetic macular edema
receptacle
    dome r.
receptive field
receptor
    r. amblyopia
    expression of chemokine r.
    r. potential
recess
    Arlt r.
    canthal r.
    optic r.
    suprapineal r.
    von Arlt r.
recession
    angle r.
    bimedial r.
    r. clamp
    conjunctival r.
    r. forceps
    r. index (RI)

    lateral rectus r.
    left inferior oblique r.
    r. of muscle
    r. of ocular muscle operation
    r. ophthalmic muscle hook
    optic muscle r.
    tendon r.
    traumatic angle r.
recession-resection (R&R)
recessive dystrophic epidermolysis
    bullosa
recess-resect (R&R)
recessus opticus
recipient bed
reciprocal innervation
reclination
recognition
    pattern r.
    symbol r.
recombinant tissue plasminogen
    activator
reconstruction
    r. of eyelid
    multiplanar r.
    ocular surface r.
    socket r.
    V-Y advancement
      myotarsocutaneous flap for upper
      eyelid r.
recording
    artifact-free r.
    oscillatory potential r.
recovery
    fluid-attenuated inversion r.
    (FLAIR)
    hyperactive immune r.
    retinal r.
    visual acuity r.
rectangle
    reading r.
rectangular blade
rectifier
    delayed r.
    inward r.
rectus
    inferior r. (IR)
    ipsilateral medial r.
    lateral r. (LR)
    r. lateralis muscle
    medial r. (MR)
    r. medialis muscle
    r. muscle of eyeball
    r. muscle pulley
    r. muscle transposition
    r. muscle transposition for paralytic
      strabismus
    superior r. (SR)
recurrent
    r. central retinitis

r. choroiditis
r. corneal erosion
r. corneal erosion syndrome
r. corneal lesion (RCL)
r. epithelial erosion
r. erosion of cornea
r. exophthalmos
r. hypopyon
r. pupillary sparing
r. visual axis opacification

recurrentis
Borrelia r.

red
r. blindness
r. cone degeneration
r. coral keratitis
r. desaturation
r. eye
r. filter
r. flash stimulus
r. free photograph
r. glare test
r. glass test
r. lens occluder
r. reflex
R. Reflex Lens Systems lens
r. rubber catheter
ruthenium r.
r. scaly plaque
r. vision

redetachment
retinal r.

red-eyed shunt syndrome
red-filter
r.-f. test
r.-f. therapy

red-free
r.-f. filter
r.-f. photography

red-green
r.-g. axis
r.-g. blindness
r.-g. glasses

redness
sectoral r.

reduced
r. eye
r. eye model
r. Snellen card
r. vergence
r. vision

reducer
McCannel ocular pressure r.
ocular pressure r.

reducing body myopathy
reductase
aldose r.
methylenetetrahydrofolate r. (MTHFR)

reduction
r. of aberration
absolute risk r.
contrast sensitivity r.
exophthalmos r.
IOP r.
precision astigmatism r.
vision r.

reduplicated cataract
reduplication of Descemet membrane
Reed-Sternberg cell
Reeh scissors
reel aspiration cannula
reepithelialization
Reese
R. muscle forceps
R. ptosis knife
R. syndrome

Reese-Ellsworth
R.-E. classification
R.-E. classification system
R.-E. group V retinoblastoma
R.-E. stage IIIA retinoblastoma

refilling
lens r.

refined refraction
refixation
Ref-Keratometer
Canon R-5+ Auto R.-K.

reflectance
radiant r.

reflected
r. color
r. light

reflecting
r. prism
r. retinoscope
r. surface

reflection
angle of r.
corneal r.
D-shaped keratometric r.
raindrop-shaped keratometric r.
shiny cellophane r.
specular r.

R

NOTES

reflection-based technique
reflective scattering
reflectivity
    internal r.
reflectometer
reflectometry
reflex
    r. accommodation
    accommodation r.
    accommodative pupillary r.
    acquired gustolacrimal r.
    r. amaurosis
    r. amblyopia
    Aschner r.
    Aschner-Dagnini r.
    attention r.
    auditory oculogyric r.
    Bechterew r.
    Bell r.
    black r.
    r. blepharospasm
    blind spot r.
    blink r.
    blunted red r.
    blunted retinoscopic r.
    cat's-eye r.
    cellophane macular r.
    cerebral cortex r.
    cerebropupillary r.
    cervicoocular r. (COR)
    Charleaux oil droplet r.
    choked r.
    ciliary r.
    ciliospinal r.
    circumpapillary light r.
    coaxially sighted corneal r.
    cochleopupillary r.
    congenital paradoxic
      gustolacrimal r.
    conjunctival r.
    consensual light r.
    consensual pupillary r.
    convergency r.
    copper-wire r.
    corneal light r.
    corneomandibular r.
    corneomental r.
    corneopterygoid r.
    corticopupillary r.
    crescentic circumpapillary light r.
    crossed r.
    cutaneous pupillary r.
    dazzle r.
    direct-light r.
    direct pupillary r.
    doll's eye r.
    emergency light r.
    eye r.
    eyeball compression r.

    eyeball-heart r.
    eye-closure r.
    eyelid-closure r.
    r. eye movement
    eye-popping r.
    fixation r.
    foveal r.
    fundal r.
    fundus r.
    fusion r.
    Gault r.
    Gifford r.
    Gifford-Galassi r.
    golden tapetal-like fundus r.
    Gunn pupillary r.
    gustatolacrimal r.
    Haab r.
    head-turning r.
    Hirschberg r.
    iridoplegia r.
    r. iridoplegia
    iris contraction r.
    juvenile r.
    lacrimal r.
    lacrimation r.
    lid r.
    lid-closure r.
    light optometer r.
    Lockwood light r.
    McCarthy r.
    myopic r.
    nasolacrimal r.
    near light r.
    oculocardiac r.
    oculocephalic r.
    oculocephalogyric r.
    oculodigital r.
    oculogyric auricular r.
    oculopharyngeal r.
    oculopupillary r.
    oculorespiratory r.
    oculosensory cell r.
    oculovestibular r.
    opticofacial winking r.
    optokinetic r.
    optomotor r.
    orbicularis pupillary r.
    otolithic-ocular r.
    palpebral oculogyric r.
    palpebromandibular r.
    paradoxical pupillary r.
    paradoxic gustolacrimal r.
    paradoxic pupillary r.
    platysmal r.
    Plitz r.
    proprioceptive head-turning r.
    proprioceptive oculocephalic r.
    pupillary light r.
    pupillary paradoxic r.

R

r. pupillometer
red r.
retinal r.
reversed pupillary r.
Ruggeri r.
senile r.
shot-silk r.
silver-wire r.
skin pupillary r.
spasm of near r.
stretch r.
supraorbital r.
synkinetic near r.
tapetal light r.
tapetal-like r.
r. tear production
r. tear secretion
threat r.
trigeminal r.
r. trigeminus
trigeminus r.
utricular r.
vestibuloocular r.
visual orbicularis r.
water-silk r.
Weiss r.
Westphal-Piltz r.
Westphal pupillary r.
white fundus r.
white pupillary r.
wink r.
yellow light r.

reflux
drug r.
r. of tears
r. vergence

reformation
r. of chamber
fornix r.
holmium bleb r. (HBR)
inferior fornix r.

refract
refractable
Refractec ViewPoint CK System
refracted light
refractile
r. body
r. crystal
r. deposit

refracting
r. angle of prism
r. medium

refraction
angle of r.
r. angle
aphakic r.
automated r.
autorefractometer r.
cycloplegic r. (CR)
cylindric r.
direct-light r.
double r.
dynamic r.
fogged manifest r.
fogging system of r.
homatropine r.
index of r. (IR, n)
law of r.
low vision r.
manifest r. (MR)
ocular r.
plane-surface r.
refined r.
r. spectacles
spherical r.
static r.
unrefined r.

refractionist
refractionometer
refractive
r. aberration
r. accommodative esotropia
r. amblyopia
r. ametropia
r. anisometropia
r. astigmatism
r. cataract surgery
r. contact lens
r. correction
r. error
r. error monitoring
R. Error Study in Children
r. eye map
r. floating implant
r. growth model
r. hyperopia
r. index
r. keratoplasty
r. keratotomy
r. laser surgery
r. lens exchange (RLE)
r. medium
r. myopia
r. outcome
r. phakic implant

NOTES

refractive *(continued)*
  r. power
  r. screening method
  r. state
refractivity
refractometer
  Abbe r.
  Canon auto r.
  Hoya HDR objective r.
  Hoya MRM objective r.
  meridional r.
  Nikon Auto Refractometer NR-1000F
  OPD-Scan r.
  Rodenstock eye r.
  8000 Supra Series auto r.
  Topcon eye r.
  Topcon RM-A2300 auto r.
  vertex r.
  Zeiss vertex r.
refractometry
  laser r.
  urine r.
refractor
  Allergan Humphrey r.
  AR 1000 r.
  automated r.
  automatic r.
  Berens r.
  Canon r.
  Castroviejo r.
  Coburn r.
  CooperVision Diagnostic Imaging r.
  Elschnig r.
  Ferris-Smith r.
  Ferris-Smith-Sewall r.
  Goldstein r.
  Graether r.
  Humphrey automatic r.
  Kirby r.
  Knapp r.
  KR 7000-P cycloplegic r.
  Kuglen r.
  Leland r.
  Marco r.
  Nidek AR-2000 Objective Automatic r.
  objective r.
  Precision r.
  Reichert r.
  Remote Vision electronic r.
  SR-IV programmed subjective r.
  subjective r.
  Topcon r.
refractory
  vernal keratoconjunctivitis r.
refrangible
Refrax corneal repair kit

Refresh
  R. contact lens comfort drops
  R. Endura eye drops
  R. Liquigel dry eye treatment
  R. Liquigel eye drops
  R. Plus
  R. Plus lubricant eye drops
  R. Plus Ophthalmic Solution
  R. PM
  R. Tears eye drops
refringence
refringency
refringent
Refsum
  R. disease
  R. syndrome
Regan-Lancaster dial
Regan low-contrast acuity chart
regard
  area of conscious r.
  object of r.
  plane of r.
  point of r.
regeneration
  aberrant r.
  r. aberration
  r. of innervation
  nerve r.
  r. of nerve
  postganglionic fiber r.
regimen
  corticosteroid-sparing r.
  medication r.
  multiple bottle r.
region
  ciliary r.
  ethmoidal r.
  infraorbital r.
  ocular r.
  orbital r.
  pretectal r.
  retrochiasmatic r.
  scutum r.
  supratemporal r.
  third framework r. (FR3)
regional
  r. block
  r. periarteritis
registration
  cyclorotational r.
  cyclotorsional r.
registry
  Australian Corneal Graft R.
regressed proliferation
regression
  myopic r.
  univariate linear r.
  univariate polytomous logistic r.
  vascular r.

regular
 r. astigmatism
 Eye Drops R.
 Vasocon R.
regulator
 OptiMed glaucoma pressure r.
 (OGPR)
rehabilitation
 optical r.
 r. technique
 visual r.
Reichert
 R. binocular indirect
 ophthalmoscope
 R. camera
 R. Ful-Vue binocular
 ophthalmoscope
 R. Ful-Vue spot retinoscope
 R. membrane
 R. noncontact tonometer
 R. ophthalmodynamometer
 R. radius gauge
 R. refractor
 R. slit lamp
 R. Zetopan microscope
Reichert-Jung Ultracut ultramicrotome
Reichling corneal scissors
reimplantation
Reinecke-Carroll lacrimal tube
reinforcement
 scleral r.
Reinverting Operating Lens System
 (ROLS)
Reis-Bücklers
 R.-B. disease
 R.-B. ring-shaped dystrophy
 R.-B. superficial corneal dystrophy
Reisinger lens-extracting forceps
Reisman sign
Reiss punctal punch
Reiter
 R. conjunctivitis
 R. disease
 R. syndrome
rejection
 allograft corneal r.
 corneal graft r.
 corneal transplant r.
 graft r.
 limbal r.
 r. line
Rekoss disc

relapsing polychondritis
relapsing/remitting multiple sclerosis
 (RR-MS)
relationship
 agonist-antagonist r.
 doctor-patient r.
 object/image r.
relative
 r. accommodation
 r. afferent pupillary defect (RAPD)
 r. amblyopia
 r. convergence
 r. divergence
 first-degree r.
 r. hemianopsia
 r. hyperopia
 near-point r.
 r. scotoma
 second-degree r.
 r. size
 r. spectacle magnification
 r. strabismus
relaxing
 r. incision
 r. retinotomy
releasable compression suture
release
 r. hallucination
 suture r.
 r. of traction for hypotony and
 vitreoretinopathy
relevant spatial frequency
reliability
 test-retest r.
reliable wave front sensor
relief
 R. Ophthalmic Solution
 symptomatic r.
REM
 rapid eye movement
remaining visual field
remedy
 novel r.
remission inducing
remnant
 globe r.
 persistent pupillary membrane r.
 pupillary membrane r.
 Weiss r.
remodeling
 corneal stromal r.
Remote Vision electronic refractor

R

NOTES

remotum
punctum r. (p.r.)
removable keratophakia lens
removal
contact lens r.
crust r.
debris r.
en bloc r.
r. of foreign body
r. of foreign body operation
lens r.
sequential suture r.
remover
Alger brush rust ring r.
Bailey foreign body r.
protein r.
ReNu 1-step daily liquid protein r.
Soft Mate protein r.
remyelination
long-term r.
Remy separator
renal
r. coloboma syndrome
r. diabetes
r. retinitis
r. retinopathy
r. ultrasound
renewed
Tears R.
renin-angiotensin system
rent
traumatic r.
Rentsch boat hook
ReNu
R. Effervescent enzymatic cleaner
R. Multi-Purpose
R. Rewetting Drops
R. 1-step daily liquid protein remover
R. 1 Step Enzymatic Cleaner
R. Thermal enzymatic cleaner
repair
Arlt epicanthus r.
Arlt eyelid r.
blepharochalasis r.
blepharoptosis r.
Fasanella-Servat ptosis r.
Jones r.
Kuhnt-Junius r.
lacrimal gland r.
levator aponeurosis r.
levator dehiscence r.
medial canthal r.
small-incision external levator r.
trichiasis r.
Wheeler halving r.
reparative giant cell granuloma

repeat
r. penetrating keratoplasty
r. treatment
repens
Dirofilaria r.
replaceable blade
replacement
lens r.
report
interventional case r.
reposited
repositioning
repositor
iris r.
Knapp iris r.
Nettleship iris r.
Sloane flap r.
reprocessing
eye movement desensitization and r. (EMDR)
reproducibility of evaluation
rescue
autologous stem cell r. (ASCR)
Rescula
research
Diabetic Retinopathy Clinical R. (DRCR)
genetic eye r.
vision r.
resection
conjunctival r.
lateral rectus muscle r.
levator r.
lid r.
Mohs microsurgical r.
muscle r.
r. of muscle
Peyman full-thickness eye-wall r.
scleral r.
wedge r.
reserve
base-in r.
base-out r.
divergence r.
fusional r.
reservoir of liquid
reshaping
overnight corneal r.
residual
r. accommodation
r. astigmatism
r. capsule
r. cortex
r. refractive error
r. vision
resilience
orbital r.

resin
    Lexan polycarbonate r.
    Medcast epoxy r.
resistance
    impact r.
    insulin r.
    outflow r.
resistive index
resolution
    r. acuity
    r. acuity perimetry
    logarithmic Minimum Angle of R.
      (logMAR)
    visual r.
Resolve/GP
resolving power
resorption
    spontaneous r.
Resource-Based Relative Value Scale
  (RBRVS)
respiratory hippus
response
    accommodation r.
    accommodative r.
    acquired immune r.
    allergic r.
    B-cell proliferative r.
    better visual r.
    cone r.
    consensual light r.
    consensual pupillary r.
    curve r.
    direct-light r.
    direct pupillary r.
    doll's eye r.
    electroretinogram flicker r.
    eosinophilic r.
    flare r.
    r. function
    immune r.
    mononuclear r.
    near r.
    neovascular r.
    partial r.
    pattern visual-evoked r. (PVER)
    polymorphonuclear r.
    pupillary near r.
    rod b-wave r.
    synkinetic near r.
    trabecular meshwork-inducible
     glucocorticoid r. (TIGR)
    vestibuloocular r. (VOR)
    vision r.

    visual-evoked r. (VER)
    visual-vestibulo-ocular r.
Restasis
restoration
    Berens-Smith cul-de-sac r.
    ocular surface r.
    r. point
ReSTOR vision implant
restrainer
    Gulani globe stabilizer and flap r.
restricted motility
restricting strand
restriction
    vertical gaze r.
restrictive syndrome
rest test
result
    false-negative r.
    false-positive r.
    visual performance r.
Retaane
retained
    r. foreign body (RFB)
    r. intraorbital metallic foreign body
    r. lens protein
retainer
    eyeglass r.
RetCam 120 fiberoptic fundus camera
reticle
    handheld magnifying r.
reticular
    r. cystoid degeneration
    r. dystrophy
    r. haze
    r. keratitis
    r. plate
reticule accommodation
reticulum
    r. cell
    r. cell lymphoma
    r. cell sarcoma
    endoplasmic r.
    extraconal fat r.
    fat r.
    rough endoplasmic r.
retina
    absent r.
    angiomatosis of r.
    arteriosclerosis of r.
    artificial silicone r.
    avascular peripheral r.
    central fovea of r.
    cerebral layer of r.

R

NOTES

retina *(continued)*
cerebral stratum of r.
cholesterol embolus of r.
ciliary part of r.
coarctate r.
coloboma of r.
concussion of r.
congenital grouped pigmentation
  of r.
deep r.
demarcation line of r.
detached r.
detachment of r.
disciform degeneration of r.
disinserted r.
disinsertion of r.
dragged r.
dysplastic r.
external limiting membrane of r.
falciform fold of r.
fat embolism of r.
flecked r.
foveal r.
ganglionic layer of r.
ganglionic stratum of r.
ganglion layer of r.
giant cyst of r.
glioma of r.
gyrate atrophy of choroid and r.
hole in r.
inferior zone of r.
inflammatory change of r.
inner molecular layer of r.
inner nuclear layer of r.
internal limiting membrane of r.
ischemic r.
juxtapapillary r.
lattice degeneration of r.
leopard r.
lipemic r.
lower r.
medial arteriole of r.
medial venulae of r.
murine r.
nasal arteriole of r.
nasal venule of r.
neovascularization of r.
nerve layer of r.
neural r.
neuroepithelial layer of r.
neurosensory r.
nuclear layer of the r.
outer nuclear layer of r.
peripheral r.
physiologic r.
pigmented layer of r.
positional abnormality of r.
postequatorial r.
primary perivasculitis of r.

primary pigmentary degeneration
  of r.
reattachment of r.
rivalry of r.
sensory r.
separation of r.
shot-silk r.
R. Society classification
stiff r.
superior zone of r.
tear of r.
temporal arteriole of r.
temporal venule of r.
temporal zone of r.
tented-up r.
thrombosis in r.
tigroid r.
upper r.
vessel abnormality of r.
watered-silk r.
yellow spot of r.

retinae
albedo r.
angiomatosis r.
arteriola medialis r.
atrophia choroideae et r.
commotio r.
cyanosis r.
ischemia r.
macula r.
ora serrata r.
pars ciliaris r.
pars iridica r.
pars nervosa r.
pars optica r.
pars pigmentosa r.
periphlebitis r.
rhytidosis r.
striae r.
torpor r.
vasa sanguinea r.
vasculitis r.
vena centralis r.

retinal
r. abiotrophy
r. acuity meter (RAM)
r. adaptation
r. anatomic structure
r. angiography
r. angioma
r. angiomatosis
r. angiomatous proliferation
r. anlage tumor
r. aplasia
r. apoplexy
r. arterial filling
r. arterial macroaneurysm
r. arterial occlusion
r. arteriole

r. arteriovenous malformation
r. artery
r. artery aneurysm
r. artery disorder
r. artery occlusion
r. artery perfusion
r. asthenopia
r. astrocytic hamartoma
r. astrocytoma
r. atresia
r. bleb
r. blindness
r. blood
r. blur spot
r. branch vein occlusion
r. break
r. burn
r. camera
r. capillaritis
r. capillary bed
r. capillary blood flow
r. capillary hemangioma
r. capillary nonperfusion
r. cavernous hemangioma
r. cell transduction
r. central artery occlusion
r. central vein occlusion
r. clouding
r. cone
r. cone dystrophy
r. correspondence
r. cryopexy
r. cryotherapy
r. crystal
r. cyst
r. cystoid space
r. degeneration slow gene
r. dehiscence
r. demarcation band
r. detachment (RD)
r. detachment hook
r. detachment pencil
r. detachment risk
r. detachment syringe
r. detachment using optical
  coherence tomography
r. dialysis
r. disease
r. disparity
r. dragging
r. drusen
r. dysplasia
r. eccentricity

r. edema
r. element
r. ellipsometer
r. embolism
r. embolus
r. epithelial pigment hyperplasia
r. error
r. excavation
r. exudate
r. fixed fold
r. flap
r. fold
r. ganglion
r. ganglion cell axon
r. ganglion cell layer
r. ganglion cell loss
r. Gelfilm implant
r. glial cell
r. glial proliferation
r. gliocyte
r. glioma
r. gliosarcoma
r. gliosis
r. hemorrhage
r. hole
r. horseshoe tear
r. hypoxia
r. ice ball
r. image
r. image size
r. imbrication
r. impact site
r. ischemia
r. isomerase
r. laser photocoagulation
r. lattice degeneration
r. lesion
r. mapping
r. microangiopathy
r. microcirculation
r. microembolism
r. microinfarct
r. micromovement
r. micropsia
r. microvasculopathy
r. migraine
r. montage
r. necrosis
r. necrosis syndrome
r. neovascular
r. nerve fiber layer (RNFL)
r. nerve fiber myelination
r. neuron

NOTES

retinal *(continued)*
r. neurotransmitter
normal-looking r.
r. periphlebitis
r. perivasculitis
r. phlebitis
r. photography
r. photoprotection
r. pigmentary dystrophy
r. pigmentation alteration
r. pigment epithelial atrophy
r. pigment epithelial defect
r. pigment epithelial hypertrophy
r. pigment epitheliitis
r. pigment epitheliopathy
r. pigment epithelium (RPE)
r. pigment epithelium dropout
r. pigment epithelium mottling
r. pigment epithelium serous detachment
r. point
r. probe sleeve
r. prophylaxis
r. prosthesis
r. quadrant neovascularization
r. racemose hemangioma
r. raphe
r. recovery
r. redetachment
r. reflex
r. rivalry
r. rod
r. rotation
r. scatter photocoagulation
r. sensitivity
r. spike
r. staphyloma
r. stress line
r. striation
r. surgery
r. tack
r. telangiectasia
r. telangiectasis
r. thickness
r. thickness abnormality
r. thickness analysis (RTA)
r. thickness analyzer (RTA)
r. thickness map
r. thinning
r. thrombosis
r. toxicity
r. translocation
r. tuft
r. vascular malformation
r. vascular microfold
r. vascular occlusion
r. vasculature
r. vasculitis
r. vasculopathy

r. vein
r. vein disorder
r. vein occlusion
r. vein sheathing
r. venous beading
r. venous circulation
r. venous nicking
r. venous obstruction
r. venous occlusion
r. venous pulse
r. venule
r. vessel
r. vessel landmark
r. vessel tortuosity
r. visual cell
r. whitening
r. wrinkling
r. zone
retinal-choroidal
r.-c. anastomosis
r.-c. dystrophy
retinal-image contrast
retinalis
lipemia r.
retinal-slip velocity
RetinaLyze System
retinascope
retinectomy
retinene isomerase
retinex theory
retinitis
acquired toxoplasmosis r.
actinic r.
AIDS-related r.
albuminuric r.
apoplectic r.
azotemic r.
candidal r.
central angiospastic r.
r. centralis serosa
central serous r.
r. circinata
circinate r.
CMV r.
Coats r.
cytomegalovirus r.
diabetic r.
r. exudativa
exudative r.
focal necrotizing r.
foveomacular r.
Ganciclovir Implant Study for Cytomegalovirus R.
gravidic r.
r. haemorrhagica
herpes simplex r.
hypertensive r.
Jacobson r.
Jensen r.

leukemic r.
metastatic r.
necrotizing r.
r. nephritica
peripheral necrotizing r.
Pick r.
r. pigmentosa (RP)
r. pigmentosa GTPase regulator
gene (RPGR)
r. pigmentosa inversa
r. pigmentosa sine pigmento
r. proliferans
proliferating r.
proliferative r.
r. punctata albescens
punctate r.
purulent r.
recurrent central r.
renal r.
rubella r.
r. sclopetaria
secondary r.
septic r.
serous r.
simple r.
solar r.
splenic r.
r. stellata
striate r.
suppurative r.
syphilitic r.
r. syphilitica
toxoplasmic r.
uremic r.
varicella-zoster r.
X-linked r.
retinoblastoma
bilateral sporadic r.
calcified r.
r. cell
exophytic r.
familial r.
r. gene
r. gene mutation
intraocular r.
r. locus
macular r.
Reese-Ellsworth group V r.
Reese-Ellsworth stage IIIA r.
sporadic r.
trilateral r.
unilateral sporadic r.
retinocerebellar angiomatosis

retinochoroid
retinochoroidal
r. atrophy
r. break
r. coloboma
r. infarction
r. layer
retinochoroidectomy
retinochoroiditis
birdshot r.
HIV-related r.
infectious r.
r. juxtapapillaris
Toxoplasma r.
toxoplasmic r.
retinochoroidopathy
birdshot r.
central serous r.
retinocortical projection
retinocytoma
retinodialysis
retinogeniculate pathway
retinogeniculostriate projection
retinograph
retinography
retinoid
retinoma
retinomalacia
Retinomax
R. 2 autorefractor
R. cordless hand-held autorefractor
R. K-Plus 2
R. K-Plus autorefractor/keratometer
R. refractometry instrument
retinometer
Heine Lambda 100 r.
Retinopan 45 camera
retinopapillitis of premature infant
retinopathy
acute anular outer r.
acute zonal occult outer r.
(AZOOR)
angiopathic r.
angiospastic r.
arteriosclerotic r.
background diabetic r. (BDR)
Bietti crystalline r.
birdshot r.
blood-and-thunder r.
r. of blood dyscrasia
bull's-eye r.
cancer-associated r. (CAR)
canthaxanthin r.

NOTES

R

retinopathy *(continued)*
    carbon monoxide r.
    carotid occlusive disease r.
    cellophane r.
    central angiospastic r.
    central disc-shaped r.
    central serous r. (CSR)
    chloroquine r.
    chloroquine/hydroxychloroquine r.
    circinate r.
    CMV r.
    compression r.
    crystalline r.
    cytomegalovirus r.
    diabetic r. (DR)
    dot-and-fleck r.
    drug abuse r.
    dysoric r.
    dysproteinemic r.
    eclamptic hypertensive r.
    eclipse r.
    electric r.
    embolic r.
    external exudative r.
    exudative r.
    familial exudative r. (FER)
    foveomacular r.
    gold dust r.
    gravidic r.
    r. hemorrhage
    hemorrhagic r.
    herpetic necrotizing r.
    high altitude r. (HAR)
    HIV r.
    hydroxychloroquine r.
    hypertensive r. (HR)
    hypotensive r.
    inflammatory r.
    ischemic r.
    Leber idiopathic stellate r.
    leukemic r.
    lipemic r.
    macular r.
    melanoma-associated r. (MAR)
    necrotizing herpetic r.
    noninfectious r.
    nonproliferative diabetic r. (NPDR)
    optic disc drusen r.
    paraneoplastic r.
    particulate r.
    pepper-and-salt r.
    pigmentary r.
    pneumatic r.
    preeclamptic hypertensive r.
    r. of prematurity (ROP)
    prematurity r.
    preproliferative diabetic r. (PPDR)
    proliferative background diabetic r.
    proliferative diabetic r. (PDR)
    proliferative lupus r.
    proliferative sickle-cell r.
    r. punctata albescens
    punctata albescens r.
    Purtscher angiopathic r.
    Purtscher-like r.
    radiation r.
    renal r.
    rubella r.
    salt-and-pepper r.
    serous r.
    sickle cell r.
    sight-threatening r.
    solar r.
    stellate r.
    surface wrinkling r.
    syphilitic r.
    tamoxifen r.
    tapetoretinal r.
    thioridazine r.
    toxic r.
    transient r.
    traumatic r.
    ultraviolet-blue photic r.
    Valsalva r.
    van Heuven anatomical
      classification of diabetic r.
    vascular r.
    venous stasis r. (VSR)
    venous stenosis r.
    vitrectomy for proliferative r.
    whiplash r.
    Wisconsin Epidemiologic Study of
      Diabetic R. (WESDR)
    X-linked juvenile r.
retinopexy
    cyanoacrylate r.
    fluid r.
    gas r.
    pneumatic r.
    prophylactic r.
    transpupillary r.
    transscleral r.
retinoschisis
    acquired r.
    age-related degenerative r.
    bullous r.
    congenital r.
    degenerative r.
    familial foveal r. (FFR)
    Goldmann-Favre r.
    juvenile r.
    juvenile X-linked r. (JXRS)
    senescent r.
    senile r.
    senile-type r.
    traumatic r.
    X-linked r. (XLRS)

X-linked juvenile r.
X-linked recessive r.

retinoscope
Copeland streak r.
Ful-Vue spot r.
Ful-Vue streak r.
Keeler r.
luminous r.
Priestley-Smith r.
reflecting r.
Reichert Ful-Vue spot r.
spot r.
streak r.

retinoscopy
Auto Ref-keratometer ARK-900
autorefractor and r.
Copeland r.
Cross r.
cylinder r.
dark r.
fogging r.
MEM r.
monocular-estimate-method
dynamic r.
noncycloplegic distance static r.
Nott r.
static r.
streak r.

retinosis
retinotomy
relaxing r.
retinotopic stimulus
retinotoxic
Retisert intravitreal implant
retractable blade
retraction
congenital myopathic eyelid r.
convergence r.
endocrine lid r.
eyelid r.
flap r.
lid r.
massive vitreous r. (MVR)
mechanical lid r.
mesencephalic lid r.
myopathic eyelid r.
neuromuscular eyelid r.
neuropathic eyelid r.
r. nystagmus
spontaneous eyelid r.
r. syndrome
thyroid lid r.
vitreous r.

retractor
Agricola lacrimal sac r.
Alexander-Ballen r.
angled iris r.
Arruga elevator r.
Arruga orbital r.
Barbie r.
Berens lid r.
Blair r.
capsule r.
Castroviejo lid r.
Coleman r.
conjunctiva r.
Converse double-ended alar r.
Conway lid r.
deep blunt rake r.
Desmarres eyelid r.
Elschnig r.
eyelid r.
Ferris-Smith r.
Ferris-Smith-Sewall r.
Fisher lid r.
flexible translimbal iris r.
Forker r.
Goldstein lacrimal sac r.
Good r.
Graether collar button micro iris r.
great big barbie r.
Grieshaber flexible iris r.
Harrington r.
Helveston big barbie tissue r.
Helveston great big barbie r.
iris r.
IrisMate flexible translimbal iris r.
Jaeger r.
Jaffe lid r.
Kaufman type II r.
Kelman iris r.
Kirby lid r.
Knapp lacrimal sac r.
Kuglen r.
lacrimal sac r.
lower lid r.
Mackool capsule r.
McGannon r.
Mueller lacrimal sac r.
Nevyas r.
Oklahoma iris wire r.
Paul lacrimal sac r.
Payne r.
Phoroptor r.
r. plication
Rizzuti iris r.

NOTES

retractor *(continued)*
    Rollet r.
    Sanchez-Bulnes lacrimal sac r.
    Sato lid r.
    Schepens orbital r.
    Schultz iris r.
    self-adhering lid r.
    self-retaining r.
    Senn r.
    Sewall r.
    Stevens muscle hook r.
    Stevenson lacrimal sac r.
    Teflon iris r.
    Thomas r.
    Ultramatic Rx Master phoroptor r.
    Visitec iris r.
    Welsh iris r.
    Wilder scleral r.

retrieval device

retriever
    Utrata r.

retroauricular complex graft

retrobulbar
    r. abscess
    r. administration
    r. akinesia
    r. alcohol injection
    r. anesthesia
    r. artery
    r. compressive lesion
    r. compressive optic neuropathy
    r. corticosteroid injection
    r. hemorrhage
    r. hemorrhage glaucoma
    r. ischemic optic neuropathy
    r. lid block
    r. needle
    r. optic neuritis
    r. space

retrochiasmal
    r. visual field defect
    r. visual field loss
    r. visual pathway

retrochiasmatic region

retrocorneal
    r. membrane
    r. nut

retrodisplacement

retroflexion of iris

retrogeniculate lesion

retrograde transsynaptic degeneration

retrohyaloid premacular hemorrhage

retroilluminate

retroillumination

retroiridian

retrolaminar

retrolental
    r. fibroplasia (RLF)
    r. space

retrolenticular

retromembranous

retroocular
    r. injection
    r. space

retroorbital headache

retroplacement

retroprosthetic membrane

retropupillary

retroscopic lens

retrospective study

retrotarsal fold

returning light beam

Reuss
    R. color chart
    R. color table

Reverdin suture needle

reversal
    r. agent
    laser presbyopia r.

reverse
    r. action window
    r. amblyopia
    r. bobbing
    r. dipping
    r. Marcus Gunn pupil
    r. optics
    r. pupillary block

reverse-cutting needle

reversed
    r. astigmatism
    r. ophthalmic artery flow (ROAF)
    r. pupillary reflex

reverse-shape implant

reversible lid speculum

Rev-Eyes

Revilliod sign

revision
    bleb r.

Revolution lens

rewetting solution

Reynold lead citrate

Rey-Osterreith Complex Figure

ReZoom multifocal refractive IOL

RFB
    retained foreign body

RGP
    rigid gas-permeable
    RGP contact lens

rhabdoid tumor

rhabdomyosarcoma
    nonorbital childhood parameningeal embryonal r.
    orbital r.

rhegmatogenous retinal detachment (RRD)

Rhein
    R. Advantage II diamond limbal-relaxing incision knife

R. Artisan lens-holding forceps
R. aspiration cannula
R. blade cleaning system
R. capsulorrhexis cystotome forceps
R. clear corneal diamond knife
R. 3D angled trapezoid diamond knife
R. 3D trapezoid diamond blade
R. fine foldable lens-insertion forceps
R. irrigation cannula
R. LASIK epithelial detaching hoe
R. LASIK epithelial detaching spatula
R. LASIK flap elevator and stromal spatula
R. LASIK flap forceps
R. LASIK flap repositioning spatula
R. reusable cautery pen

rheopheresis
Rhese position
rheumatic nodule
rheumatoid
r. hyperviscosity syndrome
r. related ulceration
r. sclerouveitis
rheumatoid-associated nuclear antigen
rhexis
runaway r.
rhinitis
acute catarrhal r.
allergic r.
atrophic r.
r. caseosa
chronic catarrhal r.
croupous r.
fibrinous r.
gangrenous r.
hypertrophic r.
membranous r.
pseudomembranous r.
purulent r.
scrofulous r.
r. sicca
syphilitic r.
tuberculous r.
rhinocanthectomy
rhinoconjunctivitis
perennial r.
r. quality of life questionnaire
seasonal r.
rhinodacryolith

rhinoorbital-cerebral mucormycosis
rhinoorbital mucormycosis
rhinophyma
rhinoplasty
rhinoscleroma
rhinosporidiosis
conjunctival r.
Rhinosporidium seeberi
rhinotomy
rhodogenesis
rhodophylactic
rhodophylaxis
rhodopsin
Rhus radicans
rhythmic nystagmus
rhytide
eyelid r.
rhytidosis retinae
RI
recession index
ribbon gauze dressing
ribbon-like keratitis
ribonucleic acid (RNA)
Ricco law
Rice pick
Richard
R. pillow
R. Products fundus camera drug organizer
Richardson methylene blue/aure II mixture
Richner-Hanhart syndrome
Ricinus communis agglutinin
rickettsial blepharitis
Ridaura
Riddoch
R. phenomenon
R. syndrome
ridge
laser r.
r. lens
mesenchymal r.
petrous r.
supraorbital r.
synaptic r.
riding bow temple
Ridley
R. anterior chamber lens implant
R. lens
R. Mark II lens implant
Riedel
R. needle
R. thyroiditis

NOTES

Rieger
>R. anomaly
>R. syndrome

rifle
>air r.

right
>r. bi-plate placement
>r. deorsumvergence
>r. deviation
>r. esotropia
>r. exotropia
>r. eye (OD)
>r. gaze
>r. gaze verticals
>r. hyperphoria
>r. hypertropia
>r. port
>r. sursumvergence

right-angle
>r.-a. deflected venule
>r.-a. prism
>r.-a. prism magnifier

right-beating nystagmus
right-eyed
right-handed cornea scissors
right/left corneoscleral scissors
rigid
>r. gas-permeable (RGP)
>r. gas-permeable contact lens
>r. pupil

rigidity
>axial r.
>low scleral r.
>mydriatic r.
>ocular r.
>scleral r.

Riley-Day syndrome
Riley-Smith syndrome
rim
>corneoscleral r.
>inferior orbital r.
>neural r.
>neuroretinal r.
>r. notching
>orbital inferior r.
>saucering of r.
>superior r.

rima, pl. **rimae**
>r. cornealis
>r. palpebrarum

rimexolone ophthalmic suspension
rimless frame
rim-to-disc ratio
ring
>abscess r.
>r. abscess
>aniridia r.
>anterior limiting r.
>anular r.

Bloomberg SuperNumb anesthetic r.
Bores twist fixation r.
capsular tension r.
cataract mask r.
r. cataract mask eye shield
centering r.
choroidal r.
ciliary r.
Cionni capsular tension r.
Coats white r.
collagenolytic trabecular r.
collagenous trabecular r.
common tendinous r.
conjunctival r.
corneal iron r.
corneal transplant centering r.
R. D chromosome syndrome
Dell fixation r.
Döllinger tendinous r.
Donders r.
endocapsular equator r.
Fine crescent fixation r.
Fine-Thornton scleral fixation r.
fixation r.
Fleischer keratoconus r.
Fleischer-Strümpell r.
Flieringa scleral fixation r.
r. forceps
Gimbel stabilization r.
Girard scleral-expander r.
glaucomatous r.
glial r.
Hansatome 8.5-mm suction r.
Hofmann-Thornton globe fixation r.
immune Wessely r.
r. infiltrate
Intacs intrastromal corneal r.
intracorneal r.
intrastromal corneal r.
r. of iris
iris r.
iron Fleischer r.
Johnston fixation r.
Kayser-Fleischer cornea r.
r. keratitis
KeraVision r.
Kraff hyperopic fixation r.
Landers irrigating vitrectomy r.
Landolt broken r.
Landolt C r.
LED-illuminated r.
r. lens expressor
lenticular r.
light reflex r.
Lowe r.
Lu-Mendez LRI guide and
>fixation r.
Martinez corneal transplant
>centering r.

Maxwell r.
McKinney fixation r.
McNeill-Goldman r.
r. melanoma
Morcher Cionni endocapsular
capsular tension r.
Morcher iris diaphragm r., type
50C, type 96G
Moretsky LASIK hinge protector
fixation r.
Nichamin fixation r.
nuclear r.
Oculaid capsular tension r.
r. perimetry
Placido r.
polymer r.
posterior limiting r.
prominent Schwalbe r.
pupil dilator r.
rust r.
Saturn r.
Schwalbe anterior border r.
scleral expander r.
scotoma r.
r. scotoma
r. of Soemmerring
Soemmerring r.
Stableyes capsular tension r.
subretinal pigment r.
suction r.
symblepharon r.
Tano r.
tantalum "O" r.
Thornton-Fine r.
Thornton fixating r.
Thornton limbal fixation r.
Tolentino r.
r. ulcer
r. ulcer of cornea
Vossius lenticular r.
Weinstein fixation r.
Weiss r.
Wessely r.
white r.
Whitten fixation r.
Zinn r.
Ringer lactate solution
ring-form congenital cataract
ringlike corneal dystrophy
28-ring Placido cone
ring-shaped
r.-s. cataract

r.-s. dystrophy
r.-s. stromal infiltrate
ring-tip forceps
Riolan muscle
Ripault sign
rip-cord suture
ripe cataract
risk
r. factor
r. factor analysis
r. factors in ARMD
glaucoma r.
ocular r.
retinal detachment r.
Scoring Tool for Assessing R.
(STAR)
Risley rotary prism
ristocetin cofactor activity
Ritch
R. contact lens
R. nylon suture laser lens
R. trabeculoplasty laser lens
Ritleng probe
Ritter fiber
rivalry
binocular r.
luminance r.
r. of retina
retinal r.
river blindness
rivus lacrimalis
Rizzuti
R. graft carrier spoon
R. iris retractor
R. lens expressor
R. rectus forceps
R. scleral fixation forceps
R. sign
Rizzuti-Spizziri cannula knife
RK
radial keratotomy
RK marker
RK-5000
ultrasound pachymeter-KMI R.
RLE
refractive lens exchange
RLF
retrolental fibroplasia
RLH
reactive lymphoid hyperplasia
RNA
ribonucleic acid
RNA III activating protein (RAP)

NOTES

RNFL
    retinal nerve fiber layer
ROAF
    reversed ophthalmic artery flow
Roaf syndrome
ROAM
    roaming optical access multiscope
roaming optical access multiscope (ROAM)
Robertson
    R. pupil
    R. sign
Roberts-SC phocomelia
Robin
    R. chalazion clamp
    R. syndrome
Robinow syndrome
Rocephin
Rochester nomogram
rocket-propelled grenade injury
rod
    r. achromatopsia
    bipolar r.
    r. b-wave amplitude
    r. b-wave response
    r. cell
    r.'s and cones
    double Maddox r.
    r. electroretinogram
    r. fiber
    r. function
    graceful swirling r.
    r. granule
    Maddox r.
    Mira silicone r.
    r. monochromasy
    r. monochromat
    r. monochromatism
    r. myopathy
    Perspex r.
    r. photoreceptor
    retinal r.
    scleral sponge r.
    semirigid silicone plastic r.
    Silastic r.
    silicone r.
    vision r.
    r. vision
rod-cone
    r.-c. amplitude
    r.-c. degeneration
    r.-c. dysfunction
    r.-c. dystrophy
    r.-c. interaction
Rodenstock
    R. eye refractometer
    R. panfunduscope
    R. panfundus lens
    R. scanning laser ophthalmoscope

    R. slit lamp
    R. system
rodent ulcer
Rodin orbital implant
roentgenogram
    orbital r.
Rolf
    R. forceps
    R. lacrimal probe
    R. lance
roll
    Fluftex gauze r.
    iris r.
    peripheral iris r.
    scleral r.
rolled-up epithelium with wavy border
roller
    r. forceps
    Lindstrom LASIK flap r.
Rollet
    R. irrigating/aspirating unit
    R. lacrimal probe
    R. retractor
    R. syndrome
rolling of eyes
ROLS
    Reinverting Operating Lens System
Romaña sign
Romberg
    R. sign
    R. syndrome
Rommel electrocautery
Romycin
RON
    radiation optic neuropathy
Rondec
    R. Drops
    R. Filmtab
    R. Syrup
Rondec-TR
rongeur
    Belz lacrimal sac r.
    biting r.
    bone r.
    Citelli r.
    Kerrison mastoid r.
    lacrimal sac r.
    Lempert r.
    single-action r.
Ronne nasal step
roof
    r. fracture
    r. of orbit
    orbital r.
root
    iris r.
    motor r.
    oculomotor r.
    sensory r.

ROP
retinopathy of prematurity
Roper alpha-chymotrypsin cannula
Roper-Hall classification
ropy mucus
Roquinimex
rosacea
acne r.
blepharitis r.
blepharoconjunctivitis r.
keratitis r.
r. keratitis
ocular r.
rosacea-meibomianitis
Rosai-Dorfman disease
Roscoe-Bunsen law
rose
r. bengal
r. bengal red solution
r. bengal stain
roseata
Rosen
R. nucleus paddle
R. phaco splitter
Rosenbach sign
Rosenbaum
R. card
R. pocket vision screener
Rosenblatt scissors
Rosenmüller
R. body
R. gland
R. node
valve of R.
R. valve
rosette
Flexner-Wintersteiner r.
Homer-Wright r.
Wintersteiner r.
Rosner tonometer
rostaporfin
rostral
r. interstitial medial longitudinal
fasciculus
r. interstitial nucleus
rotary
r. cutting tip
r. prism
rotating
r. brush
r. corneal autograft
rotating-type cutter

rotation
center of r.
corneal flap by r.
eye r.
macular translocation with
retinotomy and retinal r.
ocular r.
retinal r.
suture r.
toric intraocular lens axis r.
wheel r.
rotational
r. direction
r. nystagmus
r. test
rotator
Bechert nucleus r.
Espaillat-Deblasio nucleus r.
Jaffe-Bechert nucleus r.
Maloney nucleus r.
nucleus r.
rotatory nystagmus
Roth
R. spot
R. spot syndrome
Roth-Bielschowsky syndrome
Rothman-Gilbard corneal punch
Rothmund syndrome
Rothmund-Thomson syndrome
rotoextractor
Douvas r.
rotundum foramen
Rouget muscle
rough endoplasmic reticulum
round
r. hemorrhage
r. top bifocal
Rousseau chin-lift stabilizer
route
r. of administration
canalicular r.
external r.
topical administration r.
transconjunctival r.
Rovamycine
Roveda lid everter
roving eye movement
Rowen
R. spatula
R. white-to-white corneal gauge
Rowsey fixation cannula
Royal Australian College of
Ophthalmologists

R

NOTES

Royale intraocular lens injector
RP
> retinitis pigmentosa
> > RP hypertrophy

RP10 gene variant of retinitis pigmentosa
RPE
> retinal pigment epithelium
> > hemorrhagic RPE

RPGR
> retinitis pigmentosa GTPase regulator
> > gene

R&R
> recession-resection
> recess-resect

RRD
> rhegmatogenous retinal detachment

RR-MS
> relapsing/remitting multiple sclerosis

RSVP
> rapid serial visual presentation

RTA
> retinal thickness analysis
> retinal thickness analyzer

rub
> > Complete Moisture Plus Multi-Purpose Solution No r.

rubbing
> eye r.

rubella
> r. cataract
> congenital r.
> r. retinitis
> r. retinopathy

Rubenstein LASIK Cannula
Rubenstein-type LASIK irrigating cannula
rubeola
> r. conjunctivitis
> r. keratitis

rubeosis
> r. iridis
> r. iridis diabetica

rubeotic glaucoma
Rubinstein-Taybi syndrome
ruboxistaurin mesylate
ruby
> r. diamond knife
> r. laser

Rucker body
rudimentary eye
rudiment lens
Ruedemann lacrimal dilator
ruff
> pupillary r.

ruffed canal
Ruggeri reflex

Ruiz
> R. procedure
> R. trapezoidal keratotomy

Ruiz-Nordan trapezoidal marker
rule
> accommodation r.
> astigmatism against the r.
> astigmatism with the r.
> Behren r.
> Javal r.
> Kestenbaum r.
> Knapp r.
> Kollner r.
> Prentice r.
> Prince r.

ruler
> biometric r.
> Helveston scleral marking r.
> Hyde astigmatism r.
> Hyde-Osher keratometric r.
> Scott curved r.
> Thornton double corneal r.
> Thornton limbal incision r.

Rumex titanium instrument
Ruminson astigmatic gauge and marker
runaway rhexis
running nylon penetrating keratoplasty suture
rupture
> autosomal dominant vitellus r.
> choroidal r.
> explosive globe r.
> indirect choroidal r.
> occult scleral r.
> scleral r.
> traumatic choroidal r.

ruptured globe
Rushton ocular measurement
Russell
> R. body
> R. syndrome
> R. viper venom time

Russian
> R. forceps
> R. 4-pronged fixation hook

rust
> r. ring
> r. ring of cornea
> r. spot

ruthenium
> r. plaque
> r. red

ruthenium-106 ophthalmic plaque
Rutherford syndrome
rutidosis
Ruysch
> R. membrane
> R. tunic

ruyschiana
    membrana r.
ruyschian membrane
Rycroft
    R. cannula

R. needle
R. tying forceps

NOTES

R

S-100 protein antibody
S4 excimer laser
SA60AT intraocular lens
Sabin-Feldman dye test
Sabouraud
    S. dextrose agar
    S. medium
Sabreloc needle
Sabril
saburral
    s. amaurosis
    s. amaurosis fugax
sac
    conjunctival s.
    drainage of lacrimal s.
    Förster lacrimal s.
    lacrimal s.
    nasolacrimal s.
    tear s.
    Tenon s.
saccade
    downgaze s.
    foveating s.
    hypometric s.
    normal upward corrective s.
    ocular s.
    s. palsy
    scanning s.
    slow hypometric vertical s.
    slow-to-no s.
saccadic
    s. abnormality
    s. adaptation
    s. change
    s. contrapulsion
    s. disorder
    s. dysmetria
    s. eccentric target
    s. eye movement
    s. fixation
    s. intrusion
    s. movement of eye
    s. pulse
    s. pursuit
    s. velocity
saccadomania
sacci (*pl. of* saccus)
saccular
    s. aneurysm
    s. dilation
sacculiform
sacculus lacrimalis
saccus, pl. **sacci**
    s. conjunctivae

    s. conjunctivalis
    s. lacrimalis
Sachs tissue forceps
SAD
    seasonal affective disorder
saddle
    s. bridge
    Turkish s.
Saemisch
    S. operation
    S. section
    S. ulcer
Saenger
    S. pupil
    S. sign
SAFE
    Structure And Function Evaluation
    SAFE study
safe to drive
safety
    s. of cyclosporine
    s. eyewear
    s. glasses
    s. lens
    s. spectacles
    s. standard
Safil synthetic absorbable surgical suture
sag
    eyelid s.
SAGE
    Statpac-like Analysis for Glaucoma Evaluation
sagittal
    s. axis
    s. axis of eye
    s. axis of Fick
    s. depth
    s. height
SAI
    surface asymmetry index
Sainton sign
Sakurai-Lisch nodule
Salagen
salicylate
    physostigmine s.
saline
    Blairex sterile s.
    Ciba Vision S.
    Hydrocare preserved s.
    hypertonic s.
    Lens Plus s.
    Murine sterile s.
    phosphate-buffered s.
    Soft Mate s.

S

saline *(continued)*
    SoftWear S.
    s. solution
    sorbic acid Sorbi-Care s.
    sterile preserved s.
saline-saturated wool dressing
salivarius
    Streptococcus s.
salivary
    s. gland
    s. nucleus
Salleras procedure
salmon patch
salt
    gold s.
salt-and-pepper
    s.-a.-p. appearance
    s.-a.-p. chorioretinitis
    s.-a.-p. fundus
    s.-a.-p. retinopathy
Salus
    S. arch
    S. sign
salvage
    visual s.
Salzmann
    S. nodular corneal degeneration
    S. nodular corneal dystrophy
    S. nodule
Salz nucleus splitter
Samoan conjunctivitis
Sampaolesi line
Sanchez-Bulnes lacrimal sac retractor
Sanchez Salorio syndrome
sand
    s. dune PCO
    S. process
    s.'s of Sahara keratitis
    s.'s of Sahara syndrome
Sanders
    S. disease
    S. disorder
Sanders-Castroviejo suturing forceps
Sanders-Retzlaff-Kraff (SRK)
    Sanders-Retzlaff-Kraff formula
Sandimmune
SANDO
    sensory ataxic neuropathy with dysarthria
    and ophthalmoplegia
Sandt forceps
sandy
    s. eyes
    s. foreign body sensation
sanguineous cataract
Sanson image
SAP
    standard automated perimetry
Sappey fiber
sapphire knife

saprophytic
    s. bacteria
    s. fungus
saprophyticus
    Staphylococcus s.
sarcoid
    Boeck s.
    s. uveitis
sarcoidosis
    s. infiltration
    pediatric ocular s.
sarcoidosis-associated uveitis
sarcoma, pl. **sarcomata**
    Ewing s.
    granulocytic s.
    hemorrhagic s.
    Kaposi s.
    melanotic s.
    multifocal hemorrhagic s.
    reticulum cell s.
sarcomatosum
    ectropion s.
    glioma s.
    s. senilis
Sarfarazi dual optic intraocular lens
satellite
    s. ganglionic cell
    s. lesion
SatinCrescent tunneler
Sato
    S. cataract needle
    S. corneal knife
    S. keratoconus
    S. lid retractor
    S. operation
    S. procedure
Sattler
    S. advancement forceps
    S. layer
    S. veil
saturated color
saturation
    color s.
    oxygen s.
SaturEyes contact lens
Saturn
    S. II contact lenses
    S. ring
saturninus
    halo s.
saucering of rim
saucerization
saucer-shaped cataract
Sauer
    S. corneal débrider
    S. infant speculum
    S. suture forceps
Sauflon PW lens
Saupe cilia forceps

Sauvineau ophthalmoplegia
saw
>   Stryker s.

sayonara technique
Sayre elevator
SB
>   scleral buckle

SBS
>   shaken baby syndrome

SBV
>   single binocular vision

SC
>   scleral cautery
>   stem cell
>   subconjunctival

s̄c
>   without correction

SC60B-OUV IOL
scaffolding
>   capillary s.

scale
>   activities of daily vision s.
>   (ADVS)
>   disc damage likelihood s. (DDLS)
>   Esterman s.
>   Expanded Disability Status S.
>   (EDSS)
>   Fitzpatrick sun-sensitivity s.
>   Griffith s.
>   Indiana bleb appearance grading s.
>   Klyce-Wilson s.
>   4-level severity rating s.
>   Resource-Based Relative Value S.
>   (RBRVS)
>   Snell-Sterling visual efficiency s.
>   visual analog s. (VAS)

scalloped
>   s. border
>   s. contour
>   s. pupil

scalloping
scalpel
>   s. guard
>   s. injury
>   Microcap s.

scalp flap
scaly plaque
scan
>   artifact-free s.
>   axial CT s.
>   B s.
>   choroidal s.
>   computed tomography s.

computerized tomography s.
coronal CT s.
cross-vector A-s.
duplex s.
s. evaluation
gallium s.
isotope s.
limited gallium s.
magnetic resonance imaging s.
MRI s.
Ophthascan Mini-A s.
orbital CT s.
OTI ultrasound B & A s.
radioisotope s.
technetium s.
US-2000 echo s.

ScanMaker 4 flatbed scanner
scanner
>   Epson 3200 Perfect S.
>   Heidelberg laser tomographic s.
>   laser tomography s. (LTS)
>   ScanMaker 4 flatbed s.
>   Zeiss-Humphrey 840 UBM s.

scanning
>   s. excimer laser
>   gallium s.
>   s. laser glaucoma test
>   s. laser ophthalmoscope (SLO)
>   s. laser ophthalmoscope perimetry
>   s. laser polarimeter
>   s. laser polarimetry (SLP)
>   s. laser tomography (SLT)
>   s. prism
>   s. retinal thickness analyzer
>   s. saccade
>   s. slit confocal microscope
>   variable spot s. (VSS)

Scappa frame
scar
>   chorioretinal s.
>   corneal s.
>   disciform s.
>   disciform macular s.
>   external s.
>   fibrotic s.
>   fibrovascular s.
>   gray-white corneal s.
>   herpes simplex s.
>   linear s.
>   peripapillary s.
>   pigmented chorioretinal s.
>   s. plate

S

NOTES

scar *(continued)*
    punched-out chorioretinal s.
    vascularized s.
scarification
scarifier
    s. knife
    Kuhnt corneal s.
Scarpa staphyloma
scarring
    bulbar conjunctival s.
    conjunctival s.
    corneal s.
    episcleral s.
    ghost s.
    gossamer s.
    linear s.
    napkin-ring peripapillary s.
    quiescent stromal s.
    stromal ghost s.
    subretinal s.
scatter
    beam s.
    forward light s.
    s. laser photocoagulation
    light s.
    s. pattern
    peripheral light s.
    sclerotic s.
scattergram
scattering
    light s.
    Rayleigh s.
    reflective s.
scatterplot
SCE
    serous choroidal effusion
Scedosporium
    S. apiospermum
    S. prolificans
SCH
    suprachoroidal hemorrhage
Schaaf foreign body forceps
Schachne-Desmarres lid everter
Schaedel cross-action towel clamp
Schaffer sign
Schaumann inclusion body
schedule
    drug-dosing s.
Scheie
    S. akinesia
    S. anterior chamber cannula
    S. blade
    S. cataract-aspirating cannula
    S. cataract-aspirating needle
    S. classification
    S. electrocautery
    S. goniopuncture knife
    S. goniotomy knife

    S. operation
    S. ophthalmic cautery
    S. syndrome
    S. thermal sclerostomy
Scheie-Westcott corneal section scissors
Scheimpflug
    S. camera
    S. photography
    S. principle
    S. slit image
    S. videophotography system
Scheiner
    S. experiment
    S. principle
    S. theory
schematic eye
schenckii
    Sporothrix s.
Schepens
    S. binocular indirect
        ophthalmoscope
    S. forceps
    S. Gelfilm
    S. orbital retractor
    S. retinal detachment unit
    S. scleral depressor
    S. spoon
    S. technique
    S. thimble depressor
Schepens-Pomerantzeff ophthalmoscope
scheroma
Schilder
    S. disease
    S. encephalitis
Schiötz
    S. tonofilm
    S. tonometer
    S. tonometry
Schirmer
    S. filter paper
    S. I, II test
    S. syndrome
    S. tear quality test
    S. tear test strip
    S. test score
schisis
    s. cavity
    peripheral s.
schisis-related detachment
Schlegel lens
schleiferi
    Staphylococcus s.
Schlemm canal
Schlichting dystrophy
Schlieren phenomenon
Schmid-Fraccaro syndrome
Schmidt keratitis
Schmincke tumor

Schnabel
S. cavern
S. optic atrophy
Schnidt clamp
Schnyder
central crystalline corneal dystrophy
of S.
S. crystalline corneal dystrophy
Schocket
S. anterior chamber tube shunt
S. scleral depressor
S. tube implant
Schöler treatment
Schön theory
school myopia
Schott lid speculum
**Schubert-Bornschein congenital
stationary night blindness**
Schultz
S. fiber basket
S. iris retractor
Schumann giant type eye magnet
Schwalbe
S. anterior border ring
S. line (SL)
S. space
Schwann
S. cell
cord of S.
schwannoma
malignant s.
melanotic s.
oculomotor nerve s.
orbital s.
Schwartz-Jampel syndrome
Schwartz syndrome
Schweigger
S. capsule forceps
S. extracapsular forceps
S. hand perimeter
Schweninger-Buzzi macular atrophy
science
vision s.
scientific investigation
scimitar scotoma
scintigraphy
scintillans
synchesis s.
synchysis s.
scintillating
s. granule
s. scotoma
s. vision loss

scintillation
scintillography
lacrimal s.
scirrhencanthis
scirrhophthalmia
scissors
Aebli corneal section s.
alligator s.
anterior chamber synechia s.
Atkinson corneal s.
bandage s.
Barraquer corneoscleral s.
Barraquer vitreous strand s.
Becker corneal section spatulated s.
Berens corneal transplant s.
Berens iridocapsulotomy s.
blunt-tipped Vannas s.
Bonn iris s.
canalicular s.
capsulotomy s.
Castroviejo anterior synechia s.
Castroviejo corneal section s.
Castroviejo corneal transplant s.
Castroviejo iridocapsulotomy s.
Castroviejo keratoplasty s.
Castroviejo synechia s.
Cohan-Vannas iris s.
Cohan-Westcott s.
conjunctival s.
corneal section spatulated s.
corneoscleral right/left hand s.
curved iris s.
curved tenotomy s.
de Wecker iris s.
dissecting s.
enucleation s.
eye suture s.
Fine suture s.
Frost s.
Gill s.
Gills-Welsh s.
Gills-Welsh-Vannas angled micro s.
Girard corneoscleral s.
Grieshaber vertical cutting s.
Grieshaber vitreous s.
Halsted strabismus s.
horizontal s.
House-Bellucci alligator s.
Hunt chalazion s.
iridectomy s.
iridocapsulotomy s.
iridotomy s.
iris s.

S

NOTES

scissors *(continued)*
Irvine probe-pointed s.
Keeler intravitreal s.
keratectomy s.
keratoplasty s.
Kirby s.
Knapp iris s.
Knapp strabismus s.
Lagrange sclerectomy s.
Lawton corneal s.
left-handed cornea s.
Lister s.
Littauer dissecting s.
Littler dissecting s.
Manson-Aebli corneal section s.
Mattis corneal s.
Maunoir iris s.
Max Fine s.
Mayo s.
McClure iris s.
McGuire corneal s.
McLean capsulotomy s.
McPherson-Castroviejo corneal section s.
McPherson corneal section s.
McPherson-Vannas microiris s.
McPherson-Westcott conjunctival s.
McPherson-Westcott stitch s.
McReynolds pterygium s.
mechanized s.
micro vertical s.
micro Westcott s.
mini-keratoplasty stitch s.
mini Westcott s.
Morris vertical s.
s. motion
s. movement
MPC automated intravitreal s.
Noyes iridectomy s.
Noyes iris s.
O'Brien stitch s.
pterygium s.
ptosis s.
radial iridotomy s.
Reeh s.
Reichling corneal s.
right-handed cornea s.
right/left corneoscleral s.
Rosenblatt s.
Scheie-Westcott corneal section s.
Shield iridotomy s.
Smart s.
Spencer eye suture s.
Spring iris s.
Stevens eye s.
Stevens tenotomy s.
strabismus s.
straight tenotomy s.
superior radial tenotomy s.

Sutherland s.
Thomas s.
Thorpe s.
Thorpe-Westcott s.
Troutman-Castroviejo corneal section s.
Troutman conjunctival s.
Troutman-Katzin corneal transplant s.
Troutman microsurgical s.
Troutman suture s.
Vannas capsulotomy s.
Vannas iridocapsulotomy s.
Verhoeff s.
vibrating s.
s. vitrectomy
vitreous strand s.
Walker s.
Walker-Apple s.
Walker-Atkinson s.
Wecker iris s.
Werb s.
Westcott conjunctival s.
Westcott stitch s.
Westcott tenotomy s.
Westcott utility s.
Wilmer conjunctival s.
Wincor enucleation s.
Witherspoon vertical s.
Zaldivar iridectomy s.
scissors-shadow
SCL
soft contact lens
sclera, pl. **scleras, sclerae**
bared s.
baring of s.
blanching of s.
blue s.
buckling s.
ectasia of s.
foramen of s.
lamina cribrosa sclerae
lamina fusca sclerae
limbus of s.
massive granuloma of s.
melanosis sclerae
substantia propria sclerae
sulcus s.
white s.
scleral
s. avulsion
s. blade
s. buckle (SB)
s. buckling
s. buckling operation
s. buckling procedure
s. canal
s. canal size
s. cautery (SC)

s. channel
s. conjunctiva
s. contact lens
s. crescent
s. cyst
s. deformity
s. degeneration
s. depression
s. depressor
s. ectasia
s. erosion
s. exoplant
s. expander
s. expander ring
s. expansion band
s. expansion band procedure
s. expansion surgery
s. explant
s. explant surgery
s. fistula
s. fistulectomy operation
s. fixation light
s. flap
s. flap suture
s. framework
s. furrow
s. grip
s. hook
s. icterus
s. implant
s. indentation
s. infolding
s. lamina cribrosa
s. limbus
s. lip
s. marker
s. melting
s. miniflap
s. necrosis
s. outfolding
s. overriding
s. patch graft
s. pick
s. plexus
s. punch
s. reinforcement
s. resection
s. resection knife
s. rigidity
s. roll
s. rupture
s. search coil
s. search coil technique

s. shell
s. shell glaucoma
s. shortening clip
s. shortening operation
s. show
s. sponge rod
s. spur (SS)
s. staphyloma
s. substance
s. sulcus
s. supporter
s. tissue
s. tissue shred
s. trabecula
s. tunnel
s. tunnel abscess
s. tunnel incision
s. twist
s. twist-grip forceps
s. venous sinus
s. window
scleral-limbal-corneal incision
scleras (*pl. of* sclera)
scleratitis
sclerectasia
   partial s.
   total s.
sclerectasis
sclerectoiridectomy
sclerectoiridodialysis
sclerectome
sclerectomy
   holmium YAG laser s.
   Holth s.
   nonpenetrating deep s.
   s. punch
   thermal s.
   trabeculotome-guided deep s.
scleriasis
scleriritomy
scleritis
   anterior s.
   anular s.
   brawny s.
   deep s.
   diffuse anterior s.
   gelatinous s.
   herpes simplex s.
   idiopathic s.
   malignant s.
   necrotizing nocardial s.
   necrotizing nodular s.
   nodular s.

NOTES

S

scleritis *(continued)*
    posterior s.
    syphilitic s.
sclerochoroidal
    s. calcification
    s. thickening
sclerochoroiditis
    anterior s.
    s. anterior
    posterior s.
    s. posterior
scleroconjunctival
scleroconjunctivitis
sclerocornea
    isolated s.
    total s.
sclerocorneal
    s. junction
    s. phacoemulsification
    s. sulcus
scleroiritis
sclerokeratectomy
sclerokeratitis
sclerokeratoiritis
sclerokeratoplasty
sclerokeratosis
scleromalacia perforans
scleronyxis
sclerophthalmia
scleroplasty operation
sclerosing
    s. keratitis
    s. orbital granuloma
    s. panencephalitis chorioretinitis
    s. therapy
sclerosis, pl. **scleroses**
    arteriolar s.
    central areolar choroidal s.
    choroidal primary s.
    diffuse choroidal s.
    multiple s.
    nuclear s. (NS)
    peripapillary s.
    progressive systemic s.
    relapsing/remitting multiple s. (RR-MS)
    secondary progressive multiple s. (SP-MS)
    systemic s.
    tuberous s.
sclerostomy
    enzymatic s.
    s. needle
    posterior thermal s.
    Scheie thermal s.
    thermal s.
    trabecuphine laser s.
sclerotic
    s. cataract

    s. coat
    nuclear s. (NS)
    s. scatter
    s. scatter illumination
    s. stroma
sclerotica
    tunica s.
scleroticectomy
scleroticochoroiditis
scleroticotomy
sclerotitis
sclerotome
    Alvis-Lancaster s.
    Atkinson s.
    Curdy s.
    Lundsgaard s.
    Walker-Lee s.
sclerotomy
    anterior s.
    combined phacoemulsification and nonpenetrating deep s.
    deep s.
    foreign body s.
    23-gauge s.
    25-gauge s.
    s. operation
    s. port
    posterior s.
    s. punch
    s. removal of foreign body
    self-sealing s.
    s. with drainage
    s. with exploration
sclerotomy-related retinal break
sclerouveitis
    rheumatoid s.
sclopetaria
    chorioretinitis s.
    retinitis s.
SCMD microkeratome
SCN
    suprachiasmatic nucleus
Scobee oblique muscle hook
scolex, pl. **scoleces, scolices**
scoliosis
    ocular s.
s-cone excitation
scoop
    Arlt s.
    Daviel s.
    enucleation s.
    Kirby intraocular lens s.
    Knapp s.
    Lewis s.
    Mules s.
    Wilder s.
scope
    Bjerrum s.

tangent s.
Welch-Allyn pocket s.
scopolamine
s. HBr
s. hyoscine
score
ADVS s.
Schirmer test s.
sensitivity s.
Scoring Tool for Assessing Risk (STAR)
scotodinia
scotograph
scotoma, pl. **scotomata**
absolute s.
altitudinal s.
anular s.
arc s.
arcuate Bjerrum s.
aural s.
bitemporal hemianopic s.
Bjerrum s.
cecocentral s.
central s.
centrocecal s.
color s.
comet s.
congruous homonymous hemianopic s.
cuneate-shaped s.
double arcuate s.
eclipse s.
equatorial ring s.
false s.
flittering s.
focal s.
frame s.
glaucomatous nerve-fiber bundle s.
hemianopic s.
homonymous hemianopic s.
insular s.
ipsilateral centrocecal s.
junction s.
s. junction
junctional s.
Mariotte s.
motile s.
s. for motion
negative s.
paracentral ring s.
pericecal s.
pericentral s.
peripapillary s.

peripheral s.
physiologic s.
position s.
positive s.
quadrantic s.
relative s.
ring s.
s. ring
scimitar s.
scintillating s.
Seidel s.
sickle s.
superior arcuate s.
suppression s.
symptomatic paracentral s.
thin-rim s.
s. of Traquair
unilateral altitudinal s.
zonular s.
scotomagraph
scotomatous
scotometer
Bjerrum s.
scotometry
scotomization
scotopia
scotopic
s. adaptation
s. b wave
s. eye
s. perimetry
s. sensitivity
s. sensitivity loss
s. sensitivity syndrome
s. stimulus
s. vision
scotopsin
scotoscope
scotoscopy
Scott
S. curved ruler
S. lens-insertion forceps
scout
Optikon 2000 placido-based corneal topography system Keratron S.
scrape
corneal epithelial s.
epithelial s.
mechanical s.
post s.
scraper
diamond-dusted s.

NOTES

S

scraper *(continued)*
    diamond-dusted membrane s.
      (DDMS)
    epithelial s.
    Knolle capsule s.
    Kratz capsule s.
    Tano membrane s.
scraping
    conjunctival s.
    corneal epithelial s.
    epithelial s.
scratched contact lens
scratcher
    Jensen capsule s.
    Knolle capsule s.
    Kratz capsule s.
scratch-resistant spectacle lens
screen
    Bernell tangent s.
    Bjerrum s.
    Grey-Hess s.
    Hess diplopia s.
    Hess-Lee s.
    s. magnification
    Mitsubishi HL7955 CRT s.
    s. reader
    tangent s.
screener
    Rosenbaum pocket vision s.
    SureSight vision s.
screening
    childhood vision s.
    Modified Clinical Technique
      vision s.
    pediatric vision s.
    photo s.
    preschool s.
    suprathreshold s.
    vision s.
scrofulous
    s. conjunctivitis
    s. keratitis
    s. ophthalmia
    s. rhinitis
scroll pump
scrub
    lid s.
    OCuSoft s.
    s. typhus
scrubber
    Amoils epithelial s.
    Simcoe anterior chamber capsule s.
scurf
    lid s.
scutum region
SD
    standard deviation
SDI-BIOM wide angle viewing system

sea
    s. fan sign
    s. frond
sealant
    fibrin s.
    VH fibrin s.
sealed capsule irrigation device
seam
    pigment s.
search
    literature s.
    modified binary s. (MOBS)
Searcy
    S. anchor/fixation
    S. chalazion trephine
seasonal
    s. affective disorder (SAD)
    s. allergic conjunctivitis
    s. rhinoconjunctivitis
sebaceous
    s. adenoma
    s. cell
    s. cell carcinoma
    s. eyelid cancer
    s. gland
    s. gland carcinoma
    s. gland of conjunctiva
    s. inclusion cyst
sebaceum
    adenoma s.
seborrhea
seborrheic
    s. blepharitis
    s. debris
    s. keratosis
SEBR
    spontaneous eye blink rate
Seckel syndrome
seclusion of pupil
secobarbital sodium
second
    s. cranial nerve
    s. sight
secondary
    s. action
    s. amyloidosis
    s. angle-closure glaucoma
    s. anophthalmia
    s. astigmatism
    s. axis
    s. blepharospasm
    s. cataract
    s. childhood glaucoma
    s. curve on contact lens
    s. deviation
    s. dye test
    s. exotropia
    s. eye
    s. focal length

s. focal point
s. intraocular lens
s. inverse optic atrophy
s. keratitis
s. lens implant
s. malignant neoplasm
s. mechanism
s. membrane
s. membrane formation
s. neovascular glaucoma
s. neovascularization
s. ocular infection
s. position
s. progressive multiple sclerosis (SP-MS)
s. retinal degeneration
s. retinitis
s. strabismus
s. vitreous

second-degree relative
second-eye cataract surgery
second-grade fusion
secretion
basal tear s.
meibomian s.
oily s.
reflex tear s.
tear s.

secretogogue
secretomotor nerve
secretory epithelial cell
section
nerve cross s.
orbital s.
Saemisch s.
trigeminal nerve root s.

sectioning
noninvasively s.

sector
s. cortical cataract
s. cut
s. defect
s. iridectomy
s. iridectomy operation
s. pallor
s. palsy
s. retinitis pigmentosa

sectoral
s. iris paralysis
s. redness
s. wavelength

sectoranopia
congruous homonymous horizontal s.
congruous homonymous quadruple s.

sector-shaped defect
sedimentary cataract
SEE
Society for Excellence in Eyecare
Surgical Eye Expeditions

seeberi
Rhinosporidium s.

seeding
vitreous s.

Seeligmüller sign
seesaw
s. anisocoria
s. nystagmus

segment
anterior ocular s.
bifocal s.
capsular tension s.
compensated s.
corneal ring s.
dissimilar s.
extramedullary s.
s. height
inner s.
Intacs corneal ring s.
intramedullary s.
intrastromal corneal ring s. (ICRS)
intratemporal s.
nucleus s.
outer s.
posterior s.
prism s.

segmental
s. buckle
s. explant
s. hypoplasia
s. implant
s. iris atrophy
s. lens

segmentation
neodymium:yttrium-lithium-fluoride laser s.

Seibel
S. double-ended LASIK flap lifter and spatula
S. 3D speculum
S. LASIK flap irrigator
S. LASIK flap irrigator and squeegee cannula

S

NOTES

469

Seibel *(continued)*
S. LRI diamond knife
S. nucleus chopper
S. paracentesis valve adjuster
S. vertical safety quick chopper

Seidel
S. scotoma
S. sign
S. test

Seiff frontalis suspension set

seizure
visual s.

Selecta
S. Duet combination laser system
S. Duet glaucoma laser system
S. Duo ophthalmic laser system
S. 7000 glaucoma laser system
S. II glaucoma laser system
S. 1064 laser platform
S. Trio glaucoma laser system

selection
data s.
stepwise variable s.

selective
s. facial myectomy
s. laser trabeculoplasty (SLT)
s. photothermolysis
s. purinergic
s. transplantation

self-adhering lid retractor

self-adjusted glasses

self-adjusting
s.-a. mechanism
s.-a. suture

self-centering micromanipulator

self-fixating sideport diamond knife

self-gelling glue

self-inflicted
s.-i. blindness
s.-i. visual loss

self-management training

self-retaining
s.-r. infusion cannula
s.-r. irrigating cannula
s.-r. retractor

self-sealing
s.-s. capability
s.-s. scleral puncture
s.-s. sclerotomy
s.-s. side port

self-stabilizing vitrectomy lens

sella, pl. sellae
diaphragma sellae
empty s.
J-shaped s.
tilt of s.
s. turcica

sellar calcification

semicircular canal

semiconductor GaAIAs infrared diode laser photocoagulator

semifinished
s. blank
s. contact lens
s. glass

semilunar
s. fold
s. fold of conjunctiva

semilunaris
plica s.

semiopaque

semirigid silicone plastic rod

semiscleral contact lens

semishell implant

semisolid gel

senescent
s. cortical degenerative cataract
s. disciform macular degeneration
s. ectropion
s. elastosis
s. enophthalmos
s. entropion
s. halo
s. keratosis
s. macular exudative choroiditis
s. macular hole
s. miosis
s. nuclear degenerative cataract
s. ptosis
s. retinoschisis

senile
s. atrophy
s. chorioretinitis
s. choroidal change
s. disciform macular degeneration
s. ectropion
s. elastosis
s. entropion
s. exudative macular degeneration
s. furrow degeneration
s. guttate choroidopathy
s. halo
s. keratosis
s. lenticular myopia
s. macular exudative choroiditis
s. miosis
s. nuclear sclerotic cataract
s. reflex
s. retinoschisis
s. vitreitis

senile-type retinoschisis

senilis
arcus s.
cataract s.
choroiditis guttata s.
linea corneae s.
sarcomatosum s.

Senior-Loken syndrome

Senn retractor
senopia
Sensar
- S. acrylic intraocular lens
- S. OptiEdge AR40e IOL
- S. OptiEdge foldable acrylic IOL
- S. OptiEdge intraocular lens

sensation
- burning s.
- corneal s.
- decreased corneal s.
- s. disturbance
- foreign body s.
- gritty foreign body s.
- s. impairment
- light s.
- nociceptive s.
- sandy foreign body s.
- threshold of visual s.
- s. time

sense
- color s.
- form s.
- light s.
- stereognostic s.

sensing
- wavefront s.

sensitive
- S. Eyes
- S. Eyes daily cleaner
- S. Eyes drops
- S. Eyes Enzymatic Cleaner
- S. Eyes Plus Saline Solution
- S. Eyes saline/cleaning solution
- S. Eyes sterile saline spray

sensitivity
- s. analysis
- blur s.
- conjunctiva s.
- contrast s.
- corneal s.
- foveal s.
- increment threshold spectral s.
- light s.
- periocular drug s.
- retinal s.
- s. score
- scotopic s.
- spatial-contrast s.
- spectral s.
- s. threshold

sensor
- ocular vergence and accommodation s. (OVAS)
- oximetry s.
- pressure s.
- reliable wave front s.
- wavefront s.

Sensorcaine
- S. MPF
- S. with epinephrine

sensorial adaptation
sensorimotor disorder
sensory
- s. amblyopia
- s. ataxic neuropathy with dysarthria and ophthalmoplegia (SANDO)
- s. correspondence
- s. deprivation esotropia
- s. deprivation exotropia
- s. deprivation nystagmus
- s. detachment
- s. elevation
- s. fiber
- s. fusion
- s. nerve
- s. retina
- s. root
- s. root of ciliary ganglion
- s. stimulation
- s. system
- s. visual pathway

separable acuity
separate image test
separation
- centrifugal s.
- dichoptic s.
- fluidic ILM s.
- intraretinal s.
- s. of retina
- vitreofoveal s.
- vitreomacular s.
- vitreous s.

separator
- acrylic s.
- Akahoshi nucleus s.
- Allen stereo s.
- diamond wound s.
- disposable s.
- epithelial s.
- Kirby cylindrical zonal s.
- Kirby flat zonal s.
- Remy s.

S

NOTES

sepsis
  hematogenous s.
septa (*pl. of* septum)
septic
  s. chorioretinitis
  s. retinitis
  s. thrombosis
septica
  iridocyclitis s.
Septicon
septooptic
  s. dysplasia
  s. dysplasia syndrome
septum, pl. **septa**
  s. cavum pellucidum
  inferior orbital s.
  intermuscular s.
  orbital s.
  s. orbitale
  superior orbital s.
  tarsus orbital s.
sequela, pl. **sequelae**
  catastrophic ophthalmic s.
  postoperative s.
Sequels
  Diamox S.
sequence
  genetic s.
  linear sebaceous nevus s.
sequential
  s. measurement
  s. suture removal
sequestered space
sera (*pl. of* serum)
Serdarevic
  S. Circle of Light
  S. speculum
  S. suture adjuster
Sereine
  S. cleaner
  S. soaking and cleaning solution
  S. wetting and soaking solution
serena
  gutta s.
series
  s. 5 forceps
  Zeiss slit-lamp s.
serine protease
serious corneal complication
seropositivity rate
serosa
  retinitis centralis s.
serous
  s. chorioretinopathy
  s. choroidal detachment
  s. choroidal effusion (SCE)
  s. cyclitis
  s. cyst
  s. detachment maculopathy

s. discharge
s. iritis
s. macular detachment
s. membrane
s. pigment epithelial detachment
s. pigment epithelium
s. retinal pigment epithelium
  detachment
s. retinitis
s. retinopathy
Serpasil
serpent ulcer of cornea
serpiginous
  s. choroiditis
  s. choroidopathy
  s. corneal ulcer
  s. keratitis
  s. lesion
  s. ulceration
Serralnyl suture
Serralsilk suture
serrata
  ora s.
serrated conjunctival forceps
Serratia
  S. liquefaciens
  S. marcescens
  S. marcescens infection
serrefine
  ASSI s.
  s. clamp
  Dieffenbach s.
serum, pl. **sera**
  s. amyloid A
  s. laminin-P1
  s. lysozyme
service
  Centers for Medicare &
    Medicaid S.'s
  Lighthouse Low Vision S.
  sterilizer monitoring s.
sessile papilloma
set
  Bloomberg trabeculotome s.
  Carriazo-Barraquer instrument s.
  Catalano intubation s.
  Crawford lacrimal intubation s.
  diagnostic fitting s.
  DORC subretinal instrument s.
  Fine bimanual handpiece s.
  Jackson lacrimal intubation s.
  Jaffe laser blepharoplasty and
    facial resurfacing s.
  Jaffe lid retractor s.
  McIntyre infusion s.
  pediatric vitrectomy lens s.
  Pettigrove LASIK s.
  Price donor cornea punch s.
  Seiff frontalis suspension s.

Simcoe lens positioning s.
Steinert LASIK s.
STENTube lacrimal intubation s.
Thomas subretinal instrument s. II
Tolentino vitrectomy lens s.
variable power cross-cylinder
lens s.

seton
Ahmed drainage s.
s. drainage device
s. implantation size
s. operation

setting
field diaphragm s.
luminance s.
lux s.

setting-sun
s.-s. phenomenon
s.-s. sign

Set-Up
AMO S.-U.

seventh
s. cranial nerve
s. cranial nerve palsy

severe visual impairment and blindness (SVI/BL)

Severin
S. implant
S. lens

severity
clinical s.
disease s.
lesion s.

Sewall retractor
sewn-in lens
sew-on lens
sex-linked recessive optic atrophy
SF6
sulfur hexafluoride
SF6 gas

SFP
simultaneous foveal perception

SH
suprachoroidal hemorrhage

Shaaf cilia foreign body forceps
Shack-Hartmann aberrometry
shadow
s. graph
Purkinje s.
s. test

shadowing
acoustical s.
hollowing and s.

Shafer sign
Shaffer anterior angle classification
Shaffer-Weiss classification
shaft
cortex of hair s.
irrigating grasping forceps with curved s.
irrigating scissors with straight s.
s. vision

shagreen
anterior capsule s.
anterior mosaic crocodile s.
crocodile s.
s. pattern

shaken baby syndrome (SBS)
shallow
s. anterior chamber
s. detachment
s. socket

shallowing
anterior chamber s.
s. of chamber

sham irradiation
sham-movement vertigo
shape
eye s.
s. perception

shaped cataract
shaper
automated corneal s. (ACS)
Chiron automated corneal s.

Shapiro-Wilk test
sharp
s. hook
s. and pink (S&P)

sharp-edged IOL
Sharplan argon laser
Sharpoint
S. microsurgical knife
S. ophthalmic microsurgical suture
S. slit knife
S. spoon blade
S. Ultra-Glide corneal transplant suture
S. Ultra-Glide ophthalmic transplant suture
S. Ultra-Guide ophthalmic needle
S. UltraPlug punctum plug
S. V-lance blade

Shea
S. forceps
S. syndrome

shear force

S

NOTES

shearing
- S. cortex suction kit
- s. injury
- S. planar posterior chamber intraocular lens
- S. posterior chamber intraocular lens implant

sheath
- arachnoid s.
- bulbar s.
- dural s.
- eyeball s.
- fetal fibrovascular s.
- fibrovascular s.
- muscle s.
- nerve s.
- optic nerve s.
- pial s.
- s. syndrome

sheathing
- arteriolar s.
- halo s.
- peripheral retinal vascular s.
- perivascular s.
- retinal vein s.
- s. of retinal vessel
- vascular s.
- venous s.
- vessel s.

sheathotomy
- arteriovenous adventitial s.

Sheedy disparometer
Sheehy-Urban sliding lens adapter
sheen dystrophy
sheet
- autologous oral mucosal epithelium s.
- Barrier s.
- Eye-Pak II s.
- foil s.
- glassy s.
- ground-glass s.
- Silastic s.
- Supramid s.
- Teflon s.

sheeting
- micromesh s.

Sheets
- S. irrigating vectis
- S. lens
- S. lens glide
- S. lens-inserting forceps
- S. lens spatula

Sheets-McPherson tying forceps
shelf-type implant
shell
- s. implant
- s. prosthesis
- scleral s.

Shellgel viscoelastic solution
Shepard
- S. incision depth gauge
- S. incision irrigating cannula
- S. intraocular lens forceps
- S. intraocular lens-holding forceps
- S. intraocular utility forceps
- S. lens-inserting forceps
- S. microiris hook
- S. optical center marker
- S. radial keratotomy irrigating cannula
- S. reversed iris hook
- S. tying forceps

Shepard-Reinstein forceps
Shepherd tomahawk chopper
Sheridan-Gardiner isolated letter-matching test
Sherman card
Sherrington
- S. law
- S. law of reciprocal innervation

shield
- aluminum eye s.
- Barraquer eye s.
- Buller eye s.
- cataract mask s.
- Clear View hydrophilic s.
- collagen s.
- corneal light s.
- Cox II ocular laser s.
- dual eye s.
- Durette external laser s.
- eye s.
- face s.
- Fox aluminum s.
- Fox eye s.
- Grafco eye s.
- S. iridotomy scissors
- Jardon eye s.
- Katena scleral s.
- Mueller eye s.
- Paton eye s.
- plastic eye s.
- pressure s.
- Proshield collagen corneal s.
- ring cataract mask eye s.
- Soft Shield collagen corneal s.
- trigeminal s.
- s. ulcer
- Universal eye s.
- Visitec corneal s.
- Weck eye s.
- wrap-a-round eye s.

Shields forceps
shift
- criterion s.
- eye-head s.
- hyperopic s.

increased myopic s.
Purkinje s.
Shigella
S. flexneri
S. sonnei
shimmering
visual s.
shiny cellophane reflection
shipyard
s. conjunctivitis
s. disease
s. eye
s. keratoconjunctivitis
Shirmer basal secretion test
Shoch
S. foreign body pickup
S. suture
shock
anaphylactic s.
s. optic neuropathy
osmotic s.
shoelace stitch
Shoemaker intraocular lens forceps
short
s. ciliary nerve
s. C-loop lens
s. posterior ciliary artery
s. root of ciliary ganglion
s. sight
s. wavelength automated perimetry (SWAP)
s. wavelength autoperimetry
shortening
cicatricial s.
Shorti
S. limbal relaxing incision diamond knife
S. LRI diamond knife
short-pulse laser
short-scale contrast
shortsightedness
shotgun approach
shot-silk
s.-s. phenomenon
s.-s. reflex
s.-s. retina
show
scleral s.
Shprintzen syndrome
shred
scleral tissue s.
shredded iris

shunt
aqueous double-tubed valve s.
aqueous tube s.
Baerveldt s.
cerebral fluid s.
dural s.
Ex-PRESS mini glaucoma s.
glaucoma s.
miniature glaucoma s.
opticociliary s.
Schocket anterior chamber tube s.
s. vessel
White glaucoma pump s.
shunting
left-to-right s.
Shy-Drager syndrome
sialylated chain
sicca
blepharitis s.
keratitis s.
keratoconjunctivitis s. (KCS)
non-Sjögren keratoconjunctivitis s.
rhinitis s.
s. syndrome
transplantation of submandibular gland for keratoconjunctivitis s.
Sichel disease
sickle
s. cell anemia
s. cell disease
s. cell retinopathy
s. scotoma
sickness
s. impact profile (SIP)
simulator s.
side
s. port
s. port cannula
s. port fixation knife
s. port incision
side-biting spatula
side-cutting spatulated needle
4-sided cutting needle
sideroscope
siderosis
s. bulbi
s. conjunctivae
s. lentis
ocular s.
siderotic cataract
sidewall infusion cannula
Sieger streak
Siegrist-Hutchinson syndrome

S

NOTES

Siemens Quantum 2000 Color Doppler
Siepser
    S. endocapsular controller
    S. method
    S. sliding knot technique

sight
    s. counseling
    day s.
    far s.
    line of s.
    long s.
    near s.
    night s.
    old s.
    primary line of s.
    second s.
    short s.
    s. specific

sighted
    partially s.

sight-threatening
    s.-t. contact lens complication
    s.-t. diabetic macular edema
    s.-t. ocular inflammation
    s.-t. retinopathy
    s.-t. uveitis

sign
    Argyll Robertson pupil s.
    Arroyo s.
    ash-leaf s.
    Ballet s.
    Bárány s.
    Bard s.
    Barré s.
    Battle s.
    Bechterew s.
    Becker s.
    Bell s.
    Benson s.
    Berger s.
    Bielschowsky s.
    Bjerrum s.
    black dot s.
    black sunburst s.
    Bonnet s.
    Boston s.
    Brickner s.
    Brunati s.
    Cantelli s.
    cerebellar eye s.
    Cestan s.
    Charcot s.
    Charleaux oil droplet s.
    Chvostek s.
    Cogan lid-twitch s.
    Collier tucked lid s.
    Cowen s.
    Dalrymple s.
    digitoocular s.

Dixon Mann s.
doll's eye s.
double ring s.
s. of edema of lower eyelid
Elliot s.
Enroth s.
Epstein s.
eye-of-the-tiger s.
fish-strike s.
Gianelli s.
Gifford s.
Gower s.
Graefe s.
Griffith s.
Grocco s.
Gunn crossing s.
Hennebert s.
Hoagland s.
Hutchinson s.
Jellinek s.
Joffroy s.
Kestenbaum s.
Knies s.
Kocher s.
Lotze local s.
Macewen s.
Magendie s.
Magendie-Hertwig s.
Mann s.
Marcus Gunn pupillary s.
Marfan s.
Means s.
Metenier s.
Möbius s.
Munson s.
Nikolsky s.
ocular s.
orbicularis s.
Parrot s.
peek s.
Pick s.
Piltz s.
Prevost s.
pseudo-Graefe s.
raccoon s.
Reisman s.
Revilliod s.
Ripault s.
Rizzuti s.
Robertson s.
Romaña s.
Romberg s.
Rosenbach s.
Saenger s.
Sainton s.
Salus s.
Schaffer s.
sea fan s.
Seeligmüller s.

Seidel s.
setting-sun s.
Shafer s.
Skeer s.
Stellwag s.
Sugiura s.
Suker s.
swinging flashlight s.
T s.
Tay s.
Theimich lip s.
Topolanski s.
Tournay s.
Trousseau s.
Uhthoff s.
von Graefe s.
Watzke-Allen s.
Weber s.
Wernicke s.
white pupil s.
Widowitz s.
Wilder s.
signal
laser Doppler s.
pseudo-CSF s.
Raman s.
Signet Optical lens
signet-ring
s.-r. carcinoma
s.-r. lymphoma
significance
monoclonal gammopathy of
undetermined s. (MGUS)
Siladryl Oral
silafocon A
Silastic
S. intubation
S. plate
S. rod
S. scleral buckler implant
S. sheet
S. T-tube
sildenafil
silent
s. central retinal vein obstruction
s. cornea appearance
s. dacryocystitis
s. sinus syndrome
silica gel
silicone
s. acrylate
s. acrylate contact lens
s. brush back-flushed needle

s. button
s. circling band
s. conformer
s. contamination
s. elastomer lens
s. eye sphere
s. hemisphere
s. hydrogel contact lens
s. intraocular lens
s. introducer
s. lubricant
s. mesh implant
s. nasolacrimal intubation
s. oil
s. oil injection
s. oil instillation
s. oil tamponade
s. punctal plug
s. punctal plug therapy
s. rod
s. rod and sleeve forceps
s. sponge explant
s. sponge forceps
s. strip
S. study
s. tire
s. toric IOL
s. tube
s. tubing
silicone-covered aspiration tip
siliculose, siliquose
s. cataract
Silikon 1000 retinal tamponade
silk
s. traction suture
virgin s.
Silsoft contact lens
silver
s. compound
Gomori methenamine s. (GMS)
s. nitrate
s. nitrate solution
s. protein
s. tattoo pigment
s. wire effect
silver-wire
s.-w. arteriole
s.-w. reflex
s.-w. vessel
Simcoe
S. anterior chamber capsule
scrubber
S. corneal marker

S

NOTES

Simcoe *(continued)*
 S. cortex extractor aspiration
  cannula
 S. double-barreled
  irrigating/aspirating unit
 S. double-end lens loupe
 S. I&A system
 S. II PC aspirating needle
 S. II PC double cannula
 S. II PC lens
 S. II PC nucleus delivery loupe
 S. interchangeable tip
 S. irrigation/aspiration system
 S. lens implant forceps
 S. lens-inserting forceps
 S. lens positioning set
 S. notched spatula
 S. nucleus forceps
 S. nucleus lens loupe
 S. posterior chamber lens forceps
 S. reverse aperture cannula
 S. reverse irrigating/aspirating
  cannula
 S. scleral depressor
 S. suture needle
 S. upeop
 S. wire speculum
Similasan eye drops
simple
 s. acute conjunctivitis
 s. anisocoria
 s. color
 s. diplopia
 s. episcleritis
 s. glaucoma
 s. heterochromia
 s. hyperopic astigmatism
 s. megalocornea
 s. myopia
 s. myopic astigmatism
 s. optic atrophy
 s. plus lens
 s. retinitis
simple-central anisocoria
simplex
 epidermolysis bullosa s.
 glaucoma s.
 s. glaucoma
Simplus
 Boston S.
Simpson
 S. lacrimal probe
 S. test
simulans
 Staphylococcus s.
simulation
 computer s.
simulator
 cataract s.

 night-driving s.
 s. sickness
 video display terminal s. (VDTS)
simultanagnosia
 triad of s.
simultaneous
 s. bilateral cataract surgery
 s. color contrast
 s. foveal perception (SFP)
 s. macular perception (SMP)
 s. perception
 s. prism cover test (SPC)
Sinarest 12 Hour nasal solution
sine-wave grating
Singapore epidemic conjunctivitis
single
 s. binocular vision (SBV)
 s. cover test
 s. gene disorder
 s. lid eversion
single-action rongeur
single-armed suture
single-cut contact lens
single/double occluder
single-gene mutation
single-incision system
single-loop
 s.-l. sling design
 s.-l. technique
single-mirror goniolens
single-piece
 s.-p. acrylic IOL
 s.-p. SN60AT IOL
single-quadrant testing
single-running suture
single-stitch
 s.-s. aponeurotic tuck technique
Single-Stitch PhacoFlex
**single-stranded conformation
 polymorphism**
single-use instrument
single-vision lens
sinister
 congenital ptosis oculus s.
 oculus s. (left eye)
 tension oculus s. (TOS)
 visio oculus s. (vision of left eye)
sinistrality
sinistrocular
sinistrocularity
sinistrogyration
sinistrotorsion
Sinskey
 S. intraocular lens
 S. IOL manipulator
 S. lens-holding forceps
 S. lens hook
 S. lens-manipulating hook
 S. microiris hook

S. microlens hook
S. micro-tying forceps
S. pick
Sinskey-Wilson foreign body forceps
sinus, pl. **sinus, sinuses**
anterior chamber s.
Arlt s.
s. catarrh
cavernous s.
ethmoid s.
ethmoidal s.
frontal s.
s. headache
Maier s.
s. of Maier
s. mucocele
paranasal s.
scleral venous s.
sphenoid s.
venous s.
sinusitis
frontal s.
maxillary s.
paranasal s.
sinusoidal grating
SIP
sickness impact profile
Sipple-Gorlin syndrome
Sipple syndrome
Sisler punctum dilator
SITA
Swedish interactive thresholding
algorithm
site
retinal impact s.
sitting
s. IOP
s. measurement
situs inversus
sixth
s. cranial nerve
s. cranial nerve palsy
size
blade s.
bleb s.
burn spot s.
dark-adapted pupil s. (DAPS)
eye s.
infiltrate s.
lens s.
letter s.
mesopic pupil s.
object s.

optic disc s.
print s.
pupil s.
relative s.
retinal image s.
scleral canal s.
seton implantation s.
spot s.
Thornton guide for optical zone s.
Sjögren
S. disease
S. reticular dystrophy
S. syndrome
Sjögren-Larsson syndrome
SKBM
Summit Krumeich-Barraquer
microkeratome
SKBM microkeratome
Skeele curette
Skeer sign
skein test
skeletal abnormality
Skeleton fine forceps
skew
s. deviation
s. motion
s. pupil
skiameter
skiametry
skiascope
skiascopy
skiascotometry
SKILL
Smith-Kettlewell Institute low luminance
SKILL card
SKILL Card Test
skin
s. autograft
s. cancer compound
s. change
s. diabetes
s. flap
s. graft
s. hook
s. marking pen
overhanging eyelid s.
s. pupillary reflex
s. tension line
ski needle
skirt
vitreous s.
Sklar-Schiötz tonometer

S

NOTES

skull
>s. base tumor
>exophthalmos due to tower s.
>s. temple

sky-blue spot

SL
>Schwalbe line

slab-off
>s.-o. grinding
>s.-o. lens

Slade formed irrigation cannula

Slade-type adjustable aspirating LASIK speculum

slant
>antimongoloid s.
>S. haptic single-piece intraocular lens
>mongoloid s.
>s. muscle operation
>palpebral s.

SLE
>slitlamp examination

sleeve
>anterior segment s.
>Charles anterior segment s.
>Charles infusion s.
>clear keratin s.
>implant s.
>s. implant
>Labtician oval s.
>phaco s.
>primary hydroxyapatite-coated s.
>retinal probe s.
>s. spreading forceps
>Ultra Sleeve ultrasound s.
>ultrasound s.
>Watzke s.

sleeveless phaco tip

slide
>AO Vectographic Project-O-Chart s.
>epithelial s.
>Polaroid vectograph s.

sliding flap

slimcut blade

SlimFit
>S. ovoid intraocular lens
>S. small-incision ovoid lens

sling
>Arion s.
>s. design
>frontalis muscle s.
>s. for implant
>s. procedure
>Supramid s.
>suture s.
>tarsoligamentous s.

slippage

slit
>s. blade knife
>s. illumination

slit-beam test

slitlamp
>s. biomicroscope
>s. biomicroscopy
>s. cup
>s. examination (SLE)
>s. fluorophotometer
>s. microscope
>s. ophthalmoscopy
>s. photography

SLK
>superior limbic keratoconjunctivitis

SLO
>scanning laser ophthalmoscope

Sloan
>S. letter
>S. M system
>S. optotype
>S. reading card

Sloane
>S. Epi-Peeler
>S. flap repositor
>S. micro hoe
>S. trephine

sloping isopter

slough
>conjunctival s.

sloughing base

slow
>s. conjugate roving eye movement
>s. hypometric vertical saccade

slow-channel syndrome

slow-to-no saccade

10 SL/O Zeiss keratometer

SLP
>scanning laser polarimetry

SLT
>scanning laser tomography
>selective laser trabeculoplasty

sludging of circulation

sluggish movements of eyes and eyelids

Sly syndrome

small
>s. aperture Steri-Drape
>s. capsular bag
>s. pupil
>s. pupil cataract surgery

small-incision
>s.-i. cataract surgery
>s.-i. external levator repair
>s.-i. phacoemulsification
>s.-i. procedure
>s.-i. trabeculectomy

SmallPort phaco system

smart
> S. forceps
> S. Plug lacrimal plug
> S. scissors

smear
> conjunctival s.
> KOH s.
> Tzanck s.

smegmatis
> *Mycobacterium s.*

Smirmaul technique
Smith
> S. expressor hook
> S. intraocular capsular amputator
> S. knife
> S. lid hook
> S. modification
> S. modification of Van Lint lid block
> S. orbital floor implant
> S. speculum
> S. trabeculectomy

Smith-Fisher spatula
Smith-Green cataract knife
Smith-Indian
> S.-I. operation
> S.-I. technique

Smith-Kettlewell
> S.-K. Institute low luminance (SKILL)
> S.-K. Institute low luminance card
> S.-K. Institute low luminance card test

Smith-Leiske cross-action intraocular lens forceps
Smith-Lemli-Opitz syndrome
Smith-Magenis syndrome
Smith-Riley syndrome
SMON
> subacute myelooptic neuropathy

smooth
> s. cannula
> s. grasping forceps
> s. muscle hamartoma
> s. pursuit

smooth-edged continuous tear
smooth-pursuit movement
smooth-walled tubing
SMP
> simultaneous macular perception

SMZ-10A zoom stereo microscope

snail
> s. track degeneration
> s. tracks

snake bite-induced ptosis
snake-like
> s.-l. appearance
> s.-l. structure

snare
> Castroviejo enucleation s.
> enucleation wire s.
> s. enucleator
> Förster enucleation s.
> wire enucleation s.

Sneddon-Wilkinson disease
Snellen
> S. chart
> S. conventional reform implant
> S. entropion forceps
> S. equivalent
> S. fraction
> S. lens loupe
> S. letter
> S. letter optotype
> S. line
> S. near-vision card
> S. notation
> S. number
> S. ptosis operation
> S. reading card
> S. reform eye
> S. soft contact lens
> S. test
> S. test type
> S. vectis
> S. visual acuity

Snell law
Snell-Sterling visual efficiency scale
SnET2
> tin ethyl etiopurpurin

1-snip
> 1-s. punctum
> 1-s. punctum operation

3-snip
> 3-s. punctum
> 3-s. punctum operation

Sno-Strips
snow
> s. blindness
> s. conjunctivitis
> s. glasses

snowball opacity
snowflake cataract
snowman graft

S

NOTES

snowstorm cataract
snub-nose diamond blade
Snugfit eye patch
Snyder corneal spring forceps
soaking solution
SOCA
    Studies of the Ocular Complications in
    AIDS
society
    Canadian Ophthalmology S.
    S. of Cataract and Refractive
      Surgeons
    S. for Excellence in Eyecare
      (SEE)
    North American Neuro-
      Ophthalmology S. (NANOS)
    Ophthalmic Photographers S. (OPS)
sociodemographic variable
socket
    anophthalmic s.
    contracted s.
    s. contracture
    deep s.
    s. discharge
    s. motility
    s. prosthesis
    s. reconstruction
    shallow s.
SOD2
    superoxide dismutase 2
    SOD2 gene
sodium
    s. acetate
    s. acetate trihydrate
    s. benzoate
    s. bicarbonate
    s. biphosphate
    s. bisulfite
    s. borate
    s. carbonate
    carboxymethylcellulose s.
    cefamandole s.
    s. chloride (NaCl)
    s. chloride in solution
    s. citrate
    s. citrate dihydrate
    s. cromoglycate
    cromolyn s.
    dantrolene s.
    diclofenac s.
    ecabet s.
    s. fluorescein (NaFl)
    fluorescein s.
    flurbiprofen s.
    fomivirsen s.
    foscarnet s.
    ganciclovir s.
    s. hexametaphosphate
    hyaluronate s.

    s. hyaluronate and chondroitin
      sulfate
    s. hyaluronate solution
    s. hydroxide
    s. lauryl sulfate
    s. metabisulfite
    s. morrhuate
    naproxen s.
    nedocromil s.
    pegaptanib s.
    pentobarbital s.
    s. perborate
    phenobarbital s.
    s. phosphate
    s. propionate
    secobarbital s.
    sterile acetazolamide s.
    stibogluconate s.
    S. Sulamyd
    S. Sulamyd Ophthalmic
    sulfacetamide s.
    s. sulfate
    suramin s.
    thiopental s.
    s. thiosulfate
    triclofos s.
    valproate s.
    warfarin s.
Soemmerring
    S. crystalline swelling
    S. foramen
    S. ring
    ring of S.
    S. ring cataract
    S. spot
SOF
    superior orbital fissure
SofLens
    S. contact lens
    S. enzymatic contact lens cleaner
    S. 66 lens
SoFlex
    S. IOL
    S. series lens
SofPort
    S. AO aspheric lens
    S. easy-load injector
    S. Easy-Load lens delivery system
    S. L161 AO lens
Sof/Pro-Clean
Sofsilk nonabsorbable silk suture
soft
    s. acrylic IOL
    s. cataract
    s. contact lens (SCL)
    s. contact lens solution
    s. drusen
    s. exudate
    s. intraocular lens

s. IOL cutter
S. Mate
S. Mate Comfort Drops for Sensitive Eyes
S. Mate daily cleaning solution
S. Mate disinfection and storage solution
S. Mate Enzyme Alternative
S. Mate Enzyme Plus cleaner
S. Mate Hands Off daily cleaner
S. Mate protein remover
S. Mate saline
S. Mate Saline for Sensitive Eyes
S. Plug punctal plug
S. Shield collagen corneal shield
s. silicone sponge
s. tissue swelling
Soft-Cell eye spear
Softcon
SofTec Delivery System
soft-finger tension
SoftForm facial implant
SoftGels
HydroEye S.
SoftPlug
soft-shell technique
SoftSITE high add aspheric multifocal contact lens
soft-tipped
s.-t. cannula
s.-t. extrusion handpiece
Soft-Touch A-Probe
software
OPD-Station s.
PathFinder corneal analysis s.
posterior capsule opacification s.
tear stability analysis s.
Visulas 532 Combi s.
Visulas InterChange s.
SoftWear
S. Saline
S. Saline for Sensitive Eyes Solution
solani
Fusarium s.
Sola Optical USA Spectralite high index lens
solar
s. blindness
s. burn
s. damage
s. keratoma
s. keratosis

s. maculopathy
s. radiation
s. retinitis
s. retinopathy
solid
s. color
s. silicone with Supramid mesh implant
s. tumor
s. vision
solid-core needle with hollow tip
solid-state
diode-pumped s.-s. (DPSS)
solium
Taenia s.
Soll suture and incision marker
SOLO-care Multi-Purpose Solution
Solu-Medrol
Solurex L.A.
Solusept
solution
Acular LS ophthalmic s.
AK-Dilate ophthalmic s.
AK-Nefrin ophthalmic s.
AK-Spore S.
Akwa Tears s.
Alcon Saline Especially for Sensitive Eyes S.
Alocril ophthalmic s.
Alomide ophthalmic s.
AMO Vitrax viscoelastic s.
Amvisc Plus s.
apraclonidine ophthalmic s.
AquaLase s.
AquaSite ophthalmic s.
astringent ophthalmic s.
azelastine hydrochloride ophthalmic s.
balanced saline s.
balanced salt s. (BSS)
Barnes Hind ComfortCare soaking and wetting s.
Barnes Hind contact lens cleaning and soaking s.
Betimol beta-blocker s.
bimatoprost ophthalmic s.
BioLon s.
Bion Tears S.
Blairex sterile preserved saline s.
boric acid s.
Boston Advance Comfort Formula Conditioning S.
Boston cleaner s.

S

NOTES

solution *(continued)*

Boston Simplicity multi-action s.
brimonidine tartrate ophthalmic s.
BSS Plus ophthalmic irrigating s.
BSS sterile irrigating s.
chilled balanced salt s.
Claris Cleaning and Soaking S.
ComfortCare GP Wetting and
Soaking S.
Comfort Tears S.
Complete Comfort Plus multi-
purpose s.
ContaClair multi-purpose contact
lens s.
CooperVision balanced salt s.
Cosopt ophthalmic s.
Crolom ophthalmic s.
cromolyn sodium ophthalmic s.
Dacroise irrigating eye s.
Dakrina Ophthalmic S.
dexamethasone s.
disinfecting s.
Domeboro s.
dorzolamide hydrochloride
ophthalmic s.
dorzolamide hydrochloride-timolol
maleate ophthalmic s.
Dry Eye Therapy S.
Duovisc s.
Elestat ophthalmic s.
emedastine difurmarate
ophthalmic s.
epinastine HCl ophthalmic s.
extraocular irrigating s.
eye irrigating s.
Eye-Lube-A S.
Eye-Sed s.
Eye Stream sterile eye irrigating s.
Eye Wash s.
Feldman buffer s.
fluorescein dye and stain s.
Fluorox ophthalmic s.
Fluress ophthalmic s.
Freeman s.
gatifloxacin ophthalmic s.
Gonak ophthalmic s.
graft preservation s.
Healon s.
hyaluronic acid s.
hydrolysis of s.
hypertonic s.
HypoTears PF S.
hypotonic s.
Indocin ophthalmic s.
intraocular irrigating s.
I-Phrine Ophthalmic S.
irrigating s.
Isopto Plain S.
Isopto Tears S.

isotonic s.
Just Tears S.
ketorolac tromethamine
ophthalmic s.
ketotifen fumarate ophthalmic s.
K Sol preservation s.
Lacril Ophthalmic S.
latanoprost timolol maleate
ophthalmic s.
Lens Plus Sterile Saline S.
levofloxacin ophthalmic s.
Liquifilm Forte S.
Liquifilm Rewetting S.
Liquifilm Tears S.
Lobob Hard Contact Lens
Wetting S.
Lobob Rigid Hard Contact Lens
Soaking S.
lodoxamide tromethamine
ophthalmic s.
loteprednol etabonate ophthalmic s.
LubriTears S.
Lumigan ophthalmic s.
medocromil sodium ophthalmic s.
Miochol s.
Miostat intraocular s.
moxifloxacin HCl ophthalmic s.
multi-purpose s. (MPS)
Murine S.
Murocel ophthalmic s.
Mydfrin ophthalmic s.
mydriatic ophthalmic s.
Nature's Tears S.
nedocromil sodium ophthalmic s.
NeoDecadron S.
Neosporin Ophthalmic S.
Neo-Synephrine Ophthalmic S.
No Rub Opti-Free Express multi-
purpose disinfecting s.
Nu-Tears II S.
OcuCoat PF Ophthalmic S.
Ocupress Ophthalmic S.
ofloxacin ophthalmic s.
olopatadine HCl ophthalmic s.
olopatadine hydrochloride
ophthalmic s.
ophthalmic s.
Opti-Free Express Multi-Purpose S.
Optimum cleaning, disinfecting, and
storage s.
Opti-One Conditioning S.
Opti-One Multi-Purpose S.
Opti-Soak Conditioning S.
Optivar ophthalmic s.
osmium tetroxide s.
oxidation of s.
Patanol ophthalmic s.
pemirolast potassium ophthalmic s.
Prefrin Ophthalmic S.

preservative-free saline s.
preservatives in s.
preserved saline s.
ProConcept Wetting and
   Soaking S.
Puralube Tears S.
Pure Eyes Disinfection/Soaking S.
Pure Eyes Soaking S.
Purilens UV Disinfection S.
Quixin ophthalmic s.
Refresh Plus Ophthalmic S.
Relief Ophthalmic S.
rewetting s.
Ringer lactate s.
rose bengal red s.
saline s.
Sensitive Eyes Plus Saline S.
Sensitive Eyes saline/cleaning s.
Sereine soaking and cleaning s.
Sereine wetting and soaking s.
Shellgel viscoelastic s.
silver nitrate s.
Sinarest 12 Hour nasal s.
soaking s.
sodium chloride in s.
sodium hyaluronate s.
soft contact lens s.
Soft Mate daily cleaning s.
Soft Mate disinfection and
   storage s.
SoftWear Saline for Sensitive
   Eyes S.
SOLO-care Multi-Purpose S.
solvent s.
Soquette contact lens soaking s.
sterility of s.
Sulster S.
surfactant cleaning s.
TearGard Ophthalmic S.
Teargen Ophthalmic S.
Tearisol S.
Tears Naturale Free S.
Tears Naturale II S.
Tears Plus S.
Tears Renewed S.
timolol maleate ophthalmic gel-
   forming s.
Travatan ophthalmic s.
travoprost ophthalmic s.
Trump s.
trypan blue ophthalmic s.
Ultra Tears S.

Unicare blue and green all-in-1
   cleaning s.
Unique pH multi-urpose s.
Unisol 4 Preservative Free
   Saline S.
Vasocon-A s.
Vigamox ophthalmic s.
Visalens contact lens cleaning and
   soaking s.
Viscoat s.
viscoelastic s.
VisionBlue ophthalmic s.
Viva-Drops S.
wetting s.
Zaditor ophthalmic s.
zinc sulfate s.
Zylet ophthalmic s.
Zymar ophthalmic s.
solvent solution
somata
   amacrine cell s.
somatic cell
SON
   supraoptic nucleus
Sondermann canal
sonic pulse
SonicWAVE phacoemulsification system
sonnei
   Shigella s.
Sonogage
   S. System Corneo-Gage 20 MHz
     center frequency transducer
   S. ultrasound pachometer
sonographer
   Trans-Scan pulsed Doppler s.
sonolucent
   acoustical s.
   s. cleft
   s. lesion
Sonomed
   S. A/B-Scan system
   S. 1500 A-scan instrument
   S. A-Scan system
   S. B-1500 system
Sonometric Ocuscan
SOOF
   suborbicularis oculi fat
   SOOF lift
soothe
   S. emollient eye drops
   S. eye
SOP
   Bleph-10 SOP

S

NOTES

SOP *(continued)*
    Blephamide SOP
    Chloroptic SOP
    FML SOP
    Lacri-Lube SOP
    Pred-G SOP
Soper cone contact lens
Soquette contact lens soaking solution
sorbic
    s. acid
    s. acid Sorbi-Care saline
Sorbinil Retinopathy Trial (SRT)
Sorsby
    S. fundus dystrophy
    S. maculopathy
    S. pseudoinflammatory macular
      degeneration
    pseudoinflammatory macular
      dystrophy of S.
    S. pseudoinflammatory macular
      dystrophy
    S. syndrome
Sotos syndrome
soul blindness
sound
    lacrimal s.
source
    point s.
southern
    S. blot hybridization assay
    S. blot technique
Sovereign bifocal lens
S&P
    sharp and pink
space
    Berger s.
    Blessig s.
    circumlental s.
    episcleral s.
    Fontana s.
    intercellular s.
    interfascial s.
    interlamellar s.
    intraconal s.
    intraretinal s.
    s. of iridocorneal angle
    Kuhnt s.
    s. myopia
    object s.
    Panum fusional s.
    parafoveal cystic s.
    perichoroidal s.
    perioptic subarachnoid s.
    periscleral s.
    preseptal s.
    prezonular s.
    retinal cystoid s.
    retrobulbar s.
    retrolental s.

    retroocular s.
    Schwalbe s.
    sequestered s.
    subarachnoid s.
    subpigment epithelial s.
    subretinal s.
    suprachoroidal s.
    Tenon s.
    zonular s.
space-occupying lesion
spacer
    autogenous hard palate eyelid s.
    eyelid s.
    lower eyelid s.
Spadafora MemoryLens dialer
Spaeth classification
Spaleck forceps
Spanish silk suture
Spanlang-Tappeiner syndrome
sparganosis
    ocular s.
sparing
    foveal s.
    macular s.
    pupillary s.
    recurrent pupillary s.
Sparta microforceps
spasm
    s. of accommodation
    accommodation s.
    accommodative s.
    ciliary s.
    convergence s.
    cyclic ocular motor s.
    eyelid s.
    facial s.
    hemifacial s.
    near-reflex s.
    s. of near reflex
    nictitating s.
    oculomotor paresis with cyclic s.
    posttraumatic accommodative s.
    winking s.
spasmodic
    s. mydriasis
    s. strabismus
spasmus nutans
spastic
    s. ectropion
    s. entropion
    s. lagophthalmia
    s. miosis
    s. mydriasis
    s. paretic facial contracture
    s. pseudosclerosis
spasticity of conjugate gaze
spasticum
    ectropion s.
    entropion s.

spatial
- s. acuity
- s. discrimination
- s. information
- s. interaction
- s. localization
- s. navigation
- s. perception disorder
- s. summation

spatial-contrast sensitivity
spatially
- s. resolved value
- s. resolved wavefront aberration

spatia zonularia
spatium
- s. episclerale
- s. interfasciale
- s. intervaginale
- s. perichoroideale

spatula
- angled iris s.
- angulated iris s.
- Bangerter iris s.
- Barraquer irrigator s.
- Berens s.
- Buratto contact lens spoon and s.
- capsule fragment s.
- Carones LASEK s.
- Castroviejo cyclodialysis s.
- Castroviejo double-ended s.
- Castroviejo synechia s.
- Cleasby s.
- corneal fascia lata s.
- corneal graft s.
- Culler iris s.
- cyclodialysis s.
- double s.
- Elschnig cyclodialysis s.
- Fox LASIK s.
- French hook s.
- French lacrimal s.
- French pattern s.
- Fukasaku s.
- Gills-Welsh s.
- Guimaraes flap s.
- Guimaraes ophthalmic s.
- Hersh LASIK retreatment s.
- Hirschman s.
- hook s.
- s. hook
- iridodialysis s.
- iris s.
- Jaffe intraocular s.

- Jaffe lens s.
- Katena iris s.
- Kimura platinum s.
- Kirby angulated iris s.
- Knapp iris s.
- Knolle lens cortex s.
- Knolle lens nucleus s.
- LASEK epithelial detaching s.
- LASEK epithelial flap repositioning s.
- Lindner s.
- Lindstrom LASIK s.
- Maddox LASIK s.
- Manhattan Eye & Ear s.
- Masket phaco s.
- Maumenee vitreous sweep s.
- McIntyre s.
- McPherson s.
- McReynolds s.
- microvitreoretinal s.
- Moran enhancement s.
- needle s.
- s. needle
- nucleus s.
- Obstbaum lens s.
- Obstbaum synechia s.
- Olk vitreoretinal s.
- Pallin lens s.
- Paton double s.
- Paton single s.
- Paton transplant s.
- platinum probe s.
- s. probe
- probe s.
- Rainin clip-bending s.
- Rainin lens s.
- Rhein LASIK epithelial detaching s.
- Rhein LASIK flap elevator and stromal s.
- Rhein LASIK flap repositioning s.
- Rowen s.
- Seibel double-ended LASIK flap lifter and s.
- Sheets lens s.
- side-biting s.
- Simcoe notched s.
- Smith-Fisher s.
- s. spoon
- spoon s.
- Steinert double-ended LASIK s.
- suture pickup s.
- synechia s.

NOTES

487

spatula *(continued)*
    Tan s.
    s. temple
    Thornton malleable s.
    ultrasound s.
    vitreous sweep s.
    Wheeler iris s.
spatula/protector
spatulated needle
SPC
    simultaneous prism cover test
spear
    s. developmental cataract
    eye s.
    LASIK s.
    Merocel surgical s.
    PVA s.
    Soft-Cell eye s.
    Ultracell LASIK s.
    Weck-cel surgical s.
Spearman correlation coefficient
special
    s. sense vertigo
    s. spectacle lens
specialist
    American Society of Retina S.'s
      (ASRS)
    cornea s.
    pediatric eye s.
specialty
    ophthalmic s.
species
    halophilic noncholera *Vibrio* s.
specific
    sight s.
specimen
    formalin-fixed tissue s.
speckled corneal dystrophy
spectacle
    s. blur
    s. correction
    s. crown
    s. frame
    s. frame pad
    s. independent
    s. lens
    s. magnifier
    s. plane
spectacle-borne device
spectacle-corrected visual acuity
spectacle-free refractive correction
spectacle-induced aniseikonia
spectacle-mounted
    s.-m. camera
    s.-m. telescope
spectacles
    aphakic s.
    Bartel s.
    bifocal s.

bridge of s.
cataract s.
clerical s.
compound s.
decentered s.
divers' s.
divided s.
flat-top s.
folding s.
Franklin s.
half-eye s.
half-glass s.
Hallauer s.
hemianopic s.
industrial s.
lid crutch s.
Masselon s.
mica s.
orthoscopic s.
pantoscopic s.
periscopic s.
photochromic s.
prism s.
prismatic s.
protective s.
ptosis crutch s.
pulpit s.
refraction s.
safety s.
stenopeic s.
telescopic s.
temple of s.
tinted s.
wire frame s.
spectacular image
spectra *(pl. of* spectrum*)*
spectral-domain OCT
Spectralite Transitions lens
spectral sensitivity
SpectraMax spectrophotometer
Spectra-Pritchard 1980-PR photometer
spectrocolorimeter
Spectronic Genesys 5 spectrophotometer
spectrophotometer
    SpectraMax s.
    Spectronic Genesys 5 s.
spectroradiometer
spectroscopy
    H-magnetic resonance s.
    magnetic resonance s. (MRS)
    noncontact photo-acoustic s. (NC-
      PAS)
    Raman s.
spectrum, pl. **spectra, spectrums**
    chromatic s.
    color s.
    S. color vision meter 712
      anomaloscope
    electromagnetic s.

facioauriculovertebral s.
fortification s.
S. Lens Analysis System
ocular s.
Raman s.
visible s.
specular
s. attachment
s. glare
s. image
s. microscope
s. microscopy
s. reflection
s. reflection video-recording system
S. reflex slit lamp
speculum, pl. specula
Alfonso pediatric eyelid s.
aspirating lid s.
Azar lid s.
Barraquer-Colibri s.
Barraquer eye s.
Barraquer wire s.
basket-style scleral supporter s.
Berens s.
Brown interchangeable lid s.
Castroviejo s.
Clark s.
Cook s.
Culler s.
eye s.
eyelid s.
Feaster adjustable eyelid s.
fine-wire s.
Floyd-Barraquer wire s.
Fox s.
Gaffee s.
Ginsberg eye s.
Guell type LASIK s.
Guist s.
Guyton-Park eye s.
Guyton-Park lid s.
Hirschman s.
Jaffe lid s.
Katena s.
Keizer-Lancaster eye s.
Kershner reversible eyelid s.
Knapp eye s.
Knolle lens s.
Kratz aspirating s.
Kratz-Barraquer wire eye s.
Lancaster eye s.
Lancaster lid s.
Lancaster-O'Connor s.

Lang s.
Lester-Burch s.
lid s.
Lieberman aspirating s.
Lieberman K-Wire s.
Machat adjustable aspirating
  wire s.
Machat-type adjustable aspirating
  LASIK s.
Manche LASIK s.
Markomanolakis aspirating s.
Maumenee-Park eye s.
McKinney eye s.
McPherson s.
Mellinger s.
Metcher s.
Moria 1-piece s.
Mueller s.
Murdock eye s.
Murdock-Wiener eye s.
Murdoon eye s.
nasal s.
Pannu-Kratz-Barraquer s.
Park s.
Park-Maumenee s.
Paton single s.
Paton transplant s.
pediatric lid s.
Pierse eye s.
reversible lid s.
Sauer infant s.
Schott lid s.
Seibel 3D s.
Serdarevic s.
Simcoe wire s.
Slade-type adjustable aspirating
  LASIK s.
Smith s.
square lid s.
stop s.
Weiss s.
Williams pediatric eye s.
wire lid s.
Ziegler s.
speed
reading s.
ultra high acquisition s.
Spencer
S. chalazion forceps
S. eye suture scissors
S. silicone subimplant
Spero forceps

S

NOTES

sph.
sphere
spherical
sphenocavernous syndrome
sphenoccipital fissure
sphenofrontal suture
sphenoid
s. bone
s. door jamb
greater wing of s.
lesser wing of s.
s. sinus
s. wing meningioma
sphenoidal fissure
sphenoidalis
ala minor ossis s.
foramen s.
sphenomaxillary fissure
sphenoorbital suture
sphenopalatine ganglion
sphenorbital
sphere (sph.)
Carter s.
diopter s. (DS)
Doherty s.
s. end point
Ganzfeld s.
s. implant
s. introducer
method of the s.
Morgagni s.
Mules vitreous s.
porous hydroxyapatite s.
Pyrex eye s.
silicone eye s.
spheric
s. aberration
s. lens
spherical (sph.)
s. cornea
s. equivalent
s. equivalent lens
s. implant
s. IOL
s. lens aberration
s. refraction
s. refractive error
spherocylinder
spherocylindrical lens
spheroidal
s. degeneration
s. keratopathy
spheroid degeneration
spherometer
spherophakia
spherophakia-brachymorphia syndrome
spheroprism
sphincter
s. erosion

s. of eye
s. fiber
iris s.
s. muscle
s. muscle of pupil
s. oculi
s. oris
s. pupillae
s. tear
sphincterectomy
sphincteric
sphincterismus
sphincteritis
sphincterolysis
sphincterotomy
spicule
bone s.
spider
s. angioma
s. telangiectasia
s. vasculature
Spielmeyer-Sjögren disease
Spielmeyer-Stock disease
Spielmeyer-Vogt
S.-V. disease
S.-V. syndrome
spike
blue s.
intraocular pressure s.
IOP s.
retinal s.
spillover cell
spinal
s. canal tumor
s. miosis
s. mydriasis
spina trochlearis
spin-cast
s.-c. lens
s.-c. process
spindle
s. A, B melanoma
Axenfeld-Krukenberg s.
cataract s.
s. cataract
s. cell
s. cell melanoma
Krukenberg corneal s.
Krukenberg pigment s.
spindle-shaped
s.-s. area
s.-s. cell
spinocerebellar
s. ataxia
s. degeneration
spiral
s. field
Tillaux s.
s. of Tillaux

spiralis
>Trichinella *s.*

spiramycin
Spitz nevus
Spivack axis marker
Spizziri cannula knife
SPK
>superficial punctate keratitis

SPKT
>superficial punctate keratitis of Thygeson

splaytooth forceps
Splendore-Hoeppli phenomenon
splenic retinitis
splenium of corpus callosum
splinter disc hemorrhage
splinting
>lid s.

split-beam photographic technique
split-calvarial bone graft
split fixation
splitter
>Akahoshi nucleus s.
>beam s.
>Brierley nucleus s.
>Kraff nucleus s.
>Lindstrom Trident ophthalmic s.
>Rosen phaco s.
>Salz nucleus s.

split-thickness autograft
splitting
>foveal s.
>s. of lacrimal papilla
>s. lacrimal papilla operation
>macular s.
>Minsky intramarginal s.
>stromal s.

SP-MS
>secondary progressive multiple sclerosis

spoke-like sutural cataract
sponge
>cellulose surgical s.
>episcleral s.
>s. explant
>Fuller silicone s.
>grooved silicone s.
>s. implant
>implant s.
>Krukenberg s.
>lens s.
>Lincoff lens s.
>lint-free s.
>Merocel lint-free s.
>ophthalmic s.

>Packer tunnel silicone s.
>radial s.
>soft silicone s.
>surgical s.
>Vaiser s.
>VersaTool eye s.
>Visi-Spear eye s.
>vitrectomy s.
>Weck s.
>Weck-cel s.

spongy
>s. appearance
>s. iritis

spontaneous
>s. congenital iris cyst
>s. ectopia lentis
>s. extrusion of lens
>s. extrusion of vitreous
>s. eye blink rate (SEBR)
>s. eyelid retraction
>s. hyphema
>s. intracranial hypotension
>s. peeling
>s. resorption
>s. retinal reattachment
>s. retinal venous pulsation
>s. retrobulbar hemorrhage
>s. vitreous hemorrhage

spoon
>Alfonso-McIntyre nucleus s.
>s. blade
>Bunge evisceration s.
>Castroviejo lens s.
>cataract s.
>Culler lens s.
>Cutler lens s.
>Daviel lens s.
>Elschnig s.
>enucleation s.
>evisceration s.
>Fisher s.
>graft carrier s.
>Hess s.
>Kirby intracapsular lens s.
>Knapp lens s.
>s. knife
>LASIK aspiration s.
>lens s.
>needle s.
>s. needle
>Rizzuti graft carrier s.
>Schepens s.
>spatula s.

S

NOTES

spoon *(continued)*
    s. spatula
    Wehner s.
    Wells enucleation s.
sporadic
    s. aniridia
    s. retinoblastoma
sporangium, pl. **sporangia**
Sporanox
Sporothrix schenckii
sporotrichosis
    conjunctival s.
sports goggles
spot
    acoustic s.
    ash-leaf s.
    baring of blind s.
    birdshot s.
    Bitot s.
    blank s.
    blind s.
    blue s.
    blur s.
    Brushfield s.
    cherry-red s.
    chorioretinal atrophic s.
    cluster of pigmented s.'s
    corneal s.
    cotton-wool s. (CWS)
    cribriform s.
    depigmented s.
    dry s.
    Elschnig s.
    eye s.
    flame s.
    Förster-Fuchs black s.
    Fuchs black s.
    histo s.
    Horner-Trantas s.
    hot s.
    hypofluorescent dark s.
    iridescent s.
    leopard s.
    Lisch s.
    Mariotte blind s.
    Maurer s.
    Maxwell s.
    mongolian s.
    opacification cherry-red s.
    peripheral chorioretinal atrophic s.
    physiologic blind s.
    retinal blur s.
    s. retinoscope
    Roth s.
    rust s.
    s. size
    sky-blue s.
    Soemmerring s.
    Tay cherry-red s.

    white s.
    yellow s. (YS)
S potential
spotty corneal opacity
SPP
    standard pseudoisochromatic plate
    SPP color deficiency testing
      product
SPP2
    standard pseudoisochromatic plate part 2
    SPP2 test
Spratt mastoid curette
spray
    Sensitive Eyes sterile saline s.
    Tears Again liposome lid s.
spread
    s. function
    illusory visual s.
    pagetoid s.
    visual s.
spreader
    Athens suture s.
    conjunctiva s.
    Frederick sleeve s.
    Gill incision s.
    incision s.
    Kwitko conjunctival s.
    Suarez s.
    Wilder band s.
spring
    s. catarrh
    s. conjunctivitis
    S. iris scissors
    s. ophthalmia
    s. pupil
spring-hinge temple
springing mydriasis
springtime conjunctivitis
sprout
    angiogenic s.
spud
    Alvis foreign body s.
    curved needle eye s.
    Davis s.
    Dix foreign body s.
    Ellis foreign body s.
    eye s.
    Fisher s.
    flat eye s.
    foreign body s.
    Francis s.
    Goldstein golf-club s.
    gouge s.
    s. and gouge
    Hosford s.
    LaForce knife s.
    Levine s.
    needle s.
    O'Brien s.

Plange s.
Storz folding-handle eye s.
s. tool
Walton s.
spur
corneoscleral s.
Fuchs s.
Grunert s.
Michel s.
scleral s. (SS)
spurious cataract
Sputnik Russian razor blade
squalamine lactate
squamosa
blepharitis s.
squamous
s. cell
s. cell carcinoma
s. cell carcinoma of eyelid
s. metaplasia
s. papilloma
s. seborrheic blepharitis
square
s. lid speculum
s. prism
s. pupil
square-wave
s.-w. jerk
s.-w. pulse
squashed-tomato appearance
squeegee capsule polisher
squint
accommodative s.
angle of s.
s. angle
comitant s.
convergent s.
s. deviation
divergent s.
downward s.
Duane classification of s.
external s.
s. hook
internal s.
latent s.
noncomitant s.
s. surgery
upward s.
squinting eye
squirrel plague conjunctivitis
SR
superior rectus
Ocufit SR

SRF
subretinal fluid
SRI
surface regularity index
SR-IV programmed subjective refractor
SRK
Sanders-Retzlaff-Kraff
SRK formula
SRM
subretinal membrane
SRNV
subretinal neovascularization
SRNVM
subretinal neovascular membrane
SRP
surgical reversal of presbyopia
^{90}Sr-plaque irradiation
SRT
Sorbinil Retinopathy Trial
stereotactic radiation therapy
SS
scleral spur
SSDLP
subthreshold subfoveal diode laser
photocoagulation
S-shaped deformity
SST
Submacular Surgery Trials
ST
esotropia
Staar
S. AA 4207 lens
S. Aquaflow technique
S. implantable contact lens
S. intraocular lens
S. IOL
S. toric IOL
S. toric lens
S. 4203VF lens
S. 4207VF lens
stab
s. incision
s. incision angled blade
stability
anterior chamber s.
chamber s.
tear film s.
stabilization
dynamic s.
1-handed s.
lysozyme s.

S

NOTES

stabilizer
>   mast cell s.
>   Rousseau chin-lift s.

Stableflex anterior chamber lens

stable vision

Stableyes capsular tension ring

stage
>   Ann Arbor s.
>   s. 0 macular hole

2-staged Baerveldt glaucoma implant

2-stage procedure

1-stage reconstruction of eye socket and eyelids

staging
>   Keith-Wagener-Barker hypertensive
>   retinopathy s. (grade 1–4))

Stahl
>   S. caliper
>   S. caliper block
>   S. caliper plate
>   S. lens gauge

Stähli pigment line

stain
>   acid-fast s.
>   alizarin red s.
>   calcein-AM s.
>   calcofluor white s.
>   Diff-Quik s.
>   direct fluorescent antibody s.
>   ethidium homodimer s.
>   fluorescein s.
>   Giemsa s.
>   Gomori methenamine silver s.
>   lissamine green s.
>   Live/Dead Kit s.
>   Masson trichrome s.
>   Papanicolaou s.
>   PAS s.
>   rose bengal s.
>   trypan blue s.
>   VisionBlue trypan blue 0.06% s.

staining
>   anterior capsule s.
>   arc s.
>   arcuate s.
>   blood s.
>   blotchy positive s.
>   bright s.
>   coarse punctate s.
>   conjunctival s.
>   corneal fluorescein s.
>   corneal punctate s.
>   corneal stromal blood s.
>   crystalline lens capsule s.
>   fluorescein s.
>   focal s.
>   immunofluorescent s.
>   immunoperoxidase s.
>   3 o'clock s.

>   ocular surface vital s.
>   s. pattern
>   punctate s.
>   in situ DNA nick end-labeling s.
>   stippling and s.
>   TUNEL s.

stalk
>   optic s.

stand
>   s. magnifier
>   Mayo s.

standard
>   s. ambient light
>   American National Standards
>   Institute s.
>   ANSI s.
>   s. automated perimetry (SAP)
>   s. deviation (SD)
>   s. full-field electroretinogram
>   s. near card
>   s. notation
>   s. pseudoisochromatic plate (SPP)
>   s. pseudoisochromatic plate part 2
>   (SPP2)
>   s. pseudoisochromatic plates color
>   deficiency testing product
>   S. Pseudoisochromatic Plates Part 2
>   test
>   safety s.
>   sterility s.
>   s. thickness

standardized visual scale test (SVST)

stand-off
>   edge s.-o.

staphylococcal
>   s. allergic keratoconjunctivitis
>   s. blepharitis
>   s. blepharoconjunctivitis
>   s. conjunctivitis
>   s. hypersensitivity

Staphylococcus
>   *S. aureus*
>   *S. epidermidis*
>   *S. haemolyticus*
>   *S. hominis*
>   *S. hyicus*
>   *S. intermedius*
>   *S. lugdunensis*
>   *S. saprophyticus*
>   *S. schleiferi*
>   *S. simulans*
>   *S. warneri*

staphyloma
>   anterior corneal s.
>   anular s.
>   ciliary s.
>   congenital anterior s. (CAS)
>   s. corneae racemosum
>   corneal s.

equatorial s.
intercalary s.
peripapillary s.
posterior s.
s. posticum
projecting s.
retinal s.
Scarpa s.
scleral s.
uveal s.
staphylomatous
staphylotomy
STAR
Scoring Tool for Assessing Risk
STAR S4 ActiveTrak 3-D eye
tracking system
STAR S3 ActiveTrak excimer laser
system
STAR S4 excimer laser system
STAR S2 SmoothScan excimer
laser system
star
epicapsular lens s.
S. excimer laser
s. fold
s. lens
lens s.
Lindstrom S.
macular s.
Winslow s.
stare
hyperthyroid s.
postbasic s.
thyroid s.
Stargardt
S. and Best disease
S. dystrophy
S. maculopathy
S. syndrome
Star-Optic eye wash
Starr fixation forceps
star-shaped field
starter
Brown pocket s.
startle myoclonus
stasis, pl. **stases**
axoplasmic s.
papillary s.
venous s.
stat
S. aspirator
S. Scrub handwasher machine

state
deturgescent s.
dry eye s.
refractive s.
state-of-the-art aberrometer
static
s. accommodation insufficiency
s. automated achromatic perimetry
s. countertorsion
s. perimeter
s. refraction
s. retinoscopy
stationary
s. cataract
s. night blindness
statistic
kappa s.
statometer
Statpac-like Analysis for Glaucoma
Evaluation (SAGE)
Statpac test
status
vision-related functional s.
Stay-Brite
Stay-Wet 3
steady-state accommodation
steal syndrome
stealth
S. DBO diamond blade
S. DBO freehand diamond knife
stearate
polyoxyl 40 s.
Steele-Richardson-Olszewski
S.-R.-O. disease
S.-R.-O. syndrome
steep
s. axis
s. contact lens
steepen
steepening
corneal s.
inferior s.
videokeratographic corneal s.
steepest meridian
steerable I/A
Stefan law
Steinbrinck anomaly
Steinert
S. disease
S. double-ended claw chopper
S. double-ended LASIK spatula
S. II claw chopper
S. LASIK set

S

NOTES

495

Steinert-Deacon incision gauge
stella
  s. lentis hyaloidea
  s. lentis iridica
stellata
  retinitis s.
stellate
  s. cataract
  s. corneal laceration
  s. keratitis
  s. neuroretinitis
  s. retinopathy
Stellwag
  S. brawny edema
  S. sign
stem
  brain s.
  s. cell (SC)
  s. cell bank
  s. cell differentiation
  s. cell therapy
  s. palsy
stenochoria
stenocoriasis
stenopeic, stenopaic
  s. disc
  s. iridectomy
  s. spectacles
stenosis, pl. **stenoses**
  aqueductal s.
  carotid artery s.
  hemodynamically significant carotid
    artery s. (HSCAS)
  involutional s.
  lacrimal punctal s.
  punctal s.
  punctum s.
Stenotrophomonas maltophilia
Stenstrom ocular measurement
stent
  CellPlant s.
  lacrimal s.
  monocanalicular silicone s.
  Supramid occluding s.
stenting
  monocanalicular s.
STENTube lacrimal intubation set
step
  ComfortCare GP One S.
  corneal graft s.
  s. graft operation
  nasal s.
  Ronne nasal s.
6-step algorithm
step-down technique
Stephens soft IOL-inserting forceps
Step-Knife diamond blade knife
3-step test

stepwise
  s. fashion
  s. variable selection
stereo
  s. ophthalmoscope
  s. reindeer test
  S. Smile II stereoacuity test
  s. x-ray
stereoacuity
  variable distance s. (VDS)
stereocampimeter
  Lloyd s.
stereognostic sense
stereogram
  random-dot s. (RDS)
stereo-identical point
stereometric parameter
stereo-orthopter
stereophantoscope
stereophorometer
stereophoroscope
stereophotogrammetric profiling
stereophotography
stereopsis
  coarse s.
  Gross s.
  macular s.
  random dot s.
  s. test
stereoscope
stereoscopic
  s. acuity
  s. depth perception
  s. depth plant
  s. diagonal inverter
  s. diplopia
  s. fundus photograph
  s. imaging
  s. parallax
  s. vision
stereoscopy
stereotactic
  s. radiation therapy (SRT)
  s. radiosurgery
stereotactic radiation therapy (SRT)
stereotest
  Lang s.
  Randot Dot E s.
stereoviewer
  Donaldson s.
Steri-Drape
  S.-D. drape
  3M small aperture S.-D.
  small aperture S.-D.
sterile
  s. acetazolamide sodium
  s. adhesive bubble dressing
  s. calcium alginate swab
  s. corneal ulcer

s. endophthalmitis
s. hypopyon
s. indocyanine green kit
s. melt
s. preserved daily cleaner
s. preserved saline
s. technique
sterility
s. of solution
s. standard
sterilizer
Cox rapid dry heat transfer s.
s. monitoring service
Steriseal disposable cannula
Steritome microkeratome system
Stern-Castroviejo
S.-C. locking forceps
S.-C. suturing forceps
Sterofrin
Isopto S.
steroid
s. anti-infective ophthalmic combination drug
s. concentration
s. dependent
s. diabetes
s. glaucoma
intravitreal s.
postoperative s.
s. prophylaxis
s. therapy
steroid-induced
s.-i. cataract
s.-i. glaucoma
steroidogenic diabetes
steroid-responsive inflammatory ocular condition
Stevens
S. eye scissors
S. iris forceps
S. muscle hook retractor
S. needle holder
S. tenotomy hook
S. tenotomy scissors
Stevens-Johnson syndrome
Stevenson lacrimal sac retractor
sthenophotic
stibogluconate sodium
stick
fluorescein s.
needle s.
stickiness
morning s.

Stickler syndrome
sties (*pl. of* sty)
stiff
s. pupil
s. retina
s. retinal fold
stigmatic
s. image
s. lens
stigmatometer
stigmatometric test card
stigmatoscope
stigmatoscopy
Stiles-Crawford effect
stiletto knife
Stilling
canal of S.
S. color table
S. color test
S. plate
Stilling-Türk-Duane syndrome
stimulation
Ganzfeld s.
sensory s.
stimulator
Cam vision s.
optokinetic s.
stimulatory antibody
stimulus, pl. **stimuli**
accommodative s.
auditory s.
blue flash s.
body-referenced s.
bright-white flash s.
s. deprivation
eye-referenced s.
flash s.
flicker fusion s.
light s.
optokinetic s.
proprioceptive s.
Raman s.
red flash s.
retinotopic s.
scotopic s.
Vernier s.
visual s.
stinger
Alio-Prats irrigating s.
stinging
stippled
s. hyperfluorescence
s. pattern

NOTES

stippling and staining
stitch
    s. abscess
    bow-tie s.
    cuticular s.
    shoelace s.
    triple-throw square knot s.
    s. with twists
    zipper s.
stitch-removal forceps
stitch-removing knife
Stocker
    S. line
    S. needle
Stocker-Holt dystrophy
Stocker-Holt-Schneider dystrophy
Stokes lens
stoma, pl. **stomas, stomata**
    Fuchs s.
stone
    tear s.
stony-hard eye
stop
    Bowman needle s.
    Castroviejo corneal scissors with
      inside s.
    s. speculum
stop-and-chop phacoemulsification
  technique
storage
    Opti-Free Rinsing Disinfecting
      and S.
Storz
    S. band
    S. caliper
    S. capsule forceps
    S. cataract knife
    S. cilia forceps
    S. corneal bur
    S. corneal forceps
    S. corneal trephine
    S. corneoscleral punch
    S. folding-handle eye spud
    S. handpiece
    S. keratome
    S. keratometer
    S. lid plate
    S. microscope
    S. Microvit magnet
    S. Microvit vitrector
    S. Millennium microsurgical system
    S. Premiere Microvit
    S. radial incision marker
    S. tonometer
Storz-Atlas hand eye magnet
Storz-Bonn suturing forceps
Storz-Walker retinal detachment unit
Stoxil

strabismal
    s. deviation
    s. nystagmus
strabismic amblyopia
strabismologist
strabismometer
strabismus
    absolute s.
    accommodative s.
    alternate day s.
    alternating s.
    American Academy of Pediatric
      Ophthalmology and S.
    American Association for Pediatric
      Ophthalmology and S. (AAPOS)
    anatomic s.
    A-pattern s.
    Bielschowsky s.
    bilateral s.
    binocular s.
    Braid s.
    cicatricial s.
    comitant s.
    concomitant s.
    constant s.
    convergent s.
    cyclic s.
    s. divergence
    divergent s.
    dynamic s.
    external s.
    s. fixus
    s. forceps
    Graves s.
    s. hook
    horizontal s.
    incomitant vertical s.
    intermittent s.
    internal s.
    kinetic s.
    latent s.
    manifest s.
    mechanical s.
    mixed s.
    monocular s.
    monolateral s.
    muscular s.
    noncomitant s.
    nonconcomitant s.
    nonparalytic s.
    paralytic s.
    periodic s.
    rectus muscle transposition for
      paralytic s.
    relative s.
    s. scissors
    secondary s.
    spasmodic s.
    suppressed s.

s. surgery
unilateral s.
uniocular s.
variable s.
vertical s.
strabometer
strabometry
strabotome
strabotomy
Strachan
S. disease
S. syndrome
Strachan-Scott syndrome
straight
s. mosquito clamp
s. nonirrigating Connor wand
s. retinal probe
s. sapphire knife
s. temple
s. tenotomy scissors
s. tying forceps
straight-eyed patient
straight-line bifocal
straight-tip bipolar forceps
strain
eye s.
Strampelli lens
strand
fibrin s.
glassine s.
iris s.
lysis of restricting s.
mucin s.
mucous-like s.
mucus s.
restricting s.
stromal s.
vitreous s.
strap
Velcro head s.
strategy
dominant s.
hand-eye coordination s.
management s.
pain prevention s.
telemedicine s.
stratification
stratified squamous epithelium
Stratus OCT device
Straus curved retrobulbar needle
strawberry
s. hemangioma
s. nevus

straylight meter
streak
angioid retinal s.
angiosis s.
hypofluorescent s.
Knapp s.
lightning s.
Moore lightning s.
s. retinoscope
s. retinoscopy
Sieger s.
Verhoeff s.
Strehl ratio
strength
orbicularis s.
strephosymbolia
streptococcal
s. bacillus
s. blepharitis
Streptococcus
S. faecalis
S. pneumoniae
S. pyogenes
S. salivarius
S. viridans
streptococcus
group B s.
streptokinase
Streptomyces caespitosus
stress
hypoxic corneal s.
oxidative s.
zonular s.
stress-strain measurement
stretching
pupil s.
stretch reflex
stria, pl. **striae**
concentric s.
corneal s.
flap s.
Haab s.
Knapp s.
vertical s.
Vogt s.
striascope
striatal nigral degeneration
striate
s. keratitis
s. keratopathy
s. melanokeratosis
s. opacity

NOTES

striate *(continued)*
s. retinitis
s. visual cortex
striated glasses
striation
retinal s.
string convergence
stringy mucus
strip
color bar Schirmer s.
DET fluorescein s.
EyeClose Adhesive s.
filter paper s.
Fluorets fluorescein sodium s.
Ful-Glo fluorescein s.
gliotic s.
Lacrytest s.
marginal tear s.
s. procedure
reagent s.
Schirmer tear test s.
silicone s.
tear test s.
stripe
central reflex s.
stripper
Crawford fascial s.
fascia lata s.
stripping
cortical s.
s. membrane
stroboscopic disc
stroke-like episode
stroma, pl. **stromata**
avascular corneal s.
corneal s.
disc s.
s. of iris
iris s.
limbal s.
perilimbal s.
pigmented s.
s. plexus
sclerotic s.
vitreous s.
s. vitreum
stromal
s. anular infiltrate
s. bed
s. blood vessel
s. corneal dystrophy
s. disease
s. downgrowth
s. ectasia
s. edema
s. ghost scarring
s. haze
s. hydration
s. ingrowth

s. keratitis
s. keratouveitis
s. line
s. matrix
s. melt
s. melting
s. necrosis
s. neovascularization
s. opacity
s. photoablation
s. pocket
s. ring infiltrate
s. splitting
s. strand
s. thickness
s. thinning
s. ulcer
s. vascularization
s. wound healing
Strow corneal forceps
Struble lid everter
structural abnormality
structure
accessory visual s.
S. And Function Evaluation
(SAFE)
angle s.
Kolmer crystalloid s.
orbital s.
retinal anatomic s.
snake-like s.
strumous ophthalmia
strut
optic s.
Stryker
S. frame
S. saw
study
ACHIEVE s.
Advanced Glaucoma Intervention S.
(AGIS)
Age-Related Eye Disease S.
(AREDS)
Amblyopia Treatment S. (ATS)
Baltimore Pediatric Eye Disease S.
Beaver Dam Eye S.
Blue Mountain Eye S.
Branch Vein Occlusion S.
Central Vein Occlusion S. (CVOS)
CLAMP s.
CLEERE s.
CLEK s.
cohort s.
Collaborative Corneal
Transplantation S.'s (CCTS)
Collaborative Initial Glaucoma
Treatment S. (CIGTS)
Collaborative Longitudinal
Evaluation of Keratoconus s.

Collaborative Normal Tension
  Glaucoma S. (CNTGS)
Collaborative Ocular Melanoma S.
  (COMS)
Congenital Esotropia
  Observational S. (CEOS)
Contact Lens and Myopia
  Progression s.
Controlled High Risk Avonex
  Multiple Sclerosis Prevention S.
  (CHAMPS)
Cooperative Ocular Melanoma S.
  (COMS)
Cornea Donor S. (CDS)
Cytomegalovirus Retinitis and Viral
  Resistance S. (CRVRS)
Diabetic Retinopathy Vitrectomy S.
  (DRVS)
double-blind s.
Early Treatment Diabetic
  Retinopathy S. (ETDRS)
Early Treatment for Retinopathy of
  Prematurity s.
Egna-Neumarkt s.
Endophthalmitis Vitrectomy S.
  (EVS)
ETROP s.
European Glaucoma Prevention S.
  (EGPS)
Fluorouracil Filtering Surgery S.
  (FFSS)
Glaucoma Laser Trial Followup S.
  (GLTFS)
Herpetic Eye Disease S.
Herpetic Eye Disease S. I
Herpetic Eye Disease S. II
  (HEDS2)
Infant Aphakia Treatment S.
Krypton-Argon Regression of
  Neovascularization S. (KARNS)
Lens Opacities Case-Control S.
Longitudinal Optic Neuritis S.
  (LONS)
long-term comparative s.
Macular Photocoagulation S. (MPS)
Madurai Intraocular Lens S. IV
NEI Visual Acuity Impairment
  Survey s.
S.'s of the Ocular Complications
  in AIDS (SOCA)
Ocular Hypertension Treatment S.
  (OHTS)
PERK S.

Prism Adaptation S. (PAS)
Prospective Evaluation of Radial
  Keratotomy S.
radiologic s.
retrospective s.
SAFE s.
Temba glaucoma s.
The Berkeley Orthokeratology S.
The Silicone S.
validation s.
VALIO s.
vectographic s.
VIP S.
Vision in Preschoolers S.
Vitrectomy for Macular Hole S.
  (VMHS)
Sturge-Weber
  S.-W. disease
  S.-W. encephalotrigeminal
    angiomatosis
  S.-W. syndrome
Sturge-Weber-Dimitri syndrome
Sturm
  conoid of S.
  S. conoid
  S. interval
  interval of S.
stutzeri
  Pseudomonas s.
sty, stye, pl. **sties, styes**
  meibomian s.
  s. ophthalmic ointment
  zeisian s.
Style S2 clear-loop lens
styrene contact lens
Suarez spreader
subacute
  s. myelooptic neuropathy (SMON)
  s. necrotizing encephalomyelopathy
  s. neuroretinitis
  s. sclerosing panencephalitis
subarachnoid
  s. bleed
  s. fluid
  s. hemorrhage
  s. injection
  s. oculomotor nerve lesion
  s. oculomotor nerve palsy
  s. space
subcapsular
  s. cataract
  s. epithelium
  s. plaque

NOTES

S

subchoroidal hemorrhage
subciliary incision
subclinical
    s. diabetes
    s. optic neuritis
subconjunctival (SC)
    s. administration
    s. antibiotic
    s. chemotherapy
    s. cyst
    s. edema
    s. emphysema
    s. foreign body
    s. hemorrhage
    s. injection
    s. needle
subconjunctivitis
subcontinent
    laryngeal and ocular granulation
      tissue in children from the
      Indian s. (LOGIC)
subcortical alexia
subcutaneous
    s. amyloid
    s. fat atrophy
subduction
subdural hematoma
subepidermal calcified nodule
subepithelial
    s. corneal haze
    s. corneal opacity
    s. fibrosis
    s. keratitis
    s. nevus
    s. opacification
    s. plaque
    s. plexus
    s. punctate corneal infiltrate
subepithelialis
    keratitis punctata s.
subfoveal
    s. choroidal neovascularization
    s. lesion
    s. mass
    s. neovascular membrane
subhyaloid
    s. blood
    s. hemorrhage
subimplant
    Spencer silicone s.
subinternal limiting membrane
  hemorrhage
subjective
    S. Autorefractor-7
    s. device
    s. fixation disparity
    s. ocular comfort
    s. prism-neutralized cover test
    s. refraction test

    s. refractor
    s. testing
    s. torsion
    s. vertigo
    s. vision
subjectoscope
subluxated crystalline lens
subluxation of lens
subluxed lens
submacular
    s. fluid
    s. surgery
    S. Surgery Trials (SST)
submembrane fluid
subnormal
    s. accommodation
    s. vision
suboccipital craniectomy
suboptimal vision
suborbicularis
    s. oculi fat (SOOF)
    s. oculi fat lift
suborbital
subperiosteal
    s. abscess
    s. implant
subpigment epithelial space
subretinal
    s. aspiration cannula
    s. blood
    s. deposit
    s. fibrosis
    s. fluid (SRF)
    s. fluid cuff
    s. fluid drainage
    s. hemorrhage
    s. hydatid cyst
    s. lipid
    s. mass
    s. membrane (SRM)
    s. neovascularization (SRNV)
    s. neovascular membrane (SRNVM)
    s. pigment epithelial plaque
    s. pigment ring
    s. scarring
    s. space
subscale
    visual ability s.
subscleral
subsclerotic
subsequent hypotony
substance
    corneal s.
    s. exophthalmos
    exophthalmos-producing s. (EPS)
    s. of lens
    s. P
    scleral s.
    toxic s.

substantia
  s. corticalis lentis
  s. propria
  s. propria corneae
  s. propria sclerae
substitute
  vitreous s.
sub-Tenon
  s.-T. administration
  s.-T. anesthesia cannula
  s.-T. corticosteroid injection
  s.-T. parabulbar anesthesia
subterminale
  Clostridium s.
subthreshold
  s. light
  s. subfoveal diode laser
    photocoagulation (SSDLP)
subtilis
  Bacillus s.
subtle
  s. disc pallor
  s. mottling
subtotal
  s. orbital exenteration
  s. thyroidectomy
subtraction topography
subtype
  aggressive histologic s.
  common s.
  histologic s.
  nodular s.
subvolution
success
  anatomic s.
successive contrast
succulent vessel
suction
  s. ophthalmodynamometer
  perilimbal s.
  s. ring
  s. trephine
sudden visual loss
sudoriferous cyst
sugar cataract
sugar-induced cataract
Sugiura sign
suis
  Brucella s.
Suker sign
Sulamyd
  Sodium S.

sulbactam
sulcus, pl. **sulci**
  chiasmal s.
  ciliary s.
  corneoscleral s.
  s. fixated position
  s. fixation
  s. infraorbitalis maxillae
  infrapalpebral s.
  intramarginal s.
  iridociliary s.
  lacrimal s.
  optic s.
  orbital s.
  s. orbitales lobi frontalis
  s. sclera
  scleral s.
  sclerocorneal s.
  superior tarsal s.
  s. support
  supraorbital s.
Sulfacel 15
sulfacetamide
  s. phenylephrine
  s. and prednisolone
  s. sodium
  s. sodium and fluorometholone
sulfadiazine
sulfa drug
Sulfair
  S. 10
  S. Forte
sulfamethoxazole
Sulfamide
sulfanilamide
Sulfasuxidine
sulfate
  alkyl ether s.
  atropine s.
  chondroitin s.
  dermatan s.
  dimethyl s.
  eserine s.
  ferrous s.
  gentamicin s.
  hydroxychloroquine s.
  indinavir s.
  keratan s.
  neomycin s.
  phenelzine s.
  physostigmine s.
  polymyxin B s.
  quinine s.

NOTES

S

sulfate *(continued)*
    sodium s.
    sodium hyaluronate and
      chondroitin s.
    sodium lauryl s.
    tranylcypromine s.
    zinc s.
sulfisoxazole diolamine
sulfonamide
Sulf-10 Ophthalmic
sulfur
    s. gas
    s. hexafluoride (SF6)
sulfurhexafluoride gas
Sulphrin
Sulpred
Sulster Solution
Sulten-10
summation
    spatial s.
Summerskill operation
Summit
    S. Apex Plus excimer laser
    S. Krumeich-Barraquer
      microkeratome (SKBM)
    S. OmniMed excimer laser
    S. SVS Apex laser
    The S. HeNe aiming beam
    S. UV 200 ExciMed laser
Sumycin
sun
    s. block
    s. damage
    s. glare
sunburst
    black s.
    s. dial
    s. dial chart
    s. effect
sunburst-type lesion
sunflower cataract
Sung reverse nucleus chopper
sunrise
    S. LTK procedure
    S. LTK system
    s. syndrome
sunscreen
    optic s.
sunset
    s. fundus
    s. syndrome
sunset-glow appearance
super
    S. Field NC slit lamp lens
    s. pinky ball
    S. punctum plug
Superblade
supercilia (*pl. of* supercilium)

superciliaris
    arcus s.
superciliary
    s. arch
    s. muscle
supercilii
    musculus corrugator s.
    musculus depressor s.
supercilium, pl. **supercilia**
superduction
superficial
    s. congestion
    s. corneal line
    s. lamellar keratectomy
    s. lamellar limbo keratoplasty
    s. linear keratitis
    s. line of cornea
    s. punctate keratitis (SPK)
    s. punctate keratitis of Thygeson
      (SPKT)
    s. punctate keratopathy
    s. retinal refractile deposit
superimposed
    s. amblyopia
    s. ellipse
superinfection
    bacterial s.
    corneal s.
superior
    s. approach
    s. arcuate bundle
    s. arcuate scotoma
    arcus palpebralis s.
    arteriola macularis s.
    arteriola nasalis retinae s.
    arteriola temporalis retinae s.
    s. canaliculus
    s. cervical ganglion
    s. colliculus
    s. conjunctival fornix
    s. cornea
    s. corneal shield ulcer
    s. division palsy
    s. eyelid crease
    fissura orbitalis s.
    s. gaze
    glandula lacrimalis s.
    s. homonymous quadrantic defect
    s. lacrimal gland
    s. limbic keratoconjunctivitis (SLK)
    s. macular arteriole
    musculus tarsalis s.
    s. nasal artery
    s. nasal vein
    s. oblique extraocular muscle
    s. oblique microtremor
    s. oblique muscle and trochlear
      luxation
    s. oblique myokymia

s. oblique palsy
s. oblique tack surgery
s. oblique tendon
s. oblique tendon sheath syndrome
s. oblique transposition
s. ophthalmic vein
s. orbital fissure (SOF)
s. orbital fissure syndrome
s. orbital septum
s. palpebral furrow
s. palpebral vein
s. pole
s. polioencephalitis
s. punctum
s. quadrantanopia
s. radial tenotomy scissors
s. rectus (SR)
s. rectus bridle suture
s. rectus extraocular muscle
s. rectus forceps
s. rectus palsy
s. rim
s. salivary nucleus
s. sector iridectomy
s. tarsal muscle
s. tarsal papillary conjunctivitis
s. tarsal sulcus
s. tarsus
s. temporal artery
s. temporal vein
s. tendon of Lockwood
s. vascular arcade
vena ophthalmica s.
venula macularis s.
venula nasalis retinae s.
venula temporalis retinae s.
s. zone of retina
superiores
venae palpebrales s.
superior-hinged flap cornea
superioris
levator palpebrae s.
musculus levator palpebrae s.
supernormal vision
superonasal
s. macula
s. paracentral visual field
superotemporally
superoxide dismutase 2 (SOD2)
superpulsed laser
supertemporal bulbar conjunctiva

supertraction
conus s.
s. conus
supine IOP
supplement
antioxidant s.
ICaps TR dietary s.
MaculaRx Plus nutritional s.
MaxiVision dietary s.
nutritional s.
Ocuvite Lutein Antioxidant S.
Supplemental Therapeutic Oxygen for Prethreshold Retinopathy of Prematurity
supplementation
artificial tear s.
tear s.
supply
information s.
support
capsular s.
iris s.
sulcus s.
zonular s.
supporter
scleral s.
suppressant
aqueous s.
suppressed strabismus
suppression
s. amblyopia
central s.
facultative s.
macular s.
obligatory s.
orbital fat s.
s. scotoma
suppressor T cell
suppurativa
hyalitis s.
suppurative
s. choroiditis
s. hyalitis
s. keratitis
s. retinitis
s. ulcer
suprachiasmatic nucleus (SCN)
suprachoroid
s. lamina
s. layer
suprachoroidal
s. foreign body

S

NOTES

suprachoroidal *(continued)*
s. hemorrhage (SCH, SH)
s. space
suprachoroidea
lamina s.
supraciliaris
epicanthus s.
supraciliary canal
Supraclens
Opti-Free S.
supraduction
SupraFOIL implant
Supramid
S. bridle collagen suture
S. lens implant
S. lens implant suture
S. occluding stent
S. sheet
S. sling
Supramid-Allen implant
supranuclear
s. cataract
s. connection
s. control
s. deficiency
s. deviation
s. disorder
s. gaze center
s. input
s. lesion
s. ocular palsy
s. ophthalmoplegia
s. paresis of vertical gaze
s. pathway
supraocular
supraoptic
s. canal
s. commissure
s. nucleus (SON)
supraorbital
s. akinesia
s. arch
s. arch of frontal bone
s. artery
s. canal
s. foramen
s. incisure
s. margin of frontal bone
s. margin of orbit
s. nerve
s. neuralgia
s. notch
s. point
s. reflex
s. ridge
s. sulcus
s. vein
supraorbitale
foramen s.

supraorbitalis
incisura s.
nervus s.
suprapineal recess
suprascleral
suprasellar
s. aneurysm
s. lesion
s. meningioma
s. tumor
8000 Supra Series auto refractometer
supratemporal region
supratentorial arteriovenous malformation
suprathreshold
s. screening
s. static perimetry
Supratome microkeratome
supratrochlear nerve
supravergence
supraversion
Suprax
suprofen
suramin sodium
Surefit AC 85J lens
SureFold system
SureSight
S. autorefractor
S. vision screener
S. vision screening device
Surevue contact lens
surface
s. analgesia
anterior corneal s.
s. asymmetry index (SAI)
s. breakdown
concave reflecting s.
convex reflecting s.
curved reflecting s.
s. dyslexia
ellipsoidal back s.
s. implant
s. irregularity
s. lamellar keratoplasty
s. lubrication
modified prolate anterior s.
ocular s.
Petzval s.
s. photorefractive keratectomy
reflecting s.
s. regularity index (SRI)
s. tension
toric s.
s. wrinkling retinopathy
surfactant cleaning solution
Surgamid
surge
postocclusion s.

surgeon
> American Board of Eye S.'s (ABES)
> American College of Eye S.'s (ACES)
> Fellow of the American College of S.'s (FACS)
> Fellow of the Royal College of S.'s (FRCS)
> oculoplastic s.
> Society of Cataract and Refractive S.'s
> vitreoretinal s.

surgery
> American Society of Cataract and Refractive S. (ASCRS)
> American Society of Ophthalmic Plastic and Reconstruction S.
> angle s.
> anterior chamber refractive s.
> antiglaucoma s.
> artificial divergency s.
> asymmetric s.
> cataract s.
> ciliodestructive s.
> closed-eye s.
> coaxial microincision s.
> combined cataract/trabeculectomy s.
> corneal s.
> cosmetic oculoplastic s.
> cranioorbital s.
> cyclophotocoagulation vitreoretinal s.
> decompression s.
> decompressive s.
> Dodick laser cataract s.
> drainage implant s.
> dye-enhanced cataract s.
> endoscopic lacrimal s.
> endoscopic pigment epithelial endoscopic laser s.
> epi-LASIK s.
> extraocular muscle s.
> eyelid s.
> eye muscle s.
> eye plaque s.
> failed ptosis s.
> filtering s.
> filtration s.
> first-eye cataract s.
> fistulizing s.
> flow-based phacoemulsification s.
> foldable intraocular lens s.
> frontalis suspension s.
> glaucoma filtering s.
> glaucoma filtration s.
> horizontal muscle s.
> hyperopic LASIK s.
> idiopathic macular hole s.
> intraoperative adjustable suture s.
> keratorefractive s.
> lacrimal s.
> laser s.
> laser-filtering s.
> LASIK vision correction s.
> macular hole s.
> macular translocation s.
> microincision cataract s. (MICS)
> Mohs micrographic s.
> 2-muscle s.
> nonpenetrating filtering s.
> no-stitch phacoemulsification s.
> oculoplastic s.
> office-based s.
> open globe s.
> ophthalmic s.
> ophthalmologic s.
> orbital decompression s.
> periocular s.
> photorefractive s.
> pigment epithelial endoscopic laser s. (PEELS)
> previous cataract s.
> pterygium s.
> refractive cataract s.
> refractive laser s.
> retinal s.
> scleral expansion s.
> scleral explant s.
> second-eye cataract s.
> simultaneous bilateral cataract s.
> small-incision cataract s.
> small pupil cataract s.
> squint s.
> strabismus s.
> submacular s.
> superior oblique tack s.
> sutureless cataract s.
> sutureless pterygium s.
> symmetric s.
> vitreoretinal s.
> vitreous s.
> wavefront-guided laser eye s.
> Zyoptix customized eye s.

surgery-related
> s.-r. anxiety
> s.-r. factor

S

NOTES

Surg-E-Trol
  S.-E-T. I/A System
  S.-E-T. System irrigating/aspirating
    unit
surgical
  s. ablation pattern
  s. adjunct
  s. caliper
  s. débridement
  s. decompression
  s. decompression procedure
  s. descemetocele
  s. enzyme
  S. Eye Expeditions (SEE)
  s. gut suture
  s. intervention
  s. keratometry
  s. management protocol
  s. marking pen
  s. modification
  s. overcorrection
  s. patch grafting
  s. reversal of presbyopia (SRP)
  s. sponge
  s. trauma
  s. treatment
surgically
  s. induced astigmatism
  s. induced refractive change
Surgicraft suture needle
Surgidev
  S. PC BUV 20-24 intraocular lens
  S. suture
Surgikos disposable drape
Surgimed suture
SurgiScope
  Marco S.
Surgisol
Surgistar
  S. corneal trephine
  S. ophthalmic blade
Surodex
surplus field
sursumduction
  alternating s.
sursumvergence
  left s.
  right s.
sursumversion
survey
  Baltimore Eye S.
  Health and Activity Limitations S.
    (HALS)
survival
  ocular s.
Susac syndrome
susceptibility kill rate
suspect
  glaucoma s.

suspected keratoconus
suspension
  AK-Cide S.
  AK-Spore H.C. Ophthalmic S.
  AK-Trol S.
  Alrex ophthalmic s.
  brinzolamide ophthalmic s.
  Cortisporin Ophthalmic S.
  fluorometholone ophthalmic s.
  FML-S Ophthalmic S.
  frontalis fascia lata s.
  hydrocortisone s.
  Isopto Cetapred s.
  Lotemax ophthalmic s.
  loteprednol etabonate ophthalmic s.
  Maxitrol s.
  Metimyd s.
  nepafenac ophthalmic s.
  Poly-Dex S.
  Poly-Pred Ophthalmic S.
  Pred-G s.
  rimexolone ophthalmic s.
  Terra-Cortril Ophthalmic S.
  TobraDex ophthalmic s.
  transconjunctival frontalis s.
  Vexol 1% ophthalmic s.
  Zylet ophthalmic s.
suspensory
  s. ligament
  s. ligament of eye
Sussman
  S. lens
  S. 4-mirror gonioscope
sustained
  s. focus
  s. release intravitreal helical
    implant
sustained-release system
sustainer
  Akahoshi nucleus ring s.
sustentacular
  s. fiber
  s. tissue
Sutherland
  S. lens
  S. rotatable microsurgery instrument
  S. scissors
sutura
  s. ethmoidolacrimalis
  s. ethmoidomaxillaris
  s. infraorbitalis
  s. lacrimoconchalis
  s. lacrimomaxillaris
  s. palatoethmoidalis
  s. palatomaxillaris
sutural developmental cataract
suture
  s. abscess
  absorbable s.

adjustable s.
s. adjustment
Alcon s.
anchor s.
anchoring s.
antitorque s.
Arroyo encircling s.
Arruga encircling s.
Atraloc s.
Axenfeld s.
16-bite nylon s.
black braided nylon s.
black braided silk s.
black silk bridle s.
black silk sling s.
Bondek s.
braided silk s.
braided Vicryl s.
bridge s.
bridle s.
buried s.
canaliculus rod and s.
cardinal s.
catgut s.
cheesewiring of s.'s
chromic catgut s.
chromic collagen s.
chromic gut s.
clove-hitch s.
coated Vicryl s.
compression s.
s. of cornea operation
Dacron s.
Deknatel silk s.
Dermalon s.
Dexon s.
double-armed s.
double-running penetrating
  keratoplasty s.
Ethicon-Atraloc s.
Ethicon micropoint s.
Ethicon Sabreloc s.
everting s.
s. of eyeball operation
Faden s.
fetal Y s.
figure-of-8 s.
fixation s.
Foster s.
frontolacrimal s.
frontosphenoid s.
frontozygomatic s.
Frost s.

Gaillard-Arlt s.
groove s.
guy s.
horizontal mattress s.
infraorbital s.
interrupted nylon s.
intracameral s.
intraluminal s.
iris s.
s. of iris operation
juxtalimbal s.
lacrimoconchal s.
lacrimoethmoidal s.
lacrimomaxillary s.
lacrimoturbinal s.
lancet s.
s. lancet
s. lasso technique
s. of lens
Look s.
Mannis s.
mattress s.
McCannel s.
McLean s.
Mersilene s.
Mersilk black silk s.
Micrins microsurgical s.
Micro-Glide corneal s.
micropoint s.
mild chromic s.
monofilament nylon s.
s. of muscle operation
nonabsorbable s.
Nurolon s.
nylon 66 s.
palatomaxillary s.
s. pickup hook
pickup spatula s.
s. pickup spatula
plain catgut s.
plain collagen s.
plain gut s.
Polydek s.
polyester s.
polyglactin 910 s.
polyglycolate s.
polyglycolic acid s.
polypropylene s.
polytetrafluoroethylene s.
posterior fixation s.
postplaced s.
preplaced s.
Prolene s.

NOTES

suture *(continued)*
    Quickert s.
    releasable compression s.
    s. release
    rip-cord s.
    s. rotation
    s. rotation technique
    running nylon penetrating
      keratoplasty s.
    Safil synthetic absorbable
      surgical s.
    scleral flap s.
    s. of sclera operation
    self-adjusting s.
    Serralnyl s.
    Serralsilk s.
    Sharpoint ophthalmic
      microsurgical s.
    Sharpoint Ultra-Glide corneal
      transplant s.
    Sharpoint Ultra-Glide ophthalmic
      transplant s.
    Shoch s.
    silk traction s.
    single-armed s.
    single-running s.
    s. sling
    Sofsilk nonabsorbable silk s.
    Spanish silk s.
    sphenofrontal s.
    sphenoorbital s.
    superior rectus bridle s.
    Supramid bridle collagen s.
    Supramid lens implant s.
    surgical gut s.
    Surgidev s.
    Surgimed s.
    Swiss silk s.
    Tevdek s.
    traction s.
    transscleral s.
    twisted virgin silk s.
    Verhoeff s.
    Vicryl s.
    virgin silk s.
    white braided silk s.
    Worst s.
    Y s.
    zygomatic s.
    zygomaticofrontal s.
    zygomaticomaxillary s.
    zygomaticosphenoid s.
    zygomaticotemporal s.
SutureGroove
    S. gold eyelid weight
    S. gold eye weight implant
sutureless
    s. cataract surgery
    s. clear corneal incision

    s. pterygium surgery
    s. transconjunctival pars plana
      vitrectomy
suture-out astigmatism
suturing
    s. of eyelid
    s. forceps
    s. needle
    temporary keratoprosthesis s.
    tunnel s.
Svedberg unit
SVI/BL
    severe visual impairment and blindness
SVST
    standardized visual scale test
    corrected S.
swab
    calcium alginate s.
    eye s.
    sterile calcium alginate s.
    wooden s.
swan
    S. incision
    S. lancet
    S. syndrome
Swan-Jacob gonioprism
SWAP
    short wavelength automated perimetry
Swedish interactive thresholding
  algorithm (SITA)
sweep
    Barraquer s.
    eye s.
    iris s.
    s. view
sweet
    S. locator
    S. method
    S. original magnet
swelling
    chronic optic disc s.
    conjunctiva s.
    corneal s.
    s. of disc
    eyelid s.
    optic disc s.
    Soemmerring crystalline s.
    soft tissue s.
Swets goniotomy knife cannula
swift-cut phaco incision knife
swimmer's goggles
swimming
    s. pool conjunctivitis
    s. pool water toxicity
Swim'n Clear
swinging
    s. flashlight sign
    s. flashlight test

s. lid flap
s. light test
Swiss-cheese visual field
Swiss silk suture
switch
Prescott wireless foot s.
swollen nerve
sycosiform
syllabic blindness
Sylvian aqueduct syndrome
symblepharon
anterior s.
s. formation
inferior s.
s. lysis
posterior s.
s. ring
total s.
symblepharopterygium
symbol
s. chart
s. recognition
test s.
symmetrical
s. astigmatism
s. image blur
symmetric surgery
sympathetic
s. amaurosis
s. carotid plexus
s. heterochromia
s. hyperactivity
s. innervation failure
s. iridoplegia
s. iritis
s. nervous system
s. neuron
s. ophthalmia
s. pathway
s. uveitis
sympathetica
ptosis s.
sympathizer
sympathizing eye
sympatholytic drug
sympathomimetic eye drops
sympathoparesis
symptom
afferent visual s.
aniseikonia s.
Anton s.
Epstein s.
s. flare

habitual s.
Haenel s.
halo s.
Liebreich s.
ocular rosacea s.
rainbow s.
typical dry eye s.
Uhthoff s.
Wernicke s.
symptomatic
s. blepharospasm
s. paracentral scotoma
s. relief
synaphymenitis
synapse
photoreceptor-bipolar s.
synaptic
s. body
s. connection
s. ridge
synaptophysin antibody
synathroisis
syncanthus
synchesis scintillans
Synchrony Dual Optic Accommodating IOL
synchysis scintillans
syndectomy
syndermatotic cataract
syndesmitis
syndrome
A s.
Aarskog s.
Aase s.
accommodative effort s.
acquired Horner s.
acquired immunodeficiency s. (AIDS)
acute idiopathic blind spot enlargement s. (AIBSES)
acute retinal necrosis s.
adherence s.
adhesive s.
Adie s.
Ahlström s.
AICA s.
Aicardi s.
Alezzandrini s.
Alport s.
Alström s.
Alström-Hallgren s.
Alström-Olsen s.
alternating Horner s.

NOTES

syndrome *(continued)*

amniotic band s.
Andersen s.
Angelman s.
Angelucci s.
Angosky s.
anterior chamber cleavage s.
anterior optic chiasmal s.
antielevation s. (AES)
anti-Hu s.
antiphospholipid s.
Antley-Bixler s.
Anton s.
Anton-Babinski s.
Apert s.
aqueous misdirection s.
ARN s.
ARRON s.
arteriovenous strabismus s.
Ascher s.
ataxia-telangiectasia s.
AV strabismus s.
Axenfeld s.
Axenfeld-Rieger s.
Balint s.
Baller-Gerold s.
Bamatter s.
Bannayan s.
Bardet-Biedl s.
bare lymphocyte s.
Barlow s.
Bartter s.
basal cell nevus s.
Bassen-Kornzweig s.
Batten s.
Batten-Mayou s.
battered baby s.
battered child s.
Béal s.
Behçet s.
Behr s.
Benedikt s.
Bernard s.
Bernard-Horner s.
Bielschowsky-Jansky s.
Bielschowsky-Lutz-Cogan s.
Biemond s.
Bietti s.
big blind spot s.
bilateral uveal effusion s.
blepharophimosis ptosis s.
blepharospasm-oromandibular
   dystonia s.
blind spot s.
Bloch-Stauffer s.
Bloch-Sulzberger s.
blue rubber bleb nevus s.
Bonnet s.
Bonnet-Dechaume-Blanc s.

Bonnier s.
Bourneville s.
brachial arch s.
brittle cornea s.
Brown s.
Brown-McLean s.
Brown tendon sheath s.
Brown vertical retraction s.
Brueghel s.
Brushfield-Wyatt s.
capsular bag distention s.
capsular exfoliation s.
capsule contraction s.
CAR s.
Carpenter s.
cataract with Down s.
cat's-eye s.
cavernous sinus s.
cavernous sinus/superior orbital
   fissure s.
central scotoma s.
cerebrohepatorenal s.
cervicooculoacoustic s.
Cestan s.
Cestan-Chenais s.
Cestan-Raymond s.
Chandler s.
CHARGE s.
Charles Bonnet s. (CBS)
Charlin s.
Chédiak-Higashi s.
cherry-red spot myoclonus s.
chiasmal s.
chiasmatic s.
chronic dry eye s.
chronic smoldering toxicity s.
Churg-Strauss s.
Cianca s.
Claude-Lhermitte s.
cleavage s.
cleft s.
Coats s.
Cockayne s.
co-contraction s.
Coffin-Lowry s.
Cogan s.
Cogan-Reese s.
Cohen s.
computer vision s. (CVS)
congenital adherence s.
congenital fibrosis s.
congenital Horner s.
congenital juxtafoveolar s.
congenital rubella s.
congenital tilted disc s.
Conn s.
conotruncal anomalies face s.
Conradi s.
contact lens overwear s.

Cornelia de Lange s.
CPD s.
cranial stenosis s.
craniofacial s.
CREST s.
cri du chat s.
crocodile tears s.
Crouzon s.
Cushing s.
cutaneomucouveal s.
DAF s.
D chromosome ring s.
Degos s.
de Grouchy s.
Dejean s.
de Lange s.
de Morsier s.
de Morsier-Gauthier s.
DIDMOAD s.
diencephalic s.
DiGeorge s.
dispersion s.
distal optic nerve s.
dorsal midbrain s.
Down s.
Doyne s.
Drews s.
dry eye s. (DES)
D trisomy s.
Duane retraction s.
dural shunt s.
dyscephalic s.
dysfunctional tear s.
E s.
Eaton-Lambert s.
Edwards s.
Ehlers-Danlos s.
Eisenmenger s.
Ellingson s.
Elschnig s.
embryonic fixation s.
empty sella s.
exfoliation s. (XFS)
extrapyramidal s.
Fabry s.
Falls-Kertesz s.
Fanconi s.
fat adherence s.
fetal hydantoin s.
fetal trimethadione s.
fetal warfarin s.
fibrosis s.
Fiessinger-Leroy-Reiter s.

Fisher s.
Fitz-Hugh and Curtis s.
flaccid canaliculus s.
flecked retina s.
flocculus s.
floppy eye s.
floppy eyelid s.
Foix s.
Forssman carotid s.
Foster Kennedy s.
foveomacular cone dysfunction s.
Foville s.
Foville-Wilson s.
Franceschetti s.
Franceschetti-Klein s.
François s.
Fraser s.
Freeman-Sheldon s.
Frenkel anterior ocular traumatic s.
Frey s.
Friedenwald s.
Friedreich s.
Fuchs s.
Fuchs-Kraupa s.
GAPO s.
Gardner s.
Gass s.
Gerstmann s.
Gilbert-Behçet s.
Gillespie s.
Gitelman s.
Goldenhar s. (GS)
Goldenhar-Gorlin s.
Goldmann-Favre s.
Goltz s.
Goltz-Gorlin s.
Gorham-Stout s.
Gradenigo s.
Graefe s.
Gregg s.
Greig s.
Greither s.
Grönblad-Strandberg s.
Guillain-Barré s.
Gunn s.
Hagberg-Santavuori s.
half-moon s.
Hallermann-Streiff s.
Hallermann-Streiff-François s.
Hallervorden-Spatz s.
Hallgren s.
Haltia-Santavuori type of Batten s.
Hand-Schüller-Christian s.

S

NOTES

513

syndrome *(continued)*
Harada s.
Hay-Wells s.
Heerfordt s.
Heidenhain s.
hereditary benign intraepithelial dyskeratosis s.
hereditary hyperferritinemia-cataract s.
hereditary optic atrophy s.
heredodegenerative neurologic s.
Hermansky-Pudlak s.
Hertwig-Magendie s.
Hippel-Lindau s.
histoplasmosis s.
HLA-B27 s.
Holmes-Adie s.
Holt-Oram s.
Homer s.
Horner s.
Horner-Bernard s.
Horton s.
Hunter s.
Hunter-Hurler s.
Hurler s.
Hurler-Scheie s.
Hutchinson s.
hyperophthalmopathic s.
hyperviscosity s.
hypotony s.
hypoxic eyeball s.
ICE s.
idiopathic orbital inflammatory s. (IOIS)
idiopathic vitreomacular traction s.
immune recovery vitreitis s.
infantile nystagmus s.
infantile strabismus s.
inflammatory s.
innominate steal s.
internal capsule s.
intraoperative floppy iris s. (IFIS)
iridocorneal endothelial s.
iridocyclitis masquerade s.
iridoendothelial s.
iris-nevus s.
Irlen s.
IRVAN s.
Irvine-Gass s.
ischemic chiasmal s.
ischemic ocular s.
ischemic orbital compartment s.
Jacod s.
Jadassohn-Lewandowski s.
Jahnke s.
Jansky-Bielschowsky s.
jaw-winking s.
Jeune s.
Johnson s.

Joubert s.
Kartagener s.
Kasabach-Merritt s.
Kearns-Sayre s. (KSS)
Kehrer-Adie s.
Kennedy s.
KID s.
Kiloh-Nevin s.
Kimmelstiel-Wilson s.
Kjellin s.
Kloepfer s.
Knobloch s.
Koerber-Salus-Elschnig s.
Krause s.
Kufs s.
lacrimo-auriculo-dento-digital s.
Lambert-Eaton myasthenic s.
Langer-Giedion trichorhinophalangeal s.
Larsen s.
lateral medullary s.
Laurence-Biedl s.
Laurence-Moon s.
Laurence-Moon-Bardet-Biedl s.
Laurence-Moon-Biedl s.
Lawford s.
Leber plus s.
lens-induced UGH s.
Lenz s.
LEOPARD s.
lid imbrication s.
Li-Fraumeni s.
Löfgren s.
LOGIC s.
Lowe oculocerebrorenal s.
Lowe-Terrey-MacLachlan s.
Lyle s.
macular ocular histoplasmosis s.
Magendie-Hertwig s.
MAR s.
Marcus Gunn jaw-winking s.
Marfan s.
Marinesco-Sjögren s.
Marinesco-Sjögren-Garland s.
Marshall s.
masquerade s.
McCune-Albright s.
Meige s.
melanoma-associated retinopathy s.
Melkersson s.
Melkersson-Rosenthal s.
Meretoja s.
microtropic s.
Mietens s.
Mikulicz-Radecki s.
Mikulicz-Sjögren s.
milk-alkali s.
Millard-Gubler s.
Miller s.

Miller-Fisher s.
Milles s.
Möbius s.
Monakow s.
monofixation s.
morning glory s.
Morquio s.
Morquio-Brailsford s.
Mount-Reback s.
mucocutaneous lymph node s.
multifocal choroidopathy s.
multiple evanescent white-dot s.
 (MEWDS)
multiple lentigines s.
myasthenia s.
myasthenia-like s.
Naegeli s.
Nager s.
Nance-Horan s.
neurodegenerative s.
neuroleptic malignant s.
Nieden s.
nodulus s.
Nonne s.
Noonan s.
Nothnagel s.
nystagmus blockage s. (NBS)
ocular histoplasmosis s. (OHS)
ocular ischemic s. (OIS)
ocular motor s.
ocular-mucous membrane s.
ocular pseudoexfoliation s.
oculoauditory s.
oculobuccogenital s.
oculocerebral s.
oculocerebrorenal s.
oculocutaneous s.
oculoglandular s.
oculopalatal myoclonus s.
oculopharyngeal s.
oculorenal s.
oculorespiratory s.
OMM s.
one-and-a-half s.
optic chiasmal s.
opticocerebral s.
opticopyramidal s.
optic tract s.
orbital s.
orbital apex s.
orbital infarction s.
organoid nevus s.
osteoporosis-pseudoglioma s.

Ota nevus s.
outer retinal necrosis s.
4p- s.
9p- s.
Pallister-Hall s.
Pancoast superior sulcus s.
paraflocculus s.
paraneoplastic s.
parasellar s.
Parinaud oculoglandular s.
Parinaud-plus s.
Paterson-Brown-Kelly s.
PEHO s.
periaqueductal s.
periocular s.
Petzetakis-Takos s.
Pierre Robin s.
pigmentary dispersion s.
pigment dispersion s. (PDS)
plateau iris s.
plus-minus s.
Posner-Schlossman s.
post enucleation socket s.
posterior inferior cerebellar
 artery s.
postganglionic Horner s.
Potter s.
prechiasmal optic nerve
 compression s.
preganglionic Horner s.
presumed ocular histoplasmosis s.
 (POHS)
pretectal s.
progressive outer retinal necrosis s.
Proteus s.
pseudoexfoliation s.
pseudo-Foster Kennedy s.
pseudopresumed ocular
 histoplasmosis s.
13q- s.
Raeder paratrigeminal s.
rainbow s.
Raymond s.
Raymond-Cestan s.
recurrent corneal erosion s.
red-eyed shunt s.
Reese s.
Refsum s.
Reiter s.
renal coloboma s.
restrictive s.
retinal necrosis s.
retraction s.

S

NOTES

syndrome *(continued)*

rheumatoid hyperviscosity s.
Richner-Hanhart s.
Riddoch s.
Rieger s.
Riley-Day s.
Riley-Smith s.
Ring D chromosome s.
Roaf s.
Robin s.
Robinow s.
Rollet s.
Romberg s.
Roth-Bielschowsky s.
Rothmund s.
Rothmund-Thomson s.
Roth spot s.
Rubinstein-Taybi s.
Russell s.
Rutherford s.
Sanchez Salorio s.
sands of Sahara s.
Scheie s.
Schirmer s.
Schmid-Fraccaro s.
Schwartz s.
Schwartz-Jampel s.
scotopic sensitivity s.
Seckel s.
Senior-Loken s.
septooptic dysplasia s.
shaken baby s. (SBS)
Shea s.
sheath s.
Shprintzen s.
Shy-Drager s.
sicca s.
Siegrist-Hutchinson s.
silent sinus s.
Sipple s.
Sipple-Gorlin s.
Sjögren s.
Sjögren-Larsson s.
slow-channel s.
Sly s.
Smith-Lemli-Opitz s.
Smith-Magenis s.
Smith-Riley s.
Sorsby s.
Sotos s.
Spanlang-Tappeiner s.
sphenocavernous s.
spherophakia-brachymorphia s.
Spielmeyer-Vogt s.
Stargardt s.
steal s.
Steele-Richardson-Olszewski s.
Stevens-Johnson s.
Stickler s.

Stilling-Türk-Duane s.
Strachan s.
Strachan-Scott s.
Sturge-Weber s.
Sturge-Weber-Dimitri s.
sunrise s.
sunset s.
superior oblique tendon sheath s.
superior orbital fissure s.
Susac s.
Swan s.
Sylvian aqueduct s.
tectal midbrain s.
tegmental s.
temporal crescent s.
tendon sheath s.
Terry s.
Terson s.
Thompson s.
tight lens s. (TLS)
tilted disc s. (TDS)
Tolosa-Hunt s.
tonic pupil s.
top-of-the-basilar s.
Touraine s.
toxic anterior segment s. (TASS)
toxic strep s.
traumatic Horner s.
Treacher Collins s.
Treacher Collins-Franceschetti s.
tubulointerstitial nephritis and
  uveitis s.
UGH s.
UGH+ s.
Uhthoff s.
Ullrich s.
Ullrich-Feichtiger s.
uncal s.
Usher s.
uveal effusion s.
uveitis-vitiligo-alopecia-poliosis s.
uveocutaneous s.
uveoencephalitic s.
uveomeningeal s.
uveomeningitis s.
V s.
velocardiofacial s.
vertical retraction s.
visceral larva migrans s.
visual deprivation s.
visual paraneoplastic s.
vitreomacular traction s.
vitreoretinal choroidopathy s.
vitreoretinal traction s.
vitreous wick s.
V-K-H s.
Vogt s.
Vogt-Koyanagi s.
Vogt-Koyanagi-Harada s.

Vogt-Spielmeyer s.
von Graefe s.
von Hippel-Lindau s.
von Recklinghausen s.
Waardenburg s.
Waardenburg-Klein s.
Wagner s.
Wagner-Stickler s.
Walker-Warburg s.
Wallenberg lateral medullary s.
Warburg s.
Weber s.
Weber-Gubler s.
Weill-Marchesani s.
Weill-Reys s.
Weill-Reys-Adie s.
Werner s.
Wernicke s.
Wernicke-Korsakoff s.
Weyers-Thier s.
white dot s.
Wildervanck s.
Wilson s.
windshield wiper s.
wipe-out s.
Wolf s.
Wolfram s.
Wyburn-Mason s.
xeroderma pigmentosa s.
Zellweger s.
syndrome-associated glaucoma
synechia, pl. **synechiae**
anterior s.
anular s.
circular s.
congenital anterior s.
iridocorneal s.
iris s.
peripheral anterior s. (PAS)
posterior s.
s. spatula
total s.
total anterior s.
total posterior s.
synechial closure
synechialysis
synechiotomy
synechotome
synechotomy
syneresis of vitreous
syneretic vitreous
Synergetics
S. Awh serrated pick

S. DDMS
S. directional laser probe
S. endo illuminator
synergistic divergence
syngeneic epithelium
synkinesia
congenital oculopalpebral s.
lid-triggered s.
synkinesis
external pterygoid levator s.
facial s.
oculocephalic s.
oculomotor nerve s.
pterygoid levator s.
synkinetic
s. movement
s. near reflex
s. near response
synophrys
synophthalmia, synophthalmos,
synophthalmus
synoptophore
synoptoscope
syntenic gene
synthesis
genome s.
synthetic
S. Optics random dot butterfly test
s. penicillin
Synvisc
syphilis
acquired s.
congenital s.
ocular s.
syphilitic
s. cataract
s. chorioretinitis
s. choroiditis
s. dacryocystitis
s. episcleritis
s. iritis
s. ocular disease
s. optic perineuritis
s. retinitis
s. retinopathy
s. rhinitis
s. scleritis
s. stromal keratitis
syphilitica
retinitis s.
syringe
Anel s.
Fink-Weinstein 2-way s.

NOTES

S

syringe *(continued)*
    Fragmatome flute s.
    Fuchs retinal detachment s.
    Fuchs 2-way s.
    Goldstein anterior chamber s.
    Goldstein lacrimal s.
    Hamilton s.
    lacrimal s.
    Luer-Lok s.
    probe s.
    retinal detachment s.
    tuberculin s.
    VisionBlue s.
    2-way s.
    Yale Luer-Lok s.
syringoma
    eyelid s.
    s. tumor
syrup
    Carbodec S.
    Cardec-S S.
    Rondec S.
Systane lubricant eye drops
system
    Accurus vitreoretinal surgical s.
    advanced visual instrument s.
    Aesculap-Meditec MEL60 s.
    afocal optical s.
    Alcon closure s. (ACS)
    Alcon EyeMap EH-290 corneal
      topography s.
    Alcon Infiniti s.
    Allegretto Wave excimer laser s.
    AMO Prestige advanced cataract
      extraction s.
    AMO Prestige Phaco S.
    AMO Sovereign compact
      WhiteStar s.
    anterior eye segment analysis s.
    anterior vented gas forced
      fusion s.
    AquaLase cataract removal s.
    ArF excimer laser s.
    Automated Quantification of After-
      Cataract automated analysis s.
    autonomic nervous s.
    Badal stimulus s.
    Beaver clear cornea incision s.
    BIOM noncontact panoramic
      viewing s.
    BIOM noncontact wide-angle
      viewing s.
    Bio-Optics Bambi cell analysis s.
    Bio-Optics Bambi image analysis s.
    Bio-Optics telescope s.
    bioptic amorphic lens s.
    Blairex s.
    bleb grading s.
    boxing s.

    British N s.
    Buzard Diamond Barraqueratome
      Microkeratome S.
    Cambridge Research S.'s (CRS)
    candela videoimaging s.
    Cavitron irrigation/aspiration s.
    Cavitron-Kelman
      irrigation/aspiration s.
    central nervous s. (CNS)
    2-channel Badal optical s.
    chirped-pulse amplification s.
    Ciba TearSaver punctual gauging s.
    ClearChart digital acuity s.
    closed-loop infrared video
      tracking s.
    closed-loop s.
    Coburn irrigation/aspiration s.
    Combiline s.
    complement s.
    Complete Ophthalmic Analysis S.
      (COAS)
    Computed Anatomy Corneal
      Modeling S.
    Concentrix dual aspiration pump s.
    Corneal Modeling S.
    corneal topography s. (CTS)
    CorneaSparing LTK s.
    Cryomedical Sciences AccuProbe
      450 s.
    CryoSeal FS S.
    C-Scan corneal topography s.
    CustomCornea wavefront
      measurement s.
    DeepLight glaucoma treatment s.
    delivery s.
    dioptric s.
    Dodick laser photolysis s.
    DORC fast freeze cryosurgical s.
    DORC Hexon Illumination S. 1266
      XII
    Duet s.
    Duovisc viscoelastic s.
    EAS-1000 anterior eye segment
      analysis s.
    EMI digital imaging s.
    EpiLift epikeratome s.
    ESA s.
    excimer laser s.
    extrapyramidal s.
    Eye Cap Ophthalmic Image
      Capture S.
    EyeMap EH-290 corneal
      topography s.
    EyeSys S. 2000
    EyeSys corneal analysis s.
    EyeSys 2000 corneal topographic
      mapping s.
    EyeSys corneal topography s.
    EyeSys surface topography s.

eye-tracking s.
Fast Grind lens s.
FlapMaker microkeratome s.
full-field s.
25-gauge chandelier illumination s.
gaussian optical s.
Grieshaber power injector s.
guided trephine s. (GTS)
Hamilton repeating pipette
  dispenser s.
Hartmann-Shack wavefront sensor s.
Hexon illumination s.
Hodapp-Parrish-Anderson visual
  field staging s.
HPA visual field staging s.
Humphrey Atlas Eclipse corneal
  topography s.
Humphrey Instruments vision
  analyzer overrefraction s.
Humphrey Mastervue corneal
  topography s.
hyaloid s.
Hybriwix probe s.
Hyperion LTK s.
IMAGEnet 2000 series digital
  imaging s.
immune s.
Integre 532 delivery s.
Inverter vitrectomy s.
Iris Medical OcuLight green
  laser s.
Iris Medical OcuLight infrared
  laser s.
Iris OcuLight SLx indirect
  ophthalmoscope delivery s.
iris registration s.
irrigation/aspiration s.
Jaeger grading s.
Kappa CTD finishing s.
Kappa SP lens finishing s.
Katena quick switch I/A s.
Kellan capsular sparing s.
keratograph corneal topography s.
keratome excimer laser s.
Keratron Scout topography s.
Koeller illumination s.
Kowa fluorescein s.
lacrimal s.
LADARTracker closed-loop
  tracking s.
LADARVision 4000 excimer
  laser s.

LADARWave CustomCornea
  wavefront s.
LaFaci surgical s.
Langerman diamond knife s.
LaserScan LSX excimer laser s.
Lea s.
Legacy cataract surgical s.
lens opacities classification s.
  (LOCS)
lens-plus-eye s.
Lens Plus Oxysept S.
low-vision enhancement s. (LVES)
Mackool s.
maculopathy staging s.
Malis bipolar coagulating/cutting s.
Massachusetts XII vitrectomy s.
  (MVS)
Mastel compass-guided arcuate
  keratotomy s.
Materials Testing S.
maxwellian view optical s.
McIntyre coaxial
  irrigating/aspirating s.
McIntyre I/A s.
McIntyre III nucleus removal s.
McIntyre irrigation/aspiration s.
Medi-Duct ocular fluid
  management s.
micropigmentation s.
MicroProbe integrated laser and
  endoscope s.
MicroShape keratome s.
Microvit probe s.
midget s.
Millennium CX, LX
  microsurgical s.
Millennium transconjunctival
  standard vitrectomy 25 s.
Millennium TVS25 S.
Milli-Q water purification s.
MiraSept s.
M.I.S. multi-port illumination s.
MK-2000 keratome s.
Mojave cataract extraction s.
Monarch II intraocular lens
  delivery s.
Monarch II IOL delivery s.
Moorfields bleb grading s.
Mport lens insertion s.
M-TEC 2000 surgical s.
nasolacrimal drainage s.
Nd:YAG Photon LaserPhaco s.
Nelson grading s.

NOTES

system *(continued)*

NeoSoniX s.
Niamtu video imaging s.
Nidek combo laser s.
Nidek EC-5000 refractive laser s.
Nidek MK-2000 keratome s.
nomogram s.
ocular motor s.
Oculex drug delivery s.
oculomotor s.
Oculus BIOM noncontact lens s.
Odyssey phacoemulsification s.
OIS image digitizing s.
OIS WinStation 5000 Ophthalmic
  Imaging S.
Olson calibrated cornea trephine s.
OPD-Scan diagnostic s.
optical s.
Opti-Pure S.
optokinetic s.
Orbscan II corneal diagnostic s.
Orbscan II corneal topography s.
Orbscan II multidimensional
  diagnostic s.
Orbscan topography analysis s.
osseous s.
parasympathetic nerve s.
parasympathetic nervous s.
PAR CTS corneal topography s.
parvocellular binocular vision s.
Passport disposable injection s.
PE-400 ERG/VEP s.
PerfectCapsule s.
peripapillary choroidal arterial s.
phacoemulsification s.
Phacojack Phaco S.
Photon cataract removal s.
Photon Ocular Surgery S.
Phototome S. 2700
pial s.
Placido-disc videokeratoscopy s.
Planoscan treatment s.
postcanalicular s.
PreClean soak s.
Price corneal transplant s.
printers' point s.
pump-leak s.
pyramidal s.
QuickRinse automated instrument
  rinse s.
Quickswitch irrigation/aspiration
  ophthalmic s.
Reese-Ellsworth classification s.
Refractec ViewPoint CK S.
Reinverting Operating Lens S.
  (ROLS)
renin-angiotensin s.
RetinaLyze S.
Rhein blade cleaning s.

Rodenstock s.
Scheimpflug videophotography s.
SDI-BIOM wide angle viewing s.
Selecta Duet combination laser s.
Selecta Duet glaucoma laser s.
Selecta Duo ophthalmic laser s.
Selecta 7000 glaucoma laser s.
Selecta II glaucoma laser s.
Selecta Trio glaucoma laser s.
sensory s.
Simcoe irrigation/aspiration s.
single-incision s.
Sloan M s.
SmallPort phaco s.
SofPort Easy-Load lens delivery s.
SofTec Delivery S.
SonicWAVE phacoemulsification s.
Sonomed A/B-Scan s.
Sonomed A-Scan s.
Sonomed B-1500 s.
Spectrum Lens Analysis S.
specular reflection video-
  recording s.
STAR S4 ActiveTrak 3-D eye
  tracking s.
STAR S3 ActiveTrak excimer
  laser s.
STAR S4 excimer laser s.
STAR S2 SmoothScan excimer
  laser s.
Steritome microkeratome s.
Storz Millennium microsurgical s.
Sunrise LTK s.
SureFold s.
Surg-E-Trol I/A S.
sustained-release s.
sympathetic nervous s.
T s.
Tango SLT/YAG combination
  laser s.
tear drainage s.
tear duct s.
TMS corneal topography s.
Tomey topographic modeling s.
Tomey topography s.
Topcon CM-1000 corneal
  mapping s.
Topcon IMAGEnet digital
  imaging s.
Topographic Modeling S. (TMS)
Topographic Modeling S.-1 (TMS-
  1)
Topographic Modeling S.-2 (TMS-
  2)
Topographic Scanning S. (TopSS)
TopSS/AngioScan s.
TopSS topographic scanning s.
T-PRK laser s.
trocar-cannula s.

Ultrasound Biomicroscope S.
Unfolder Sapphire implantation s.
UniPulse 1040 Surgical CO_2
  laser s.
United Sonics J shock phaco
  fragmentor s.
Venturi-Flo valve s.
VERIS III s.
vertebrobasilar s.
vestibular s.
ViewPoint CK s.
Vision Analyzer/Overrefraction S.
Vision Master excimer laser s.
Visitec surgical vitrectomy s.
visual-evoked response imaging s.
  (VERIS)
visual sensory s.
Visulab S.
Visx Star 3 excimer laser s.
Visx Star II stromal
  photoablation s.
Visx Star S2 excimer laser s.
Visx 20/20 version 4.01 vision
  keycard s.
Visx WaveScan wavefront s.
vortex s.
Wallach Ophthalmic Cryosurgery S.
water-based tinting s.
WaveFront S.
Wave phacoemulsion s.
WaveScan WaveFront S.
Wheeler cyclodialysis s.
WhiteStar power modulation s.

wide-angle viewing s.
Wilmer Cataract Photo-grading S.
Wisconsin age-related maculopathy
  grading s.
xenon illumination s.
YC 1400 Ophthalmic YAG
  laser s.
Zaldivar limbal-relaxing incision s.
Zeiss DAS-1 hydrophobic s.
Zeiss fiberoptic illumination s.
zoom s.
Zyoptix excimer laser s.

systemic
  s. administration
  s. amyloidosis
  s. arterial hypertension
  s. autoimmune disease
  s. bacterial endophthalmitis
  s. corticosteroid
  s. corticosteroid therapy
  s. drug
  s. glucocorticoid
  s. hyperosmolar agent
  s. immunomodulatory therapy
  s. lupus erythematosus
    choroidopathy
  s. marker of inflammation
  s. medication
  s. myopathy
  s. myositis
  s. pathology
  s. sclerosis

NOTES

T

tension
    T lens
    T sign
    T system
T+
    increased tension
TA
    temporal arteritis
tabes dorsalis
tabetic optic atrophy
table
    Reuss color t.
    Stilling color t.
    600XLE mobile surgery t.
table-mounted autorefractor
tablet
    Carbiset T.
    Carbiset-TR T.
    Carbodec TR T.
    Ocuvite Lutein t.
    PBZ t.
    PBZ-SR t.
Tac-40
tachistesthesia
tachistoscope
tack
    retinal t.
taco test
tacrolimus
tactile tension
tadpole pupil
tadpole-shaped pupil
Taenia solium
tag
    vitreoretinal t.
tagged image file format (TIFF)
Taillefer valve
Takahashi iris retractor forceps
Takata laser
Takayasu
    idiopathic arteritis of T.
talantropia
Talbot
    T. law
    T. unit
talc
TALK
    total anterior lamellar keratoplasty
talking word processor
tamoxifen retinopathy
tamponade
    gas t.
    intraocular t.

intraocular silicone oil t.
    long-acting gas t.
    silicone oil t.
    Silikon 1000 retinal t.
tandem scanning confocal microscope
tangent
    t. perimetry
    t. scope
    t. screen
    t. screen testing
tangential
    t. illumination
    t. incision
Tangier disease
Tango SLT/YAG combination laser system
Tanne
    T. corneal cutting block
    T. corneal punch
    T. guillotine-style punch
Tano
    T. diamond dusted needle
    T. double-mirror peripheral vitrectomy lens
    T. eraser
    T. membrane scraper
    T. micro serrated forceps
    T. ring
Tan spatula
tantalum
    t. clip
    t. mesh
    t. mesh implant
    t. "O" ring
TAO
    thyroid-associated ophthalmopathy
TAP
    tension by applanation
tap
    anterior chamber t.
    aqueous t.
    choroidal t.
    vitreous t.
tap-biopsy
tape
    Blenderm t.
    brow t.
    optokinetic t.
    Transpore eye t.
taper-cut needle
tapered-shaft punctum plug
taper-point needle
tapetal light reflex
tapetal-like reflex

T

tapetochoroidal
t. degeneration
t. dystrophy
tapetoretinal
t. degeneration
t. retinopathy
tapetoretinopathy
tapetum
t. lucidum
t. nigrum
t. oculi
taping
eyelid t.
tapioca iris melanoma
tapir
bouche de t.
target
accommodative t.
Air Force test grid t.
fixation t.
intracellular t.
monocular fixation t.
saccadic eccentric t.
von Graefe t.
tarsadenitis
tarsal
t. angle
t. artery
t. asthenopia
t. canal
t. cartilage
t. conjunctiva
t. cyst
t. ectropion
t. gland
t. laceration
t. membrane
t. muscle
t. plate
t. portion of eyelid
t. sandwich technique
t. strip procedure
t. strip tarsorrhaphy
tarsales
glandulae t.
tarsalis
epicanthus t.
tarsectomy
Blaskovics t.
Kuhnt t.
tarsi (*pl. of* tarsus)
tarsitis
tuberculous t.
tarsocheiloplasty
tarsochiloplasty
tarsoconjunctival
t. composite graft
t. flap

t. gland
t. pedicle
tarsoligamentous sling
tarsomalacia
tarsoorbital
tarsophyma
tarsoplasia
tarsoplasty
tarsorrhaphy
tarsal strip t.
tarsotomy
transverse t.
tarsus, pl. tarsi
inferior t.
t. orbital septum
t. osseus
superior t.
tinea tarsi
Taser penetrating ocular injury
task
reading t.
TASS
toxic anterior segment syndrome
tattoo
t. of cornea operation
t. pigment
tattooing
corneal t.
lamellar t.
medical t.
t. needle
Tauranol
Tavist
Tavist-1
Tay
T. cherry-red spot
T. choroiditis
T. disease
T. sign
Tay-Sachs disease
Tazarotene
Tazorac
TBUT
tear breakup test
TCB
transconjunctival blepharoplasty
TCD
transcranial Doppler
T-cell
T-c. activation
T-c. inhibitor
T-c. lymphoma
TCF
total conjunctival flap
TDME
tractional diabetic macular edema
TDS
tilted disc syndrome

TdT
  terminal deoxynucleotidyl transferase
tear
  T.'s Again eye drops
  T.'s Again gel drops
  T.'s Again liposome lid spray
  T.'s Again MC
  T.'s Again Night & Day gel
  T.'s Again preservative-free drops
  Akwa T.'s
  Androgen T.
  artificial t.'s (AT)
  Bion T.'s
  blended artificial t.'s
  bloody t.'s
  t. breakup
  t. breakup test (TBUT)
  breakup time of t.
  t. break-up time
  t. breakup time test
  circular t.
  t. clearance rate
  Clerz 2 artificial t.'s
  Comfort T.'s
  conjunctival t.
  crocodile t.'s
  t. drainage
  t. drainage system
  t. duct
  t. duct patency
  t. duct system
  t. evaporation
  t. exchange
  t. film
  t. film breakup time
  t. film debris
  t. film disorder
  t. film instability
  t. film lubrication
  t. film osmolarity
  t. film stability
  t. film test
  fishmouth t.
  flap t.
  t. flow
  t. fluorescein clearance
  t. function test
  t. gas
  giant retinal t. (GRT)
  t. gland
  horseshoe t.
  iatrogenic retinal t.
  iris sphincter t.

  Isopto T.'s
  Just T.'s
  t. lake
  t. layer
  Liquifilm T.'s
  low viscosity artificial t.'s
  t. of meniscus
  Milroy Artificial T.'s
  t. mixing
  mucin of t.
  t. mucus ferning
  Murine T.'s
  Muro T.'s
  Natural T.'s
  T.'s Naturale
  T.'s Naturale Forte
  T.'s Naturale Free
  T.'s Naturale Free lubricant eye
    drops
  T.'s Naturale Free Solution
  T.'s Naturale II lubricant eye
    drops
  T.'s Naturale II Polyquad eye
    drops
  T.'s Naturale II Solution
  T.'s Naturale lubricant eye drops
  T.'s Naturale PM lubricant eye
    drops
  T.'s Naturale PM lubricant eye
    ointment
  T.'s Naturale silicone punctum
    plug
  T.'s Natural Forte lubricant eye
    drops
  nonpreserved artificial t.
  operculated retinal t.
  t. osmolarity
  T.'s Plus
  T.'s Plus lubricant eye drops
  T.'s Plus Solution
  t. pool
  preservative-free artificial t.'s
  t. production
  t. protein
  t. protein deposit
  t. pump
  Puralube T.'s
  t. quality
  t. quantity
  reflux of t.
  T.'s Renewed
  T.'s Renewed lubricant ointment
  T.'s Renewed Solution

T

NOTES

tear *(continued)*
    t. of retina
    retinal horseshoe t.
    t. sac
    t. secretion
    t. secretion classification
    smooth-edged continuous t.
    sphincter t.
    t. stability analysis software
    t. stone
    t. supplementation
    t. test strip
    traction-related t.
    t. turnover
    Ultra T.'s
    Visine T.'s
    vitreous cells as indicator of
       retinal t.
    t. volume
teardrop pupil
Tear-Efrin
Tearfair
tear-film disturbance
TearGard Ophthalmic Solution
Teargen
    T. II lubricant eye drops
    T. Ophthalmic Solution
tear-induced retinal detachment
tearing
    t. child
    nonreflex t.
Tearisol Solution
TearSaver punctum plug
Tearscope
    Keeler T.
    T. Plus photographer
    T. Plus tear film kit
tear-secreting gland
technetium scan
technician
    certified paraoptometric t. (CPOT)
technique
    air-bubble dissection t.
    Armaly-Drance t.
    aseptic injection t.
    aspiration t.
    Atkinson t.
    automated tissue delamination t.
    bare scleral t.
    big bubble t.
    bimanual t.
    blue field stimulation t.
    Blumenthal nucleus delivery t.
    Boyden chamber t.
    Brockhurst t.
    Buratto t.
    capsule forceps t.
    chip-and-flip phacoemulsification t.
    CK conventional pressure t.

    closed-dissection t.
    conjunctival advancement t.
    contact lens fitting t.
    cost-ineffective current screening t.
    crack-and-flip phacoemulsification t.
    Crawford t.
    cross-cylinder t.
    divide-and-conquer t.
    double pentagon t.
    excimer laser surgical t.
    feeder-frond t.
    femtosecond laser t.
    finger iridectomy t.
    flicker fusion frequency t.
    flip-and-chop t.
    fluorometric t.
    frequency doubling t.
    frontalis sling t.
    Gibson t.
    glaucoma filtration t.
    Goldmann kinetic t.
    Goldmann static t.
    high-tension suturing t.
    Hughes modification of Burch t.
    hyperopic LASIK t.
    immunohistochemical t.
    injection t.
    iris fixation t.
    iris-suture t.
    Kaplan-Meier estimation t.
    karate chop t.
    Kaufman-Capella cryopreservation t.
    Knoll refraction t.
    Lambda phacoemulsification t.
    laser-scrape t.
    lens insertion t.
    letterbox t.
    Light Touch t.
    masquerade t.
    Maurice corneal depot t.
    McCannel suture t.
    McReynolds t.
    microlymphocytotoxicity t.
    microphacoemulsification t.
    Miyake t.
    Miyake-Apple posterior video t.
    mustache t.
    needle-and-syringe t.
    O'Brien akinesia t.
    open-sky t.
    ophthalmic vitreous surgical t.
    phacochop t.
    Phakonit nucleus division t.
    piezoelectric transducer t.
    preferential-looking t.
    push-plus refraction t.
    Quickert 3-suture t.
    radioimmunoassay t.
    reflection-based t.

rehabilitation t.
sayonara t.
Schepens t.
scleral search coil t.
Siepser sliding knot t.
single-loop t.
single-stitch aponeurotic tuck t.
Smirmaul t.
Smith-Indian t.
soft-shell t.
Southern blot t.
split-beam photographic t.
Staar Aquaflow t.
step-down t.
sterile t.
stop-and-chop phacoemulsification t.
suture lasso t.
suture rotation t.
tarsal sandwich t.
transillumination t.
transocular t.
transpupillary t.
transscleral suture fixation t.
tumbling t.
tunnel surgical t.
Tzanck t.
Van Lint modified t.
vertical chopping t.
von Graefe t.
zonular-friendly t.

Technolas
T. 217 excimer laser
T. 217 laser-based technology
T. 217z excimer laser

technologist
certified ophthalmic t. (COT)
certified ophthalmic medical t.
(COMT)

technology
frequency doubling t. (FDT)
imaging t.
in-lab lens casting t.
nerve fiber t.
objective noninvasive t.
power modulation t.
Technolas 217 laser-based t.
wavefront t.
WhiteStar power modulation t.

Technomed
T. C-Scan
T. C-Scan videokeratoscope

Tecnis
T. acrylic IOL

T. foldable intraocular lens
T. foldable IOL
T. Z9000 lens
tectal midbrain syndrome
tectonic
t. corneal graft
t. epikeratoplasty
t. keratoplasty
Teflon
T. block
T. implant
T. injection catheter
T. iris retractor
T. plate
T. plug
T. sheet
tegmental syndrome
teichopsia
Tek-Clear accommodating intraocular lens
Telachlor
telangiectasia
calcinosis cutis, Raynaud
phenomenon, esophageal motility
disorder, sclerodactyly, and t.
(CREST)
essential t.
foveal t.
generalized essential t. (GET)
hereditary hemorrhagic t.
idiopathic acquired retinal t.
macular t.
retinal t.
spider t.
telangiectasis
bilateral juxtafoveal t. (BJT)
idiopathic juxtafoveal retinal t.
idiopathic perifoveal t. (IPT)
retinal t.
telangiectatic
t. blood vessel
t. glioma
Teldrin
telebinocular
telecanthus
telehopsias
telemedical evaluation
telemedicine strategy
teleopsia
telephoto effect
telepresence environment
telescope
afocal t.

NOTES

T

527

telescope *(continued)*
    Eschenbach monocular t.
    Galilean t.
    Hopkins rod lens t.
    implantable miniaturized t. (IMT)
    monocular t.
    spectacle-mounted t.
telescopic
    t. lens
    t. spectacles
Telfa
    T. pad
    T. plastic film dressing
Teller
    T. acuity card
    T. visual acuity
Temba glaucoma study
TEMoo mode beam laser
template
temple
    cable t.
    curl t.
    hockey-end t.
    t. length
    library t.
    loafer t.
    paddle t.
    riding bow t.
    skull t.
    spatula t.
    t. of spectacles
    spring-hinge t.
    straight t.
    Venturi adjusted t.
temporal
    t. arteriole of retina
    t. arteritis (TA)
    t. artery
    t. artery biopsy
    t. artery pallor
    t. bone
    t. bulbar conjunctiva
    t. canthus
    t. catchment angle
    t. crescent
    t. crescent syndrome
    t. hemianopsia
    t. island of visual field
    t. lobe
    t. lobe field defect
    t. lobe unilateral cerebral
      hemisphere lesion
    t. loop
    t. macula
    medial superior t. (MST)
    middle t. (MT)
    t. modulation perimetry
    t. optic disc pallor
    t. peaking

    t. pit
    t. raphe
    t. self-sealing clear corneal incision
    t. vascular arcade
    t. venule of retina
    t. wedge
    t. zone
    t. zone of retina
temporalis muscle
temporary
    t. balloon buckle
    t. diabetes
    t. intracanalicular collagen implant
    t. keratoprosthesis (TKP)
    t. keratoprosthesis suturing
    t. prism
temporooccipital artery
temporoparietal lobe
tenacious
    t. distance fusion
    t. proximal fusion
tendency-oriented perimetry (TOP)
tendinous insertion
tendon
    t. advancement
    Brown t.
    canthal t.
    lateral canthal t.
    levator t.
    Lockwood t.
    medial canthal t.
    t. recession
    t. sheath syndrome
    superior oblique t.
    tenotomy of ocular t.
    t. tucker
    Zinn t.
tendo oculi
tendotomy *(var. of* tenotomy)
tenectomy
Tennant
    T. Anchorflex AC lens
    T. implant
    T. lens-inserting forceps
    T. titanium suturing forceps
    T. tying forceps
Tennant-Colibri corneal forceps
Tennant-Troutman superior rectus
   forceps
Tenner
    T. lacrimal cannula
    T. titanium suturing forceps
Tenon
    T. capsule
    T. fascia bulbi
    T. fibroblast
    T. flap
    T. membrane
    T. patch graft

T. sac
T. space
tenonectomy
tenonitis
tenonometer
tenontotomy
tenoplasty
cyanoacrylate tissue adhesive augmented t.
Tenormin
tenosynovitis
tenotome
tenotomist
tenotomize
tenotomy, tendotomy
Arroyo t.
Arruga t.
curb t.
free t.
graduated t.
t. hook
intrasheath t.
t. of ocular tendon
t. operation
Z marginal t.
tensile strength of vessel
Tensilon
T. implant
T. test
tension (T)
applanation t. (AT)
t. by applanation (TAP)
t. of eye
finger t.
hard-finger t.
increased t. (T+)
intraocular oxygen t.
normal t. (TN)
normal-finger t.
ocular t. (Tn)
t. oculus sinister (TOS)
soft-finger t.
surface t.
tactile t.
t. test
zonular t.
tensor insertion
tented-up retina
tenting
geometric t.
tentorial nerve
Tenzel
T. elevator

T. forceps
T. rotational cheek flap
Terak
T. Ophthalmic Ointment
T. with polymyxin B sulfate ointment
teratogenic association
teratoma
orbital t.
terfenadine
Terg-A-Zyme
terminal
t. bulb
t. deoxynucleotidyl transferase (TdT)
t. deoxynucleotidyl transferase-mediated dUTP-digoxigenin nick-end labeling (TUNEL)
terminaux
bouton t.
terminus
incision t.
Terra-Cortril Ophthalmic Suspension
Terramycin
polymyxin B and T.
T. w/polymyxin B Ophthalmic Ointment
terreus
Aspergillus t.
Terrien marginal degeneration
Terry
T. astigmatome
T. keratometer
T. silicone capsule polisher
T. syndrome
Terry-Schanzlin astigmatome
Terson
T. capsule forceps
T. extracapsular forceps
T. syndrome
tertiary
t. position
t. vitreous
tertius palpebra
tessellated fundus
Tessier
T. classification
T. clefting
test
active force generation t.
Adams desaturated D15 t.
afterimage t.
alternate cover t. (ACT)

T

NOTES

test *(continued)*

alternate cover-uncover t.
alternating light t.
Ames t.
Amsler t.
anaglyph t.
anomaloscope plate t. (APT)
Arabic eye t.
a-wave t.
Bagolini striated glasses t.
Bailey-Lovie near t.
Bárány caloric t.
basic secretion t.
Behçet skin puncture t.
Bence Jones t.
Benton Facial Recognition T.
Berens 3-character t.
Berens pinhole and dominance t.
Berkeley glare t.
Bielschowsky-Parks head-tilt 3-step t.
Bielschowsky 3-step head-tilt t.
binocular visual acuity t.
biochrome t.
biometry t.
biopter t.
blindness t.
Bonferroni t.
breakup time t.
brightness acuity t. (BAT)
Bruchner t.
butterfly t.
caloric irrigation t.
t. card
cardinal field t.
Catford visual acuity t.
3-character t.
child-friendly VDS t.
chi-squared test
cocaine t.
color bar Schirmer tear t.
color comparison t.
color vision t.
Color Vision Testing Made Easy t. (CVTMET)
complement fixation t.
t. condition
confrontation visual field t.
contour stereo t.
contrast sensitivity t. (CST)
corneal impression t. (CIT)
corneal staining t.
cotton thread tear t.
cover t.
cover-uncover t.
critical flicker fusion t.
cross cover t.
CRS Color Vision T.
cytogenetic t.

dark-room t.
DEM t.
denervation supersensitivity t.
developmental eye movement t.
D-15 Hue Desaturated Panel t.
direct chlamydial immunofluorescence t.
dissimilar image t.
dissimilar target t.
t. distance
Dix-Hallpike t.
4-dot t.
double Maddox rod t.
dry eye t. (DET)
duction t.
duochrome t.
Dupuy-Dutemps dacryocystorhinostomy dye t.
dye disappearance t. (DDT)
E t.
edrophonium chloride t.
Ehrmann t.
t. eye
Eyecuity wireless visual acuity t.
Farnsworth-Munsell 100-hue color vision t.
Farnsworth panel D15 t.
FastPac 24-2 t.
Fisher exact t.
fistula t.
flashlight t.
flicker fusion frequency t.
flicker perimetry t.
fluorescein angiogram t.
fluorescein clearance t. (FCT)
fluorescein dilution t.
fluorescein dye disappearance t.
fluorescein instillation t.
fluorescein strip t.
fluorescent antibody t.
fly t.
FM-100 hue t.
fog t.
forced duction t.
forced generation t.
forward traction t.
Foucault knife-edge t.
Fridenberg stigmatometric t.
Fridenberg stigometric card t.
Friedman t.
Frisby-Davis 2 distance stereoacuity t.
functional acuity contrast t. (FACT)
Getman-Henderson-Marcus visual manipulation t.
glare t.
glaucoma hemifield t. (GHT)
Goldmann visual field t.

Graefe t.
Gray oral reading t.
Grooved Pegboard t.
Haidinger brush t.
hair bulb incubation t.
hand-motion visual acuity t.
hand-movement visual acuity t.
haploscopic t.
Hardy-Rand-Ritter t.
Harrington-Flocks t.
head-tilt t.
Hering t.
Hering-Bielschowsky after-image t.
Herpchek herpes simplex virus t.
Hess screen t.
hiding Heidi facial expressions t.
higher visual function t.
Hirschberg t.
Holladay contrast acuity t.
Holmgren color t.
Holmgren wool skein t.
Hooper Visual Organization T.
  (HVOT)
HOTV visual acuity t.
housefly t.
HRR pseudoisochromatic t.
28-Hue de Roth t.
90-hue discrimination t.
100-hue t.
Humphrey 24-2 glaucoma
  hemifield t.
ice pack t.
illumination t.
interference visual acuity t.
intravenous thyrotropin-releasing
  hormone t.
Ishihara t.
Jaeger visual t.
Jenning t.
Jones I, II dye t.
Keystone multi-stereo t.
Keystone view stereopsis t.
King-Devick saccade t.
Kirby-Bauer disc sensitivity t.
Kodak Surecell Chlamydia t.
Kolmogorov-Smirnov t.
Krimsky prism t.
Kruskal-Wallis t.
Kveim t.
lacrimal irrigation t.
lactoferrin t.
Lactoplate t.
Lagrange t.

Lancaster red-green t.
Lancaster screen t.
Landolt C optotype t.
lantern t.
Lanthony desaturated D15 t.
t. letter
letter t.
Lighthouse distance visual acuity t.
light projection t.
light-stress t.
line t.
linear visual acuity t.
log rank t.
lupus erythematosus cell t.
macular computerized
  psychophysical t. (MCPT)
Maddox rod t.
Maddox wing t.
magnetic field-search coil t.
major amblyoscope t.
Mann-Whitney U t.
Mantoux t.
Marcus Gunn t.
Marlow t.
Mauthner t.
McNemar chi-squared t.
Mecholyl t.
Mentor B-VAT II BVS contour
  circles distance stereoacuity t.
Mentor B-VAT II BVS random
  dot E distance stereoacuity t.
microhemagglutination t.
MicroTrac direct specimen t.
Minnesota low-vision reading t.
mirror rocking t.
Mollon-Reffin minimal t.
monocular confrontation visual
  field t.
Mr. Color t.
mydriatic provocative t.
Nagel t.
near vision t.
neostigmine t.
neutral density filter t.
New York Lighthouse acuity t.
nudge t.
nystagmus t.
t. object
objective prism-neutralized cover t.
Octopus 201 perimeter t.
Ocugene glaucoma genetic t.
ocular motility t.
oculocephalic t.

T

NOTES

test *(continued)*
  ophthalmic t.
  Optec 3000 contrast sensitivity t.
  optic disc hemifield t.
  optokinetic t.
  ornithine tolerance t.
  Otis-Lennon School Ability T. (OLSAT)
  parallax t.
  Parks-Bielschowsky 3-step head-tilt t.
  Park 3-step t.
  passive forced duction t.
  P&C t.
  Pearson chi-square t.
  Pease-Allen Color t.
  Pepper Visual Skills for Reading t.
  perimeter corneal reflex t.
  peripheral detection t.
  photostress t.
  pilocarpine t.
  pinhole and dominance t.
  planned comparison t.
  Polaroid 3D Vectograph t.
  preschool Randot stereoacuity t.
  preschool visiting screening t.
  primary dye t.
  prism t.
  prism adaptation t. (PAT)
  prism and alternate cover t. (PACT)
  4 prism base-out t.
  prism and cover t.
  prism dissociation t.
  prism-neutralized cover t.
  prism shift t.
  prism vergence t.
  Prostigmin t.
  provocative t.
  pseudoisochromatic color t.
  pupil cycle induction t.
  Rabinowitz-McDonnell t.
  random dot E stereoacuity t.
  Randot Stereo Smile t.
  rapid plasma reagin t.
  Raven progressive matrices t.
  Rayleigh color matching t.
  reading speed t.
  red-filter t.
  red glare t.
  red glass t.
  rest t.
  rotational t.
  Roth 28-hue t.
  Sabin-Feldman dye t.
  scanning laser glaucoma t.
  Schirmer I, II t.
  Schirmer tear quality t.
  secondary dye t.

  Seidel t.
  separate image t.
  shadow t.
  Shapiro-Wilk t.
  Sheridan-Gardiner isolated letter-matching t.
  Shirmer basal secretion t.
  Simpson t.
  simultaneous prism cover t. (SPC)
  single cover t.
  skein t.
  SKILL Card T.
  slit-beam t.
  Smith-Kettlewell Institute low luminance card t.
  Snellen t.
  SPP2 t.
  standardized visual scale t. (SVST)
  Standard Pseudoisochromatic Plates Part 2 t.
  Statpac t.
  3-step t.
  stereopsis t.
  stereo reindeer t.
  Stereo Smile II stereoacuity t.
  Stilling color t.
  subjective prism-neutralized cover t.
  subjective refraction t.
  swinging flashlight t.
  swinging light t.
  t. symbol
  Synthetic Optics random dot butterfly t.
  taco t.
  tear breakup t. (TBUT)
  tear breakup time t.
  tear film t.
  tear function t.
  Tensilon t.
  tension t.
  thyroid function t. (TFT)
  thyrotropin-releasing hormone t.
  Titmus stereo t.
  Titmus stereoacuity t.
  Titmus vision t.
  TNO stereo t.
  traction t.
  transillumination t.
  TRH t.
  triiodothyronine suppression t.
  tumbling E t.
  t. type
  tyrosinase t.
  University of Waterloo Colored Dot T. (UWCDot)
  useful field of view t.
  VDS t.
  vertical prism t.
  Vistech 6500 contrast t.

visual manipulation t.
Visuscope motor t.
Visuscope sensory t.
Washington University road t.
  (WURT)
water-drinking t.
water provocative t.
Watzke-Allen t.
W4D t.
Welland t.
Werner t.
Wernicke t.
Westcott t.
Wilbrand prism t.
Wilcoxon matched pairs t.
Wilcoxon signed rank t.
Wirt stereo t.
Wirt stereopsis t.
Wirt vision t.
Worth 4-dot near flashlight t.
Zone-Quick tear t.

tester

APT-5 Color Vision T.
Baylor-Video Acuity T. (BVAT)
Mentor B-VAT II video acuity t.
Miller-Nadler glare t.
Phoroptor vision t.
Prio video display terminal
  vision t.
Topcon vision t.
Vistech Multivision Contrast T.
  8000

testing

Allen figure acuity t.
antenatal t.
Bruchner reflex t.
confrontation visual field t.
contrast sensitivity t.
cranial nerve t.
dark-room t.
diagnostic t.
4-diopter base-out prism t.
double-quadrant t.
extraocular muscle t.
filter glasses for color t.
forced duction t.
hypothesis t.
kinetic visual field t.
lacrimal t.
levator function t.
macular photostress t.
near acuity t.
near vision t.

pathergy t.
provocative t.
pursuit t.
quick estimation by sequential t.
  (QUEST)
rapid antibiotic susceptibility t.
  (RAST)
single-quadrant t.
subjective t.
tangent screen t.
visual acuity t.
visual field t.
zippy estimating by sequential t.
Zone-Quick tear volume t.

test-retest

t.-r. analysis
t.-r. correlation
t.-r. reliability
t.-r. variability

tetani

Clostridium t.

tetanus prophylaxis
tetany

t. cataract
zonular t.

tetartanopia
tetartanopsia
Tetcaine
tetraborate

potassium t.

tetracaine hydrochloride
Tetracon
tetracycline
tetraethylammonium chloride
tetrafilcon A
tetrahydrozoline hydrochloride
tetranopsia
Tetrasine Extra Ophthalmic
tetrasodium

diquafosol t.

tetrastichiasis
tetroxide

osmium t.

Tevdek suture
texaphyrin

lutetium t. (lu-tex)

text blindness
TFT

thyroid function test

TG-140 needle
thalamolenticular
thalamopeduncular

NOTES

thalamus
optic t.
Thalomid
Thal procedure
thaw-freeze
Thayer-Martin plate
THC:YAG laser
Theimich lip sign
Thelazia callipaeda
thelaziasis
Theobald probe
theobromae
Lasiodiplodia t.
Theodore keratoconjunctivitis
theory
accommodative arching t.
Alhazen t.
color t.
Helmholtz t.
Hering t.
Ladd-Franklin t.
migration t.
molecular dissociation t.
opponent colors t.
retinex t.
Scheiner t.
Schön t.
trichromatic color t.
Unna abtropfung t.
Wollaston t.
Young-Helmholtz color vision t.
therapeutic
t. contact lens
t. dacryocystorhinostomy
t. decision-making
t. equivalence
t. iridectomy
t. neuroprotective antiglaucoma drug
therapy
adjuvant t.
alkylating agent t.
antiallergy t.
antifungal t.
antiglaucoma t.
antiretroviral t.
antiviral t.
argon laser t.
cidofovir t.
cobalt t.
combination t.
corticosteroid t.
cytokine t.
developmental vision t.
3-dimensional conformal fractionated
radiation t.
diode laser t.
disease-modifying t.
dry eye t.
external beam radiation t.

fluorescein-potentiated argon laser t.
(FPAL)
ganciclovir t.
gene t.
highly active antiretroviral t.
(HAART)
hydroxychloroquine t.
hyperbaric oxygen t.
immunoadsorption t.
immunomodulatory t.
laser t.
localized carboplatin t.
long-term suppressive t.
maximum tolerated medical t.
Mini-Drops eye t.
miotic t.
mydriatic-cycloplegic t.
occlusion t.
optimal medical t. (OMT)
palliative t.
pencil push-up t.
photocoagulation t.
photodynamic t. (PDT)
PhotoPoint laser t.
radiation t.
red-filter t.
sclerosing t.
silicone punctal plug t.
stem cell t.
stereotactic radiation t. (SRT)
steroid t.
systemic corticosteroid t.
systemic immunomodulatory t.
thrombolytic t.
topical anticataract t.
topical ocular hypotensive t.
topical secretogogue t.
topography-guided t.
Tranquileyes eye hydrating t.
transcorneal oxygen t.
vision rehabilitation t.
vision restoration t.
TheraTears
T. liquid gel
T. lubricant eye drops
thermal
t. adhesion
t. burn
t. cataract
t. cautery
t. effect
t. injury
t. keratoplasty (TKP)
t. punctal occlusion
t. sclerectomy
t. sclerostomy
thermally altered collagen
thermocautery

thermocycler
> Touchdown t.

thermokeratoplasty
> laser t. (LTK)

thermoluminescence detector (TLD)

thermosclerectomy

thermosclerostomy

thermosclerotomy

thermotherapy
> adjuvant microwave t.
> microwave plaque t.
> transpupillary t. (TT, TTT)

The Silicone Study

thick
> t. cornea
> t. lens

thickening
> sclerochoroidal t.

thickness
> central corneal t. (CCT)
> t. of contact lens
> contact lens t.
> corneal t.
> flap t.
> lipid layer t.
> mean foveal t.
> t. measurement
> retinal t.
> standard t.
> stromal t.

Thiel-Behnke corneal dystrophy

thimerosal

thin
> t. bleb
> t. cornea
> t. lens

thinning
> choroidal t.
> corneal t.
> peripheral corneal t.
> retinal t.
> stromal t.

ThinProfile eyelid implant

thin-rim scotoma

thioglycate broth

thiomalate
> gold sodium t.

thiopental sodium

thioridazine
> t. hydrochloride
> t. retinal toxicity
> t. retinopathy

thiosulfate
> sodium t.

third
> t. cranial nerve
> t. cranial nerve palsy
> t. framework region (FR3)
> t. order neuron

third-grade fusion

Thomas
> T. brush
> T. cryoextractor
> T. cryoprobe
> T. cryoptor
> T. fixation forceps
> T. irrigating-aspirating cannula
> T. operation
> T. retractor
> T. scissors
> T. subretinal instrument set II

Thompson syndrome

Thorazine

Thornton
> T. arcuate blade
> T. double corneal ruler
> T. fixating ring
> T. fixation forceps
> T. guide for optical zone size
> T. limbal fixation ring
> T. limbal incision ruler
> T. malleable spatula
> T. needle
> T. optical center marker
> Thorton optic zone marker
> T. triple micrometer knife
> T. tri-square blade

Thornton-Fine ring

Thorpe
> T. caliper
> T. conjunctival forceps
> T. corneal forceps
> T. foreign body forceps
> T. 4-mirror vitreous fundus laser lens
> T. scissors
> T. slit lamp
> T. surgical gonioscope

Thorpe-Westcott scissors

Thrasher lens implant forceps

thread
> mucous t.

threat reflex

threshold
> absolute t.

T

NOTES

threshold *(continued)*
    achromatic t.
    brightness difference t.
    chromatic contrast t.
    color-contrast t.
    t. disease
    displacement t.
    t. effect
    final t.
    light differential t.
    t. limit value (TLV)
    minimum light t.
    prebleached dark-adapted t.
    quantitative static t.
    sensitivity t.
    t. stage III of retinopathy of prematurity (TS III ROP)
    tolerance t.
    visual t.
    t. of visual sensation
thromboangiitis obliterans
thromboembolic episode
thrombolytic therapy
thrombosed artery
thrombosis
    carotid artery t.
    cavernous sinus t.
    orbital vein t.
    t. in retina
    retinal t.
    septic t.
thromboxane receptor antagonist
thrombus, pl. **thrombi**
    fibrin t.
through-the-lid contact ultrasound
thrush
    lid t.
thumb occluder
Thurmond
    T. nucleus-irrigating cannula
    T. pachymetry marker
Thygeson
    T. chronic follicular conjunctivitis
    T. disease
    punctate keratitis of T.
    superficial punctate keratitis of T. (SPKT)
    T. superficial punctate keratitis
    T. superficial punctate keratopathy
thymic hypoplasia
thymidine analog
thymoxamine hydrochloride
Thymoxid
thyroid
    t. exophthalmos
    t. eye disease
    t. function test (TFT)
    t. gland disorder
    t. lid retraction

    t. ophthalmopathy
    t. orbitopathy
    t. stare
thyroid-associated ophthalmopathy (TAO)
thyroidectomy
    subtotal t.
thyroiditis
    Hashimoto t.
    Riedel t.
thyroid-related orbitopathy
thyroid-releasing hormone (TRH)
thyrotoxic
    t. exophthalmos
    t. myopathy
thyrotoxicosis ophthalmoplegia
thyrotropic exophthalmos
thyrotropin-releasing
    t.-r. hormone
    t.-r. hormone test
thyroxine, thyroxin
TIA
    transient ischemic attack
Tiapridex
tic
    t. douloureux
    local t.
    motor t.
ticarcillin
ticrynafen ointment
TIFF
    tagged image file format
tight
    t. contact lens
    t. lens syndrome (TLS)
    t. orbit
TIGR
    trabecular meshwork-inducible glucocorticoid response
        TIGR gene
tigré
    fundus t.
tigroid
    t. background
    t. fundus
    t. retina
Tilavist
Tillaux
    extraocular muscles of T.
    spiral of T.
    T. spiral
Tillyer bifocal lens
tilt
    compensatory head t.
    optical t.
    pantoscopic t.
    t. of sella
    visual t.

tilted
- t. disc
- t. disc syndrome (TDS)
- t. vision

tilting
- IOL t.
- t. lens
- t. lens atresia

time
- breakup t. (BUT)
- b-wave implicit t.
- death-to-preservation t.
- edge-light pupil cycle t.
- fading t.
- implicit t.
- lacrimal transit t.
- not invasive break-up t.
- phaco t.
- photostress recovery t. (PRT)
- Russell viper venom t.
- sensation t.
- tear break-up t.
- tear film breakup t.
- t. trade-off utility
- tumor doubling t.
- variable rise t.

Timentin
Timex TMX optical eyewear
timolol
- t. gellan
- t. hemihydrate
- t. maleate
- t. maleate ophthalmic gel-forming solution
- t. and pilocarpine

Timoptic
- T. Ocudose
- T. Ophthalmic

Timoptic-XE Ophthalmic
TIMP3 gene
Timpilo
T-incision
tinea tarsi
tin ethyl etiopurpurin (SnET2)
tinnitus
- gaze-evoked t.

tint
- eyelash t.

tinted
- t. contact lens
- t. spectacles
- t. vision

tinting of spectacle lens

tip
- Binkhorst t.
- central dissecting t.
- t. cleaner caddie
- diathermy t.
- disposable Keratoplast t.
- dissecting t.
- endolaser probe t.
- flared ABS t.
- Girard irrigating t.
- guillotine cutting t.
- Keeler lancet t.
- Keeler micro round t.
- Keeler micro spear t.
- Keeler puncture t.
- Keeler razor t.
- Keeler triple facet t.
- Kelman t.
- Kelman-Mackool flare t.
- Keratoplast t.
- Luer syringe t.
- Microtip phaco t.
- Mitchell viscoelastic removal I/A t.
- nonaspirating ultrasonic phaco chopper t.
- olive t.
- phaco t.
- pointed cystotome t.
- rotary cutting t.
- silicone-covered aspiration t.
- Simcoe interchangeable t.
- sleeveless phaco t.
- solid-core needle with hollow t.
- Welsh flat olive-t.

tire
- 276 t.
- implant t.
- t. implant
- silicone t.
- Watzke t.

tissue
- t. adhesive
- adipose t.
- t. bed
- collagen t.
- conjunctiva-associated lymphoid t.
- conjunctival mucosa-associated lymphoid t.
- connective t.
- corneal stroma t.
- cutaneous t.
- donor t.
- ectopic t.

NOTES

tissue *(continued)*
    epibulbar t.
    epiciliary proliferative t.
    episcleral t.
    eye t.
    t. forceps
    frozen t.
    human allograft t.
    hypergranulation t.
    hyperreflective t.
    iris t.
    limbal t.
    McCarey-Kaufman preserved
      donor t.
    mesoblastic t.
    t. microarray
    mucosa-associated lymphoid t.
      (MALT)
    nonfixed t.
    nuclear t.
    orbital adipose t.
    pericanalicular connective t.
    t. plasminogen
    t. plasminogen activator (TPA,
      tPA)
    posterior corneal t.
    pterygial t.
    scleral t.
    sustentacular t.
    transplantation of posterior
      corneal t.
    uveal t.
tissue-engineered cornea
tissue-specific pericyte
titanium
    t. miniplate
    t. needle
    t. suturing forceps
Titmus
    T. stereoacuity test
    T. stereo fly
    T. stereo test
    T. vision test
TKP
    temporary keratoprosthesis
    thermal keratoplasty
TLD
    thermoluminescence detector
TLS
    tight lens syndrome
TLV
    threshold limit value
TM
    trabecular meshwork
TMS
    Topographic Modeling System
      TMS corneal topography system

TMS-1
    Topographic Modeling System-1
      TMS-1 videokeratoscope
TMS-2
    Topographic Modeling System-2
      TMS-2 computer-assisted
        videokeratoscope
      TMS-2 computerized corneal
        topographer
TN
    normal tension
Tn
    ocular tension
TNO stereo test
tobacco-alcohol amblyopia
tobacco amblyopia
TobraDex
    T. ophthalmic
    T. ophthalmic ointment
    T. ophthalmic suspension
Tobralcon
tobramycin and dexamethasone
Tobrasol
Tobrex Ophthalmic
Todd
    T. cautery
    T. electrocautery
    T. gouge
    T. paralysis
tolazoline
Tolentino
    T. prism lens
    T. ring
    T. vitrectomy lens
    T. vitrectomy lens set
    T. vitreous cutter
tolerability
    ocular t.
tolerance threshold
Tolman micrometer
Tolosa-Hunt syndrome
Tomas
    T. iris hook
    T. suture hook
tomato-ketchup fundus
tome
    Laschal precision suture t.
    precision suture t.
Tomey
    T. autorefractor
    T. autotopographer
    T. ConfoScan confocal microscope
    T. refractive workstation
    T. retinal function analyzer
    T. TMS-1 photokeratoscope
    T. topographic modeling system
    T. topography system
tomodensitometry

tomograph
  Heidelberg retina t. (HRT)
  Heidelberg retina t. II (HRT-II)
tomography
  axial t.
  carbonic anhydrase t.
  complex motion t.
  computed t. (CT)
  confocal scanning laser t.
  CSL t.
  3D i-Scan ultrasound t.
  Heidelberg retinal t.
  helical computed t.
  Humphrey model 2000 optical
    coherence t.
  ocular coherence t.
  optical coherence t. (OCT)
  optical coherence t.-3 (OCT3)
  optic coherence t.
  orbital t.
  retinal detachment using optical
    coherence t.
  scanning laser t. (SLT)
Tomycine
TON
  traumatic optic neuropathy
tonic
  t. accommodation
  t. convergence
  t. downward deviation
  t. lid
  t. pupil
  t. pupil syndrome
  t. upward deviation
  t. vergence
tonicity agent
tonofilm
  Schiötz t.
tonogram
tonograph
tonography
Tonomat applanation tonometer
tonometer
  air-puff contact t.
  air-puff noncontact t.
  Alcon t.
  Allen-Schiötz t.
  AO Reichert Instruments
    applanation t.
  applanation t.
  Barraquer applanation t.
  Barraquer operating room t.
  Berens t.

  biprism applanation t.
  Carl Zeiss t.
  Challenger digital applanation t.
  Coburn t.
  Digilab t.
  Draeger t.
  Durham t.
  electronic t.
  Gartner t.
  Goldmann t.
  Goldmann applanation t. (GAT)
  Harrington t.
  impression t.
  indentation t.
  Intermedics intraocular t.
  Keeler Pulsair t.
  Lombart t.
  low-weight t.
  Mackay-Marg electronic t.
  Maklakoff t.
  Mueller electronic t.
  noncontact t. (NCT)
  OBF t.
  Pach-Pen XL t.
  Perkins applanation t.
  pneumatic t.
  portable PT100 noncontact t.
  pressure phosphene t.
  ProTon portable t.
  Pulsair t.
  Reichert noncontact t.
  Rosner t.
  Schiötz t.
  Sklar-Schiötz t.
  Storz t.
  Tonomat applanation t.
  Tono-Pen XL t.
tonometry
  applanation t. (AT)
  automatic t.
  digital t.
  indentation t.
  Schiötz t.
Tono-Pen
  Oculab T.-P.
  T.-P. XL
  T.-P. XL tonometer
tonsil
  cerebellar t.
Tooke
  T. corneal knife
  T. cornea-splitting knife

NOTES

tool

lens simulation sales t.

spud t.

3-toothed forceps

toothed forceps

TOP

tendency-oriented perimetry

Topamax

Topcon

T. aspheric lens

T. chart projector

T. CM-1000 corneal mapping system

T. eye refractometer

T. 50IA camera

T. IMAGEnet digital imaging system

T. keratometer

T. KR-7500 auto-kerato-refractometer

T. LM P5 digital lensometer

T. noncontact morphometric analysis

T. perimeter

T. refractor

T. RM-A2300 auto refractometer

T. RM8000B table-mounted autorefractor

T. SL-7E photo slip lamp

T. SL-E Series slit lamp

T. SL-1E slit lamp

T. SP-1000 noncontact specular microscope

T. TRC-501A fundus camera

T. TRC-50VT retinal camera

T. TRC-50X retinal camera

T. TRV-50VT fundus camera

T. vision tester

topical

t. administration route

t. androgen agonist

t. anesthesia

t. anesthetic

t. anesthetic eye drops

t. anticataract therapy

t. application

t. cycloplegic

t. drug

t. 5-fluorouracil

t. glucocorticoid

t. hyperosmolar agent

NeoDecadron T.

t. ocular antihypertensive agent

t. ocular hypotensive therapy

t. secretogogue therapy

t. treatment

topiramate

TOPO

topographic simulated keratometric power

top-of-the-basilar syndrome

topogometer

topographer

AstraMax stereo t.

Atlas 995 t.

Atlas corneal t.

CT 200 corneal t.

Dicon CT 200 corneal t.

Keratron corneal t.

Keratron scout t.

Medmont E300 t.

TMS-2 computerized corneal t.

topographic

t. agnosia

t. anatomy

t. astigmatism

t. disorientation

t. echography

t. electroretinography

T. Modeling System (TMS)

T. Modeling System-1 (TMS-1)

T. Modeling System-2 (TMS-2)

t. scanning/indocyanine green angiography combination instrument

T. Scanning System (TopSS)

t. simulated keratometric power (TOPO)

topographical electroretinogram

topographically

t. guided therapeutic laser in situ keratomileusis

t. guided therapeutic LASIK

topography

ablation planner t.

color-coded corneal t.

computer-assisted corneal t. (CACT)

computerized corneal t.

confocal laser scanning t.

corneal t.

elevation t.

eye t.

EyeSys Technologies corneal t.

Holladay Diagnostic Summary t.

Humphrey Systems ablation planner t.

optic disc t.

Orbscan corneal t.

subtraction t.

TopSS scanning laser retinal t.

topography-guided

t.-g. ablation

t.-g. LASIK

t.-g. therapy

Topolanski sign

Topolyzer
Allegretto Wave T.
topometer
C-Scan color-ellipsoid t.
ToPreSite
TopSS
Topographic Scanning System
TopSS scanning laser
ophthalmoscope
TopSS scanning laser retinal
topography
TopSS topographic scanning system
TopSS/AngioScan system
Toradol
T. Injection
T. Oral
torcula
toric
t. ablation
back surface t.
t. contact lens
t. intraocular lens
t. intraocular lens axis rotation
posterior t.
t. spectacle lens
t. surface
toricity
Toric-Optima series lens
torn iris
toroidal contact lens
torpor retinae
torque
muscle t.
torsiometer
torsion
Listing t.
ocular t.
subjective t.
torsional
t. deviation
t. diplopia
t. movement
t. nystagmus
t. oscillopsia
torticollis
ocular t.
tortuosity
familial arteriolar t.
retinal vessel t.
t. of retinal vessel
vascularized t.
venous t.
vessel t.

Torulopsis glabrata
TOS
tension oculus sinister
total
t. anterior lamellar keratoplasty
(TALK)
t. anterior synechia
t. astigmatism
t. blindness
t. cataract
t. colorblindness
t. conjunctival flap (TCF)
t. exudative detachment
t. eye analysis
t. hydrophthalmia
hypermetropia, t. (Ht)
t. hyperopia (Ht)
t. hyphema
t. iridectomy
t. keratoplasty
t. ophthalmoplegia
t. posterior synechia
t. sclerectasia
t. sclerocornea
t. steady-state tear flow
t. symblepharon
t. synechia
t. vitrectomy
totalis
ophthalmoplegia t.
Toti
T. operation
T. procedure
toto
eye removed in t.
touch
corneal endothelial t.
iridocorneal t.
3-point t.
vitreous t.
Touchdown thermocycler
Touchlite zoom lens
Touraine syndrome
Tournay
T. phenomenon
T. sign
Touton giant cell
towelette
DisCide disinfecting t.
toxemic retinopathy of pregnancy
toxic
t. amaurosis
t. amblyopia

NOTES

toxic *(continued)*
  t. anterior segment syndrome (TASS)
  t. cataract
  t. diabetes
  t. epidermal necrolysis
  t. follicular conjunctivitis
  t. maculopathy
  t. optic neuropathy
  t. reaction
  t. retinal metallosis
  t. retinopathy
  t. strep syndrome
  t. substance
toxicity
  amiodarone t.
  chloroquine t.
  chloroquine/hydroxychloroquine t.
  corneal t.
  hydroxychloroquine t.
  light t.
  ocular t.
  phenothiazine t.
  photic retinal t.
  retinal t.
  swimming pool water t.
  thioridazine retinal t.
toxic-nutritional disease
toxicogenic conjunctivitis
toxin
  botulin t. (BTX)
  botulinum A t.
  botulinum t. A
  botulinum t. type F
toxin-induced myopathy
Toxocara canis
toxocariasis
  t. endophthalmitis
  ocular t.
Toxoplasma
  T. chorioretinitis
  T. gondii
  T. gondii infection
  T. retinochoroiditis
toxoplasmic
  t. choroiditis
  t. retinitis
  t. retinochoroiditis
  t. uveitis
toxoplasmosis
  t. chorioretinitis
  congenital t.
  fulminant ocular t.
  ocular t.
  punctate outer retinal t.
Toynbee corpuscle
TPA, tPA
  tissue plasminogen activator
    intravitreal TPA

T-PRK
  tracker-assisted photorefractive keratectomy
  T-PRK laser
  T-PRK laser system
trabecula, pl. **trabeculae**
  anterior chamber t.
  corneoscleral t.
  scleral t.
trabecular
  t. aspiration
  t. fiber
  t. membrane
  t. membrane pigment
  t. meshwork (TM)
  t. meshwork-inducible glucocorticoid response (TIGR)
  t. network
  t. outflow
trabeculectomy
  ab externo t.
  Cairns t.
  external t.
  t. flap
  initial t.
  t. operation
  Pearce t.
  phaco t.
  small-incision t.
  Smith t.
trabeculitis glaucoma
trabeculodialysis
trabeculodysgenesis
trabeculopexy
  argon laser t. (ALT)
trabeculoplasty
  argon laser t. (ALTP)
  diode laser t. (DLT)
  laser t. (LTP)
  pneumatic t.
  selective laser t. (SLT)
trabeculopuncture
trabeculotome
  Harms t.
  McPherson t.
trabeculotome-guided deep sclerectomy
trabeculotomy probe
trabeculotomy-trabeculectomy
  combined t.-t.
trabeculum
trabecuphine laser sclerostomy
Tracey
  T. aberrometer
  T. wavefront image
trachoma, pl. **trachomata**
  Arlt t.
  t. body
  brawny t.
  cicatrizing t.

follicular t.
t. gland
gland t.
granular t.
inactive t.
MacCallan classification of t.
prosthesis-induced t.
Türck t.
World Health Organization
  classification of t.
trachoma-inclusion conjunctivitis (TRIC)
trachomatis
  Chlamydia t.
trachomatous
  t. conjunctivitis
  t. dacryocystitis
  t. keratitis
  t. pannus
tracing
  optical ray t.
  ray t.
track
  bear t.'s
  corneal paracentesis t.
  filtration t.
  polar bear t.'s
  snail t.'s
tracker
  Purkinje image t.
tracker-assisted
  t.-a. photorefractive keratectomy (T-
    PRK)
  t.-a. PRK laser
tracking
  pursuit t.
tract
  accessory nucleus of optic t.
  geniculocalcarine t.
  leiomyoma of uveal t.
  optic t.
  uveal t.
traction
  anterior loop t.
  t. band
  diabetic t.
  epiretinal membrane t.
  foveal t.
  macular t.
  t. macular detachment
  Moss t.
  peripheral vitreoretinal t.
  posterior hyaloid t.
  t. retinal detachment

t. suture
t. test
vessel t.
vitreomacular t.
vitreopapillary t.
vitreoretinal t.
vitreous t.
tractional
  t. diabetic macular edema (TDME)
  t. force
  t. retinal degeneration
  t. retinal detachment (TRD)
traction-related tear
traditional IOL
trained retinal locus
training
  optometric vision t.
  self-management t.
  vision t.
tramadol
tranexamic acid
Tranquileyes eye hydrating therapy
transantral orbital decompression
TransBleph implant
transcaruncular-transconjunctival
  approach
transciliary
  t. filtration
  t. filtration procedure
transconjunctival
  t. aqueous oozing
  t. blepharoplasty (TCB)
  t. cryopexy
  t. frontalis suspension
  t. lower eyelid blepharoplasty
  t. route
  t. sutureless vitrectomy
transcorneal oxygen therapy
transcranial Doppler (TCD)
transcript
  latency associated t. (LAT)
transcutaneous electrical nerve
  stimulation of macula
transducer
  Neuroguard pulsed wave t.
  Ocuscan 400 t.
  pressure t.
  Sonogage System Corneo-Gage 20
    MHz center frequency t.
  UBM t.
  vector array t.
transducin

NOTES

transduction
retinal cell t.
transepithelial photoablation
transfer
t. function
gene t.
transferase
terminal deoxynucleotidyl t. (TdT)
transferred ophthalmia
transfixion
t. of iris
t. of iris operation
transformation
keratocyte t.
transformed migraine
transgene expression
transient
t. ametropia
t. blindness
t. congestion
t. early exophthalmos
t. hypotony
t. ischemic attack (TIA)
t. keratopathy
t. layer of Chievitz
t. monocular visual loss
t. myopia
t. neonatal myasthenia
t. obscuration of vision
t. optic disc edema
t. photopsia
t. retinopathy
t. unilateral dilation
t. unilateral mydriasis
t. vertebrobasilar ischemia
t. visual obscuration
transillumination
iris t.
t. technique
t. test
transilluminator
Finnoff t.
transition
t. lens
t. zone
transitional zone
translimbal
translocated eye
translocation
balanced t.
foveal t.
full macular t.
macular t.
t. needle
retinal t.
translucent
transmembrane glycoprotein
transmissibility
oxygen t. (Dk/L)

transmission
t. electron microscope
t. electron microscopy
ephaptic t.
light t.
transmitted light
transneuronal degeneration
transocular technique
transorbital leukotomy
transparency
corneal t.
transparent ulcer of cornea
trans pars plana
transplant
corneal t.
lamellar corneal t.
McReynolds pterygium t.
ocular muscle t.
penetrating corneal t.
transplantation
amniotic membrane t.
t. antigen
autologous chondrocyte t.
t. of cornea
corneal t.
endothelial cell t.
epithelial t.
limbal autograft t. (LAT)
limbal-conjunctival autograft t.
(LCAT)
limbal stem-cell t.
t. of muscle operation
organ t.
photoreceptor t.
t. of posterior corneal tissue
selective t.
t. of submandibular gland for
keratoconjunctivitis sicca
transplanted cornea
Transpore eye tape
transposition
medial rectus t.
muscle t.
rectus muscle t.
superior oblique t.
vertical muscle t.
transpunctal endocanalicular approach
transpupillary
t. cyclophotocoagulation
t. laser
t. retinopexy
t. technique
t. thermotherapy (TT, TTT)
Trans-Scan pulsed Doppler sonographer
transscleral
t. cryopexy
t. cryotherapy
t. diathermy

t. fixation of dislocated intraocular lens
t. laser cyclophotocoagulation
t. neodymium:yttrium-aluminum-garnet cyclophotocoagulation for glaucoma
t. retinal photocoagulation
t. retinopexy
t. suture
t. suture fixation
t. suture fixation technique
transsclerally sutured posterior chamber lens (TS-SPCL)
transsphenoidal encephalocele
transsynaptic degeneration
transverse
t. axis of Fick
t. suture of Krause
t. tarsotomy
transvitreal
transzonular vitreal injection cannula
Trantas dot
tranylcypromine sulfate
trap
t. incision
laser t.
trap-door
t.-d. fracture
t.-d. scleral buckle operation
trapezoid
t. angled CVD diamond knife
t. blade
t. single-plane clear corneal incision
trapezoidal keratotomy
Traquair
T. island
junctional scotoma of T.
scotoma of T.
trauma, pl. **traumas, traumata**
air bag-associated t.
antecedent t.
t. at birth
birth ocular t.
blunt t.
corneal t.
eye t.
eyelid t.
focal t.
intraocular foreign body t.
massive orbital t.
occult penetrating orbitocranial t.
ocular t.

orbital t.
orbitocranial t.
penetrating t.
periocular t.
prenatal ocular t.
prevalence of ocular t.
previous t.
surgical t.
traumatic
t. amblyopia
t. angle recession
t. aniridia
t. atrophy
t. choroidal rupture
t. choroiditis
t. corneal abrasion
t. corneal cyst
t. degenerative cataract
t. endophthalmitis
t. glaucoma
t. gliosis
t. Horner syndrome
t. hyphema
t. iritis
t. microhyphema
t. mydriasis
t. myopathy
t. optic neuropathy (TON)
t. ptosis
t. pupillary miosis
t. rent
t. retinopathy
t. retinoschisis
t. scleral cyst
t. wound dehiscence
traumatized eye
Travatan ophthalmic solution
travoprost ophthalmic solution
TRC-SS2 stereoscopic fundus camera
TRD
tractional retinal detachment
Treacher
T. Collins-Franceschetti syndrome
T. Collins syndrome
treating herpetic anterior uveitis
treatment
antimicrobial t.
argon laser retinal t.
corticosteroid t.
customized ablation t.
dye-enhanced feeder vessel t.
empirical steroid t.
external beam radiation t.

NOTES

treatment *(continued)*
    focal laser t.
    laser capsulotomy t.
    Ocular Microcirculation View
      Analysis T. (OMVAT)
    off-label t.
    t. option
    t. parameter
    PhotoPoint t.
    t. plan
    postoperative t.
    t. protocol
    Refresh Liquigel dry eye t.
    repeat t.
    Schöler t.
    surgical t.
    topical t.
    t. zone laser ablation
tree
    vascular t.
trematode infection
trematodiasis
tremor
    head t.
    immunosuppressant-induced head t.
    oculopalatal t.
tremulous
    t. cataract
    t. iris
trepanation
    t. of cornea
    corneal t.
trephinating
trephination
    elliptical t.
    excimer laser t.
    host t.
    nonmechanical t.
    open-sky t.
    partial-thickness t.
trephine
    Arroyo t.
    Arruga lacrimal t.
    automated t.
    automatic t.
    Bard-Parker t.
    Barraquer t.
    Barron epikeratophakia t.
    Barron-Hessburg corneal t.
    Barron radial vacuum t.
    t. blade
    bone t.
    bone-biting t.
    Boston t.
    Caldwell suction t.
    Castroviejo corneal transplant t.
    Castroviejo improved t.
    chalazion t.

    corneal prosthesis t.
    Davis t.
    disposable t.
    Elliot corneal t.
    Elschnig t.
    epithelial t.
    Gradle corneal t.
    Grieshaber calibrated t.
    Grieshaber corneal t.
    Guyton corneal transplant t.
    handheld t.
    Hanna t.
    Hessburg-Barron disposable
      vacuum t.
    Hessburg-Barron suction t.
    Katena t.
    King corneal t.
    lacrimal t.
    LASEK alcohol well and
      epithelial t.
    lid t.
    Martinez disposable corneal t.
    M-brace corneal t.
    Moria t.
    Mueller electric corneal t.
    Olson calibrated cornea t. (OCCT)
    Ophtec 9.0 mm t.
    Paton corneal t.
    Pharmacia corneal t.
    punch t.
    razor-blade t.
    Searcy chalazion t.
    Sloane t.
    Storz corneal t.
    suction t.
    Surgistar corneal t.
    Troutman tenotomy t.
    Walker t.
    Weck t.
Treponema
    T. pallidum
    T. pallidum hemagglutination
treponemal antibody
TRH
    thyroid-releasing hormone
    TRH test
triad
    Charcot t.
    Hutchinson t.
    near t.
    t. of retinal cone
    t. of simultanagnosia
trial
    A T. of Bifocals in Myopic
      Children with Esophoria
    t. case
    t. case and lens
    t. clip

Complications of Age-Related Macular Degeneration Prevention T. (CAPT)
t. contact lens
Correction of Myopia Evaluation T. (COMET)
Cytomegalovirus Retinitis Retreatment T. (CRRT)
Diabetes Control and Complications T.
Early Manifest Glaucoma T. (EMGT)
Foscarnet-Ganciclovir Cytomegalovirus Retinitis T. (FGCRT)
t. frame
Ganciclovir-Cidofovir Cytomegalovirus Retinitis T. (GCCRT)
Glaucoma Laser T. (GLT)
HPMPC Peripheral Cytomegalovirus Retinitis T.
Ischemic Optic Neuropathy Decompression T. (IONDT)
Monoclonal Antibody Cytomegalovirus Retinitis T. (MACRT)
Sorbinil Retinopathy T. (SRT)
Submacular Surgery T.'s (SST)

triamcinolone
t. acetonide
intravitreal t.

triangle
Arlt t.
color t.
fitting t.
frontal t.
Wernicke t.

triangular capsulotomy
Tri-Beeled trapezoidal keratome
tributary vein occlusion
TRIC
trachoma-inclusion conjunctivitis
tricarbocyanine dye
trichiasis repair
trichilemmoma
Trichinella spiralis
trichodysplasia
trichofolliculoma tumor
trichoma
trichomatosis
trichomatous
trichophytosis

trichosis carunculae
trichroic
trichroism
trichromacy
trichromat
trichromatic, trichromic
t. color theory
trichromatism
anomalous t.
trichromatopsia
anomalous t.
trichromic (*var. of* trichromatic)
triclofos sodium
tricurve contact lenses
trifacet blade
trifacial neuralgia
trifluoperazine hydrochloride
trifluorothymidine
trifluperidol hydrochloride
trifluridine eye drops
trifocal
executive t.
t. glasses
t. lens
trigeminal
t. denervation
t. herpes zoster dermatitis
t. nerve (NV)
t. nerve root section
t. neuralgia
t. neuropathic keratopathy
t. pain
t. reflex
t. sensory ganglion
t. shield
trigeminus
nervus t.
reflex t.
t. reflex
trigger mechanism
trigone
Mueller t.
trihydrate
sodium acetate t.
triiodothyronine suppression test
trilamellar
trilateral retinoblastoma
trimethidium methosulfate
trimethoprim and polymyxin B
triopathy
Tri-Ophtho
triparanol
tripelennamine

T

NOTES

triple
- t. facet-tip needle
- t. procedure
- t. symptom complex
- t. vision

triple-agent immunosuppression
triple-throw square knot stitch
triplokoria, triptokoria
triplopia
tripod fracture
Tri-Port sub-Tenon anesthesia cannula
triptokoria (*var. of* triplokoria)
Triptone Caplets
triradiate line
Tris-borate buffer
trisector
- Alfonso nucleus ophthalmic t.

trisodium phosphonoformate hexahydrate
Trisol
tristichia
tritan axis
tritanomalous
tritanomaly
tritanope
tritanopia
tritanopic
Tri-Thalmic HC
trocar
- beveled t.
- Veirs t.

trocar-cannula system
trochlea
- t. musculi obliqui superioris bulbi
- t. of superior oblique muscle

trochlear
- t. fossa
- t. fovea
- t. hamulus
- t. muscle
- t. nerve
- t. nerve lesion
- t. nerve nucleus
- t. nerve palsy
- t. tubercle

trochlearis
- fossa t.
- fovea t.
- nervus t.
- spina t.

Trokel lens
troland
tromethamine
- ketorolac t.
- lodoxamide t.

Tropheryma whippelii
trophic
- t. change
- t. defect
- t. keratitis
- t. keratopathy
- t. retinal degeneration
- t. ulceration of cornea

tropia
- alternating t.
- constant monocular t.
- t. deviation
- horizontal t.
- intermittent t.
- vertical t.

tropica
- *Leishmania t.*

Tropicacyl
tropical
- t. optic neuropathy
- t. polyhexamethylene biguanide

tropicalis
- *Candida t.*

tropicamide
- hydroxyamphetamine and t.

tropic deviation
tropometer
troposcope
Trousseau sign
Troutman
- T. blade holder
- T. cannula
- T. conjunctival scissors
- T. corneal dissector
- T. corneal knife
- T. implant
- T. lens loupe
- T. microsurgical scissors
- T. needle holder
- T. nonincisional lamellar dissector
- T. operation
- T. punch
- T. rectus forceps
- T. suture scissors
- T. tenotomy trephine
- T. tying forceps

Troutman-Barraquer
- T.-B. corneal fixation forceps
- T.-B. corneal utility forceps

Troutman-Castroviejo
- T.-C. corneal fixation forceps
- T.-C. corneal section scissors

Troutman-Katzin corneal transplant scissors
Troutman-Llobera fixation forceps
Troutman-Tooke corneal knife
true
- t. exfoliation
- t. hemianopsia
- t. image
- t. visual acuity (TVA)

Trump solution
truncated contact lens
truncation

trunk
> facial nerve t.

Trupower aspherical lens
TruPro lacrimal cannula
Trusopt
TruVision lens
trypan
> t. blue
> t. blue ophthalmic solution
> t. blue stain

Trypanosoma
trypanosomiasis
trypsin-digested explant
trypticase soy broth
TSC
> tuberous sclerosis complex

T-sign
TS III ROP
> threshold stage III of retinopathy of
> prematurity

TS-SPCL
> transsclerally sutured posterior chamber
> lens

Tsuneoka irrigating chopper
TT
> transpupillary thermotherapy

TTT
> transpupillary thermotherapy

T-tube
> cul-de-sac irrigation T-t.
> Houser cul-de-sac irrigator T-t.
> lacrimal duct T-t.
> polyethylene T-t.
> Pyrex T-t.
> Silastic T-t.
> vinyl T-t.

tube
> Ahmed glaucoma drainage t.
> Ahmed glaucoma valve t.
> Ahmed shunt t.
> angled suction t.
> anterior chamber t.
> Baerveldt glaucoma implant t.
> Baerveldt shunt t.
> Bowman t.
> corneal t.
> Crawford t.
> encircling polyethylene t.
> endotracheal t.
> Eppendorf t.
> Frazier suction t.
> fusion t.
> Houser cul-de-sac irrigator t.

> Jones Pyrex t.
> Jones tear duct t.
> large-bore aspiration t.
> laser t.
> Luer t.
> microfuge t.
> Molteno shunt t.
> Monoka t.
> neural t.
> Plexiglas t.
> polyethylene t.
> Pyrex t.
> Questek laser t.
> Quickert-Dryden t.
> Reinecke-Carroll lacrimal t.
> silicone t.
> vinyl t.

tuber
> frontal t.

tubercle
> t. bacillus
> caseating t.
> lacrimal t.
> lateral orbit t.
> lateral orbital t.
> lateral palpebral t.
> optic disc t.
> trochlear t.
> Whitnall t.

tubercular retinal vasculitis
tuberculin syringe
tuberculoma
> optochiasmatic t.

tuberculosis
> t. conjunctivitis
> intraocular t.
> *Mycobacterium t.*

tuberculous
> t. dacryocystitis
> t. iritis
> t. keratitis
> t. phlyctenulosis
> t. rhinitis
> t. tarsitis
> t. uveitis

tuberous
> t. sclerosis
> t. sclerosis complex (TSC)

tube-shunt procedure
tubing
> bicanalicular t.
> fluted spiral t.
> t. introducer forceps

NOTES

tubing *(continued)*
    silicone t.
    smooth-walled t.
    viscodissector t.
Tübinger
    T. perimeter
    T. perimetry
tubular
    t. vision
    t. visual field
tubulointerstitial nephritis and uveitis syndrome
tuck
    eyelid t.
    iris t.
    left superior oblique t.
    t. procedure
tucked lid of Collier
tucker
    Bishop tendon t.
    Burch-Greenwood tendon t.
    tendon t.
Tudor-Thomas graft
tuft
    cystic retinal t.
    neovascular t.
    retinal t.
    vitreoretinal t.
    zonular-traction retinal t.
tularemia
    oculoglandular t.
tularemic conjunctivitis
tularensis
    conjunctivitis t.
    Francisella t.
Tulevech cannula
tulle gras dressing
Tullio phenomenon
tumbling
    t. E cube
    t. E test
    t. procedure
    t. technique
    t. technique operation
tumor
    anemone cell t.
    t. apex
    apical t.
    benign t.
    brain t.
    Brooke t.
    carcinoid t.
    t. cell
    cerebellar astrocytoma t.
    cerebellopontine angle t.
    chiasmal t.
    choristoma t.
    choroidal melanocytic t.
    collision t.

compressive optic nerve t.
congenital limbal corneal dermoid t.
conjunctival lymphoid t.
craniofacial fibroosseous t.
cystic hydrocystoma t.
dermoid t.
t. doubling time
ependymoma t.
epithelial t.
t. of eyelid
eyelid t.
fibroosseous t.
fossa t.
Grawitz t.
hair follicle t.
histiocytic t.
t. of interior of eye
interior eye t.
intraocular t.
intrasellar t.
Koenen t.
lacrimal gland epithelial t.
lymphoid t.
lymphoproliferative t.
malignant epithelial t.
malignant eyelid t.
medulloblastoma t.
melanocytic iris t.
mesenchymal t.
t. metastasis
metastasis of t.
metastatic choroidal t.
metastatic orbital t.
mixed t.
mucinous adenocarcinoma t.
t. necrosis factor
neurogenic t.
nonepithelial t.
ocular adnexal t.
t. of optic nerve
optic nerve t.
orbital t.
Pancoast t.
papilliform t.
phakomatous choristoma t.
pilomatrixoma t.
pituitary t.
plasma cell t.
pleomorphic spindle cell t.
primitive neuroectodermal t. (PNET)
Rathke pouch t.
retinal anlage t.
rhabdoid t.
Schmincke t.
skull base t.
solid t.
spinal canal t.

suprasellar t.
syringoma t.
trichofolliculoma t.
vascular t.
Warthin t.
waxy t.
Wilms t.
Zimmerman t.
tumor-free margin
tunable dye laser
TUNEL
terminal deoxynucleotidyl transferase-
mediated dUTP-digoxigenin nick-end
labeling
TUNEL assay
TUNEL staining
tungsten-halogen lamp
tunic
Brücke t.
fibrous t.
fibrovascular t.
Ruysch t.
vascular t.
tunica
t. albuginea oculi
t. conjunctiva
t. conjunctiva palpebrarum
t. fibrosa bulbi
t. interna bulbi
t. nervea
t. sclerotica
t. sensoria bulbi
t. uvea
t. vasculosa bulbi
t. vasculosa lentis
t. vasculosa oculi
tunnel
t. cauterization
t. dissection
t. enlargement
t. field
t. groove
t. incision
t. location
t. paracentesis
scleral t.
t. surgical technique
t. suturing
t. vision
tunneled implant
tunneler
crescent scleral t.
SatinCrescent t.

turbidity-reducing unit
turbo-tip of phacoemulsification unit
turcica
sella t.
Türck trachoma
Turkish saddle
Turk line
turnover
epithelial t.
tear t.
turricephaly
tutamina oculi
Tutoplast
TVA
true visual acuity
tweezers
jeweler's t.
laser t.
optic t.
twelfth nerve palsy
twilight
t. blindness
t. vision
twin cone
twirling method
twist
t. fixation hook
scleral t.
stitch with t.'s
twisted virgin silk suture
twitch
Cogan lid t.
eyelid t.
Tycos manometer
tying forceps
tying/stitch removal forceps
tyloma conjunctivae
tylosis ciliaris
tyloxapol
Tyndall
T. effect
T. phenomenon
type
t. 1, 2 choroidal neovascularization
t. 1, 2 diabetes
Jaeger test t.
t. 1 herpes simplex virus
point system test t.
Snellen test t.
test t.
typhlology
typhlosis

T

NOTES

typhus
      epidemic t.
      scrub t.
typical
      t. achromatopsia
      t. coloboma
      t. drusen
      t. dry eye symptom
typoscope
tyramine hydrochloride

Tyrell iris hook
tyrosinase-negative type oculocutaneous albinism
tyrosinase-positive type oculocutaneous albinism
tyrosinase test
tyrosinemia type I, II, III
Tzanck
      T. smear
      T. technique

UBM
ultrasonic biomicroscope
ultrasound biomicroscope
ultrasound biomicroscopy
UBM measurement
UBM transducer
UCVA
uncorrected visual acuity
UEA-1
Ulex europaeus agglutinin 1
UGH
uveitis, glaucoma, hyphema
UGH syndrome
UGH+ syndrome
Uhthoff
U. phenomenon
U. sign
U. symptom
U. syndrome
UL
upper lid
ulcer
acne rosacea corneal u.
ameboid u.
anular u.
bacterial infectious corneal u.
catarrhal corneal u.
central corneal u.
chronic serpiginous u.
community-acquired corneal u.
conjunctival u.
contact lens-induced peripheral u.
(CLPU)
corneal u.
dendriform u.
dendritic herpes simplex corneal u.
descemetocele u.
fascicular u.
fungal corneal u.
geographic herpes simplex
corneal u.
herpes simplex corneal u.
herpetic u.
hypopyon u.
infectious corneal u.
Jacob u.
marginal catarrhal u.
marginal corneal u.
metaherpetic u.
Mooren corneal u.
noncentral u.
oval-shaped vernal u.
peripheral corneal u.
pneumococcal u.
pneumococcus u.

ring u.
rodent u.
Saemisch u.
serpiginous corneal u.
shield u.
sterile corneal u.
stromal u.
superior corneal shield u.
suppurative u.
vernal shield u.
visually insignificant infectious
corneal u.
von Hippel internal corneal u.
xerophthalmic u.
ulcerated lesion
ulceration
u. of cornea
frank corneal u.
geographic u.
herpes epithelial tropic u.
indolent u.
Mooren u.
necrotizing sclerocorneal u. (NSU)
perilimbal u.
peripheral corneal u.
rheumatoid related u.
serpiginous u.
ulcerative keratitis
ulcerogranuloma
ulceromembranous
ulcerosa
blepharitis u.
ulcus serpens corneae
ulectomy
***Ulex europaeus* agglutinin 1 (UEA-1)**
Ullrich-Feichtiger syndrome
Ullrich syndrome
Ultex
U. bifocal
U. lens
Ultima
Dioptron U.
U. 2000 photocoagulator
Ultra
U. mag lens
U. Sleeve ultrasound sleeve
U. Tears
U. Tears Solution
U. view SP slit lamp lens
Ultracaine
Ultracell LASIK spear
ultra high acquisition speed
ultra-high-resolution ophthalmic imaging
ultra-high-speed ophthalmic imaging
Ultra-Image A-scan

U

Ultra-Lase
ultra-late phase
Ultram
Ultramatic
>U. Project-O-Chart (UPOC)
>U. Project-O-Chart projector
>U. Rx Master Phoroptor
>U. Rx Master phoroptor retractor

ultramicrotome
>Reichert-Jung Ultracut u.

Ultrapred
UltraPulse laser
Ultrascan Digital 2000 contact
>**ultrasound A-scan**

Ultra-select nitinol guide wire
UltraShaper Keratome
Ultrasharp round blade microKnife AU
>**681-21-3**

ultrasmall incision implant
ultrasonic
>u. biomicroscope (UBM)
>u. cataract-removal lancet
>u. cataract-removal lancet needle
>u. insonification
>u. micrometer
>u. pachymetry

ultrasonogram
>A-scan u.
>B-scan u.
>Doppler u.
>gray-scale u.

ultrasonographic biomicroscopy
ultrasonography
>A-scan u.
>B-scan u.
>contact B-scan u.
>CooperVision u.
>Doppler u.
>water-bath u.

ultrasound
>Acuson u.
>Alcon Digital B 2000 u.
>Axisonic II u.
>u. biomicroscope (UBM)
>U. Biomicroscope System
>u. biomicroscopy (UBM)
>B-scan u.
>CooperVision u.
>3D i-Scan ophthalmic u.
>Doppler u.
>high-gain digital u.
>kinetic u.
>ocular u.
>Ocuscan A-scan biometric u.
>u. pachometer
>u. pachymeter-KMI RK-5000
>renal u.
>u. sleeve

>u. spatula
>through-the-lid contact u.

UltraTears
ultra-thin surgical blade
ultraviolet (UV)
>u. A (UVA)
>u. A light
>u. B (UVB)
>u. blocker
>u. burn
>u. filter
>u. fluorescence photography
>u. keratoconjunctivitis
>u. keratopathy
>u. radiation
>u. radiation exposure
>u. ray ophthalmia

ultraviolet-blue photic retinopathy
ultraviolet-induced injury
UltraVue lens
Ultrazyme enzymatic cleaner
umbilicated cataract
umbrella
>u. iris
>u. punctum plug

umbrella-like pattern
unaberrated chart
unable to close eyelid
Unasyn
uncal syndrome
uncinate
>u. procedure
>u. process of lacrimal bone

unclosed macular hole
uncomplicated graft
unconventional outflow
uncorrected visual acuity (UCVA)
uncrossed diplopia
uncut spectacle lens
underaction
>congenital superior oblique u.

undercorrection
underlying
>u. conus
>u. cornea

undertaking
>visually complex u.

underwater diathermy unit
undine
undissociated alkaloid
undulatory nystagmus
unequal retinal image
Unfolder Sapphire implantation system
ung
>ointment

unguis
>os u.
>pterygium u.

unharmonious ARC

Unicare blue and green all-in-1 cleaning solution
Unicat diamond knife
unifocal
  u. helioid choroiditis
  u. optic nerve lesion
uniform BSS flow
unilateral
  u. acute idiopathic maculopathy
  u. altitudinal scotoma
  u. arcus
  u. conjunctivitis
  u. corneal lattice dystrophy
  u. hearing loss
  u. hemianopia
  u. hemianopsia
  u. lesion
  u. microtremor
  u. papilledema
  u. proptosis
  u. ptosis of eyelid
  u. sporadic retinoblastoma
  u. strabismus
unilocular hemianopia
uniocular
  u. cataract
  u. hemianopsia
  u. strabismus
Uniplanar style PC II lens
UniPulse 1040 Surgical CO$_2$ laser system
Unique pH multi-purpose solution
UniShaper Keratome
Unisol
  U. Plus
  U. 4 Preservative Free Saline Solution
unit
  Alcon cryosurgical u.
  Alcon irrigating/aspirating u.
  Alcon 20,000 Legacy u.
  Alcon 10,000 Master u.
  Alcon phacoemulsification u.
  Ångström u.
  AO Reichert Instruments Ful-Vue diagnostic u.
  Bishop-Harman irrigating/aspirating u.
  Bovie electrocautery u.
  Bovie electrosurgical u.
  Bovie retinal detachment u.
  Bracken irrigating/aspirating u.
  Charles irrigating/aspirating u.

  Coburn irrigation/aspiration u.
  Cooper I&A u.
  Cooper irrigating/aspirating u.
  CooperVision irrigating/aspirating u.
  CooperVision irrigation/aspiration u.
  cryosurgical u.
  diathermy u.
  Dougherty irrigating/aspirating u.
  Drews irrigating/aspirating u.
  Fox irrigating/aspirating u.
  Frigitronics cryosurgical u.
  Gass irrigating/aspirating u.
  Gibson irrigating/aspirating u.
  Girard ultrasonic u.
  Hyde irrigating/aspirating u.
  Hyde irrigator/aspirator u.
  Intermedics Phaco I/A u.
  Iolab irrigating/aspirating u.
  irrigation/aspiration u.
  Irvine irrigating/aspirating u.
  Keeler cryosurgical u.
  Kelman cryosurgical u.
  Kelman irrigating/aspirating u.
  Kelman phacoemulsification u.
  lacrimal functional u.
  u. of light
  log u.
  u. of luminous flux
  u. of luminous intensity
  Mallett u.
  McIntyre irrigating/aspirating u.
  microcautery u.
  Mira diathermy u.
  mobile eye u.
  near Mallett u.
  neonatal intensive care u.
  N$_2$O cryosurgical u.
  u. of ocular convergence
  ocutome vitrectomy u.
  Phaco Cavitron irrigating/aspirating u.
  Phaco Emulsifier Cavitron u.
  Rollet irrigating/aspirating u.
  Schepens retinal detachment u.
  Simcoe double-barreled irrigating/aspirating u.
  Storz-Walker retinal detachment u.
  Surg-E-Trol System irrigating/aspirating u.
  Svedberg u.
  Talbot u.
  turbidity-reducing u.
  turbo-tip of phacoemulsification u.

U

NOTES

unit *(continued)*
    underwater diathermy u.
    Visitec aspiration u.
    Visitec irrigating/aspirating u.
    Visitec vitrectomy u.
unitas
    oculi u.
United Sonics J shock phaco fragmentor system
unity conjugacy planes
univariant analysis
univariate
    u. linear regression
    u. polytomous logistic regression
universal
    U. conformer
    U. eye shield
    U. II forceps
    U. implant
    U. lens-folding forceps
    U. Pathfinder knife
    U. phaco chopper/manipulator
    U. slit lamp
    U. soft tip cannulated sliding extrusion needle
universale
    angiokeratoma corporis diffusum u.
university
    U. of Waterloo chart
    U. of Waterloo Colored Dot Test (UWCDot)
Univis
    U. bifocal
    U. lens
UniVisc
Univision low-vision microscopic lens
Unizyme enzymatic cleaner
Unna abtropfung theory
unoprostone
    u. isopropyl
    u. isopropyl ester
unpegged hydroxyapatite implant
unrecognized risk factor
unrefined refraction
unsafe to drive
unstable tear film
unstained
    u. lens
    u. wet mount
unwanted migration of pigment
unzipper
    Katzen flap u.
up
    base up (BU)
UPA
    urokinase-type plasminogen activator
up-and-down staircases procedure
upbeating nystagmus
upbeat nystagmus

updrawn pupil
upgaze paralysis
UPOC
    Ultramatic Project-O-Chart
    UPOC projector
upper
    u. blepharoplasty
    u. canaliculus
    u. eyelid
    u. hemianopsia
    u. lid (UL)
    u. palpebral conjunctiva
    u. punctum
    u. retina
    u. tarsal conjunctiva
upside-down
    u.-d. ptosis
    u.-d. reversal of vision
uptake
    lacrimal gland gallium u.
upward
    u. gaze
    u. squint
Uram E2 compact MicroProbe laser
urate band keratopathy
uratic
    u. conjunctivitis
    u. iritis
uremic
    u. amaurosis
    u. amblyopia
    u. optic neuropathy
    u. retinitis
Uribe orbital implant
urica
    cornea u.
    keratitis u.
urinary
    u. GAG assay
    u. glycosaminoglycan measurement assay
urine refractometry
urogastrone
urokinase-type plasminogen activator (UPA)
Urrets-Zavalia retinal surgical lens
US-2000 echo scan
USC marker
useful field of view test
Usher syndrome
UTAS 2000 electroretinography instrument
utility
    time trade-off u.
Utrata
    U. capsulorrhexis forceps
    U. foldable lens cutter
    U. retriever

Utrata-Kershner capsulorrhexis cystotome forceps
utricular reflex
UV
 ultraviolet
  UV blocking filter
  UV change
  UV damage
  UV exposure
  UV keratitis
  UV keratoconjunctivitis
  UV Nova Curve lens
  UV radiation protection
UVA
 ultraviolet A
UV-absorbing IOL
UVB
 ultraviolet B
uvea
 tunica u.
uveae
 ectropion u.
 entropion u.
uveal
 u. atrophy
 u. coat
 u. coloboma
 u. effusion
 u. effusion syndrome
 u. entropion
 u. framework
 u. juvenile xanthogranuloma
 u. melanocyte
 u. melanocytic proliferation
 u. melanoma
 u. metastasis
 u. neurofibroma
 u. nevus
 u. osteoma
 u. staphyloma
 u. tissue
 u. tract
 u. tract hamartoma
 u. tract hemangioma
uvealis
 pars u.
uveitic
 u. band keratopathy
 u. glaucoma
 u. phase
uveitis, uveitides, pl. **uveitides**
 anterior u.
 aspergillosis u.

 bacterial u.
 Behçet u.
 bilateral u.
 candidal u.
 childhood u.
 chronic anterior u. (CAU)
 endogenous u.
 excessive rebound u.
 fibrous u.
 Förster u.
 Fuchs u.
 fungal u.
 u., glaucoma, hyphema
 granulomatous anterior u.
 herpes simplex u.
 heterochromic u.
 HLA-B27-associated u.
 hypopyon u.
 immune recovery u.
 u. intermedia
 intermediate u.
 Kirisawa u.
 lens-induced u.
 leptospiral u.
 nongranulomatous anterior u.
 parasitic u.
 pediatric u.
 peripheral u.
 phacoanaphylactic u.
 phacoantigenic u.
 phacogenic u.
 phacolytic u.
 phacotoxic u.
 posterior u.
 postoperative anterior u.
 protozoan u.
 psoriatic u.
 sarcoid u.
 sarcoidosis-associated u.
 sight-threatening u.
 sympathetic u.
 toxoplasmic u.
 treating herpetic anterior u.
 tuberculous u.
 viral u.
 vitiligo u.
 Vogt-Koyanagi bilateral u.
 zoster u.
uveitis-vitiligo-alopecia-poliosis syndrome
uveocutaneous syndrome
uveoencephalitic syndrome
uveoencephalitis
uveomeningeal syndrome

U

NOTES

uveomeningitis syndrome
uveomeningoencephalitis
uveoparotitis
uveoplasty
uveoretinitis
uveoscleral outflow

uveoscleritis
Uvex lens
UV-induced fluorescence
UV-mediated ocular damage
UWCDot
    University of Waterloo Colored Dot Test

V
volume
V exotropia
V pattern
V syndrome
Va_{cc}
corrected visual acuity
Vac
Vaper V. II
vaccinia
blepharoconjunctivitis v.
v. gangrenosa
generalized v.
v. infection
keratitis v.
ocular v.
progressive v.
vaccinial keratitis
vacciniforme
hydroa v.
vaccinulosa
keratitis post v.
vacuolar configuration
vacuole
autophagic v.
cortical v.
nonmembrane-bound v.'s
Vac-Up
vacuum
Venturi-type live v.
vacuum-based pump
vacuum-centering guide
vagus nerve paralysis
***Vahlkampfia* cyst**
Vaiser sponge
valacyclovir
Valcyte
valdecoxib
valganciclovir HCl
validation study
Valilab electrocautery
VALIO
Verteporfin with Altered Light in Occult
VALIO study
valproate sodium
Valsalva
V. maneuver
V. retinopathy
Valtrex
value
Abbe v.
C v.
Dk v.
equivalent oxygen percentage v.
Hertel v.
keratometry v.
negative predictive v.
ocular hemodynamic v.
Orbscan v.
pachymetry v.
positive predictive v.
predictive v.
prismatic dioptric v.
spatially resolved v.
threshold limit v. (TLV)
value-based medicine
valve
Ahmed glaucoma v. (AGV)
Ahmed glaucoma biplate v.
Béraud v.
Bianchi v.
Bochdalek v.
filtering v.
Foltz v.
v. of Hasner
Hasner v.
Huschke v.
Krause v.
Krupin v.
Krupin-Denver v.
Rosenmüller v.
v. of Rosenmüller
Taillefer v.
VA magnetic orbital implant
Van
V. Herick filtration
V. Herick modification
V. Lint akinesia
V. Lint anesthesia
V. Lint block
V. Lint flap
V. Lint injection
V. Lint modified technique
van
v. den Berg stray-light meter
v. der Hoeve disease
v. Heuven anatomical classification of diabetic retinopathy
Vancocin
vancomycin
vanillism
vanishing bone disease
Vannas
V. capsulotomy
V. capsulotomy scissors
V. iridocapsulotomy scissors
Vantage ophthalmoscope
Vaper Vac II
VAQ
Visual Activities Questionnaire

variabilis
  erythrokeratodermia v. (EKV)
variability
  test-retest v.
variable
  v. distance stereoacuity (VDS)
  v. duty cycle
  eye-related v.
  v. power cross-cylinder lens set
  v. repetition rate (VRR)
  v. rise time
  sociodemographic v.
  v. spot scanning (VSS)
  v. strabismus
variance
  analysis of v. (ANOVA)
varians
  metamorphopsia v.
variant
  genetic v.
  Heidenhain v.
  Miller-Fisher v.
  morphologic v.
variation
  coefficient of v.
  diurnal v.
  missense v.
varicella
  v. iridocyclitis
  v. keratitis
  v. zoster ophthalmicus
  v. zoster virus (VZV)
varicella-zoster retinitis
varices (*pl. of* varix)
varicoblepharon
varicose ophthalmia
varicula
Varilux
  V. lens implant
  V. Pangamic thin plastic lens
varix, pl. **varices**
  conjunctival v.
  orbital v.
  vortex vein v.
VAS
  visual analog scale
vasa sanguinea retinae
vascular
  v. abnormality
  v. arcade
  v. cataract
  v. cerebellar disease
  v. channel
  v. circle of optic nerve
  v. coat of eyeball
  v. congestion
  v. dilatation
  v. disorder
  v. endothelial cell

v. endothelial growth factor
  (VEGF)
  v. filling defect
  v. frond
  v. funnel
  v. hamartoma
  v. inhibition
  v. keratitis
  v. lamina of choroid
  v. loop
  v. network
  v. occlusion
  v. occlusive disease
  v. optical disc swelling without
    visual loss
  v. plexus
  v. regression
  v. retinopathy
  v. sheathing
  v. tree
  v. tumor
  v. tunic
vascularity
  bleb v.
  intrinsic v.
vascularization
  conjunctival v.
  corneal v.
  stromal v.
vascularized
  v. plaque
  v. scar
  v. tortuosity
vasculature
  abnormal v.
  choroidal v.
  disc v.
  perimacular v.
  persistent fetal v.
  retinal v.
  spider v.
vasculitis
  benign retinal v.
  granulomatous v.
  hypocomplementemic urticarial v.
    (HUV)
  idiopathic retinal v.
  leukocytoclastic v.
  limbal v.
  necrotizing v.
  obstructive retinal v.
  orbital v.
  v. retinae
  retinal v.
  tubercular retinal v.
vasculogenesis
  fetal v.
vasculonebulous keratitis
vasculopathic downbeat nystagmus

vasculopathy
exudative idiopathic polypoidal choroidal v.
idiopathic polypoidal choroidal v. (IPCV)
occlusive retinal v.
polypoidal choroidal v. (PCV)
radiation-induced v.
radiogenic v.
retinal v.
vasoactive amine
Vasocidin Ophthalmic
Vasocine
VasoClear
V. A
V. Ophthalmic
Vasocon
V. Regular
V. Regular Ophthalmic
Vasocon-A
V.-A Ophthalmic
V.-A solution
vasoconstrictor
vasodilator
vasopermeability
Vasosulf Ophthalmic
vault
lens v.
vaulting of contact lens
VBIO
video binocular indirect ophthalmoscope
VC
acuity of color vision
VCA
Vision Council of America
VDA
visual discriminatory acuity
VDS
variable distance stereoacuity
VDS test
VDTS
video display terminal simulator
VE
visual efficiency
VECP
visual-evoked cortical potential
vection
circular v.
vectis
Anis irrigating v.
anterior chamber irrigating v.
aspirating/irrigating v.
Drews-Knolle reverse irrigating v.

irrigating anterior chamber v.
irrigating/aspirating v.
Look irrigating v.
plastic disposable irrigating v.
Sheets irrigating v.
Snellen v.
vectograph chart
vectographic study
vector
v. analysis
v. array transducer
Fourier-transformed v.
VEGF
vascular endothelial growth factor
veil
dimple v.
pigmented v.
Sattler v.
vitreous v.
veiling glare
vein
angular v.
anterior ciliary v.
anterior conjunctival v.
aqueous v.
Ascher v.
branch retinal v. (BRV)
central retinal v. (CRV)
choriovaginal v.
choroid v.
ciliary v.
cilioretinal v.
conjunctival v.
endophlebitis of retinal v.
episcleral v.
facial v.
frontal diploic v.
Galen v.
inferior nasal v.
inferior ophthalmic v.
inferior palpebral v.
inferior temporal v.
Kuhnt postcentral v.
lacrimal v.
muscular v.
nasofrontal v.
nicking of retinal v.
occlusion of branch v.
occlusion of retinal v.
ophthalmic v.
ophthalmomeningeal v.
opticociliary shunt v.
palpebral v.

V

NOTES

vein *(continued)*
    posterior ciliary v.
    posterior conjunctival v.
    retinal v.
    superior nasal v.
    superior ophthalmic v.
    superior palpebral v.
    superior temporal v.
    supraorbital v.
    vortex v.
Veirs
    V. cannula
    V. trocar
Velcro head strap
velocardiofacial syndrome
velocimeter
    Doppler v.
    laser Doppler v.
velocimetry
    laser Doppler v.
velocity
    v. error
    retinal-slip v.
    saccadic v.
velonoskiascopy
velum, pl. **vela**
    corneal v.
Velva Kleen
VEM
    vergence eye movement
vena, pl. **venae**
    v. angularis
    v. centralis retinae
    venae choroideae oculi
    v. diploica frontalis
    v. facialis
    v. lacrimalis
    v. nasofrontalis
    v. ophthalmica inferior
    v. ophthalmica superior
    v. ophthalmomeningea
    v. vorticosae
venography
    magnetic resonance v. (MRV)
    orbital v.
venomanometry
venous
    v. beading
    v. congestion
    v. engorgement
    v. hemangioma
    v. loop
    v. occlusive disease
    v. pulsation
    v. sheathing
    v. sheath patch
    v. sinus
    v. stasis
    v. stasis retinopathy (VSR)

    v. stenosis retinopathy
    v. tortuosity
vented gas forced infusion (VGFI)
venter frontalis musculi occipitofrontalis
ventricle
    cerebral v.
ventriculography
Venturi
    V. adjusted temple
    V. aspiration vitrectomy device
    V. effect
    V. pump
Venturi-Flo valve system
Venturi-type live vacuum
venula, pl. **venulae**
    v. macularis inferior
    v. macularis superior
    v. nasalis retinae inferior
    v. nasalis retinae superior
    v. temporalis retinae inferior
    v. temporalis retinae superior
venule
    v. banking
    macular v.
    retinal v.
    right-angle deflected v.
VEP
    visual-evoked potential
VER
    visual-evoked response
vera
    polycoria v.
Verga lacrimal groove
vergence
    v. eye movement (VEM)
    v. facility
    fusional v.
    v. of lens
    negative vertical v.
    power v.
    reduced v.
    reflux v.
    tonic v.
    vertical v.
    zero v.
Verhoeff
    V. capsule forceps
    V. lens expressor
    V. scissors
    V. streak
    V. suture
VERIS
    visual-evoked response imaging system
    VERIS III system
Verisyse phakic IOL
vermiform
    v. contraction
    v. movement

vermis
    cerebellar v.
    dorsal v.
vernal
    v. catarrh
    v. conjunctivitis
    v. keratoconjunctivitis (VKC)
    v. keratoconjunctivitis refractory
    v. shield ulcer
Vernier
    V. optometer
    V. stimulus
    V. visual acuity
verruca vulgaris papilloma
VersaTool eye sponge
version
    ductions and v.'s (D&V)
    v. movement
vertebral angiography
vertebrobasilar
    v. artery
    v. artery insufficiency
    v. system
    v. vascular abnormality
Verteporfin with Altered Light in Occult (VALIO)
vertex, pl. **vertices**
    v. of distance
    front v.
    v. of power
    v. refractometer
vertical
    v. axis
    v. axis of eye
    v. axis of Fick
    v. chopping technique
    v. comitant deviation
    v. diplopia
    v. divergence
    v. divergence position
    v. duction
    v. forceps
    v. fusional vergence amplitude
    v. fusion range
    v. gaze
    v. gaze center
    v. gaze paresis
    v. gaze restriction
    v. hemianopsia
    v. illumination
    v. laxity
    v. meridian
    v. movement

    v. muscle
    v. muscle transposition
    v. myoclonus
    v. nystagmus
    v. parallax
    v. phoria
    v. plane
    v. prism bar
    v. prism test
    v. rectus muscle
    v. retraction syndrome
    right gaze v.'s
    v. strabismus
    v. strabismus fixus
    v. stria
    v. tropia
    v. vergence
    v. vertigo
verticillata
    cornea v.
vertiginous
vertigo
    benign paroxysmal positional v. (BPPV)
    objective v.
    ocular v.
    sham-movement v.
    special sense v.
    subjective v.
    vertical v.
vertometer
vesicle
    chorionic v.
    clear lid v.
    compound v.
    cornea v.
    corneal v.
    lens v.
    lenticular v.
    lid v.
    multilocular v.
    ocular v.
    ophthalmic v.
    optic v.
    pinocytotic v.
vesicula ophthalmica
vesicular
    v. involvement
    v. keratitis
    v. keratopathy
vesiculation
    eyelid v.
vesiculosus linear endothelial

V

NOTES

V-esotropia
vessel
    v. abnormality of retina
    anomalous v.
    choroidal v.
    ciliary v.
    collateral v.
    congested v.
    conjunctival v.
    v. constriction
    dilated episcleral v.
    disc neurovascular v.
    episcleral v.
    episcleral blood v.
    feeder v.
    frond of v.
    ghost v.
    v. landmark measurement
    nasal v.
    neovascular iris v.
    opticociliary shunt v.
    orbital v.
    perilimbal conjunctival v.
    retinal v.
    v. sheathing
    sheathing of retinal v.
    shunt v.
    silver-wire v.
    stromal blood v.
    succulent v.
    telangiectatic blood v.
    tensile strength of v.
    v. tortuosity
    tortuosity of retinal v.
    v. traction
vestibular
    v. cortex
    v. disorder
    v. nerve
    v. nucleus
    v. nystagmus
    v. organ
    v. pupillary reaction
    v. system
vestibulocerebellar ataxia
vestibulocochlear
vestibuloocular
    v. reflex
    v. response (VOR)
vestibulotoxicity
    gentamicin-induced v.
Vexol 1% ophthalmic suspension
V-exotropia
VF
    visual field
VF-14 questionnaire
VFC
    viscous fluid controller

VFQ
    Visual Function Questionnaire
VFQ-25
    25-Item Visual Function Questionnaire
VGFI
    vented gas forced infusion
V-groove gauge
VH
    vitreous hemorrhage
    VH fibrin sealant
VHF
    visual half-field
VI
    visual impairment
vial
    multiple-dose v.
Vibramycin
vibrating scissors
Vibratome
vibratory nystagmus
Vibrio vulnificus
Vickers
    V. forceps
    V. needle holder
Vicodin
vicrosurgery
Vicryl suture
VID
    visible iris diameter
vidarabine
Vidaurri
    V. double irrigation cannula
    V. irrigator
video
    v. binocular indirect ophthalmoscope (VBIO)
    v. display terminal simulator (VDTS)
    v. keratography
    v. specular microscope
videoendoscope
    fiberoptic v.
videokeratograph
    EyeSys v.
videokeratographer
    Humphrey 992 v.
videokeratographic corneal steepening
videokeratography
    computer-assisted v.
    computerized corneal v.
    v. pattern
videokeratoscope
    computer-assisted v.
    EyeSys v.
    Keratron v.
    Technomed C-Scan v.
    TMS-1 v.
    TMS-2 computer-assisted v.
videometer

videooculographic image
videooculography
vidian
    v. nerve
    v. neuralgia
    v. neurectomy
Vieth-Müller
    V.-M. horopter
    V.-M. circle
view
    axial v.
    Caldwell v.
    coronal v.
    field of v.
    Miyake v.
    sweep v.
    Waters v.
ViewPoint CK system
vigabatrin
Vigamox ophthalmic solution
Villasenor ultrasonic pachymeter
villus, pl. **villi**
vinyl
    v. T-tube
    v. tube
violet
    v. haptic
    v. vision
    visual v.
    v. wavelength
VIP
    Vision in Preschoolers
    VIP Study
Vira-A Ophthalmic
viral
    v. blepharitis
    v. capsid antigen
    v. conjunctivitis
    v. infection
    v. interstitial keratitis
    v. keratoconjunctivitis
    v. ocular disease
    v. uveitis
viral-induced demyelination
Virchow corpuscle
virgin
    v. silk
    v. silk suture
viridans
    Streptococcus v.
Viridis Lite photocoagulator
Viroptic Ophthalmic

virtual
    v. focus
    v. image
    v. point
    v. reality head-mounted display
    V. Reality Symptom Questionnaire (VRSQ)
    V. Retinal Display (VRD)
virulence
    microbial v.
virus
    alpha herpes v.
    BK v.
    cornea herpes zoster v.
    cytomegalic inclusion v.
    Epstein-Barr v. (EBV)
    herpes simplex v. (HSV)
    herpes simplex v. type I
    herpes zoster v.
    human immunodeficiency v. (HIV)
    human T-lymphotropic v.
    influenza v.
    JC v.
    v. keratoconjunctivitis
    lymphocytic choriomeningitis v.
    molluscum v.
    Newcastle disease v.
    type 1 herpes simplex v.
    varicella zoster v. (VZV)
virustatics
Visalens
    V. contact lens cleaning and soaking solution
    V. Wetting
Visante OCT
VISC
    vitreous infusion suction cutter
visceral
    v. larva migrans (VLM)
    v. larva migrans syndrome
    v. myopathy
viscoadaptive agent
viscoanesthesia
Viscoat solution
viscocanalostomy
viscodelamination
viscodissection
viscodissector
    v. tubing
    vitreoretinal v.
viscoelastic
    v. agent
    CoEase v.

NOTES

V

viscoelastic *(continued)*
    v. material
    Optimize v.
    v. product
    v. solution
Visco expression cannula
Viscoflow cannula
Viscolens lens
viscosimeter
    capillary tube plasma v.
viscosity
    high v.
viscosity-increasing agent
viscosurgical device
viscous
    v. fluid controller (VFC)
    Neo-Synephrine V.
    v. ochre fluid
    v. xanthochromic fluid
Visculose
Visian
    V. implantable collamer lens
    V. IOL
visibility
    v. acuity
    v. curve
visible
    v. drusen
    v. iris diameter (VID)
    v. spectrum
Visi-Drape
    V.-D. Elite ophthalmic drape
    V.-D. mini aperture drape
    V.-D. mini incise drape
Visiflex drape
visile
Visine
    V. AC
    Advanced Relief V.
    V. Extra Ophthalmic
    V. L.R.
    V. LR Ophthalmic
    V. Original
    V. Tears
    V. Tears PF
Visine-A
visio
    v. oculus dextra (vision of right eye) (VOD)
    v. oculus sinister (vision of left eye)
vision
    6/6 v.
    20/20 v.
    achromatic v.
    acuity of color v. (VC)
    ambulatory v.
    v. analyzer
    V. Analyzer/Overrefraction System

artificial v.
baseline v.
best corrected v.
binocular v.
binocular single v. (BSV)
blue v.
blurred v.
blurring of v.
botulism-induced blurred v.
V. Care enzymatic cleaner
central island of v.
central keyhole of v.
cerebral tunnel v.
chromatic v.
color v. (CV)
colored v.
cone v.
v. correction
V. Council of America (VCA)
counting fingers v.
crystal clear v.
day v.
decreasing v.
v. deprivation myopia
dichromatic v.
dimness of v.
direct v.
distance v.
distortion of v.
double v. (DV)
duplicity theory of v.
v., each eye (VOU)
eccentric v.
extramacular binocular v.
facial v.
false v.
field of v.
finger v.
finger-counting v.
fluctuating v.
form v.
foveal v.
functional v.
glare v.
green v.
half v.
halo v.
hand-motion v. (HMV)
haploscopic v.
hazy v.
Helmholtz theory of color v.
Hering theory of color v.
improved v.
indirect v.
iridescent v.
keyhole v.
line of v.
linear v.
loss of v.

v. loss
low v.
macular binocular v.
V. Master excimer laser system
misty v.
monocular v.
motion v.
multiple v.
naked v. (Nv)
near v.
night v.
no light perception v.
obscure v.
organ of v.
oscillating v.
painless blurred v.
painless progressive loss of v.
peripheral v.
persistence of v.
phantom v.
photopic v.
Pick v.
pinhole v.
V. in Preschoolers (VIP)
V. in Preschoolers Study
pseudoscopic v.
rainbow v.
reading v.
red v.
reduced v.
v. in reduced illumination
v. reduction
v. rehabilitation therapy
v. research
residual v.
v. response
v. restoration therapy
v. rod
rod v.
v. science
scotopic v.
v. screening
shaft v.
single binocular v. (SBV)
solid v.
stable v.
stereoscopic v.
subjective v.
subnormal v.
suboptimal v.
supernormal v.
V. Tech lens
tilted v.

tinted v.
v. training
transient obscuration of v.
triple v.
tubular v.
tunnel v.
twilight v.
upside-down reversal of v.
violet v.
word v.
yellow v.
VisionBlue
    V. ophthalmic agent
    V. ophthalmic solution
    V. syringe
    V. trypan blue 0.06% stain
vision-compromising lesion
vision-correcting contact lens
vision-limiting complication
vision-related
    v.-r. functional status
    v.-r. quality of life
vision-threatening
    v.-t. complication
    v.-t. vitreous hemorrhage
Visi-Spear eye sponge
Visitec
    V. angled lens hook
    V. aspiration unit
    V. capsule polisher curette
    V. Company lens
    V. corneal shield
    V. corneal suture manipulating hook
    V. cortex extractor
    V. double-cutting cystotome
    V. intraocular lens dialer
    V. iris retractor
    V. irrigating/aspirating cannula
    V. irrigating/aspirating unit
    V. lens pusher
    V. manipulator
    V. micro double-iris hook
    V. microhook
    V. microiris hook
    V. nucleus removal loupe
    V. RK zone marker
    V. straight lens hook
    V. surgical vitrectomy system
    V. vitrectomy unit
Visolett magnifier
Visometer
    Lotmar V.

V

NOTES

Vista
    Blue V.
Vistacon
Vistakon contact lens
Vistaquel
Vistaril
Vistazine
Vistech
    V. 6500 contrast test
    V. Multivision Contrast Tester 8000
    V. wall chart
Vistide
visual
    v. aberration
    v. ability subscale
    V. Activities Questionnaire (VAQ)
    v. acuity
    v. acuity decrease
    v. acuity recovery
    v. acuity testing
    v. agnosia
    v. allesthesia
    v. analog scale (VAS)
    v. angle
    v. aphasia
    v. association area
    v. attentiveness
    v. autism
    v. axis
    v. axis opacification
    v. behavior
    v. blackout
    v. cell
    v. challenge
    v. cone
    v. confusion
    v. corkscrew defect
    v. cortex
    v. cycle
    v. deprivation syndrome
    v. development
    v. direction
    v. disability
    v. discomfort
    v. discrimination
    v. discriminatory acuity (VDA)
    v. disturbance
    v. dysfunction
    v. efficiency (VE)
    v. electrophysiology
    v. ergonomics
    v. extinction
    v. field (F, VF)
    v. field change
    v. field criteria
    v. field damage
    v. field defect
    v. field finding
    v. field fluctuation
    v. field improvement
    v. field index
    v. field loss
    v. field progression
    v. field testing
    v. function
    v. function evaluation
    V. Function Questionnaire (VFQ)
    v. half-field (VHF)
    v. hallucination
    v. halo
    v. image
    v. impairment (VI)
    v. inattention
    v. line
    v. manipulation test
    v. memory
    v. metacognition
    v. metrics
    v. neglect
    v. orbicularis reflex
    v. organ
    v. outcome
    v. parameter
    v. paraneoplastic syndrome
    v. pathway
    v. pathway disease
    v. perception
    v. performance measure
    v. performance result
    v. perseveration
    v. pigment
    v. plane
    v. point
    v. preservation
    v. process
    v. prognosis
    v. projection
    v. psychophysics
    v. purple
    v. radiation
    v. rehabilitation
    v. resolution
    v. salvage
    v. seizure
    v. sensory system
    v. shimmering
    v. side effect
    v. spread
    v. stimulus
    v. threshold
    v. tilt
    v. violet
    v. white
    v. yellow
    v. zone
visual-deprivation amblyopia

visual-evoked
v.-e. cortical potential (VECP)
v.-e. potential (VEP)
v.-e. response (VER)
v.-e. response imaging system (VERIS)
visualization
contrast v.
double-contrast v.
visually
v. complex undertaking
v. evoked potential mapping
v. impaired child
v. impaired driver
v. insignificant infectious corneal ulcer
v. significant cataract
visual-motor integration
visual-spatial agnosia
Visual-Tech machine
visual-vestibulo-ocular response
Visucam nonmydriatic fundus camera
Visudyne
Visulab System
Visulas
V. argon C laser
V. argon/YAG laser
V. 532 Combi software
V. Combi 532/YAG laser
V. InterChange software
V. 532 laser
V. Nd:YAG laser
V. 690s PDT laser
V. YAG C, E, S laser
V. YAG II plus laser
VisuMed MEL60 laser
visuoauditory
visuognosis
visuopsychic
visuosensory
visuospatial disorder
Visuscope
V. motor
V. motor test
V. ophthalmoscope
V. sensory test
Visuskop
Visutron
Visx
V. contoured ablation method
V. Contoured Ablation Pattern
V. 2020 excimer laser
V. procedure

V. refractive planner
V. S2, S3 excimer laser
V. Star 3 excimer laser system
V. Star II stromal photoablation system
V. Star Reticule aiming beam
V. Star S3 ActiveTrak laser
V. Star S2 excimer laser system
V. Star S2 laser
V. Twenty/Twenty excimer laser
V. 20/20 version 4.01 vision keycard system
V. WaveScan
V. WaveScan wavefront system
Vit-A-Drops
VitaLase Er:YAG laser
vital dye
VitalEyes
vitallium
v. implant
v. miniplate
vitamin
v. A deficiency
v. A palmate
ICaps ocular v.
Ocuvite PreserVision v.'s
vitelliform
v. degeneration of macula
v. macular degeneration
v. macular dystrophy
v. maculopathy
v. retinal dystrophy
vitelline macular degeneration
vitelliruptive
v. degeneration
v. macular dystrophy
vitellirupture
vitiliginous
v. chorioretinitis
v. choroiditis
vitiligo, pl. vitiligines
v. iridis
perilimbal v.
v. uveitis
Vitrase
Vitrasert intravitreal implant
Vitravene
Vitrax
vitrea
lamina v.
membrana v.
vitreal
v. bleed

V

NOTES

vitreal *(continued)*
    v. hemorrhage
    v. lamina
    v. liquefaction
    v. membrane
vitrectomy
    anterior v.
    automated v.
    closed-system pars plana v.
    complete v.
    conventional pars plana v.
    core v.
    inside-out core v.
    v. instrument
    lens-sparing v.
    V. for Macular Hole Study
     (VMHS)
    manual v.
    no-suture v.
    open-sky v.
    pars plana Baerveldt tube insertion
     with v.
    pars plana posterior v.
    partial v.
    pneumatic v.
    port v.
    3-port pars plana v.
    posterior v.
    v. for proliferative retinopathy
    scissors v.
    v. sponge
    v. for subretinal cyst
    sutureless transconjunctival pars
     plana v.
    total v.
    transconjunctival sutureless v.
    Weck-cel v.
vitrector
    Alcon v.
    automated v.
    CooperVision v.
    Frigitronics v.
    guillotine v.
    Kaufman type II v.
    mechanical v.
    Microvit v.
    Storz Microvit v.
vitrector-cut anterior capsulectomy
vitrectorhexis
    anterior v.
vitrein
vitreitis
    dense v.
    idiopathic v.
    immune recovery v.
    senile v.
vitreocapsulitis
vitreociliary glaucoma
vitreofoveal separation

vitreolysis
    YAG v.
vitreomacular
    v. interface
    v. separation
    v. traction
    v. traction syndrome
Vitreon sterile intraocular fluid
vitreopapillary traction
vitreophage
    Kaufman v.
vitreoretinal (VR)
    v. adhesion
    v. aspirate
    v. attachment
    v. choroidopathy syndrome
    v. condensation
    v. contusion
    v. degeneration
    v. disorder
    v. dysplasia
    v. infusion cutter
    v. interface
    v. interface abnormality
    v. micropick
    v. pathology
    v. surgeon
    v. surgery
    v. tag
    v. traction
    v. traction syndrome
    v. tuft
    v. viscodissector
vitreoretinochoroidopathy
vitreoretinopathy
    anterior proliferative v. (APVR)
    closed-funnel v.
    erosive v.
    exudative v.
    familial exudative v. (FEVR)
    proliferative v. (PVR)
    proliferative diabetic v. (PDVR)
    release of traction for hypotony
     and v.
vitreoschisis
vitreotapetoretinal dystrophy
vitreous
    v. abscess
    absent v.
    anterior v.
    v. aspirating needle
    v. aspiration
    v. aspiration biopsy
    v. base
    v. block
    v. block glaucoma
    v. blood
    v. breakthrough hemorrhage
    v. bulge

v. cavity
v. cell
v. cells as indicator of retinal tears
v. cellular reaction
v. chamber
v. chamber of eye
v. clarity
v. clouding
v. coloboma
coloboma of v.
v. condensation
v. contraction
core v.
cortical v.
v. culture
detached v.
v. detachment
v. face
v. fiber
v. floater
v. fluff
v. fluorophotometry
v. foreign body
v. foreign body forceps
v. gel
v. haze
v. hemorrhage (VH)
v. hernia
v. herniation
v. humor
hyperplastic primary v.
v. inflammation
v. infusion suction cutter (VISC)
knuckle of loose v.
v. lacuna
v. lamina
liquified v.
loss of v.
v. loss
v. membrane
micelles in v.
v. microsurgery
v. neovascularization
v. opacification
v. opacity
organized v.
v. pencil
v. penetration
persistent anterior hyperplastic primary v.
persistent hyperplastic primary v. (PHPV)

persistent hypertrophic primary v. (PHPV)
persistent posterior hyperplastic primary v.
persistent primary hyperplastic v.
posterior v.
v. presentation
primary persistent hyperplastic v.
v. prolapse
puff of loose v.
v. retraction
secondary v.
v. seeding
v. separation
v. skirt
spontaneous extrusion of v.
v. strand
v. strand scissors
v. stroma
v. substitute
v. surgery
v. sweep spatula
syneresis of v.
syneretic v.
v. tap
tertiary v.
v. touch
v. traction
v. transplant needle
v. veil
v. wick syndrome
vitreous-aspirating cannula
vitreum
corpus v.
stroma v.
vitreus
humor v.
vitritis
vitronectin bind
vitrosin
Viva-Drops
V.-D. eye drops
V.-D. Solution
VKC
vernal keratoconjunctivitis
V-K-H
Vogt-Koyanagi-Harada
V-K-H syndrome
V-lance
V-l. blade
V-l. blade/knife
V-lancet knife

V

NOTES

VLM
 visceral larva migrans
VMD2 gene
VMHS
 Vitrectomy for Macular Hole Study
VOD
 visio oculus dextra (vision of right eye)
Vogel formula
Vogt
 V. cataract
 V. cornea
 V. degeneration
 V. disease
 limbal girdle of V.
 limbal palisades of V.
 V. line
 V. operation
 palisades of V.
 V. stria
 V. syndrome
 white limbal girdle of V.
 V. white limbal girdle
Vogt-Koyanagi
 V.-K. bilateral uveitis
 V.-K. syndrome
Vogt-Koyanagi-Harada (V-K-H)
 V.-K.-H. disease
 V.-K.-H. syndrome
Vogt-Spielmeyer
 V.-S. disease
 V.-S. syndrome
volitantes
 muscae v.
Volk
 V. aspheric lens
 V. conoid lens implant
 V. coronoid lens
 V. G Series lens
 V. high-resolution aspherical lens
 V. Minus noncontact adapter
 V. 3 mirror ANF+ lens
 V. 3 mirror gonio fundus laser lens
 V. Plus noncontact adapter cap and equipment
 V. quadraspheric lens
 V. retinal scale adapter
 V. SuperMacula 2.2 focal laser lens
 V. SuperQuad 160 contact lens
 V. SuperQuad 160 panretinal lens
 V. Transequator lens
 V. ultra field aspherical lens adapter
 V. yellow filter adapter
Volkmann cataract
Voltaren Ophthalmic
volume (V)
 choroidal blood v. (ChBVol)

 orbital v.
 tear v.
voluntary
 v. convergence
 v. convergency
 v. eye movement
 v. nystagmus
 v. saccadic oscillation
volvulosis
volvulus
 Onchocerca v.
von
 v. Arlt recess
 v. Gierke disease
 v. Graefe cataract knife
 v. Graefe cautery
 v. Graefe cystotome
 v. Graefe electrocautery
 v. Graefe fixation forceps
 v. Graefe iris forceps
 v. Graefe knife needle
 v. Graefe muscle hook
 v. Graefe operation
 v. Graefe prism dissociation method
 v. Graefe sign
 v. Graefe strabismus hook
 v. Graefe syndrome
 v. Graefe target
 v. Graefe technique
 v. Graefe tissue forceps
 v. Helmholtz eye model
 v. Hippel angioma
 v. Hippel disease
 v. Hippel internal corneal ulcer
 v. Hippel-Lindau disease
 v. Hippel-Lindau syndrome
 v. Hippel operation
 v. Kossa method
 v. Noorden incision
 v. Recklinghausen disease
 v. Recklinghausen syndrome
VOR
 vestibuloocular response
voriconazole
vortex, pl. **vortices**
 v. corneal dystrophy
 Fleischer v.
 v. keratopathy
 v. lentis
 v. pattern
 v. system
 v. vein
 v. vein varix
vortex-like clump
vorticosae
 vena v.
Vossius lenticular ring

VOU
    vision, each eye
V-pattern
        V-p. esotropia
        V-p. exotropia
VR
    vitreoretinal
VRD
    Virtual Retinal Display
VRR
    variable repetition rate
VRSQ
    Virtual Reality Symptom Questionnaire
VSG 2/3F graphic card
V-slit lamp

VSR
    venous stasis retinopathy
VSS
    variable spot scanning
Vuero meter
vulnificus
        v. keratitis
        Vibrio v.
V-Y advancement myotarsocutaneous flap for upper eyelid reconstruction
Vygantas-Wilder retinal drainage probe
VZV
    varicella zoster virus
        VZV dendrite
        VZV disciform lesion

NOTES

V

Waardenburg-Jonkers
    corneal dystrophy of W.-J.
    dystrophy of W.-J.
Waardenburg-Klein syndrome
Waardenburg syndrome
Wachendorf membrane
Wadsworth-Todd cautery
Wagner
    W. disease
    W. epiretinal membrane dissector
    W. hereditary vitreoretinal
      degeneration
    W. hyaloid retinal degeneration
    W. syndrome
    W. vitreoretinal dystrophy
Wagner-Stickler syndrome
waking ptosis
Waldeau fixation forceps
Waldeyer gland
Walker
    W. coagulator
    W. electrode
    W. lid everter
    W. micro pin
    W. scissors
    W. trephine
Walker-Apple scissors
Walker-Atkinson scissors
Walker-Lee sclerotome
Walker-Warburg syndrome
wall
    confluent lipid w.
    eye w.
    w. push maneuver
Wallach
    W. cryosurgery freezer
    W. cryosurgical pencil
    W. Ophthalmic Cryosurgery System
3-wall decompression
Wallenberg lateral medullary syndrome
wallerian degeneration
wall-eye
wall-eyed bilateral internuclear
    ophthalmoplegia (WEBINO)
Walser corneoscleral punch
Walton
    W. punch
    W. spud
wand
    angled Connor w.
    Connor angled w.
    Connor curved w.
    Connor straight irrigating w.
    Connor straight nonirrigating w.
    curved Connor w.

    Powell w.
    straight nonirrigating Connor w.
Wang lens
Warburg syndrome
wardrobe
    eyewear w.
warfarin sodium
warm compress
warmed fluid
warm-same
    cold-opposite, w.-s. (COWS)
warneri
    Staphylococcus w.
warpage
    contact lens-induced w.
    corneal w.
war-related injury
wart
    Hassall-Henle w.
    Henle w.
Warthin tumor
wartlike body
Wasca aberrometer
wash
    Eye W.
    Irrigate eye w.
    Lavoptik eye w.
    Star-Optic eye w.
Washington University road test
    (WURT)
washout
    anterior chamber w.
    color w.
water
    w. cell
    w. content
    w. fissure
    w. provocative test
water-based tinting system
water-bath ultrasonography
water-contact angle
water-drinking test
watered-silk retina
water-silk reflex
Waters view
watertight closure
watery
    w. discharge
    w. eye
Watt stave bender
Watzke
    W. band
    W. forceps
    W. sleeve
    W. tire

W

Watzke-Allen
> W.-A. sign
> W.-A. test

wave
> A w.
> w. aberration map
> B w.
> C w.
> continuous w. (CW)
> D w.
> heat-causing radiofrequency w.
> radiofrequency w.
> scotopic b w.
> The W. phacoemulsion system

wave-edge knife
waveform
> blood flow velocity w. (BFVW)
> pendular-jerk w.

wavefront
> w. aberration function
> w. aberrometer
> w. ablation pattern
> w. analysis
> convergent w.
> w. error
> w. map
> w. sensing
> w. sensor
> w. technology

wavefront-corrected IOL
wavefront-guided
> w.-g. ablation
> w.-g. laser eye surgery
> w.-g. LASIK

WaveFront System
wavelength
> sectoral w.
> violet w.

WaveScan
> Visx W.
> W. WaveFront System

waxy
> w. exudate
> w. lesion
> w. tumor

2-way
> 2-w. cataract-aspirating cannula
> 2-w. syringe
> 2-w. towel clip

W4D
> Worth 4-dot
> W4D test

WDSCL
> well-differentiated small-cell lymphoma

weakness
> zonular w.

wear
> enzymatic cleaner for extended w.

> orthokeratology lens w.
> protective sports eye w.

wearer
> contact lens w.

Weaver
> W. chalazion forceps
> W. trocar introducer

Weber
> W. knife
> W. law
> W. paralysis
> W. sign
> W. syndrome

Weber-Elschnig lens loupe
Weber-Gubler syndrome
web eye
WEBINO
> wall-eyed bilateral internuclear
> ophthalmoplegia

Webster needle holder
Weck
> W. eye shield
> W. knife
> W. microscope
> W. sponge
> W. trephine

Weck-cel
> W.-c. sponge
> W.-c. surgical spear
> W.-c. vitrectomy

Wecker iris scissors
wedge
> Livingston peribulbar w.
> w. resection
> temporal w.

Weeks
> W. bacillus
> W. needle

weeping eczematous lesion
Wegener granulomatosus conjunctivitis
WEH/CHOP
> Wills Eye Hospital/Children's Hospital of
> Philadelphia

Wehner spoon
Weibel-Palade body
Weigert ligament
weight
> birth w.
> Blinkeze external lid w.
> EyeClose external eyelid w.
> gold w.
> SutureGroove gold eyelid w.

Weil
> W. disease
> W. lacrimal cannula

Weil-Felix reaction
Weill-Marchesani syndrome
Weill-Reys-Adie syndrome
Weill-Reys syndrome

Weinstein
    W. fixation ring
    W. fixation ring and flap lifter
Weiss
    W. reflex
    W. remnant
    W. ring
    W. speculum
Welch
    W. Allyn SureSight autorefractor
    W. 4-drop device
Welch-Allyn
    W.-A. halogen penlight
    W.-A. ophthalmoscope
    W.-A. pocket scope
welchii
    Clostridium w.
welder's
    w. conjunctivitis
    w. keratoconjunctivitis
well
    alcohol w.
    LASEK alcohol w.
Welland test
well-centered IOL
well-differentiated small-cell lymphoma (WDSCL)
Wells enucleation spoon
Welsh
    W. cortex extractor
    W. cortex stripper cannula
    W. flat olive-tip
    W. flat olive-tip double cannula
    W. iris retractor
    W. pupil-spreader forceps
Werb
    W. right-angle probe
    W. scissors
Werdnig-Hoffmann disease
Werner
    W. syndrome
    W. test
Wernicke
    W. encephalopathy
    W. pupil
    W. radiation
    W. reaction
    W. sign
    W. symptom
    W. syndrome
    W. test
    W. triangle

Wernicke-Korsakoff
    W.-K. psychosis
    W.-K. syndrome
WESDR
    Wisconsin Epidemiologic Study of Diabetic Retinopathy
Wesley-Jessen lens
Wessely ring
West
    W. gouge
    W. Indian amblyopia
    W. lacrimal cannula
    W. lacrimal sac chisel
Westcott
    W. conjunctival scissors
    W. stitch scissors
    W. tenotomy scissors
    W. test
    W. utility scissors
Westergren method
Western
    W. blot
    W. immunoblotting analysis
Westphal
    W. phenomenon
    W. pupillary reflex
Westphal-Piltz
    W.-P. phenomenon
    W.-P. reflex
Westphal-Strümpell disease
wet
    w. ARMD
    w. cell
    w. dressing
    w. eye
    w. form
    w. form of age-related macular degeneration
    Lens W.
    w. mount
wet-field
    w.-f. cautery
    w.-f. diathermy
    w.-f. electrocautery
Wet-N-Soak
    W.-N.-S. Plus
wetting
    w. agent
    w. angle
    w. angle of contact lens
    Liquifilm W.
    w. solution
    Visalens W.

W

NOTES

Weyers-Thier syndrome
WF
   wide field
Whatman No. 1 qualitative-type filter paper
Wheeler
   W. blade
   W. cyclodialysis system
   W. cystotome
   W. discission knife
   W. eye sphere implant
   W. halving repair
   W. iris spatula
   W. method
   W. operation
   W. procedure
wheel rotation
whiplash retinopathy
whippelii
   Tropheryma w.
Whipple
   W. disc
   W. disease
white
   w. braided silk suture
   calcofluor w.
   w. cell
   w. dot
   w. dot syndrome
   w. of eye
   w. fundus reflex
   W. glaucoma pump shunt
   w. laser
   w. laser lesion
   w. light
   w. light tandem-scanning confocal microscope
   w. limbal girdle of Vogt
   w. pediatric cataract
   w. petroleum
   w. pigment
   w. pupil
   w. pupillary reflex
   w. pupil sign
   w. retinal necrosis
   w. ring
   w. ring of cornea
   w. sclera
   w. spot
   w. stromal infiltrate
   visual w.
   w. without pressure
white-centered hemorrhage
white-eyed blowout fracture
whitening
   ischemic retinal w.
   retinal w.
white-on-white perimetry

WhiteStar
   W. power modulation system
   W. power modulation technology
white-to-white measurement
Whitnall
   W. ligament
   W. sling operation
   W. tubercle
Whitney superior rectus forceps
Whitten fixation ring
whole-globe enucleation
whorled corneal opacities
whorling
   corneal w.
whorl lens
whorl-like configuration
wick
   filtering w.
wicking glue patch
wide-angle
   w.-a. glaucoma
   w.-a. viewing system
wide field (WF)
wide-field eyepiece
widening
   palpebral fissure w.
widespread diffuse corneal edema
Widmark conjunctivitis
Widowitz sign
width
   angle w.
   anterior chamber angle w.
   curve w.
   orbital w.
Wieger ligament
Wiener
   W. corneal hook
   W. keratome
   W. scleral hook
Wies
   W. chalazion forceps
   W. operation
   W. procedure
Wilbrand prism test
Wilcoxon
   W. matched pairs test
   W. signed rank test
wild
   W. lens
   W. operating microscope
Wilde forceps
Wilder
   W. band spreader
   W. cystotome
   W. cystotome knife
   W. lacrimal dilator
   W. lens loupe
   W. scleral depressor
   W. scleral retractor

W. scoop
W. sign
Wildervanck syndrome
**Wilkerson intraocular lens-insertion
forceps**
Williams
W. pediatric eye speculum
W. probe
Willis
circle of W.
Wills
W. Eye Hospital
W. Eye Hospital/Children's Hospital
of Philadelphia (WEH/CHOP)
W. Hospital utility forceps
W. utility eye forceps
Wilmer
W. Cataract Photo-grading System
W. conjunctival scissors
W. Eye Institute
W. Ophthalmological Institute
Wilms tumor
Wilson
W. degeneration
W. disease
W. syndrome
Wiltmoser optical arm
Wincor enucleation scissors
wind-blown contaminant
window
clear w.
w. defect
reverse action w.
scleral w.
windshield wiper syndrome
wing cell
winking
jaw w.
w. spasm
wink reflex
Winslow star
Winter Helping Hand
Wintersteiner rosette
wipe débridement
wipe-out
w.-o. phenomenon
w.-o. syndrome
Wipes-SPF
Lid W.-S.
wire
cheese w.
w. enucleation snare
w. frame spectacles

Kirschner w.
w. lid speculum
w. mesh implant
Ultra-select nitinol guide w.
wire-loop keratoscope
wiring
copper w.
interosseous w.
Wirt
W. stereopsis test
W. stereo test
W. vision test
Wisconsin
W. age-related maculopathy grading
system
W. Epidemiologic Study of
Diabetic Retinopathy (WESDR)
wise
W. iridotomy laser lens
W. iridotomy-sphincterotomy laser
lens
with
w. contact lenses (c̄cl)
w. correction (cc)
w. motion
Witherspoon vertical scissors
without
w. correction (s̄c)
w. glasses
with-the-rule (WTR)
w.-t.-r. astigmatism
wobbly eye
Wolfe
W. forceps
W. graft
W. method
Wolfram syndrome
Wolfring
accessory lacrimal gland of W.
gland of W.
W. lacrimal gland
Wolf syndrome
Wollaston
W. doublet
W. theory
Wood
W. lamp
W. lens
W. light examination
wooden swab
Woods Concept lens
wool saturated in saline dressing

W

NOTES

word
>w. blindness
>w. vision

working lens

workstation
>Light Blade laser w.
>Tomey refractive w.

workup
>preoperative w.

World Health Organization classification of trachoma

worse eye

Worst
>W. Claw lens
>W. goniotomy lens
>W. implantation forceps
>W. medallion lens
>W. pigtail probe
>W. Platina iris-fixated lens
>W. suture

Wort circle

Worth
>W. amblyoscope
>W. concept of fusion
>W. 4-dot (W4D)
>W. 4-dot near flashlight test
>W. strabismus forceps

wound
>w. apposition
>w. closure
>w. dehiscence
>w. edge
>full-thickness corneal w.

>w. gape
>gunshot w.
>w. healing phenomenon
>w. management
>ocular gunshot w.
>open-sky cataract w.
>penetrating scleral w.
>puncture w.

wrap-a-round eye shield

Wratten filter

wreath
>ciliary w.
>w. pattern stromal infiltrate

Wright
>W. fascia needle
>W. ophthalmic needle

wrinkle filler

wrinkling
>epithelial w.
>macular surface w.
>w. membrane
>w. PCO
>retinal w.

writer
>braille w.

WTR
>with-the-rule
>WTR astigmatism

Wundt-Lamansky law

WURT
>Washington University road test

Wyburn-Mason syndrome

Wydase

X
exophoria
X cell

x
axis of cylindric lens
x axis
4x 4 gauze dispenser
Xalatan
Xalcom
xanthelasma
x. around eyelid
florid x.
x. palpebrarum
xanthelasmatosis bulbi
xanthism
xanthochromic fluid
xanthocyanopsia
xanthogranuloma
juvenile x. (JXG)
juvenile iris x.
necrobiotic x.
uveal juvenile x.
xanthogranulomatosis
xanthokyanopy
xanthoma
x. elasticum
x. palpebrarum
x. planum
xanthomatosis
x. bulbi
cerebrotendinous x.
xanthophane
xanthophyll pigment
xanthopsia, xanthopia
xanthopsin
X-Chrom contact lens
Xe
xenon
xenon (Xe)
x. arc
x. arc photocoagulation
x. arc photocoagulator
x. endoillumination
x. illumination system
xenophthalmia
xeroderma
x. of Kaposi
x. pigmentosa syndrome
x. pigmentosum
xeroma
xerophthalmia
xerophthalmic ulcer
xerophthalmus
xeroscope grid distortion

xerosis
x. conjunctivae
conjunctival x.
x. of cornea
corneal x.
Corynebacterium x.
xerotic
x. degeneration
x. keratitis
X-esotropia
X-exotropia
XFS
exfoliation syndrome
Xibrom
X-linked
X-l. achromatopsia
X-l. blue cone monochromatism
X-l. cone
X-l. cone dystrophy
X-l. congenital cataract
X-l. congenital night blindness
X-l. fashion
X-l. inheritance
X-l. juvenile retinopathy
X-l. juvenile retinoschisis
X-l. recessive retinoschisis
X-l. retinitis
X-l. retinitis pigmentosa (XLRP)
X-l. retinoschisis (XLRS)
XLRP
X-linked retinitis pigmentosa
XLRS
X-linked retinoschisis
Xomed Surgical Products
XP
exophoria
X-pattern
X-p. esotropia
X-p. exotropia
x-ray
orbital x-r.
polytome x-r.
stereo x-r.
x-ray-induced cataract
Xsorb punctal plug
X-strabismus
XT
exotropia
X(T)
intermittent exotropia
Xylocaine with epinephrine
xylosoxidans
Alcaligenes x.

X

Y

Y cell
Y hook
Y suture

y

y axis

YAG

yttrium-aluminum-garnet
YAG cyclocryotherapy
YAG laser
YAG laser capsulotomy
YAG laser cyclophotocoagulation
YAG laser disruption
YAG posterior capsulotomy
YAG vitreolysis

Yaghouti LASIK polisher
Yale

Y. Luer-Lok
Y. Luer-Lok needle
Y. Luer-Lok syringe

Yamagishi viscocanalostomy cannula
Yannuzzi fundus laser lens
Yasuma protocol
Yates correction
YC 1400 Ophthalmic YAG laser system
year

quality-adjusted life y. (QALY)

yellow

y. blindness
y. dye laser
indicator y.
y. light reflex
y. point
y. spot (YS)
y. spot of retina
y. vision
visual y.

yellow-mutant oculocutaneous albinism
yellow-ochre hemorrhage
yellow-white choroidal mass
yield

lens to y.

yoke

y. movement
y. muscle

Yorktown-style designer series display
Youens lens
Young-Helmholtz color vision theory
Young theory of light
YS

yellow spot

Y-suture of crystalline lens
yttrium-aluminum-garnet (YAG)

y.-a.-g. laser

Z

Z axis of Fick
Z band
Z marginal tenotomy
Z myotomy

Zaditen
Zaditor ophthalmic solution
Zaldivar

Z. anterior procedure (ZAP)
Z. degree gauge
Z. iridectomy forceps
Z. iridectomy scissors
Z. knife
Z. limbal-relaxing incision system
Z. LRI marker
Z. micro acrylic lens implantation forceps
Z. reverse capsulorrhexis forceps

Z-alpha lens
ZAP

Zaldivar anterior procedure
ZAP diamond knife

Z-axis elevation
zeaxanthin
Zeeman effect
Zeis

gland of Z.
Z. gland

zeisian

z. gland
z. sty

Zeiss

Z. carbon arc slit lamp
Z. cine adapter
Z. DAS-1 hydrophobic system
Z. FF450 fundus camera
Z. fiberoptic illumination system
Z. goniolens
Z. gonioscope
Z. IOL Master laser interferometer
Z. LA 110 projection Lensmeter
Z. lens
Z. OM-3 operating microscope
Z. operating field loupe
Z. ophthalmoscope
Z. OpMi-6 FR microscope
Z. photocoagulator
Z. slit-lamp series
Z. vertex refractometer
Z. Visulas 532, 532s laser
Z. Visulas 690s laser
Z. Visulas YAG II laser

Zeiss-Barraquer

Z.-B. cine microscope
Z.-B. surgical microscope

Zeiss-Comberg slit lamp
Zeiss-Gullstrand loupe
Zeiss-Humphrey 840 UBM scanner
Zeiss-Nordenson fundus camera
Zellballen pattern
Zellweger syndrome
Zenapax
zenarestat
Zephiran
Zernike

Z. algorithm
Z. coefficient
Z. decomposition
Z. polynomial

zero

z. optical power
z. power lens
z. vergence

Zestril
zidovudine
Ziegler

Z. blade
Z. cautery
Z. cilia forceps
Z. electrocautery
Z. iris knife needle
Z. knife
Z. lacrimal dilator
Z. probe
Z. puncture
Z. speculum

Zimmerman tumor
Zinacef
zinc

z. acetate
z. bacitracin
bacitracin z.
z. sulfate
z. sulfate solution

Zincfrin
Zinn

anulus of Z.
circle of Z.
Z. circlet
Z. corona
Z. ligament
Z. membrane
Z. ring
Z. tendon
zone of Z.
zonule of Z.
Z. zonule

Zinn-Haller arterial circle
zipped angle
zipper stitch

Z

zippy estimating by sequential testing
Zithromax
zithromycin
Zöllner
  Z. figure
  Z. line
zona, pl. **zonae**
  z. ciliaris
  z. ophthalmica
zonal granuloma
zone
  ablation z.
  anterior optic z.
  apical z.
  z. B-cell lymphoma
  blur z.
  Bowman z.
  capillary-free z.
  central steep z.
  choroidal watershed z.
  ciliary z.
  z. of contact lens
  z. of discontinuity
  z. 1 disease
  extravisual z.
  fissure z.
  foveal avascular z. (FAZ)
  interpalpebral z.
  junctional z.
  lens z.
  limbal z.
  markers for z.
  nasal z.
  neutral z.
  nuclear z.
  null z.
  optical z. (OZ)
  z. of penetration
  posterior optical z. (POZ)
  pupillary z.
  retinal z.
  temporal z.
  transition z.
  transitional z.
  visual z.
  z. of Zinn
Zone-Quick
  Z.-Q. tear test
  Z.-Q. tear volume testing
zonula, pl. **zonulae**
  z. adherens
  z. ciliaris
  z. occludens
zonular
  z. attachment
  z. band
  z. damage
  z. dialysis
  z. disruption

  z. fiber
  z. keratitis
  z. nuclear cataract
  z. pulverulent cataract
  z. scotoma
  z. space
  z. stress
  z. support
  z. sutural cataract
  z. tension
  z. tetany
  z. weakness
zonulares
  fibrae z.
zonular-friendly technique
zonularia
  spatia z.
zonular-traction retinal tuft
zonule
  ciliary z.
  defective z.
  lens z.
  loose z.
  missing z.
  Zinn z.
  z. of Zinn
zonulitis
zonulolysis, zonulysis
  Barraquer z.
  enzymatic z.
zonulotomy
zonulysis
zoom
  Z. and Sniper sports goggles
  z. system
zoster
  z. sine herpete
  z. uveitis
Zostrix
Zovirax
Zuckerkandl dehiscence
Zurich suturing forceps
Z-View aberrometer
zygoma
zygomatic
  z. bone
  z. foramen
  z. foramen of Arnold
  z. fracture
  z. nerve
  z. suture
zygomaticofacial
  z. canal
  z. foramen
  z. nerve
zygomaticofrontal suture
zygomaticomaxillary suture
zygomaticoorbital
  z. artery

z. foramen
z. process
z. process of maxilla
zygomaticosphenoid suture
zygomaticotemporal
z. canal
z. foramen
z. nerve
z. suture
zygomaticus
nervus z.

zygomycosis
Zylet
Z. ophthalmic solution
Z. ophthalmic suspension
Zymar ophthalmic solution
Zyoptix
Z. customized eye surgery
Z. excimer laser system
Z. Infinity laser
Zyrtec
Zywave II aberrometer

NOTES

Z

587

Contents: The Appendices

Anatomical Illustrations

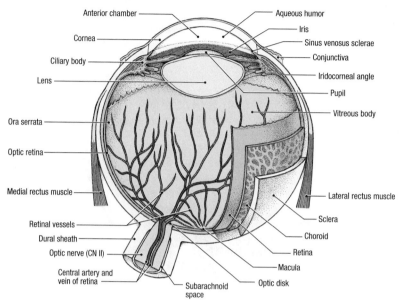

Structure of the eye.

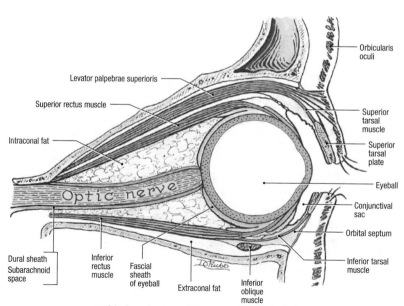

Orbital contents and upper eyelid, sagittal view.

Appendix 1

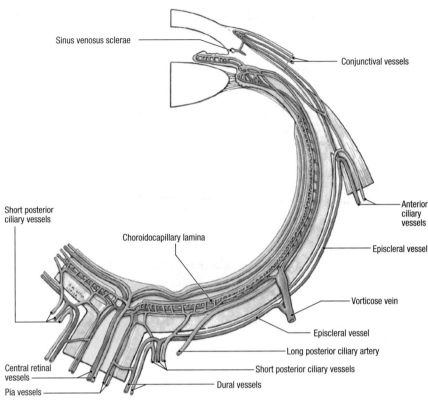

Blood supply to the eyeball.

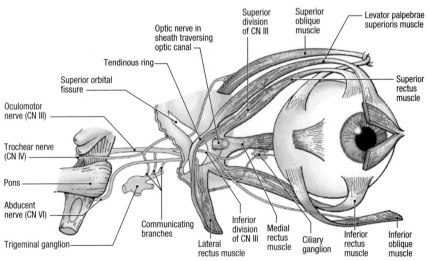

Distribution of ocular cranial nerves.

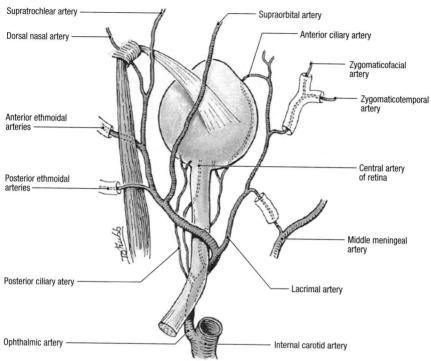

Supratrochlear artery

Dorsal nasal artery

Anterior ethmoidal arteries

Posterior ethmoidal arteries

Posterior ciliary atery

Ophthalmic artery

Supraorbital artery

Anterior ciliary artery

Zygomaticofacial artery

Zygomaticotemporal artery

Central artery of retina

Middle meningeal artery

Lacrimal artery

Internal carotid artery

Ophthalmic arteries.

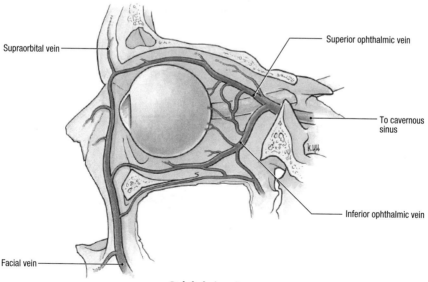

Supraorbital vein

Facial vein

Superior ophthalmic vein

To cavernous sinus

Inferior ophthalmic vein

Ophthalmic veins.

A3

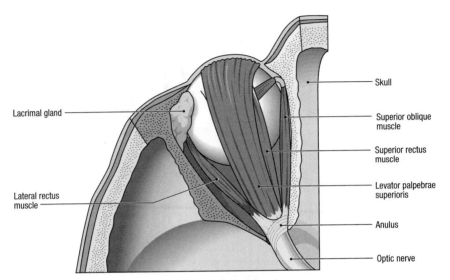

Skull

Lacrimal gland

Superior oblique muscle

Superior rectus muscle

Levator palpebrae superioris

Lateral rectus muscle

Anulus

Optic nerve

Orbital cavity, superior view.

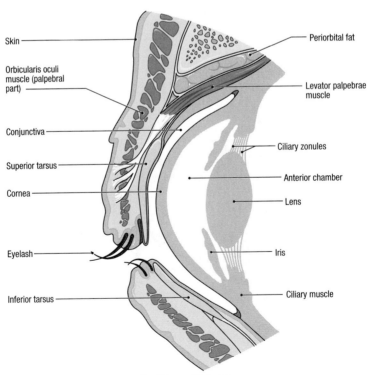

Skin

Periorbital fat

Orbicularis oculi muscle (palpebral part)

Levator palpebrae muscle

Conjunctiva

Ciliary zonules

Superior tarsus

Anterior chamber

Cornea

Lens

Eyelash

Iris

Inferior tarsus

Ciliary muscle

Eyelids, sagittal view.

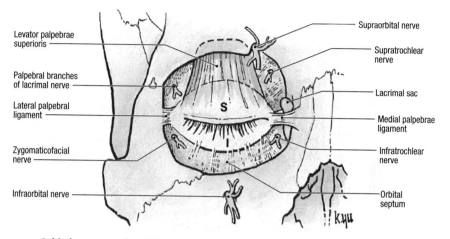

Orbital septum and eyelid, anterior view. (S) Superior and (I) inferior tarsal plates.

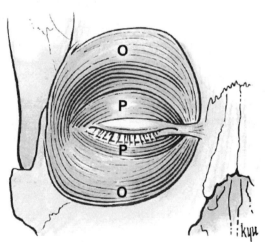

Orbicularis oculi, anterior view. (O) Orbital parts of the orbicularis oculi, (P) palpebral parts of the orbicularis oculi.

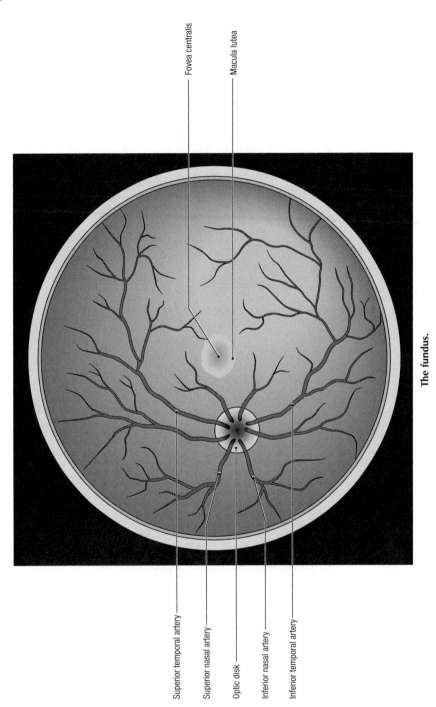

Fovea centralis

Macula lutea

Superior temporal artery

Superior nasal artery

Optic disk

Inferior nasal artery

Inferior temporal artery

The fundus.

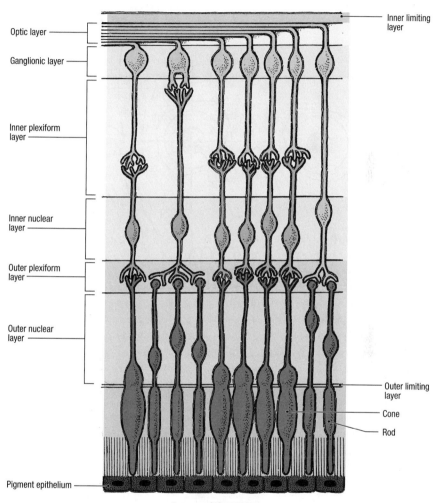

Inner limiting layer

Optic layer

Ganglionic layer

Inner plexiform layer

Inner nuclear layer

Outer plexiform layer

Outer nuclear layer

Outer limiting layer

Cone

Rod

Pigment epithelium

Layers of the retina.

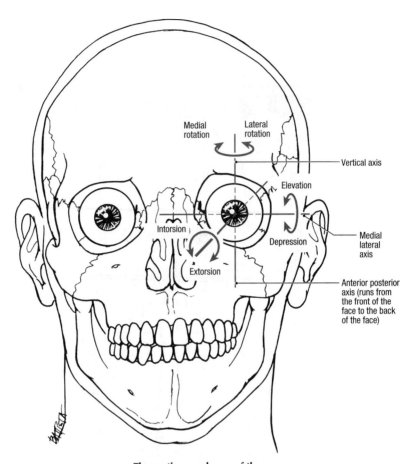

The motions and axes of the eye.

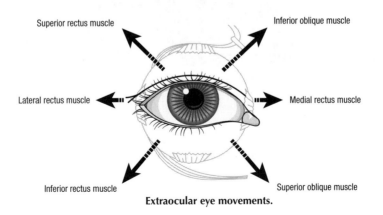

Extraocular eye movements.

Movements of the Eyes and the Muscles Employed

Sideways motion (ab- and adduction)	Vertical motion	Oblique motion	Rolling motion
Dextroversion	**Elevation (lifting)**	**Dextroelevation**	**Extorsion (outward rolling)**
Right eye: lateral rectus	Superior rectus	Right eye: superior rectus	Inferior rectus
Left eye: medial rectus	Inferior oblique	Left eye: inferior oblique	Inferior oblique
Levoversion	**Depression (lowering)**	**Dextrodepression**	**Intorsion (inward rolling)**
Right eye: medial rectus	Inferior rectus	Right eye: inferior rectus	Superior rectus
Left eye: lateral rectus	Inferior oblique	Left eye: superior oblique	Superior oblique
		Levoelevation	
		Left eye: superior rectus	
		Right eye: inferior oblique	
		Levodepression	
		Left eye: inferior rectus	
		Right eye: superior oblique	

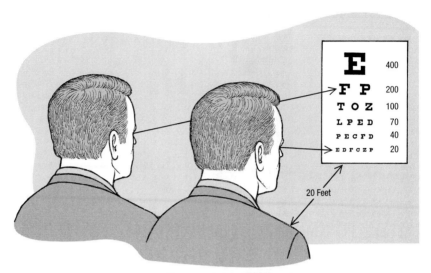

Snellen test of visual acuity.

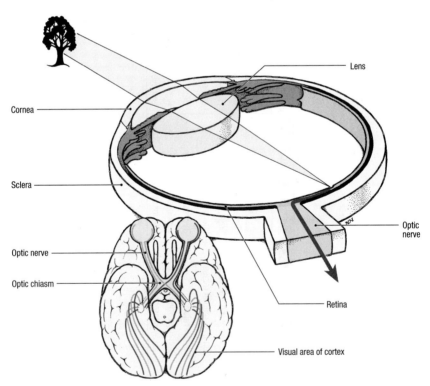

Vision. Light passes through the cornea and is focused onto the retina by the lens. Cells in the retina then transmit this information through the optic nerve to the visual area of the cortex.

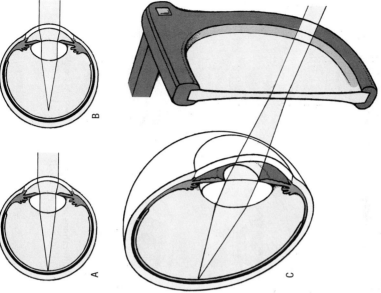

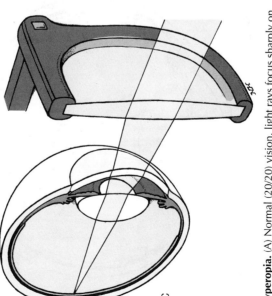

Myopia. (A) Normal (20/20) vision, light rays focus sharply on retina. (B) Myopic (nearsighted) vision, light rays from a distance come to a sharp focus in front of the retina. (C) Myopia corrected by eyeglasses with concave lenses.

Hyperopia. (A) Normal (20/20) vision, light rays focus sharply on retina. (B) Hyperopic (farsighted) vision, light rays from close objects come to a sharp focus behind the retina. (C) Hyperopia corrected by eyeglasses with convex lenses.

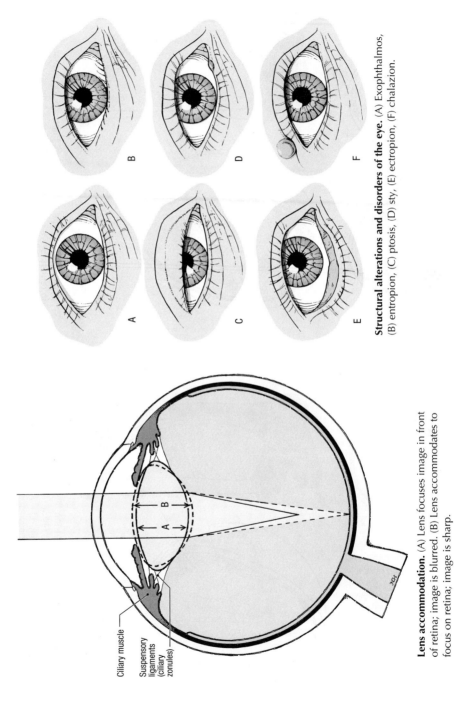

Structural alterations and disorders of the eye. (A) Exophthalmos, (B) entropion, (C) ptosis, (D) sty, (E) ectropion, (F) chalazion.

Lens accommodation. (A) Lens focuses image in front of retina; image is blurred. (B) Lens accommodates to focus on retina; image is sharp.

Ciliary muscle

Suspensory ligaments (ciliary zonules)

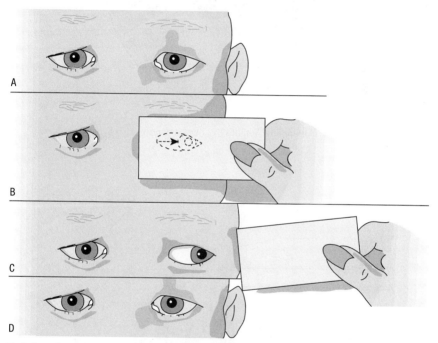

Technique for cover test to test for exophoria (misalignment). (A) Child's eyes appear to be in good alignment. (B) Left eye is then covered for 5 seconds. (C) When card is removed, left eye moves back to alignment. (D) This "drifting" indicates a misalignment.

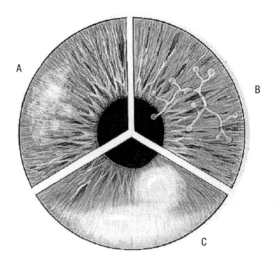

Corneal ulcers. (A) Marginal keratitis, (B) herpes dendrite, (C) hypopyon ulcer.

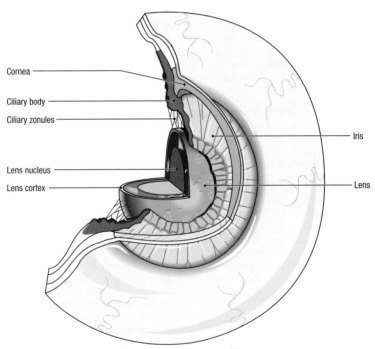

Cornea

Ciliary body

Ciliary zonules

Iris

Lens nucleus

Lens cortex

Lens

Cataract. Note opacity of lens.

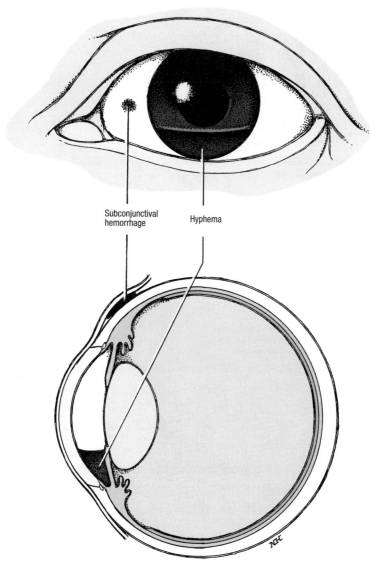

Hyphema (anterior chamber hemorrhage) and subconjunctival hemorrhage.

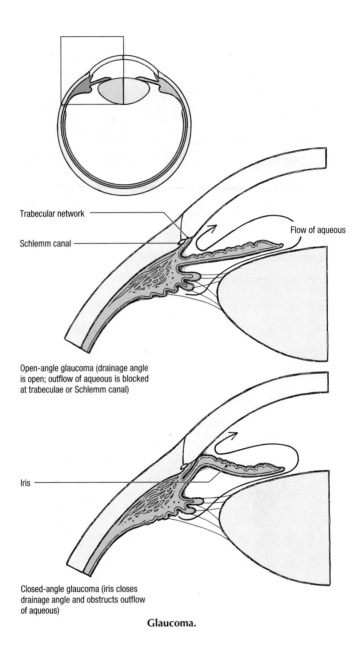

Trabecular network

Schlemm canal

Flow of aqueous

Open-angle glaucoma (drainage angle
is open; outflow of aqueous is blocked
at trabeculae or Schlemm canal)

Iris

Closed-angle glaucoma (iris closes
drainage angle and obstructs outflow
of aqueous)

Glaucoma.

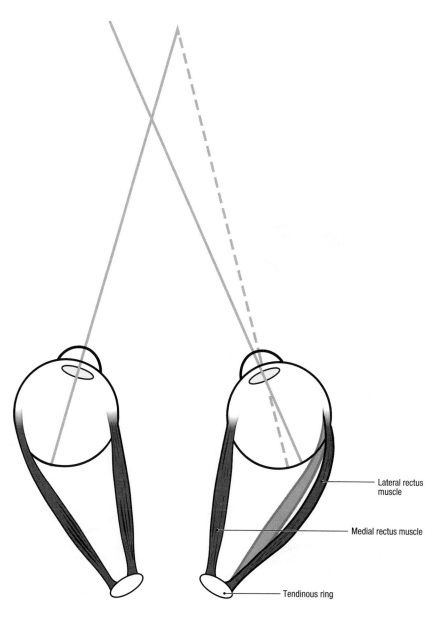

Lateral rectus
muscle

Medial rectus muscle

Tendinous ring

Diagram of the condition of strabismus, where one eye cannot focus with the other.
View of eyeballs and their musculature from above with lines of vision indicated. Note
that right eye has an elongated muscle that does not allow it to turn the eyeball far
enough to focus on a point in the distance.

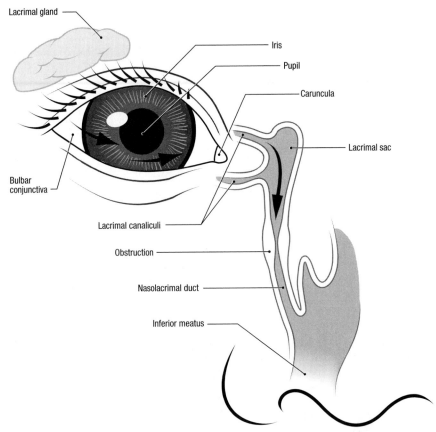

Obstructed lacrimal apparatus. Tears are secreted by the lacrimal gland. Tears, after passing over the eyeball, drain into the lacrimal sac. The nasolacrimal duct is obstructed, preventing tears from emptying into the inferior meatus of the nose and causing inflammation.

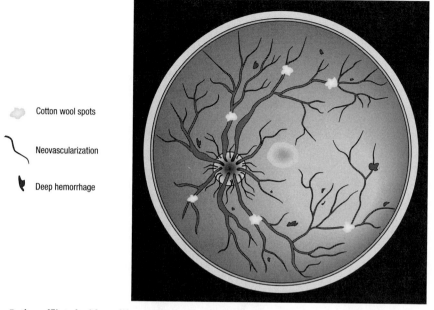

Cotton wool spots

Neovascularization

Deep hemorrhage

Retina afflicted with proliferative diabetic retinopathy as seen through an ophthalmoscope.

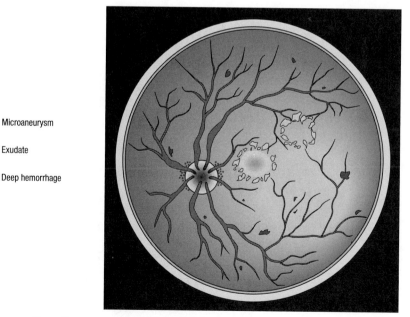

Microaneurysm

Exudate

Deep hemorrhage

The retina as seen through an ophthalmoscope. Retina shows various characteristics associated with background diabetic retinopathy.

Anatomical Illustrations

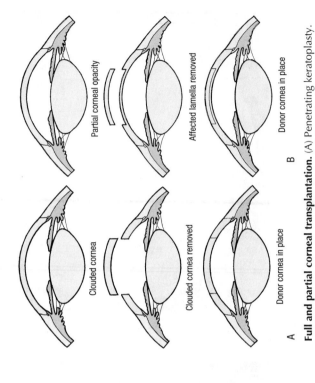

Full and partial corneal transplantation. (A) Penetrating keratoplasty. A full-thickness (7 to 8 mm) disk is removed from the host and replaced with a matching full-thickness button from the donor. (B) Lamellar keratoplasty. A thin layer of corneal tissue is excised from the host eye, sparing the stroma and entire endothelium.

A
- Clouded cornea
- Clouded cornea removed
- Donor cornea in place

B
- Partial corneal opacity
- Affected lamella removed
- Donor cornea in place

Intraocular lens implant insertion into the anterior chamber of the eye.

- Iris
- Incision
- Lens implant

Appendix 2
Cranial Nerves

1. Nerves of the Head and Neck Region

Nerve	Origin	Course	Innervation
Abducent	Pons	Intradural on clivus; traverses cavernous sinus and superior orbital fissure to enter orbit	Lateral rectus
Ansa cervicalis	Hypoglossal	Descends on external surface of carotid sheath	Omohyoid, sternohyoid, and sternothyroid
Deep petrosal	Internal carotid plexus	Traverses cartilages of foramen lacerum, joins greater petrosal nerve at entrance of pterygoid canal	Lacrimal gland, mucosa of nasal cavity, palate, and upper pharynx
Glossopharyngeal	Rostral end of medulla	Exits cranium via jugular foramen, passes between superior and middle constrictors of pharynx to tonsillar fossa, enters posterior third of tongue	Somatic to stylopharyngeus; visceral to parotid gland; sensory of posterior tongue, pharynx, tympanic cavity, auditory tube, carotid body, and sinus
Great auricular	Cervical plexus	Ascends over sternocleidomastoid; anterior and parallel to external jugular	Skin of auricle, adjacent scalp, and over angle of jaw
Greater occipital	Medial branch of posterior ramus of spinal nerve C2	Pierces deep muscles of neck and trapezius to ascend posterior scalp to vertex	Posterior scalp
Greater petrosal	Genu of facial nerve	Exits facial canal via hiatus for greater petrosal nerve	Pterygoid ganglion for innervation of lacrimal, nasal, palatine, and upper pharyngeal mucous glands

(continued)

Nerve	Origin	Course	Innervation
Hypoglossal	Between pyramid and olive of myelencephalon	Hypoglossal canal, medial to angle of mandible, between mylohyoid and hypoglossus to muscles of tongue	Intrinsic and extrinsic muscles of tongue
Intermediate	Facial nerve	Acoustic meatus to distal end of facial nerve	Pterygopalatine and submandibular ganglia via greater petrosal nerve, chorda tympani; tongue and palate
Lesser occipital	Cervical plexus	Parallel to anterosuperior border of sterno-cleidomastoid	Skin of posterior surface of auricle and adjacent scalp
Lesser petrosal	Tympanic plexus	Tympanic cavity to middle cranial fossa; sphenopetrosal fissure or foramen ovale	Otic ganglion for secretomotor innervation of parotid gland
Long thoracic	Anterior rami	Distally on external surface of serratus anterior	Serratus anterior
Nerve to mylohyoid	Inferior alveolar nerve	Inferior alveolar nerve of mandibular foramen to groove on medial aspect of ramus of mandible	Mylohyoid and anterior belly of digastric muscle
Nerve to tensor tympani	Otic ganglion	Cartilaginous portion of pharyngotympanic tube to semicranial of tensor tympani	Tensor tympani
Nerve to tensor veli palatini	Anterior mandibular nerve	Branch of nerve to medial pterygoid	Tensor veli palatini
Olfactory	Olfactory cells in olfactory epithelium of roof of nasal cavity	Foramen of cribriform plate to ethmoid, to olfactory bulbs	Olfactory mucosa; sense of smell
Phrenic	Cervical plexus	Superior thoracic aperture between mediastinal pleura and pericardium	Diaphragm; pericardial sac, mediastinal pleura, diaphragmatic peritoneum

(*continued*)

Nerve	Origin	Course	Innervation
Posterior inferior nasal	Greater palatine	Greater palatine canal through plate of palatine bone meatuses	Mucosa of inferior concha and walls of inferior and middle
Subclavian	Brachial plexus	Posterior to clavicle, anterior to brachial plexus and subclavian artery	Subclavius; sternoclavicular joint
Supraclavicular, lateral, intermediate, and medial	Cervical plexus	Center or posterior border of sternocleido-mastoid; fan out as they descend into lower neck, upper thorax, and shoulder	Skin of lower anterolateral neck, uppermost thorax, and shoulder
Supraorbital	Frontal nerve	Supraorbital foramen, breaks up into small branches of forehead	Mucous membrane of frontal sinus, conjunctivae, and skin
Suprascapular	Brachial plexus	Posterior triangle of neck; under superior transverse scapular ligament	Supraspinatus, infraspinatus muscles; superior and posterior glenohumeral joint
Supratrochlear	Facial nerve	Supraorbital nerve, divides into two or more branches	Skin in middle of forehead to hairline
Transverse cervical	Cervical plexus	Posterior border of sternocleido-mastoid muscle, runs anteriorly across muscle	Skin overlying anterior triangle of neck
Trochlear	Dorsolateral aspect of mesocephalon below inferior colliculus	Passes around brainstem to enter dura in edge of tentorium close to posterior clinoid process; runs in lateral wall of cavernous sinus, entering orbit via superior orbital fissures	Superior oblique muscle
Upper subscapular	Brachial plexus	Posteriorly enters subscapularis	Superior portion of subscapularis

2. Nerves of the Facial Region

Nerve	Origin	Course	Innervation
Auriculotemporal	Mandibular nerve	Passes between neck of mandible and external acoustic meatus to accompany superficial temporal artery	Skin anterior to auricle, posterior temporal region, tragus, helix of auricle, exterior acoustic meatus, upper tympanic membrane
Buccal	Mandibular nerve	Infratemporal fossa, passes anteriorly to reach cheek	Skin and mucosa of cheek, buccal gingiva
Chorda tympani	Facial nerve	Traverses tympanic cavity, passes between incus and malleus; exits temporal bone via petrotympanic fissure; enters infratemporal fossa, merges with lingual nerve	Submandibular and sublingual glands; taste sensation from anterior tongue
Deep temporal	Mandibular nerve	Temporal fossa to temporalis muscle	Temporalis; periosteum of temporal fossa
External nasal	Anterior ethmoidal nerve	Runs in nasal cavity and emerges on face between nasal bone and lateral nasal cartilage	Skin on dorsum of nose, including tip of nose
Facial	Posterior border of pons	Runs through internal acoustic meatus and facial canal of petrous part of temporal bone, exiting via stylomastoid foramen; intraparotid plexus	Stapedius, posterior belly of digastric, stylohyoid facial and scalp muscles; skin of external acoustic meatus
Greater palatine	Branch of pterygopalatine ganglion (maxillary nerve)	Passes inferiorly through greater palatine canal and foramen	Palatine glands; mucosa of hard palate

(continued)

Nerve	Origin	Course	Innervation
Inferior alveolar	Terminal branch of posterior mandibular nerve	Lateral and medial pterygoid muscles of infratemporal fossa to enter mandibular canal of mandible	Lower teeth, periodontium, periosteum, and gingiva of lower jaw
Infraorbital	Terminal branch of maxillary nerve	Runs in floor of orbit and emerges at infraorbital foramen	Skin of cheek, lower lid, lateral side of nose and inferior septum and upper lip, upper premolar incisors and canine teeth; mucosa of maxillary sinus and upper lip
Lesser palatine	Pterygopalatine ganglion (maxillary nerve)	Passes inferiorly through palatine canal and lesser palatine foramen	Glands of soft palate; mucosa of soft palate
Lingual	Terminal branch of posterior mandibular nerve	Joins chorda tympani, passes anteroinferiorly between lateral and medial pterygoid muscles, oral cavity	Submandibular ganglion and submandibular and sublingual salivary glands
Mandibular	Trigeminal ganglion	Foramen ovale to infratemporal fossa, divides into anterior and posterior trunks, ramifying into smaller branches, bifurcating into lingual and inferior alveolar nerve	Muscles of mastication, mylohyoid, anterior belly of digastric, tensor tympanic, tensor veli palatini; skin overlying mandible, teeth, gingiva, tongue, and temporo-mandibular joint
Masseteric	Mandibular nerve	Passes laterally through mandibular notch	Masseter; temporo-mandibular joint
Maxillary	Trigeminal nerve	Anteriorly through foramen rotundum, to pterygopalatine fossa, sends roots to pterygoid ganglion (maxillary nerve); continues anteriorly through infraorbital fissures as infraorbital nerve	Pterygopalatine ganglion, lacrimal gland, mucosal glands of nasal cavity, palate, and upper pharynx; skin overlying maxillary mucosa of posteroinferior nasal cavity, maxillary sinus, upper half of mouth (teeth, gingiva and mucosa of palate, vestibule and cheek)

(continued)

Cranial Nerves

Nerve	Origin	Course	Innervation
Mental	Terminal branch of inferior alveolar nerve	Mandibular canal at mental foramen	Skin of chin; skin and mucosa of lower lip
Nasopalatine	Pterygopalatine ganglion (maxillary nerve)	Exits pterygopalatine fossa via sphenopalatine foramen; runs anteroinferiorly across nasal septum, to incisive foramen to palate	Mucosal glands of nasal septum; mucosa of nasal septum, anterior-most hard palate
Nerve to lateral and medial pterygoid	Anterior mandibular nerve	Arises in infratemporal fossa, inferior to foramen ovale	Lateral and medial pterygoid muscles
Nerve to pterygoid canal	Formed by merger of greater and deep petrosal nerves	Traverses pterygoid canal, to pterygoid ganglion in pterygoid fossa	Pterygopalatine ganglion
Nerve to stapedius	Facial nerve	Arises as facial nerve, descends posterior to muscle in facial canal	Stapedius
Pharyngeal	Pterygopalatine ganglion	Passes posteriorly through palatovaginal canal	Supplies mucosa of nasopharynx posterior to the pharyngo-tympanic tubes
Superior alveolar	Maxillary nerve	Posteriorly emerges from pterygo-maxillary fissure into infratemporal fossa to posterior aspect of maxilla; Middle and anterior: arises from infraorbital nerve of maxillary sinus, descends walls of sinus	Mucosa of maxillary sinus, maxillary teeth and gingiva

(*continued*)

Nerve	Origin	Course	Innervation
Trigeminal	Lateral surface of pons by two roots: motor and sensory	Crosses medial part of crest of petrous part of temporal bone, trigeminal cave of dural mater lateral to body of sphenoid and cavernous sinus; motor root passes ganglion to become part of mandibular nerve	Motor: somatic; muscles of mastication, mylohyoid, anterior belly of digastric, tensor tympanic, tensor veli palatini; Sensory: dura of anterior and middle cranial fossa, skin of face, teeth, gingiva, mucosa of nasal cavity, paranasal sinuses, and mouth
Zygomatic	Maxillary nerve	Arises in floor of orbitdivides into two temporal nerves, traverses foramina of same; communicating branch joins lacrimal nerve	Skin over zygomatic arch, anterior temporal region; conveys secretory postsynaptic parasympathetic fibers from pterygopalatine ganglion to lacrimal gland

3. Nerves of the Eye Region

Nerve	Origin	Course	Innervation
Ciliary, long and short	Nasociliary nerve; short ciliary ganglion	Passes to posterior aspect of eyeball	Cornea, conjunctiva; ciliary body and iris
Deep petrosal	Internal carotid plexus	Traverses cartilage of foramen lacerum to join greater petrosal nerve at entrance to pterygoid canal	Conveys the post-synaptic sympathetic fibers destined for the lacrimal gland and mucosa of the nasal cavity, palate, and upper pharynx
Frontal	Ophthalmic nerve	Crosses orbit on superior aspect of levator palpebrae superioris; divides into supraorbital and supratrochlear branches	Skin of forehead, scalp, eyelid, and nose; conjunctiva of upper lid and mucosa of frontal sinus
Infratrochlear	Nasociliary nerve	Follows medial wall of orbit to upper eyelid	Skin, conjunctiva, lining of upper eyelid

(continued)

Nerve	Origin	Course	Innervation
Lacrimal	Ophthalmic nerve	Palpebral fascia of upper eyelid near lateral angle of eye	Small area of skin and conjunctiva of lateral part of upper eyelid
Nasociliary	Ophthalmic nerve	Arises in superior orbital fissure, antero-medially across retrobulbar orbit, providing sensory root to ciliary ganglion; terminates as infratrochlear nerve	Ciliary ganglion (short) coveys postsynaptic sympathetic and para-sympathetic to ciliary body and iris; tactile sensation for eyeball; mucous membrane of ethmoid cells, antero-superior nasal cavity; skin of dorsum and apex of nose
Oculomotor	Interpeduncular fossa of mesencephalon	Dura of posterior clinoid process, lateral wall of cavernous sinus, enters orbit through superior orbital fissure and divides into superior and inferior branches	All extraocular muscles, except superior oblique and lateral rectus; presynaptic parasym-pathetic fibers to ciliary ganglions for ciliary body and sphincter pupillae
Ophthalmic	Trigeminal ganglion	Anteriorly in lateral wall of cavernous sinus to enter orbit through superior orbital fissure, branching into frontal, nasociliary, and lacrimal nerve	General sensation from eyeball; mucous mem-brane of ethmoid cells, frontal sinus, dura of anterior cranial fossa, falx cerebri, and tentor-ium cerebelli, antero-superior nasal cavity; skin of forehead, upper lid, and dorsum and apex of nose
Optic	Ganglion cells of retina	Exits orbit via optic canals; fibers from nasal half of retina cross to contralateral side at chiasm; passes via optic tracts to geniculate bodies, superior colliculus and pretectum	Vision from retina
Posterior ethmoidal	Nasociliary	Leaves orbit via posterior ethmoid foramen	Supplies ethmoid and sphenoid paranasal sinuses

Sample Reports

ARGON LASER TRABECULOPLASTY

PREOPERATIVE DIAGNOSIS: Open angle glaucoma, right eye.

POSTOPERATIVE DIAGNOSIS: Open angle glaucoma, right eye.

OPERATION: Argon laser trabeculoplasty, right eye.

ANESTHESIA: Topical.

PROCEDURE: The patient was brought to the laser room in satisfactory condition with appropriate informed consent of the risks, benefits, and alternatives of the procedure having been explained, including pain, glaucoma, decreased vision, need for further surgery, and bleeding. Drops of Iopidine and pilocarpine had been placed while in the holding area. The patient was seated at the slit lamp apparatus and the head positioned and secured. The argon laser aiming beam was focused carefully using a trabeculoplasty lens. Laser shots were placed along the trabecular meshwork approximately every 2 to 3 laser spot widths apart for 180 degrees of the trabecular meshwork. The spot width was 50 microns and the duration of one laser shot was 0.1 second. A total of 60 shots were given consisting of 600 to 800 millijoules. A satisfactory reaction at the trabecular meshwork was considered to be a blanching or bubble production at the point of laser application. The patient's head was released and drops of Iopidine were instilled.

Postoperative instructions were reviewed, which included alerting the patient to possible symptoms of elevated intraocular pressure in the operated eye. Followup examination in the office was prescribed to occur 1 to 3 hours after the procedure.

BILATERAL UPPER LID BLEPHAROPLASTY

PREOPERATIVE DIAGNOSIS: Bilateral upper lid dermatochalasis.

POSTOPERATIVE DIAGNOSIS: Bilateral upper lid dermatochalasis.

PROCEDURE PERFORMED: Bilateral upper lid blepharoplasty.

OPERATIVE REPORT: The surgical procedure was done in the outpatient clinic. The periorbital regions were prepped in sterile fashion. The patient was then put into the sitting position and the incision sites were marked. The measured amount of surgical excision tissue was 8 mm to 10 mm in both upper lids at the highest point. I should note that this fellow has fairly prominent brows and he was advised that surgical blepharoplasty might not result in as complete result as he was expecting. The patient was then placed in supine position and 2% local anesthetic with epinephrine was injected into each upper lid after the instillation of tetracaine eye drops. A total of 2.5 mL was used for each upper lid. The patient was then draped. Attention was turned to the right side, where an incision was made using the 15-blade extending through skin. Westcott scissors were then used to undermine the orbicularis muscle. The tissue was removed using sharp dissection as well as Colorado needle on the cautery. A cold pack was applied.

A similar procedure was done with the left upper lid. Bleeding was controlled using electrocautery. A cold saline gauze pad was applied.

I then returned to the right upper lid where the lid shape was formed using three 5-0 plain interrupted sutures. The skin margin was then approximated using a running 5-0 Ethilon suture. The wound was clean and dry. I then turned my attention to the left upper lid, where again the lid margin was formed using three 5-0 plain interrupted sutures and following with skin closure of a running subcuticular 5-0 Ethilon suture. The wound was clean and dry.

Tobrex ointment was applied to both wound margins. The patient was instructed to remain head up at 45 degrees and to use a cold pack for 10 to 15 minutes every couple of hours for the next 48 hours while awake. He was instructed to not take any aspirin postoperatively, but to use plain Tylenol for discomfort. There was some excessive bleeding at that time of the surgery; however, the wounds were clean and dry postoperatively. He was able to obtain a closure of his lids with minimal effort. The patient was discharged in satisfactory condition. He will be followed in the office in 5 days' time.

DACRYOCYSTITIS RHINOSTOMY AND REPAIR OF CANALICULAR ATRESIA

PREOPERATIVE DIAGNOSES:

1. Chronic dacryocystitis, right side.

2. Canalicular atresia, upper and lower canaliculus, right side.

POSTOPERATIVE DIAGNOSES:

1. Chronic dacryocystitis, right side.

2. Canalicular atresia, upper and lower canaliculus, right side.

OPERATION:

1. Dacryocystitis rhinostomy of right side.

2. Repair of canalicular atresia, upper and lower canaliculus, right side, with placement of lacrimal microtube.

ANESTHESIA: Local infiltrative with monitored anesthesia care.

INDICATIONS: This 36-year-old gentleman notes constant epiphora since birth. He is also noted to have a mass of the right lacrimal fossa and episodic discharge.

PROCEDURE: After informed consent was obtained, the patient was taken to the operating room and placed supine on the operating room table. Previously, a gentian violet marking pen had been used to mark the furthest clinical extent of the atretic canaliculi, both upper and lower. In addition, the caruncle was marked out should a conjunctivodacryocystorhinostomy with lacrimal Jones tube placement be necessary. The patient received appropriate preoperative monitoring and sedation, and a solution of 2% lidocaine with 1:100,000 epinephrine in a 50/50 mixture with 0.75% bupivacaine was given subcutaneously in the area of the previously demarcated dacryocystorhinostomy incision. The anterior ethmoidal nerve was also blocked utilizing 2 mL of this same solution by injecting 10 mm superior to the medial canthal tendon on the right side in the medial orbit. The lateral wall of the nose was also infiltrated with this same solution as was the anterior head of the middle turbinate. The head of the middle turbinate was also packed in the area of the middle meatus of the nose with a 4% cocaine-soaked gauze. General endotracheal tube anesthesia had been obtained without incident. The surgeon performed the surgical scrub. Upon his return, the patient was prepped and draped in usual sterile fashion for ophthalmic surgery. A hard corneal shield was placed before the cornea of the right eye after a series of 0.5% topical tetracaine drops had been applied.

The reconstruction of the atretic canaliculi was performed first. Examination of the upper and lower canaliculi revealed distal atresia of the upper and lower canaliculus. A cutdown was performed over the more proximal segment of canaliculi and a sterile safety pin was used to dilate the very atretic segment of canaliculus. A quadruple 0-Bowman probe was then used to cannulate the atretic canaliculus. Care was taken to avoid creating a false track; however, the course of the track marked out the presumed course of the atretic but functional canaliculi, both upper and lower. A similar procedure was performed on the lower after the upper had been completed. Further dilation was performed with a pediatric punctum dilator. After this, a triple 0-Bowman probe was placed and stenosis was noted at the level of the common canaliculus through the inferior punctum. A double 0- and then single 0-Bowman probe were advanced through the remaining portion of the canaliculus to the level of the hard stop of the nasal bone. Irrigation at this point produced reflux. There was no ability to decompress the lacrimal sac. Further dilatation was performed so that a #1-Bowman probe could be admitted through both the superior and inferior atretic canaliculi.

Attention was next directed to the dacryocystorhinostomy portion of the procedure. A #15-Bard-Parker blade was used to incise the previously demarcated dacryocystorhinostomy site. A hemostat was used to spread the fibers of the orbicularis muscle, and the sharp edge of a Freer periosteal elevator was used to strip periosteum down to the level of periorbita. A very enlarged lacrimal sac was noted, and the lacrimal sac was reflected laterally to allow for exposure of the bony nasolacrimal fossa. While retracting the lacrimal sac, a large amount of green to brown mucopurulent debris was then expressed through the superior portion of the sac. This was cultured. This allowed for further inspection of the nasolacrimal fossa, which was noted to be markedly enlarged from the normal diameter. The medial wall of the lacrimal sac was then sent for biopsy. The rhinostomy was then begun by in-fracturing at the level of the lacrimal maxillary suture. A Kerrison punch was used to enlarge the rhinostomy to a final diameter of 15 mm. Superiorly, the rhinostomy had been enlarged so that no bony edge was closer than 5 mm to the exit of the common canaliculus. Hemostasis had been achieved with direct digital pressure, Bovie cautery, and topical thrombin-soaked Gelfoam. The area was then packed with the Gelfoam soaked in topical thrombin.

Attention was directed back to the now reconstructed canaliculi. A 0-Bowman probe was inserted through the superior canaliculus, through the common canaliculus to exit the medial portion of the lacrimal sac. In a similar fashion, a double 0-Bowman probe was passed through the inferior canaliculus. The anterior lacrimal sac flap was fashioned with sharp Westcott scissors, as was the posterior lacrimal sac flap. The nasal mucosa was then incised with cutting cautery, fashioning an anterior and posterior H-flap. The cocaine-soaked gauze was removed from the right naris. Alignment of the rhinostomy through the lacrimal sac and common canaliculus was noted to be adequate. The lacrimal probes were removed and a Guibor tube was placed through the superior and inferior canaliculus, through the rhinostomy to exit the right naris. The posterior lacrimal sac and posterior nasal mucosal flap were noted to align without tension. The rhinostomy was then packed with Gelfoam soaked in topical thrombin. The anterior flaps were closed with an interrupted 4-0 chromic suture in a horizontal mattress fashion. The deep layers of the orbicularis muscle were closed with a 5-0

Vicryl suture. The skin layers were closed with a series of interrupted mini-vertical mattress sutures. The nose was further packed with a nasal tampon coated with Maxitrol ointment at the tip and soaked in topical thrombin. The Guibor tube had been tied upon itself in the nose. The lacrimal microtube tension was adjusted in the medial canthus. The single dental roll and an eye patch were placed. The patient was extubated without incident and moved to the recovery room in stable condition.

ECTROPION, CANTHOPEXY, AND UPPER AND LOWER LID 3-SNIP PROCEDURE

PREOPERATIVE DIAGNOSIS: Bilateral lower lid ectropion with punctal stenosis and lateral canthal dystopia.

POSTOPERATIVE DIAGNOSIS: Bilateral lower lid ectropion with punctal stenosis and lateral canthal dystopia.

OPERATIONS PERFORMED:

1. Bilateral lower lid medial ectropion.

2. Bilateral lateral canthopexy.

3. Upper and lower lid 3-snip procedure bilaterally.

ANESTHESIA: Neuroleptanesthesia and local.

PROCEDURE: This patient was brought to the operating room and given neuroleptanesthesia. The entire face and orbital areas were prepped and draped in usual sterile fashion. Xylocaine 2% with adrenaline mixed in equal parts with 0.5% Marcaine plain was infiltrated around all 4 puncta, into the medial lower lids, and into the lateral lower lid and lateral canthal region. A punctal dilator was used to dilate the puncta on all 4 lids. A 3 snip procedure was then carried out with Vannas scissors on all 4 puncta. The right lower lid was pulled downwards. The horizontal ellipse of conjunctiva, lower lid retractors, and orbital septum was removed 4 mm below the punctum for a horizontal length of 4 mm straddling the punctum and avoiding the canaliculus. Hemostasis was assured with bipolar cautery. A double arm 6-0 chromic suture was passed such that each arm went through the upper edge of the ellipse, one medial and one lateral to the punctum, again avoiding the canaliculus. Each arm was then brought out through the apex of the ellipse, and through the skin, 11-mm below the punctum. The two arms were tied to each other over the skin, thus correcting the medial ectropion. Following this, a similar procedure was carried out on the medial left lower lid.

The right lateral canthal dystopia was then addressed. A lateral canthotomy and inferior cantholysis was performed and a tarsal strip was fashioned with the excess lid. Hemostasis was obtained with meticulous bipolar cautery. A 5-0 Prolene suture was passed horizontally obliquely upwards through the periosteum just inside the lateral orbital rim twice then back and forth through the tarsal strip and tied and cut short. A separate interrupted suture of the same material was placed through these structures and also tied and cut short. The lateral canthal angle was reformed with a 6-0 silk suture left long. The canthotomy wound was closed with further interrupted 6-0 silk sutures, one of which imbricated the canthal angle from the suture to keep it away from the eye. Following this, a similar procedure was carried out on the left side; that is, a lateral canthopexy via tarsal strip procedure.

At the end of the case, both eyelids were in excellent position. Vision was unchanged and hemostasis was excellent. Antibiotic ointment was placed on the wounds and in the eyes. He tolerated the procedure extremely well and left the operating room in good condition.

ENUCLEATION OF THE EYE

OPERATION: Enucleation of right eye.

PROCEDURE: The patient was brought to the operating room and prepped and draped in the usual fashion. The left eye was approached and a 360 degree conjunctival peritomy was performed with Westcott scissors. Wet-field cautery was used for hemostasis during the procedure. Dissection took place in all four quadrants to loosen the Tenon capsule from the scleral adhesions.

Next, the rectus muscles were isolated in turn and cut with cautery. Finally, the oblique muscles were isolated and cut with cautery, and then a large curved hemostat was placed on the optic nerve. The optic nerve was then cut with curved scissors, and the eye removed from the socket. There was about a 0.25 cm stump of optic nerve attached to the globe, and the clamp was left on the remaining optic nerve segment for hemostasis. After approximately 5 minutes, this was removed and hemostasis was noted to be excellent. The enucleated eye was sent for pathology.

Finally, the implant ball was placed into the socket and the Tenon capsule was closed with 4 0 Vicryl suture in an interrupted fashion in two different layers. The conjunctiva was closed with 8 0 Vicryl suture in a running fashion with meticulous closure.

A conformer was placed into the conjunctival sac and Maxitrol ointment placed in the socket. The patient had subconjunctival injections of Decadron and gentamicin, and a pad and Fox shield were placed over the eye.

EXTRACAPSULAR CATARACT EXTRACTION WITH INSERTION OF INTRAOCULAR LENS

OPERATION: Extracapsular cataract extraction with insertion of an intraocular lens, left eye.

PROCEDURE: Prior to surgery, a Honan intraocular pressure reducer balloon was placed over the left eye. The balloon pressure was then inflated to 30 mmHg and allowed to remain in place for 45 minutes prior to surgery. The patient was taken to the operating room, where local anesthesia was administered with lidocaine 2% with epinephrine for a Nadbath lid block. Retrobulbar anesthesia and akinesia were achieved with an equal mixture of Marcaine 0.75% with epinephrine and lidocaine 4% along with Wydase. The patient was then prepped and draped in the usual sterile ophthalmic manner and attention was directed to the left eye.

A lid speculum was inserted between the lids, and the intraocular pressure was measured with a Schiotz tonometer. The remainder of the procedure was conducted through the use of the Weck ophthalmic microscope.

The eye was stabilized with a 4-0 black silk superior rectus traction suture and was subsequently deflected downward. A limbal peritomy was performed with Westcott scissors from 10 o'clock around to 2 o'clock. Eraser bipolar cautery was utilized to effect hemostasis. A scleral incision was made 2 mm superior to the superior limbus with a 6610 Beaver blade to one-half the depth of the sclera for 12 mm in length. The dissection was then carried posteriorly from the base of the incision into clear cornea. A #75 Beaver blade was utilized to create a stab wound into clear cornea at 2 o'clock to provide an access port. A keratome was utilized to enter the anterior chamber through the base of the corneoscleral wound at 10 o'clock.

Healon was injected into the anterior chamber through a cystitome needle. The needle was subsequently used to effect an anterior capsulotomy, and capsule forceps were utilized to effect a circular tear capsulorrhexis capsulotomy. Balanced salt solution was injected underneath the capsule to dissect the nucleus free from the capsule.

The 10 o'clock incision was then enlarged with right and left cutting corneoscleral scissors to 12 mm in length. Through the use of a lens loop and Colibri forceps, the nucleus was expressed through the wound. Two interrupted 10-0 nylon sutures were then inserted through the corneoscleral wound, dividing the wound into equal thirds.

A Cavitron irrigation and aspiration tip was inserted through the wound and lens cortical material irrigated and aspirated. Following this, the posterior capsule was noted to be intact and Healon was injected into the anterior chamber.

An IOLAB posterior chamber intraocular lens, Model G-708G of 22 diopters lens power, had previously been soaked in balanced salt solution. The lens was flushed with fresh balanced salt solution and coated with Healon. Angled McPherson tying forceps were then used to insert the lens through the scleral incision with the inferior foot of the haptic passing beneath the anterior capsule at 6 o'clock. Long-angled McPherson tying forceps were then used to place the superior foot of the haptic through the pupil behind the anterior capsule at 12 o'clock. A Sinskey hook was utilized to rotate the lens and ensure its stability. Miochol was injected into the anterior chamber to constrict the pupil.

Balanced salt solution was then utilized to deepen the chamber and firm up the eye. Additional 10-0 nylon interrupted sutures were utilized to close the corneoscleral wound. At the completion of the maneuver, the wound was watertight. The eye evidenced normal pressure and the pupil was round, central, and lay immediately over the haptic of the posterior chamber lens. The conjunctival wound was coapted with bipolar cautery. Gentamicin and Celestone, 0.5 mL each, were separately injected through the inferior conjunctival cul-de-sac into the sub-Tenon space. The Barraquer lid speculum was removed, Maxitrol ointment instilled, and a patch and Fox shield placed over the eye.

HYPERTROPIA REPAIR

PREOPERATIVE DIAGNOSIS: Right hypertropia secondary to right superior oblique palsy.

POSTOPERATIVE DIAGNOSIS: Right hypertropia secondary to right superior oblique palsy.

OPERATION: A 5-mm resection of right superior rectus muscle and myectomy of the right inferior oblique muscle.

PROCEDURE: The patient was taken to the operating room. After intravenous sedation with Versed and fentanyl, she was given a peribulbar injection of Marcaine and Wydase. A pressure-lowering device was placed in the eye for 10 minutes to achieve hypotony. The area around both eyes were prepared with iodine and water and draped in the usual fashion as a sterile field. The right conjunctival cul-de-sac was irrigated with dilute Betadine solution. A lid speculum was placed in the right palpebral fissure.

An incision was made in the inferotemporal bulbar conjunctiva of the right eye. The right inferior and right lateral rectus muscles were identified through this incision and retracted. A muscle hook was then placed into the inferotemporal orbit, and the inferior oblique muscle was retrieved. This muscle was secured on two hemostats. The muscle between the hemostat was excised with the ends of the muscle cauterized. The stumps were then released into the orbit. The conjunctiva was closed with a running 6-0 Vicryl suture.

Attention was then turned to the superior bulbar conjunctiva where an incision was made between the 10 o'clock and the 2 o'clock position at the limbus. Relaxing incisions were made posteriorly at the 2 o'clock and 10 o'clock positions. The superior rectus muscle was isolated with blunt and sharp dissection and secured with a muscle hook. Additional anesthesia was given with a local infiltration on the muscle with 2% Xylocaine. Two 6-0 Vicryl sutures were placed through the temporal and nasal margins of the muscle. These sutures were drawn taut and tied. The muscle was then reinserted and resutured to the globe with the same sutures at a point 5 mm posterior to the original insertion. The stump on the insertion site was cauterized. The conjunctiva was then closed with interrupted 6-0 Vicryl sutures.

At the conclusion of the procedure, TobraDex ointment was instilled, the conjunctiva was closed, and a monocular patch was applied. The patient tolerated the procedure well and left the operating room in good condition.

HYPHEMA IRRIGATION

PREOPERATIVE DIAGNOSIS: Hyphema OS.

POSTOPERATIVE DIAGNOSIS: Hyphema OS.

OPERATION: Irrigation of hyphema OS.

INDICATIONS: Uncontrolled intraocular pressure after hyphema post cataract surgery.

HISTORY: The patient underwent apparent uneventful trabeculectomy in the left eye in January 1998. Although the surgery was uneventful, the following day he had an almost total hyphema. No surgical intervention was done but his intraocular pressure was controlled with medication, and eventually the intraocular pressure became well-controlled by the trabeculectomy, although a fibrous plaque was left on his lens because of the absorbed blood. Ironically, he underwent cataract surgery with posterior chamber intraocular lens implant in this eye to restore the vision and to be able to obtain a fundus view because of his diabetic retinopathy. The procedure was uneventful and a foldable posterior chamber lens was implanted. At the end of the surgery the eye looked perfect. The following day he presented to the office with an almost total hyphema in the left eye and an intraocular pressure of 73. He stated that morning he had noticed some discomfort in the eye and change in his vision. Because of the fact that it took so long for the eye to attain a functional status, as with his first hyphema, it was elected to irrigate the hyphema immediately.

PROCEDURE: He was given some intravenous sedation by the anesthesiologist and then given topical anesthesia with 1% Xylocaine with epinephrine and tetracaine. The previous cataract incision was opened with a 2.5 mm keratome. The IA tip of the Legacy machine was used to irrigate some of the blood from the anterior chamber. Intracameral Xylocaine was also used for anesthesia. Some of the blood could not be aspirated but was actually removed with capsulorrhexis forceps after some Viscoat had been placed in the anterior chamber. Several attempts were made to irrigate the blood that seemed to be trapped in the superior chamber; whether it had originated in this area or near the trabeculectomy site was possible but could not be determined with certainty. At this point, irrigation removed no more blood and forceps removed no more blood. It was elected to terminate the procedure at this point. Most of the optic of the lens was clean. Whether rebleeding would occur was impossible to say. The incision was closed with one interrupted 10-0 nylon suture. The anterior chamber was then reformed with BSS. Then 40 mg of triamcinolone was injected subconjunctivally at the nasal inferior fornix. The speculum was removed, and a light patch and shield were applied. The patient tolerated the procedure well and was returned to the recovery room in good condition.

PARS PLANA VITRECTOMY, MEMBRANE PEELING, SCLERAL BUCKLE, ENDOLASER, AND GAS–FLUID EXCHANGE

OPERATION: Pars plana vitrectomy for complex retinal detachment, membrane peeling, scleral buckle, endolaser, and gas-fluid exchange.

PROCEDURE: Following informed consent and the identification of the patient, the patient was brought into the operating room, alert and in stable condition. Regional anesthesia and akinesia were obtained using a mixture of Marcaine, lidocaine, and Wydase given in a retrobulbar block. The patient was then prepped and draped in the usual sterile fashion for ophthalmic procedure. The lid speculum was placed. A conjunctival peritomy was performed to 360 degrees using Westcott scissors and 0.12 forceps. Stevens scissors were used to dissect in each of the four quadrants. A muscle hook was used to grasp the inferior rectus muscle and the muscle was then bridled using 4-0 black silk suture. Each of the four rectus muscles was bridled in a similar fashion. Once all of the muscles were isolated and each muscle was cleaned using a Q-tip, 4-0 white silk suture bites were placed in each of the four quadrants in preparation for placing the scleral buckle. A Ruby blade was used to enter the eye 4 mm posterior to the surgical limbus infratemporally and a trocar cannula infusion system was put into position and the position checked with a light pipe prior to turning the infusion on. Additional sclerotomies were made supratemporally and supranasally using the Ruby blade, also 4 mm posterior to the surgical lumbus. The light pipe and ocutome were then inserted through the sclerotomy sites and the cortical vitreous was removed from the posterior surface in the lens to the anterior surface of the retina.

The retina was noted to be detached and there was noted to be a large open macular hole present. In addition, there were membranes present on the surface of the retina, creating a star-fold infratemporally. A Michel pick was used to raise membranes from the surface of the retina and peel back the posterior hyaloid to approximately the equator. The ocutome probe was used to remove remaining vitreous from the eye. Subretinal fluid was drained through a macular hole and also through a small retinotomy that was made near the supratemporal arcade. At this time, a 287 scleral buckle element was placed for 360 degrees around the eye and the four pre-placed sutures were then tightened and tied, with the notch rotated posteriorly. The ends of the buckle were tied together using 4-0 white silk suture. Scleral plugs were placed into the sclerotomy sites prior to placing the buckle. An air-fluid exchange was then performed and the retina was noted to flatten nicely. Additional drainage of fluid was performed through the retinotomy site. Several minutes were allowed to pass for additional fluid to accumulate and this fluid was removed using active suction. Active suction was also used prior to the gas–fluid exchange to raise portions of the posterior hyaloid. Once the retina was completely flattened, approximately 500 endolaser spots were placed along the buckle and around the retinotomy site. A gas–gas exchange was then performed using SF 6 gas. The sclerotomy sites were closed using 7-0 Vicryl suture material. The conjunctiva was closed using 6-0 plain suture material. All of the bridle sutures were removed prior to closing of the conjunctiva. Subconjunctival injection of Ancef and dexamethasone was performed. Atropine drops were placed topically on the eye and the eye was then patched in closed position with an eye shell placed on top. The patient tolerated the procedure well and was transferred to the recovery room in stable condition.

PENETRATING KERATOPLASTY

OPERATION: Penetrating keratoplasty, 7.75 mm in a 7.5-mm bed, right eye.

PROCEDURE: After clearance from the anesthesiologist and using topical anesthesia with 0.75% bupivacaine, the right eye was prepped and draped in the usual fashion and massage was done until the bulb and orbit were soft. The Goldmann-McNeil blepharostat was inserted and sutured to the episclera with Vicryl suture. The recipient cornea was measured and a 7.75 mm trephine was selected for the donor, which was prepared in the usual fashion. A 7.5 mm trephine was then used for the recipient until penetration occurred. Additional deepening of the outer quadrants was done with a Supersharp. Curved corneal scissors to the right and left were used to completely excise the recipient button. The fluid centrally was cleaned up with cellulose sponges. The pupil was enlarged by first creating snip incisions with Vannas scissors and then extending these, and small amounts of capsule and cortical material were also excised. A very small amount of bleeding occurred, but this stopped spontaneously. The Healon was then placed, as well as Miochol, and the donor corneal button was transferred to the operative field, where it was secured in position using 4 interrupted 10-0 nylon sutures followed by a 10-0 nylon suture in running fashion with the knot superiorly. Prior to tying this, the interrupted sutures were removed, the running suture tension was adjusted, and a permanent knot was created and buried in recipient stroma. The suture tension was adjusted further. The intraocular Healon was evacuated and replaced with balanced salt solution, and the wound was assessed with saline sponges and found to be watertight and in good position with a deep anterior chamber and no evidence of vitreous to the wound. The blepharostat was removed and subconjunctival injections of gentamicin, Ancef, and Celestone were given and a drop of Betagan 0.5% was instilled. A semi-pressure patch and shield were placed over the operated eye and the patient was brought to the recovery room in good condition.

PHACOEMULSIFICATION AND LENS IMPLANT

PREOPERATIVE DIAGNOSIS: Senile cataract, right eye.

POSTOPERATIVE DIAGNOSIS: Senile cataract, right eye.

OPERATION: Phacoemulsification and lens implant, right eye.

PROCEDURE: The patient was taken to the operating room and placed under IV sedation. The patient was prepped in the usual sterile manner. Van Lint akinesia and retrobulbar anesthesia were performed with a combination of 2% Xylocaine and 0.75% Marcaine in equal volumes with 1 mL of Wydase added. For 5 minutes a Honan balloon was placed in the right globe after 5% Betadine solution was placed in the inferior cul-de-sac. The patient was prepped and draped in the usual manner. A Lieberman speculum was placed in the right eye and superior and inferior fornices were irrigated with balanced salt solution. A 4-0 silk traction suture was placed in the superior rectus muscle, tied and draped above. Conjunctival peritomy was fashioned. Hemostasis was done with wet-field cautery. A 19 blade was used to create a paracentesis at the 2:30 position. Viscoat was placed in the anterior chamber. A 6.0-mm scleral tunnel was dissected in the anterior cornea. A 2.6 keratome was used to enlarge the internal incision. Healon was placed in the chamber and a 5.0-mm capsulorrhexis was fashioned. Hydrodissection and hydrodelineation were performed with a balanced salt solution attached to a Pierce needle. The phaco tip was then introduced into the eye and 4 troughs down to the depth of the posterior plate were sculpted at 90 degrees to one another. Segments were then separated sequentially with secondary phaco power. Irrigation aspiration was used to remove residual cortical material. A 5.2 keratome was used to enlarge the internal incision. Healon was placed in the chamber and a plus 23 diopter lens was inserted and dialed into the horizontal position. All viscoelastic material was removed from the anterior chamber. At the conclusion of the case, the anterior chamber was deep. The implant was in perfect position. The iris was constricted beyond the optic. The conjunctival peritomy was closed with wet-field cautery. Pilocarpine 2% x 2 was placed. Maxitrol ophthalmic ointment was placed. Patch and shield were placed. The patient was taken to the recovery room in good condition.

COURSE AND CONDITION: Uneventful, the patient was sent to recovery.

ESTIMATED BLOOD LOSS: Negligible.

SPECIMEN: Lens to pathology.

PTERYGIA REMOVAL AND PLACEMENT OF CONJUNCTIVAL GRAFT

PREOPERATIVE DIAGNOSIS: Invasive pterygia, right eye.

POSTOPERATIVE DIAGNOSIS: Invasive pterygia, right eye.

OPERATION: Pterygia removal with placement of autologous free-floating conjunctival grafts (nasal and temporal).

ANESTHESIA: Intravenous anesthesia.

INDICATIONS: The patient is referred for evaluation and treatment of severe invasive pterygia nasally and temporally in both eyes. The diagnosis is confirmed. The patient desires removal of these invasive and destructive lesions and is felt to be an excellent candidate for the same. He was electively admitted through the outpatient unit at this time for the above-indicated desired procedure OD.

PROCEDURE: He was taken to the operating room and placed on the operating table in the supine position. An IV was started and separate amounts of fentanyl and Pentothal administered intravenously. After a suitable plane of anesthesia was obtained, 4.5 mL of standard retrobulbar medication was injected in a peribulbar fashion around the right eye, which was then prepped and draped in the usual sterile fashion. Clean sterile drapes were then placed over the patient's right eye. A blepharostat was placed between lids of the right eye. The operating microscope was then swung in position over the patient's right eye, and the entire procedure was done under direct visualization with the operating microscope. The pterygia were easily visualized arising from the medial and temporal interpalpebral bulbar conjunctiva and encroaching onto the cornea for approximately 3.0 to 3.5 mm temporally and 2.5 to 3.0 mm nasally. The head of the nasal lesion was grasped with 0.12 corneal forceps, elevated vertically off the plane of the cornea with the plane of dissection obtained at the level of the Bowman membrane, and a superficial keratectomy was performed to peel the lesion back to the level of the limbus. It was then undermined on the bulbar conjunctiva with West-cott scissors and the base was completely excised. The temporal lesion was removed in an identical fashion. Hand-held thermocautery was used to obtain hemostasis in both beds. The edge of the cut conjunctiva was then reapproximated to the underlying episcleral tissues with interrupted 8-0 Vicryl sutures x 7 in both nasal and temporal beds. This resulted in a bare scleral defect measuring 5 mm horizontally and 7 mm vertically on both sides. Locking Castroviejo forceps were placed at the 2 o'clock position and the eye was rotated infratemporally to expose the superior nasal intermuscular quadrant. A 6 x 9 mm ellipse was drawn in this virgin bulbar conjunctiva. It was undermined with 2% Xylocaine with 1:100,000 epinephrine, and then the conjunctiva was removed, preserving the underlying Tenon capsule. The conjunctival graft was then rotated medially into the nasal site and sutured with interrupted 8-0 Vicryl sutures x 8. The Castroviejo forceps were then placed at the 10 o'clock position, and the eye was rotated inferonasally, exposing the supratemporal intermuscular quadrant. Again, a 6 x 9 mm ellipse was drawn in like fashion with thermocautery unit, undermined with Xylocaine, excised with Westcott scissors, rotated into the recipient bed, and sutured into the site with interrupted 8-0 Vicryl sutures x 8.

At the end of the procedure, sponge and needle counts were correct. The conjunctival grafts were in good order with no blood, air, or fluid under the graft. The edges were approximated well. There was no undue tension in any direction on the grafts, and they were in good order. Homatropine ophthalmic drops were placed by instillation in this eye. Maxitrol ophthalmic drops were placed by instillation, and Steri-Drapes and blepharostat were removed. The eye was dressed with a soft patch and Fox shield. The patient was then placed on a gurney and returned to the outpatient area, discharged in satisfactory postoperative condition.

The patient will have one month of convalescence. During that time, his sutures will be dissolving on their own and he will be tapered off medication. He initially will be restricting activity such that he will not rub, scratch, or itch the eye; in any way get the eye wet or dirty; or be exposed to excessively dirty or dusty environments. He is to use Advil or extra-strength Tylenol for pain relief but avoid aspirin-containing products for at least 48 hours. He is to leave the Fox shield and patch on the right eye at all times until he is seen in the office 24 hours after the procedure for patch removal and institution of topical medications. He and his family understand these postoperative stipulations well and will be compliant with them. I anticipate he will have dramatic improvement in his ocular motility status with hopeful total prevention of recurrence of the recurrent pterygia and taking of the graft.

PTOSIS REPAIR

OPERATION: Repair of ptosis, right and left eyes.

PROCEDURE: The patient was brought into the operating room. The eyes were prepped and draped for bilateral eyelid surgery. Tetracaine was applied to both eyes. The upper lid crease was demarcated with a marking pen on both upper lids. The excess upper eyelid skin tissue was then demarcated with a marking pen. Intravenous sedation was given. Lidocaine 2% with epinephrine was used to infiltrate both upper eyelids. Adequate anesthesia was achieved.

The right eye was addressed first. Utilizing a #15 Bard Parker blade, an incision was made along the lid crease. The incision was then carried along through the superior margin of the demarcated upper eyelid excess tissue. Utilizing sharp dissection as well as the unipolar cutting and coagulating Bovie, the eyelid skin and orbicularis were removed. Areas of thinning of the intramuscular septum with prolapsed fat were addressed. The prolapsed fat was excised where indicated. Hemostasis was achieved with unipolar Bovie. A 4 x 4 moistened saline sponge was placed over the right upper eyelid. Attention was then directed to the left upper eyelid. The excess upper lid skin was removed in a similar fashion. Hemostasis was achieved with a Bovie. Closure was then performed of the right upper eyelid. Several supratarsal fixation sutures were placed to address the ptosis. The skin was then closed with a running 6-0 Prolene suture. The left eye was closed in a similar fashion. The patient tolerated the procedure well. The drapes were removed. Maxitrol ointment was placed in each eye. The patient was transferred to the recovery area in stable condition.

RETINAL DETACHMENT

PREOPERATIVE DIAGNOSIS: Left retinal detachment.

POSTOPERATIVE DIAGNOSIS: Left retinal detachment.

OPERATION: Left scleral buckle.

ANESTHESIA: Neuroleptanesthesia.

PROCEDURE: The patient was brought to the operating room, where he received a left retrobulbar injection mixed with Xylocaine and Marcaine. The left eye was prepped and draped in the usual fashion. A lid speculum was inserted. A standard 360-degree limbal conjunctival peritomy was made with a relaxing incision nasally and temporally to rectus muscles with #2-0 silk tie, and direct ophthalmoscopy was performed. The patient was noted to have an inferior macula with retinal detachments and retinal breaks at the 3 o'clock and 4 o'clock position. These were treated with confluent cryotherapy, and the break was localized 11.5 mm from the limbus. A 240 band was directed on the eye, anchored 11.5 mm from the limbus nasally and 12 mm temporally. Subretinal fluid was drained inferotemporally within the bed of the buckle. Subretinal fluid drained well and the buckle was tightened with no need for intraocular gas, air, or fluid. There were no complications noted. The end of the band was trimmed up from the mucosa with 7-0 Vicryl suture. Pred Forte, Ocuflox, and atropine drops were applied. A patch and shield were applied. The patient will be nursed lying flat on his back in the postoperative period.

TRABECULECTOMY

PREOPERATIVE DIAGNOSIS: Poorly controlled open angle glaucoma left eye.

POSTOPERATIVE DIAGNOSIS: Poorly controlled open angle glaucoma left eye.

OPERATION: Trabeculectomy left eye.

INDICATIONS: Poorly controlled intraocular pressure in a patient who is poorly compliant with medications.

PROCEDURE: The patient was given Versed and fentanyl intravenously. She was given a retrobulbar block OS with 2% Xylocaine with Wydase. She was then prepped and draped for surgery in the usual manner.

The lids OS were retracted with the speculum. Superior rectus suture of 4-0 silk was placed with the operating microscope in position. The Alcon V-lance was used to make an entrance into the anterior chamber at the 11:30 position; the conjunctiva in the supertemporal quadrant was ballooned up using a 30-gauge needle and balanced saline solution. Blunt scissors were used to open the conjunctiva and Tenon capsule in the supertemporal quadrant, and dissection was carried up to the limbus bluntly. The anterior part of the conjunctival flap was retracted with 8-0 silk sutures. The sclera in the supertemporal quadrant was marbleized with the bipolar cautery. The trabeculectomy flap with the base at the limbus was outlined with ophthalmic cautery and then incised along the cautery lines with a #75-Beaver blade. Then the Alcon crescent knife was used to make a lamellar dissection in the eighth section of the triangle in the sclera well into clear cornea. The anterior chamber was entered with a 75-blade, and a block of clear-colored tissue was excised with the trabeculectomy punch. A peripheral iridectomy was made with the Vannas scissors. There was a small amount of bleeding encountered originally but this eventually stopped; one drop of 10% phenylethyl was used to help stop the bleeding. The apex of the scleral flap was tacked and was sutured down loosely with one 10-0 nylon suture. The run-off from the trabeculectomy site was tested by injecting balanced saline solution into the anterior chamber and it was seen to be excellent. Prior to the performance of the iridectomy, Miochol was irrigated into the anterior chamber. The conjunctiva was then closed using running interlocking 9-0 Vicryl suture. The superior rectus suture was then removed. The anterior chamber was deepened with balanced saline solution. Then 0.3 mL of 5-fluorouracil was injected subconjunctivally in the inferior fornix. A sterile dressing and atropine were applied at the cornea. The speculum was removed and a light patch then applied. The patient tolerated the procedure well and was returned to the outpatient area in good condition.

Appendix 4
Common Terms by Procedure

Argon Laser Trabeculoplasty
argon laser aiming beam
argon laser trabeculoplasty
blanching
bubble production
Iopidine
laser shots
open angle glaucoma
pilocarpine
slit lamp apparatus
spot width
trabecular meshwork
trabeculoplasty lens

Bilateral Upper Lid Blepharoplasty
blepharoplasty
Colorado needle
dermatochalasis
electrocautery
epinephrine
Ethilon suture
orbicularis muscle
periorbital region
tetracaine
Tobrex ointment
Westcott scissors

Dacryocystitis Rhinostomy and Repair of Canalicular Atresia
anterior ethmoidal nerve
atretic canaliculi
Bard-Parker blade
Bovie cautery
Bowman probe
canalicular atresia
canaliculus
chronic dacryocystitis

cocaine-soaked gauze
common canaliculus
conjunctivodacryocystorhinostomy
cutdown
cutting cautery
dacryocystitis rhinostomy
dacryocystorhinostomy incision
epiphora
Freer periosteal elevator
Guibor tube
hard corneal shield
hard stop
H-flap
horizontal mattress fashion
inferior punctum
in-fracturing
Kerrison punch
lacrimal fossa
lacrimal Jones tube
lacrimal maxillary suture
lacrimal microtube
lacrimal sac
Maxitrol ointment
medial canthal tendon
middle meatus
middle turbinate
mini-vertical mattress sutures
mucopurulent debris
nasal tampon
nasolacrimal fossa
orbicularis muscle
pediatric punctum dilator
periorbita
superior canaliculus
thrombin-soaked Gelfoam
topical tetracaine drops
Westcott scissors

Ectropion, Canthopexy, and Upper and Lower Lid 3-Snip Procedure

adrenaline
bipolar cautery
canaliculus
canthal angle
canthal dystopia
cantholysis
canthopexy
canthotomy
double-arm chromic suture
ectropion
hemostasis
horizontal ellipse
imbricated
lid retractor
Marcaine
neuroleptanesthesia
orbital rim
orbital septum
periosteum
Prolene suture
punctal dilator
punctal stenosis
punctum
tarsal strip
Vannas scissors
Xylocaine

Enucleation of the Eye

conformer
conjunctival peritomy
conjunctival sac
curved hemostat
curved scissors
Decadron
enucleation
Fox shield
gentamicin
hemostasis
implant ball
Maxitrol ointment

oblique muscles
optic nerve
rectus muscles
scleral adhesions
subconjunctival injection
Tenon capsule
Westcott scissors
wet-field cautery

Extracapsular Cataract Extraction with Insertion of Intraocular Lens

access port
akinesia
angled McPherson tying forceps
anterior capsulotomy
anterior chamber
balanced salt solution
balloon pressure
Barraquer lid speculum
Beaver blade
bipolar cautery
capsule forceps
Cavitron irrigation and aspiration tip
Celestone
circular tear capsulorrhexis
    capsulotomy
coapted
Colibri forceps
conjunctival cul-de-sac
corneoscleral wound
cystitome needle
epinephrine
eraser bipolar cautery
extracapsular cataract extraction
Fox shield
gentamicin
haptic
Healon
Honan intraocular pressure reducer
    balloon
inferior foot
intraocular lens

intraocular pressure
IOLAB posterior chamber intraocular
 lens
keratome
lens cortical material
lens loop
lid speculum
lidocaine
limbal peritomy
long-angled McPherson tying forceps
Marcaine
Maxitrol ointment
Miochol
Nadbath lid block
posterior capsule
retrobulbar anesthesia
right and left cutting corneoscleral
 scissors
Schiotz tonometer
scleral incision
Sinskey hook
stab wound
sub-Tenon space
superior limbus
superior rectus traction suture
Weck ophthalmic microscope
Westcott scissors
Wydase

Hypertropia Repair

Betadine solution
conjunctival cul-de-sac
fentanyl
hypertropia
hypotony
inferior oblique muscle
inferior rectus muscle
inferotemporal bulbar conjunctiva
inferotemporal orbit
lateral rectus muscle
lid speculum
Marcaine
monocular patch

muscle hook
myomectomy
palpebral fissure
peribulbar injection
relaxing incisions
superior bulbar conjunctiva
superior oblique palsy
superior rectus muscle
TobraDex ointment
Versed
Wydase
Xylocaine

Hyphema Irrigation

anterior chamber
capsulorrhexis forceps
epinephrine
fibrous plaque
hyphema
IA tip
intracameral
intraocular pressure
keratome
Legacy machine
nasal inferior fornix
subconjunctivally
tetracaine
trabeculectomy
triamcinolone
Viscoat
Xylocaine

Pars Plana Vitrectomy, Membrane Peeling, Scleral Buckle, Endolaser, and Gas–Fluid Exchange

active suction
air–fluid exchange
akinesia
Ancef
atropine drops
black silk suture
bridle sutures

complex retinal detachment
conjunctival peritomy
cortical vitreous
dexamethasone
endolaser spots
eye shell
gas–fluid exchange
gas–gas exchange
inferior rectus muscle
lid speculum
lidocaine
light pipe
macular hole
Marcaine
membrane peeling
Michel pick
muscle hook
ocutome probe
pars plana vitrectomy
posterior hyaloid
retinotomy
retrobulbar block
Ruby blade
scleral buckle
scleral plugs
sclerotomy site
SF-6 gas
Stevens scissors
subconjunctival injection
subretinal fluid
supratemporal arcade
surgical lumbus
trocar cannula infusion system
Westcott scissors
white silk suture bites
Wydase

Penetrating Keratoplasty
Ancef
balanced salt solution
Betagan
blepharostat
bupivacaine

Celestone
cellulose sponges
curved corneal scissors
donor corneal button
episclera
gentamicin
Goldmann-McNeil blepharostat
Healon
Miochol
nylon sutures
penetrating keratoplasty
recipient button
recipient cornea
recipient stroma
saline sponges
semi-pressure patch
snip incisions
subconjunctival injections
Supersharp
suture tension
trephine
Vannas scissors
Vicryl suture

Phacoemulsification and Lens Implant
balanced salt solution
Betadine solution
capsulorrhexis
conjunctival peritomy
Healon
hemostasis
Honan balloon
hydrodelineation
hydrodissection
inferior cul-de-sac
inferior fornix
keratome
Lieberman speculum
Marcaine
Maxitrol
paracentesis
phaco tip

phacoemulsification
Pierce needle
pilocarpine
retrobulbar anesthesia
scleral tunnel
silk traction suture
superior fornix
superior rectus muscle
Van Lint akinesia
Viscoat
viscoelastic material
wet-field cautery
Wydase
Xylocaine

Pterygia Removal and Placement of Conjunctival Graft

autologous free-floating conjunctival graft
bare scleral defect
blepharostat
Bowman membrane
bulbar conjunctiva
conjunctival graft
corneal forceps
epinephrine
episcleral tissues
fentanyl
Fox shield
hand-held thermocautery
homatropine ophthalmic drops
interpalpebral bulbar conjunctiva
invasive pterygia
locking Castroviejo forceps
Maxitrol ophthalmic drops
nasal bed
operating microscope
pentothal
peribulbar fashion
recipient bed
retrobulbar medication
Steri-Drapes

superficial keratectomy
temporal bed
Tenon capsule
Vicryl sutures
virgin bulbar conjunctiva
Westcott scissors
Xylocaine

Ptosis Repair

Bard-Parker blade
epinephrine
hemostasis
intramuscular septum
lidocaine
marking pen
Maxitrol ointment
moistened saline sponge
orbicularis
prolapsed fat
Prolene suture
ptosis
sharp dissection
supratarsal fixation sutures
tetracaine
unipolar cutting and coagulating Bovie
upper lid crease

Retinal Detachment

atropine
confluent cryotherapy
direct ophthalmoscopy
lid speculum
limbal conjunctival peritomy
limbus
macula
Marcaine
neuroleptanesthesia
Ocuflox
Pred Forte
relaxing incision
retinal break
retinal detachment
retrobulbar injection

scleral buckle
subretinal fluid
Vicryl suture
Xylocaine

Trabeculectomy

5-fluorouracil
Alcon crescent knife
Alcon V-lance
anterior chamber
atropine
balanced saline solution
Beaver blade
bipolar cautery
blunt scissors
cautery lines
conjunctiva
conjunctival flap
fentanyl
inferior fornix
iridectomy
lamellar dissection
limbus

marbleized
Miochol
open angle glaucoma
operating microscope
ophthalmic cautery
peripheral iridectomy
phenylethyl
retrobulbar block
run-off
scleral flap
silk sutures
speculum
superior rectus suture
supertemporal quadrant
Tenon capsule
trabeculectomy flap
trabeculectomy punch
trabeculectomy site
Vannas scissors
Versed
Vicryl suture
Wydase
Xylocaine

Appendix 5
Drugs by Indication

ALLERGIC DISORDERS (OPHTHALMIC)
Adrenal Corticosteroid
  HMS Liquifilm®
  medrysone

ANESTHESIA (OPHTHALMIC)
Local Anesthetic
  Flucaine® [US]
  Fluoracaine® [US]
  proparacaine and fluorescein

ANGIOGRAPHY (OPHTHALMIC)
Diagnostic Agent
  AK-Fluor [US]
  Angiscein® [US]
  Diofluor™ [Can]
  fluorescein sodium
  Fluorescite® [US/Can]
  Fluorets® [US/Can]
  Fluor-I-Strip-AT® [US]
  Fluor-I-Strip® [US]
  Ful-Glo® [US]

BLEPHARITIS
Antifungal Agent
  Natacyn® [US/Can]
  natamycin

BLEPHAROSPASM
Ophthalmic Agent, Toxin
  Botox® Cosmetic [US/Can]
  Botox® [US]
  botulinum toxin type A

CATARACT
Adrenergic Agonist Agent
  Neo-Synephrine® Ophthalmic [US]
  phenylephrine

CHORIORETINITIS
Adrenal Corticosteroid
  A-HydroCort® [US]
  A-methapred® [US]
  Apo-Prednisone® [Can]
  Aristocort® Forte Injection [US]
  Aristocort® Intralesional Injection [US]
  Aristocort® Tablet [US/Can]
  Aristospan® Intraarticular Injection [US/Can]
  Aristospan® Intralesional Injection [US/Can]
  betamethasone (systemic)
  Celestone® Soluspan® [US/Can]
  Celestone® [US]
  Cortef® Tablet [US/Can]
  cortisone acetate
  Cortone® [Can]
  Decadron® [US/Can]
  Deltasone® [US]
  Depo-Medrol® [US/Can]
  Dexamethasone Intensol® [US]
  dexamethasone (systemic)
  DexPak® TaperPak® [US]
  Diodex® [Can]
  hydrocortisone (systemic)
  Hydrocortone® Phosphate [US]
  Kenalog® Injection [US/Can]
  Medrol® [US/Can]
  methylprednisolone
  Orapred™ [US]
  Pediapred® [US/Can]
  PMS-Dexamethasone [Can]
  Prednicot® [US]
  prednisolone (systemic)
  Prednisol® TBA [US]
  prednisone
  Prednisone Intensol™ [US]
  Prelone® [US]

Solu-Cortef® [US/Can]
Solu-Medrol® [US/Can]
Sterapred® DS [US]
Sterapred® [US]
triamcinolone (systemic)
Winpred™ [Can]
PMS-Dexamethasone [Can]
Prednicot®

CMV RETINITIS
Antiviral Agent
Valcyte™ [US/Can]
valganciclovir

CONJUNCTIVITIS (ALLERGIC)
Adrenal Corticosteroid
HMS Liquifilm® [US]
medrysone
Antihistamine
Alavert™ [US-OTC]
Aler-Dryl [US-OTC]
Aller-Chlor® [US-OTC]
Allerdryl® [Can]
AllerMax® [US-OTC]
Allernix [Can]
Apo-Dimenhydrinate® [Can]
Apo-Hydroxyzine® [Can]
Apo-Loratadine® [Can]
Atarax® [US/Can]
azatadine
Banophen® [US-OTC]
Benadryl® Allergy [US-OTC/Can]
Benadryl® Dye-Free Allergy [US-OTC]
Benadryl® Injection [US]
brompheniramine
chlorpheniramine
Chlorphen [US-OTC]
Chlor-Trimeton® [US-OTC]
Chlor-Tripolon® [Can]
Claritin® Hives Relief [US-OTC]
Claritin® Kids [Can]
Claritin® [US-OTC/Can]
clemastine
cyproheptadine
Dayhist® Allergy [US-OTC]
dexchlorpheniramine
Diabetic Tussin® Allergy Relief [US-OTC]
dimenhydrinate
Dimetapp® Children's ND [US-OTC]
Diphen® AF [US-OTC]
Diphenhist [US-OTC]
diphenhydramine
Diphen® [US-OTC]
Dramamine® [US-OTC]
Genahist® [US-OTC]
Gravol® [Can]
Hydramine® [US-OTC]
hydroxyzine
Hyrexin-50® [US]
levocabastine
Livostin® [US/Can]
loratadine
Nolahist® [US-OTC/Can]
Novo-Dimenate [Can]
Novo-Hydroxyzin [Can]
Novo-Pheniram® [Can]
olopatadine
Patanol® [US/Can]
Periactin® [Can]
phenindamine
PMS-Diphenhydramine [Can]
PMS-Hydroxyzine [Can]
Siladryl® Allergy [US-OTC]
Silphen® [US-OTC]
Tavist® Allergy [US-OTC]
Tavist® ND [US-OTC]
Vistaril® [US/Can]
Antihistamine/Decongestant Combination
Andehist NR Drops [US]
Carbaxefed RF [US]
carbinoxamine and pseudoephedrine

Carboxine-PSE [US]
Hydro-Tussin™-CBX [US]
Palgic®-DS [US]
Palgic®-D [US]
Pediatex™-D [US]
Rondec® Drops [US]
Rondec® Tablets [US]
Rondec-TR® [US]
Sildec [US]
Antihistamine, H1 Blocker, Ophthalmic
Apo-Ketotifen® [Can]
Emadine® [US]
emedastine
ketotifen
Novo-Ketotifen [Can]
Zaditen® [Can]
Zaditor™ [US/Can]
Antihistamine, Ophthalmic
Astelin® [US/Can]
azelastine
Optivar® [US]
Corticosteroid, Ophthalmic
Alrex® [US/Can]
Lotemax® [US/Can]
loteprednol
Mast Cell Stabilizer
Alamast™ [US/Can]
Alocril™ [US/Can]
nedocromil (ophthalmic)
pemirolast
Nonsteroidal Antiinflammatory Drug
(NSAID)
Acular LS™ [US]
Acular® P.F. [US]
Acular® [US/Can]
ketorolac
Ophthalmic Agent, Miscellaneous
Alamast™ [US/Can]
pemirolast
Phenothiazine Derivative
Phenadoz™ [US]
Phenergan® [US/Can]
promethazine

CONJUNCTIVITIS (BACTERIAL)
Antibiotic, Ophthalmic
Iquix® [US]
Levaquin® [US/Can]
levofloxacin
Quixin™ [US]

CONJUNCTIVITIS (VERNAL)
Adrenal Corticosteroid
HMS Liquifilm® [US]
medrysone
Mast Cell Stabilizer
Alomide® [US/Can]
lodoxamide tromethamine

CORNEAL EDEMA
Lubricant, Ocular
Muro 128® [OTC]
sodium chloride

CYCLOPLEGIA
Anticholinergic Agent
AtroPen® [US]
Atropine
Atropine-Care® [US]
Buscopan® [Can]
Cyclogyl® [US/Can]
cyclopentolate
Cylate® [US]
Diopentolate® [Can]
Dioptic's Atropine Solution [Can]
Diotrope® [Can]
homatropine
Isopto® Atropine [US/Can]
Isopto® Homatropine [US]
Isopto® Hyoscine [US]
Minim's Atropine Solution [Can]
Mydriacyl® [US/Can]
Opticyl® [US]
Sal-Tropine™ [US]
scopolamine

Tropicacyl® [US]
tropicamide

DRY EYES
Ophthalmic Agent, Miscellaneous
  Akwa Tears® [US-OTC]
    AquaLase™ [US]
  AquaSite® [US-OTC]
  artificial tears
  balanced salt solution
  Bion® Tears [US-OTC]
  BSS® Plus [US/Can]
  BSS® [US/Can]
  carbopol 940 (Canada only)
  carboxymethylcellulose
  Celluvisc™ [Can]
  collagen implants
  Eye-Stream® [Can]
    hydroxypropyl cellulose
  HypoTears PF [US-OTC]
  HypoTears [US-OTC]
  Isopto® Tears [US]
    Lacrisert® [US/Can]
  Liquifilm® Tears [US-OTC]
  Moisture® Eyes PM [US-OTC]
  Moisture® Eyes [US-OTC]
  Murine® Tears [US-OTC]
  Murocel® [US-OTC]
  Nature's Tears® [US-OTC]
  Nu-Tears® II [US-OTC]
  Nu-Tears® [US-OTC]
  OcuCoat® PF [US-OTC]
  OcuCoat® [US-OTC]
  Puralube® Tears [US-OTC]
  Refresh® Liquigel [US-OTC]
  Refresh® Plus [US-OTC/Can]
  Refresh® Tears [US-OTC]
  Refresh® [US-OTC]
  Soft Plug® [US]
  Teardrops® [Can]
  Teargen® II [US-OTC]
  Teargen® [US-OTC]
  Tearisol® [US-OTC]

Tears Again® Gel Drops™ [US-OTC]
Tears Again® Night and Day™ [US-OTC]
Tears Again® [US-OTC]
Tears Naturale® Free [US-OTC]
Tears Naturale® II [US-OTC]
Tears Naturale® [US-OTC]
Tears Plus® [US-OTC]
Tears Renewed® [US-OTC]
Theratears® [US]
Ultra Tears® [US-OTC]
Viva-Drops® [US-OTC]

EPISCLERITIS
Adrenal Corticosteroid
  HMS Liquifilm® [US]
  medrysone

ESOTROPIA
Cholinesterase Inhibitor
  echothiophate iodide
  Phospholine Iodide® [US]

EYE INFECTION
Antibiotic/Corticosteroid, Ophthalmic
  AK-Trol® [US]
  AntibiOtic® Ear [US]
  bacitracin, neomycin, polymyxin B, and hydrocortisone
  Blephamide® [US/Can]
  Cortimyxin® [Can]
  Cortisporin® Cream [US]
  Cortisporin® Ointment [US/Can]
  Cortisporin® Ophthalmic [US]
  Dexacidin® [US]
  Dexacine™ [US]
  Dioptimyd® [Can]
    Dioptrol® [Can]
    FML-S® [US]
  Maxitrol® [US/Can]
  NeoDecadron® [US]
  neomycin and dexamethasone

neomycin, polymyxin B, and
  dexamethasone
neomycin, polymyxin B, and
  hydrocortisone
neomycin, polymyxin B, and
  prednisolone
PediOtic® [US]
Poly-Pred® [US]
Pred-G® [US]
prednisolone and gentamicin
sulfacetamide and prednisolone
sulfacetamide sodium and
  fluorometholone
TobraDex® [US/Can]
tobramycin and dexamethasone
Vasocidin® [US/Can]
Antibiotic, Ophthalmic
  Akne-Mycin® [US]
  AK-Poly-Bac® [US]
  AK-Sulf® [US]
  AKTob® [US]
  Alcomicin® [Can]
  Apo-Erythro Base® [Can]
  Apo-Erythro E-C® [Can]
  Apo-Erythro-ES® [Can]
  Apo-Erythro-S® [Can]
  Apo-Oflox® [Can]
  Apo-Tetra® [Can]
  Apo-Tobramycin® [Can]
  A/T/S® [US]
  Baciguent® [US/Can]
    BaciiM® [US]
  bacitracin
  bacitracin and polymyxin B
  bacitracin, neomycin, and polymyxin
    B
  Betadine® First Aid Antibiotics +
    Moisturizer [US-OTC]
  Bleph®-10 [US]
  Carmol® Scalp [US]
  Cetamide™ [Can]
  chloramphenicol
    Chloromycetin® [Can]

Chloromycetin® Sodium Succinate
  [US]
Ciloxan® [US/Can]
ciprofloxacin
Cipro® [US/Can]
Cipro® XL [Can]
Cipro® XR [US]
Diochloram® [Can]
Diogent® [Can]
Diomycin® [Can]
Diosulf™ [Can]
E.E.S.® [US/Can]
Erybid™ [Can]
Eryc® [US/Can]
Eryderm® [US]
Erygel® [US]
EryPed® [US]
Ery-Tab® [US]
Erythrocin® [US]
Erythromid® [Can]
erythromycin
Floxin® [US/Can]
Garamycin® [Can]
Genoptic® [US]
Gentak® [US]
gentamicin
Iquix® [US]
Klaron® [US]
Levaquin® [US/Can]
levofloxacin
LID-Pack® [Can]
Minim's Gentamicin 0.3% [Can]
Nebcin® [Can]
neomycin, polymyxin B, and
  gramicidin
Neosporin® Neo To Go® [US-OTC]
Neosporin® Ophthalmic Ointment
  [US/Can]
Neosporin® Ophthalmic Solution
  [US/Can]
Neosporin® Topical [US-OTC]
Neotopic® [Can]
Nu-Erythromycin-S [Can]

Nu-Tetra [Can]
Ocuflox® [US/Can]
Ocusulf-10 [US]
ofloxacin
Optimyxin® [Can]
Optimyxin Plus® [Can]
Ovace™ [US]
oxytetracycline and polymyxin B
PCE® [US/Can]
Pentamycetin® [Can]
PMS-Erythromycin [Can]
PMS-Polytrimethoprim [Can]
PMS-Tobramycin [Can]
Polycidin® Ophthalmic Ointment
    [Can]
Polysporin® Ophthalmic [US]
Polysporin® Topical [US-OTC]
Polytrim® [US/Can]
Quixin™ [US]
Romycin® [US]
SAB-Gentamicin [Can]
Sans Acne® [Can]
Sodium Sulamyd® [US/Can]
Sulf-10® [US]
sulfacetamide
Sumycin® [US]
Terramycin® w/Polymyxin B
    Ophthalmic [US]
tetracycline
Theramycin Z® [US]
TOBI® [US/Can]
tobramycin
Tobrex® [US/Can]
Tomycine™ [Can]
trimethoprim and polymyxin B
Wesmycin® [US]

EYE IRRITATION

Adrenergic Agonist Agent
AK-Con™ [US]
Albalon® [US]
Allersol® [US]
Clear Eyes® ACR [US-OTC]

Clear Eyes® [US-OTC]
naphazoline
Naphcon Forte® [Can]
Naphcon® [US-OTC]
phenylephrine and zinc sulfate
Privine® [US-OTC]
VasoClear® [US-OTC]
Vasocon® [Can]
Zincfrin® [US-OTC/Can]

Ophthalmic Agent, Miscellaneous
Akwa Tears® [US-OTC]
AquaSite® [US-OTC]
artificial tears
Bion® Tears [US-OTC]
HypoTears PF [US-OTC]
HypoTears [US-OTC]
Isopto® Tears [US]
Liquifilm® Tears [US-OTC]
Moisture® Eyes PM [US-OTC]
Moisture® Eyes [US-OTC]
Murine® Tears [US-OTC]
Murocel® [US-OTC]
Nature's Tears® [US-OTC]
Nu-Tears® II [US-OTC]
Nu-Tears® [US-OTC]
OcuCoat® PF [US-OTC]
OcuCoat® [US-OTC]
Puralube® Tears [US-OTC]
Refresh® Tears [US-OTC]
Refresh® [US-OTC]
Teardrops® [Can]
Teargen® II [US-OTC]
Teargen® [US-OTC]
Tearisol® [US-OTC]
Tears Again® [US-OTC]
Tears Naturale® Free [US-OTC]
Tears Naturale® II [US-OTC]
Tears Naturale® [US-OTC]
Tears Plus® [US-OTC]
Tears Renewed® [US-OTC]
Ultra Tears® [US-OTC]
Viva-Drops® [US-OTC]

EYELID INFECTION
Antibiotic, Ophthalmic
  mercuric oxide
  Ocu-Merox®
Pharmaceutical Aid
  boric acid

GIANT PAPILLARY CONJUNCTIVITIS
Mast Cell Stabilizer
  Crolom® [US]
  cromolyn sodium
  Opticrom® [US/Can]

GLAUCOMA
Adrenergic Agonist Agent
  dipivefrin
  epinephrine
  Mydfrin® [US/Can]
  Neo-Synephrine® Ophthalmic [US]
  Ophtho-Dipivefrin™ [Can]
  Phenoptic® [US]
  phenylephrine
  PMS-Dipivefrin [Can]
  Propine® [US/Can]
Alpha2-Adrenergic Agonist Agent, Ophthalmic
  Alphagan® P [US/Can]
  apraclonidine
  brimonidine
  Iopidine® [US/Can]
  PMS-Brimonidine Tartrate [Can]
  ratio-Brimonidine [Can]
Beta-Adrenergic Blocker
  Alti-Timolol [Can]
  Apo-Levobunolol® [Can]
  Apo-Timol® [Can]
  Apo-Timop® [Can]
  Betagan® [US/Can]
  betaxolol
  Betimol® [US]
  Betoptic® S [US/Can]
  Blocadren® [US]
  carteolol
  Cartrol® Oral [Can]
  dorzolamide and timolol
  Gen-Timolol [Can]
  Istalol™ [US]
  levobunolol
  metipranolol
  Novo-Levobunolol [Can]
  Nu-Timolol [Can]
  Ocupress® Ophthalmic [Can]
  Optho-Bunolol® [Can]
  OptiPranolol® [US/Can]
  Phoxal-timolol [Can]
  PMS-Levobunolol [Can]
  PMS-Timolol [Can]
  Tim-AK [Can]
  timolol
  Timoptic® OcuDose® [US]
  Timoptic® [US/Can]
  Timoptic-XE® [US/Can]
Carbonic Anhydrase Inhibitor
  acetazolamide
  Apo-Acetazolamide® [Can]
  Apo-Methazolamide® [Can]
  Azopt® [US/Can]
  brinzolamide
  Daranide® [US/Can]
  Diamox® [Can]
  Diamox® Sequels® [US]
  dichlorphenamide
  dorzolamide
  dorzolamide and timolol
  methazolamide
  Trusopt® [US/Can]
Cholinergic Agent
  carbachol
  Carbastat® [Can]
  Diocarpine [Can]
  Isopto® Carbachol [US/Can]
  Isopto® Carpine [US/Can]
  Miostat® [US/Can]
  pilocarpine
  pilocarpine and epinephrine

Pilocar® [US]
Pilopine HS® [US/Can]
Cholinesterase Inhibitor
echothiophate iodide
Eserine® [Can]
Isopto® Eserine [Can]
Phospholine Iodide® [US]
physostigmine
Diuretic, Osmotic
Amino-Cerv™ [US]
Aquacare® [US-OTC]
Aquaphilic® With Carbamide [US-OTC]
Carmol® 10 [US-OTC]
Carmol® 20 [US-OTC]
Carmol® 40 [US]
Carmol® Deep Cleaning [US]
DPM™ [US-OTC]
Gormel® [US-OTC]
Kerlac® [US]
Lanaphilic® [US-OTC]
mannitol
Nutraplus® [US-OTC]
Osmitrol® [US/Can]
Rea-Lo® [US-OTC]
Resectisol® [US]
UltraMide 25™ [Can]
Ultra Mide® [US-OTC]
urea
Ureacin® [US-OTC]
Uremol® [Can]
Urisec® [Can]
Vanamide™ [US]
Ophthalmic Agent, Miscellaneous
bimatoprost
glycerin
Osmoglyn® [US]
Rescula® [US]
unoprostone
Prostaglandin
latanoprost
Xalatan® [US/Can]
Prostaglandin, Ophthalmic

Travatan® [US/Can]
travoprost

GLIOMA
Antineoplastic Agent
CeeNU® [US/Can]
lomustine
Antiviral Agent
interferon alfa-2b and ribavirin
combination pack
Rebetron® [US/Can]
Biological Response Modulator
interferon alfa-2b
interferon alfa-2b and ribavirin
combination pack
Intron® A [US/Can]
Rebetron® [US/Can]

GONOCOCCAL OPHTHALMIA NEONATORUM
Topical Skin Product
silver nitrate

HYPERTENSION (OCULAR)
Alpha2-Adrenergic Agonist Agent,
Ophthalmic
Alphagan® P [US/Can]
brimonidine
PMS-Brimonidine Tartrate [Can]
ratio-Brimonidine [Can]
Beta-Adrenergic Blocker
Apo-Levobunolol® [Can]
Betagan® [US/Can]
levobunolol
Novo-Levobunolol [Can]
Optho-Bunolol® [Can]
PMS-Levobunolol [Can]

INTRAOCULAR PRESSURE
Ophthalmic Agent, Miscellaneous
glycerin
Osmoglyn® [US]

IRIDOCYCLITIS
Adrenal Corticosteroid
  HMS Liquifilm® [US]
  medrysone
Anticholinergic Agent
  Buscopan® [Can]
  Diotrope® [Can]
  Isopto® Hyoscine [US]
  Mydriacyl® [US/Can]
  Opticyl® [US]
  Scopace™ [US]
  scopolamine
  Tropicacyl® [US]
  tropicamide

KERATITIS
Adrenal Corticosteroid
  Flarex® [US/Can]
  fluorometholone
  FML® Forte [US/Can]
  FML® [US/Can]
  PMS-Fluorometholone [Can]
Anticholinergic Agent
  Diotrope® [Can]
  Mydriacyl® [US/Can]
  Opticyl® [US]
  Tropicacyl® [US]
  tropicamide
Mast Cell Stabilizer
  Crolom® [US]
  cromolyn sodium
  Opticrom® [US/Can]

KERATITIS (EXPOSURE)
Ophthalmic Agent, Miscellaneous
  Akwa Tears® [US-OTC]
  AquaSite® [US-OTC]
  artificial tears
  Bion® Tears [US-OTC]
  HypoTears PF [US-OTC]
  HypoTears [US-OTC]
  Isopto® Tears [US]
  Liquifilm® Tears [US-OTC]

Moisture® Eyes PM [US-OTC]
Moisture® Eyes [US-OTC]
Murine® Tears [US-OTC]
Murocel® [US-OTC]
Nature's Tears® [US-OTC]
Nu-Tears® II [US-OTC]
Nu-Tears® [US-OTC]
OcuCoat® PF [US-OTC]
OcuCoat® [US-OTC]
Puralube® Tears [US-OTC]
Refresh® Tears [US-OTC]
Refresh® [US-OTC]
Teardrops® [Can]
Teargen® II [US-OTC]
Teargen® [US-OTC]
Tearisol® [US-OTC]
Tears Again® [US-OTC]
Tears Naturale® Free [US-OTC]
Tears Naturale® II [US-OTC]
Tears Naturale® [US-OTC]
Tears Plus® [US-OTC]
Tears Renewed® [US-OTC]
Ultra Tears® [US-OTC]
Viva-Drops® [US-OTC]

KERATITIS (FUNGAL)
Antifungal Agent
  Natacyn® [US/Can]
  natamycin

KERATITIS (HERPES SIMPLEX)
Antiviral Agent
  trifluridine
  Viroptic® [US/Can]

KERATITIS (VERNAL)
Antiviral Agent
  trifluridine
  Viroptic® [US/Can]
Mast Cell Stabilizer
  Alomide® [US/Can]
  lodoxamide tromethamine

KERATOCONJUNCTIVITIS (VERNAL)
Mast Cell Stabilizer
  Alomide® [US/Can]
  lodoxamide tromethamine

MACULAR DEGENERATION
Ophthalmic Agent
  verteporfin
  Visudyne® [US/Can]

MIOSIS
Alpha-Adrenergic Blocking Agent
  dapiprazole
  Rev-Eyes™ [US]
Cholinergic Agent
  acetylcholine
  carbachol
  Carbastat® [Can]
  Diocarpine [Can]
  Isopto® Carbachol [US/Can]
  Isopto® Carpine [US/Can]
  Miochol-E® [US/Can]
  Miostat® [US/Can]
  pilocarpine
  pilocarpine and epinephrine
  Pilocar® [US]
  Pilopine HS® [US/Can]
Nonsteroidal Antiinflammatory Drug (NSAID)
  Alti-Flurbiprofen [Can]
  Ansaid® [US/Can]
  Apo-Flurbiprofen® [Can]
  flurbiprofen
  Froben® [Can]
  Froben-SR® [Can]
  Novo-Flurprofen [Can]
  Nu-Flurprofen [Can]
  Ocufen® [US/Can]

MYDRIASIS
Adrenergic Agonist Agent
  AK-Dilate® [US]
  Mydfrin® [US/Can]
  Neo-Synephrine® Ophthalmic [US]
  Phenoptic® [US]
  phenylephrine
Anticholinergic/Adrenergic Agonist
  Cyclomydril® [US]
  cyclopentolate and phenylephrine
  Murocoll-2® [US]
  phenylephrine and scopolamine
Anticholinergic Agent
  atropine
  Atropine-Care® [US]
  Cyclogyl® [US/Can]
  cyclopentolate
  Cylate® [US]
  Diopentolate® [Can]
  Dioptic's Atropine Solution [Can]
  Diotrope® [Can]
  homatropine
  Isopto® Atropine [US/Can]
  Isopto® Homatropine [US]
  Minim's Atropine Solution [Can]
  Mydriacyl® [US/Can]
  Opticyl® [US]
  Tropicacyl® [US]
  tropicamide

NEURITIS (OPTIC)
Adrenal Corticosteroid
  A-HydroCort® [US]
  A-methaPred® [US]
  Apo-Prednisone® [Can]
  Aristocort® Forte Injection [US]
  Aristocort® Intralesional Injection [US]
  Aristocort® Tablet [US/Can]
  Aristospan® Intraarticular Injection [US/Can]
  Aristospan® Intralesional Injection [US/Can]
  betamethasone (systemic)
  Celestone® Soluspan® [US/Can]

Celestone® [US]
Cortef® Tablet [US/Can]
cortisone acetate
Cortone® [Can]
Decadron® [US/Can]
Deltasone® [US]
Depo-Medrol® [US/Can]
Dexamethasone Intensol® [US]
dexamethasone (systemic)
DexPak® TaperPak® [US]
Diodex® [Can]
hydrocortisone (systemic)
Hydrocortone® Phosphate [US]
Kenalog® Injection [US/Can]
Medrol® [US/Can]
methylprednisolone
Orapred™ [US]
Pediapred® [US/Can]
PMS-Dexamethasone [Can]
Prednicot® [US]
prednisolone (systemic)
Prednisol® TBA [US]
prednisone
Prednisone Intensol™ [US]
Prelone® [US]
Solu-Cortef® [US/Can]
Solu-Medrol® [US/Can]
Sterapred® DS [US]
Sterapred® [US]
triamcinolone (systemic)
Winpred™ [Can]

OCULAR INJURY
Nonsteroidal Antiinflammatory Drug
  (NSAID)
  flurbiprofen
  Ocufen® Ophthalmic [US/Can]

OCULAR REDNESS
Adrenergic Agonist Agent
  AK-Dilate® [US]
  AK-Nefrin® [US]
  Albalon® [US]

Allersol® [US]
Claritin® Allergic Decongestant
  [Can]
Clear Eyes® ACR [US-OTC]
Clear Eyes® [US-OTC]
Dionephrine® [Can]
Eye-Sine™ [US-OTC]
Formulation R™ [US-OTC]
Genasal [US-OTC]
Geneye® [US-OTC]
Medicone® [US-OTC]
Murine® Tears Plus [US-OTC]
Mydfrin® [US/Can]
naphazoline
Naphcon Forte® [Can]
Naphcon® [US-OTC]
Neo-Synephrine® Ophthalmic [US]
Optigene® 3 [US-OTC]
oxymetazoline
Phenoptic® [US]
phenylephrine
Privine® [US-OTC]
Relief® [US-OTC]
tetrahydrozoline
VasoClear® [US-OTC]
Vasocon® [Can]
Visine® Advanced Relief [US-OTC]
Visine® L.R. [US-OTC]
Visine® Original [US-OTC]
Antihistamine/Decongestant
  Combination
  Albalon®-A Liquifilm [Can]
  naphazoline and antazoline
  naphazoline and pheniramine
  Naphcon-A® [US-OTC/Can]
  Opcon-A® [US-OTC]
  Vasocon-A® [US-OTC/Can]
  Visine-A™ [US-OTC]

OPHTHALMIC DISORDERS
Adrenal Corticosteroid
  A-HydroCort® [US]
  AK-Pred® [US]

A-methapred® [US]
Apo-Prednisone® [Can]
Aristocort® Forte Injection [US]
Aristocort® Intralesional Injection
   [US]
Aristocort® Tablet [US/Can]
Aristospan® Intraarticular Injection
   [US/Can]
Aristospan® Intralesional Injection
   [US/Can]
betamethasone (systemic)
Celestone® Soluspan® [US/Can]
Celestone® [US]
Cortef® Tablet [US/Can]
corticotropin
cortisone acetate
Cortone® [Can]
Deltasone® [US]
Depo-Medrol® [US/Can]
dexamethasone (ophthalmic)
Diopred® [Can]
Econopred® Plus [US]
Econopred® [US]
Flarex® [US/Can]
fluorometholone
FML® Forte [US/Can]
FML® [US/Can]
H.P. Acthar® Gel [US]
Hydeltra-T.B.A.® [Can]
hydrocortisone (systemic)
Hydrocortone® Phosphate [US]
Inflamase® Forte [US/Can]
Inflamase® Mild [US/Can]
Kenalog® Injection [US/Can]
Maxidex® [US/Can]
Medrol® [US/Can]
methylprednisolone
Novo-Prednisolone [Can]
PMS-Fluorometholone [Can]
Pred Forte® [US/Can]
Pred Mild® [US/Can]
Prednicot® [US]
prednisolone (ophthalmic)

prednisone
Prednisone Intensol™ [US]
Sab-Prenase® [Can]
Solu-Cortef® [US/Can]
Solu-Medrol® [US/Can]
Sterapred® DS [US]
Sterapred® [US]
triamcinolone (systemic)
Winpred™ [Can]

OPHTHALMIC SURGERY
Nonsteroidal Antiinflammatory Drug
   (NSAID)
   Cataflam® [US/Can]
   Voltaren Ophthalmic® [US]
   Voltare Ophtha® [Can]

OPHTHALMIC SURGICAL AID
Ophthalmic Agent, Miscellaneous
   Cellugel® [US]
   GenTeal® Mild [US-OTC]
   GenTeal® [US-OTC/Can]
   Gonak™ [US-OTC]
   Goniosoft™ [US]
   hydroxypropyl methylcellulose
   Tears Again® MC [US-OTC]

RETINOBLASTOMA
Antineoplastic Agent
   Cosmegen® [US/Can]
   cyclophosphamide
   Cytoxan® [US/Can]
   dactinomycin
   Procytox® [Can]

REYE SYNDROME
Ophthalmic Agent, Miscellaneous
   glycerin
   Osmoglyn® [US]

STRABISMUS
Cholinesterase Inhibitor
   echothiophate iodide

Phospholine Iodide® [US]
Ophthalmic Agent, Toxin
  Botox® [US]
  botulinum toxin type A

SURGICAL AID (OPHTHALMIC)

Ophthalmic Agent, Viscoelastic
  chondroitin sulfate and sodium
    hyaluronate
  sodium hyaluronate
  Viscoat® [US]

UVEITIS

Adrenal Corticosteroid
  rimexolone
  Vexol® [US/Can]
Adrenergic Agonist Agent
  AK-Dilate® [US]
  AK-Nefrin® [US]
  Dionephrine® [Can]
  Formulation R™ [US-OTC]
  Medicone® [US-OTC]
  Mydfrin® [US/Can]
  Neo-Synephrine® Ophthalmic [US]
  Phenoptic® [US]
  phenylephrine
  Relief® [US-OTC]
Anticholinergic Agent
  AtroPen® [US]
  atropine
  Atropine-Care® [US]
  Buscopan® [Can]
  Dioptic's Atropine Solution [Can]
  homatropine
  Isopto® Atropine [US/Can]
  Isopto® Homatropine [US]
  Isopto® Hyoscine [US]

Minim's Atropine Solution [Can]
Sal-Tropine™ [US]
scopolamine

XEROPHTHALMIA

Ophthalmic Agent, Miscellaneous
  Akwa Tears® [US-OTC]
  AquaSite® [US-OTC]
  artificial tears
  Bion® Tears [US-OTC]
  HypoTears PF [US-OTC]
  HypoTears [US-OTC]
  Isopto® Tears [US]
  Liquifilm® Tears [US-OTC]
  Moisture® Eyes PM [US-OTC]
  Moisture® Eyes [US-OTC]
  Murine® Tears [US-OTC]
  Murocel® [US-OTC]
  Nature's Tears® [US-OTC]
  Nu-Tears® II [US-OTC]
  Nu-Tears® [US-OTC]
  OcuCoat® PF [US-OTC]
  OcuCoat® [US-OTC]
  Puralube® Tears [US-OTC]
  Refresh® Tears [US-OTC]
  Refresh® [US-OTC]
  Teardrops® [Can]
  Teargen® II [US-OTC]
  Teargen® [US-OTC]
  Tearisol® [US-OTC]
  Tears Again® [US-OTC]
  Tears Naturale® Free [US-OTC]
  Tears Naturale® II [US-OTC]
  Tears Naturale® [US-OTC]
  Tears Plus® [US-OTC]
  Tears Renewed® [US-OTC]
  Ultra Tears® [US-OTC]
  Viva-Drops® [US-OTC]

Notes

Notes

Notes

Notes

Notes

Notes

Notes

Notes

Notes

Notes